ADVANCES IN VETERINARY SCIENCE AND COMPARATIVE MEDICINE

VOLUME 27

ADVISORY BOARD

W. I. B. Beveridge
J. H. Gillespie
W. R. Hinshaw

C. E. Hopla
Norman D. Levine
C. A. Mitchell

W. R. Pritchard

CONTRIBUTORS TO THIS VOLUME

Babiker Abbas
Gary B. Anderson
Douglas F. Antczak
Roy Barzilai
S. M. Dennis
W. Jean Dodds
John B. Gratzek
A. G. Hendrickx
K. Huston

H. W. Leipold
Mark J. Newman
K. Perk
Hans P. Riemann
J. M. Rowland
Arnon Shimshony
Keith R. Solomon
W. Jape Taylor
Gerrit Uilenberg

ADVANCES IN VETERINARY SCIENCE AND COMPARATIVE MEDICINE

Edited by

CHARLES E. CORNELIUS
*California Primate Research Center
University of California
Davis, California*

CHARLES F. SIMPSON
*College of Veterinary Medicine
University of Florida
Gainesville, Florida*

Volume 27

1983

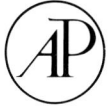

ACADEMIC PRESS
A Subsidiary of Harcourt Brace Jovanovich, Publishers
New York London
Paris San Diego San Francisco São Paulo Sydney Tokyo Toronto

COPYRIGHT © 1983, BY ACADEMIC PRESS, INC.
ALL RIGHTS RESERVED.
NO PART OF THIS PUBLICATION MAY BE REPRODUCED OR
TRANSMITTED IN ANY FORM OR BY ANY MEANS, ELECTRONIC
OR MECHANICAL, INCLUDING PHOTOCOPY, RECORDING, OR ANY
INFORMATION STORAGE AND RETRIEVAL SYSTEM, WITHOUT
PERMISSION IN WRITING FROM THE PUBLISHER.

ACADEMIC PRESS, INC.
111 Fifth Avenue, New York, New York 10003

United Kingdom Edition published by
ACADEMIC PRESS, INC. (LONDON) LTD.
24/28 Oval Road, London NW1 7DX

LIBRARY OF CONGRESS CATALOG CARD NUMBER: 53-7098
ISBN 0-12-039227-5

PRINTED IN THE UNITED STATES OF AMERICA

83 84 85 86   9 8 7 6 5 4 3 2 1

CONTENTS

CONTRIBUTORS ix
PREFACE xi
ERRATUM xiii

Histocompatibility Polymorphisms of Domestic Animals
MARK J. NEWMAN AND DOUGLAS F. ANTCZAK

  I. Introduction 2
 II. Structure and Function of the Major Histocompatibility System ... 4
III. Histocompatibility Systems of Dogs 18
 IV. Histocompatibility Systems of Swine 32
  V. Histocompatibility Systems of Cattle 43
 VI. Histocompatibility Systems of Horses 54
VII. Histocompatibility Systems of Sheep and Goats 61
VIII. Histocompatibility Systems of Cats 63
 IX. Conclusions 63
     References 66

Sickled Red Cells in the Cervidae
W. JAPE TAYLOR

  I. Introduction 77
 II. Production and Behavior of Sickled Cells 80
III. Molecular Mechanisms of Sickling 83
 IV. Primary Structure and Genetics of the Hemoglobins 90
  V. Summary 94
     References 95

Corticosteroid Teratogenicity
J. M. ROWLAND AND A. G. HENDRICKX

  I. Introduction 99
 II. Interspecies Comparison of Corticosteroid Teratogenicity 100
III. Factors Determining Corticosteroid-Induced Cleft Palate 111
 IV. Conclusion 123
     References 124

Embryo Transfer in Domestic Animals
Gary B. Anderson

I. Introduction 129
II. History 130
III. Applications of Embryo Transfer to Large Animals 132
IV. Current Embryo Transfer Technology 138
V. Future Developments in Embryo Transfer 154
    References 156

Immune-Mediated Diseases of the Blood
W. Jean Dodds

I. Introduction 163
II. Clinical Signs 165
III. Diagnosis 166
IV. Findings 173
V. Predisposing Factors 178
VI. Management and Treatment 190
VII. Prevention 194
    References 195

Bovine Congenital Defects
H. W. Leipold, K. Huston, and S. M. Dennis

I. Introduction 198
II. Definitions 199
III. Nature and Effect 199
IV. Frequency 201
V. Causes 203
VI. Kansas Genetic Disease Program 215
VII. Specific Defects 217
VIII. Conclusions 256
    References 258

Acaricide Resistance In Ticks
Keith R. Solomon

I. Introduction 273
II. Occurrence and Geographic Location of Tick Resistance 277
III. Acaricide Resistance in Single-Host Ticks 277

IV. Acaricide Resistance in Multihost Ticks 282
   V. Methods for Determining Resistance to Acaricides 284
  VI. Mechanisms of Resistance 288
 VII. Management of Resistance 290
      References 293

Control And Therapy of Fish Diseases
John B. Gratzek

   I. Background 297
  II. Veterinary Medicine and Fish Disease Control 298
      References 321

Avian Lymphoproliferative Diseases and Their Virus Associations
K. Perk

   I. Introduction 325
  II. Classification 326
 III. Avian Retroviruses 327
  IV. Clinical and Pathological Features 330
   V. Epidemiology, Virology, and Oncogenesis 336
  VI. Relationship of LPD to RE 342
 VII. Concluding Comments 343
      References 343

Rift Valley Fever
Arnon Shimshony and Roy Barzilai

   I. Introduction and History 347
  II. The Etiological Agent 349
 III. The Host 366
  IV. Epidemiological Features 390
   V. Prevention and Control Measures 408
      References 416

Heartwater (*Cowdria ruminantium* Infection): Current Status
Gerrit Uilenberg

   I. Introduction 428
  II. The Causal Agent 436

III.	Transmission	440
IV.	Distribution	444
V.	Susceptibility	445
VI.	Epidemiology	452
VII.	The Disease	457
VIII.	Diagnosis	460
IX.	Immunity	464
X.	Therapy	467
XI.	Prevention	469
XII.	Heartwater in the Western Hemisphere	473
	References	475

Diagnosis and Control of Bovine Paratuberculosis (Johne's Disease)

HANS P. RIEMANN AND BABIKER ABBAS

I.	Introduction	481
II.	The Host–Parasite Relationship in Johne's Disease	483
III.	The Diagnosis of Johne's Disease	485
IV.	Efforts toward Control of Johne's Disease	495
V.	Summary	501
	References	503

INDEX	507
CONTENTS OF RECENT VOLUMES	515

CONTRIBUTORS

Numbers in parentheses indicate the pages on which the authors' contributions begin.

BABIKER ABBAS, Department of Epidemiology and Preventive Medicine, University of California, Davis, California 95616 (479)

GARY B. ANDERSON, Department of Animal Science, University of California, Davis, California 95616 (129)

DOUGLAS F. ANTCZAK, James A. Baker Institute for Animal Health, New York State College of Veterinary Medicine, Cornell University, Ithaca, New York 14853 (1)

ROY BARZILAI, Israel Institute for Biological Research, Ness Ziona, Israel (347)

S. M. DENNIS, Department of Pathology, College of Veterinary Medicine, Kansas State University, Manhattan, Kansas 66506 (197)

W. JEAN DODDS, Division of Laboratories and Research, New York State Department of Health, Albany, New York 12201 (163)

JOHN B. GRATZEK, Department of Medical Microbiology, College of Veterinary Medicine, University of Georgia, Athens, Georgia 30602 (297)

A. G. HENDRICKX, California Primate Research Center, University of California, Davis, California 95616 (99)

K. HUSTON,[1] Department of Pathology, College of Veterinary Medicine, Kansas State University, Manhattan, Kansas 66506 (197)

H. W. LEIPOLD, Department of Pathology, College of Veterinary Medicine, Kansas State University, Manhattan, Kansas 66506 (197)

MARK J. NEWMAN, James A. Baker Institute for Animal Health, New York State College of Veterinary Medicine, Cornell University, Ithaca, New York 14853 (1)

K. PERK, The Hebrew University of Jerusalem, Rehovot Campus, Rehovot 761000, Israel (325)

HANS P. RIEMANN, Department of Epidemiology and Preventive Medicine, University of California, Davis, California 95616 (479)

[1]Present address: Ohio Agricultural Research and Development Center, Wooster, Ohio 44691.

J. M. ROWLAND, California Primate Research Center, University of California, Davis, California 95616 (99)

ARNON SHIMSHONY, Veterinary Services and Animal Health, Beit Dagan 50250, Israel (347)

KEITH R. SOLOMON, Department of Environmental Biology, University of Guelph, Guelph, Ontario, N1G 2W1 Canada (273)

W. JAPE TAYLOR, Department of Medicine, University of Florida College of Medicine, Gainesville, Florida 32610 (77)

GERRIT UILENBERG, Institute for Tropical Veterinary Medicine and Protozoology, Faculty of Veterinary Medicine, State University of Utrecht, 3572 BP Utrecht, The Netherlands (425)

PREFACE

This volume of *Advances in Veterinary Science and Comparative Medicine* contains scholarly presentations on a variety of topics of interest to the scientific community. Subjects discussed in the several chapters include avian lymphoproliferative diseases and their virus associations, heartwater, sickle red cells in Cervidae, immune-mediated diseases of the blood, histocompatibility polymorphisms of domestic animals, control and therapy of fish diseases, corticosteroid teratogenicity, acaricide resistance in ticks, embryo transfer in domestic animals, bovine paratuberculosis, and bovine congenital defects.

Studies of avian lymphoproliferative diseases provide insights into molecular genetics and genetic engineering. Avian leukemia viruses are models to analyze the interaction of viruses with various types of differentiating cells.

Heartwater, or cowdriosis, is an infectious disease of African ruminants transmitted by ticks of the genus *Amblyoma*. It is caused by the rickettsia *Cowdria ruminatium*. Research on heartwater in the Caribbean is just beginning.

Hemoglobin polymerizes within the red cells from most species of deer when exposed to oxygen and an elevated pH. The typical sickle cell in deer is virtually identical in shape, mechanical fragility, and viscosity to the human sickle cell.

The immune-mediated diseases of man and animals constitute a group of poorly understood disorders in which antibodies are produced against tissues of the body. The opportunity for recovery is best if the causative agent can be identified and removed.

Research on histocompatibility systems has increased dramatically during the past decade. The pig and dog have served as models of organ grafting in transplantation studies. Therefore, the major histocompatibility systems of these two animals have received the most attention.

Disease control in fish follows the same health management practices followed with other types of animals. Antimicrobials, vaccines, and bacterins are commonly used.

Ticks are probably the most important problem affecting livestock in the subtropical and temperate regions of the world. Continued use of acaricides in an indiscriminate manner may lead to the build up of a stable resistance that could persist.

The highly technical methods of embryo transfer currently used in cattle will soon be extended to other species. In addition, the production of clones in domestic animals may soon be a reality using techniques such as nuclear transplantation.

Corticosteroids have been extensively studied as teratogenic agents since 1950 when it was found that administration of cortisone to pregnant mice caused cleft palates in offspring. It is now known that corticosteroids in all mammalian species that have been studied produce a wide spectrum of abnormalities. This demonstrated teratogenicity raises the question of possible human teratogenicity.

An update of information concerning Rift Valley fever, bovine paratuberculosis (Johne's disease), and bovine congenital defects is also included in this volume.

C. E. CORNELIUS
C. F. SIMPSON

ERRATUM

ADVANCES IN VETERINARY SCIENCE AND COMPARATIVE MEDICINE VOLUME 26

The subtitle on the spine of this volume should read

THE RESPIRATORY SYSTEM

as on the halftitle and title pages.

ADVANCES IN
VETERINARY SCIENCE AND
COMPARATIVE MEDICINE

VOLUME 27

Histocompatibility Polymorphisms of Domestic Animals

MARK J. NEWMAN AND DOUGLAS F. ANTCZAK

James A. Baker Institute for Animal Health, New York State College of Veterinary Medicine, Cornell University, Ithaca, New York

I.	Introduction	2
II.	Structure and Function of the Major Histocompatibility System	4
	A. Genetic Structure	4
	B. Molecular Structure and Tissue Distribution	6
	C. Population Structure	8
	D. Immunological Function of MHS Molecules	9
	E. Non-MHS–Linked Immune Response Genes	14
	F. Nonimmunological Functions of the MHS	15
	G. Detection of MHS Polymorphisms	15
III.	Histocompatibility Systems of Dogs	18
	A. Introduction	18
	B. DLA: Class I Antigens	18
	C. DLA: Class II Antigens	21
	D. Immune Response Genes	27
	E. Functional Studies of the DLA System	27
	F. Non-DLA Lymphocyte Alloantigens and Genes Linked to DLA	31
	G. International Workshops on Canine Immunogenetics	31
IV.	Histocompatibility Systems of Swine	32
	A. Introduction	32
	B. SLA: Class I Antigen Definition, Serology, and Genetics	32
	C. SLA: Class II Antigens	34
	D. Miniature Pigs	35
	E. Biochemical Characterization of SLA Antigens	36
	F. Histocompatibility Studies	37
	G. Tissue Distribution of SLA Antigens	39
	H. Antigens Shared by Erythrocytes and Lymphocytes	40
	I. Non-MHS Lymphocyte Alloantigens	41
	J. Genes Linked to SLA	42
	K. Association of Production Traits with SLA Antigens	42
V.	Histocompatibility Systems of Cattle	43
	A. Introduction	43

	B.	Are Bovine Erythrocyte Antigens Expressed on Lymphocytes?	43
	C.	Class I Antigens	45
	D.	Class II Antigens	50
	E.	Non-MHS Lymphocyte Alloantigens and Linkage of the BoLA Region to Other Genetic Markers	52
	F.	The BoLA System and Disease Associations	53
	G.	BoLA and HLA Cross-Reactivity	54
VI.	Histocompatibility Systems of Horses		54
	A.	The ELA Region	54
	B.	Non-ELA Lymphocyte Alloantigens	56
	C.	Histocompatibility and Pregnancy in Horses	58
	D.	ELA and Combined Immunodeficiency Disease	60
VII.	Histocompatibility Systems of Sheep and Goats		61
	A.	Histocompatibility Systems of Sheep	61
	B.	Histocompatibility Systems of Goats	62
VIII.	Histocompatibility Systems of Cats		63
IX.	Conclusions		63
	References		66

I. Introduction

The genes that control the successful engraftment or rejection of transplanted tissues and organs in mammals are collectively known as histocompatibility genes. At least 45 histocompatibility genes have been identified in experimental studies in mice (Klein, 1975), and similar numbers are thought to exist in other species. The products of these genes are known as histocompatibility or transplantation antigens.

Histocompatibility genes can be divided into three categories. The strong or major histocompatibility genes occur in tight linkage in a genetic region called the major histocompatibility system (MHS). Collectively, histocompatibility differences at MHS genes constitute the most important barrier to allograft survival. The weak or minor histocompatibility genes are scattered throughout the genome. Individually, their contribution to graft rejection is small (Klein, 1975). A third category of histocompatibility genes has recently been described. These code for the medial histocompatibility antigens, so called because they share properties of both MHS and minor histocompatibility antigens (Fischer-Lindahl and Langhorne, 1981). This article will concentrate primarily on the genes of the MHS.

The purpose of this article is twofold: (1) to provide a short description of the structure and function of the MHS of mammals and (2) to summarize the extent of characterization of histocompatibility systems in seven species of veterinary importance. These are the dog, pig, cow, horse, sheep, goat, and cat. The MHS of the chicken has been the subject of several recent reviews (Longenecker and Mosmann, 1981; Briles and Briles, 1982) and will not be covered.

The specialized vocabulary adopted by histocompatibility researchers has long been a barrier to the transplantation of ideas across disciplines. Hence, we have devoted considerable time to definition (and sometimes re-definition) of terms in this article.

Several unique characteristics of the MHS have served to make this system a focus for immunogenetic research. First, the MHS has a distinct chromosomal organization that is very similar in all mammalian species thus far examined (Götze, 1977; Gill et al., 1978). This evolutionary conservation of genetic structure suggests that the MHS has functions that have proved worth preserving. Second, the genes of the MHS are extremely polymorphic: they occur in a very large number of allelic forms. This polymorphism has also apparently been maintained throughout species diversification (Bodmer, 1972). Third, in the artificial situation of tissue and organ transplantation, the gene products of the MHS have an overriding importance as antigens. It has been estimated that approximately 1 of every 10 T lymphocytes can respond to a full MHS-incompatible graft (Wilson et al., 1968; Binz and Wigzell, 1975; Ford et al., 1975), whereas the frequency of lymphocytes reactive to minor histocompatibility antigens (Ford and Simonsen, 1971) or nonhistocompatibility antigens (Lefkovitz, 1974) is several orders of magnitude lower. This bias of the T-cell repertoire toward the recognition of foreign MHS antigens has been termed "alloaggression," an expression that well describes the violence of immunological reactions toward MHS antigens. Finally, there is the question of the true biological function of the genes of the MHS. Although all of the functions of the MHS are not known, several important immunological traits have been demonstrated to be controlled or influenced by genes of the MHS, both experimentally and at the clinical level.

Any attempt to understand the MHS must address three important questions that are directed at the characteristics just outlined:

1. Why are the transplantation reactions that are directed against antigens of the MHS so violent?
2. How do the MHS genes and their products operate at the cellular level to regulate immune responses?
3. Why does the MHS exist in such a highly polymorphic state?

The answers to these questions are not yet fully understood, but it is possible to address them in general terms. This requires some knowledge of the genetic and molecular structure of the mammalian MHS.

The MHS of humans and of the laboratory animal species has been reviewed extensively (Klein, 1975, 1979; Snell *et al.*, 1976; Götze, 1977; Bodmer, 1978; Svejgaard *et al.*, 1979). We have attempted to summarize here only the most important aspects of the biology of major histocompatibility systems.

II. Structure and Function of the Major Histocompatibility System

A. GENETIC STRUCTURE

The MHS is a chromosomal region that contains several genes with related functions (gene families). The exact number of genes within the MHS and its true boundaries are not precisely known and have been defined arbitrarily. In both human and mouse at least 10 genes that are considered to be part of the MHS proper have been identified.

Figure 1 shows a schematic diagram of the most important genes contained within the MHS. Some or all of the loci pictured have been described in all mammals that have been investigated (Götze, 1977), although the exact order of these loci varies between species. The MHS genes have been assigned to one of three categories, based on the structural and/or functional characteristics of their gene products. The categories are called simply Class I, Class II, or Class III (Klein, 1979). It is now believed that the genes within the different gene families have arisen by the process of gene duplication from a single primordial gene of each type. Three loci coding for Class I molecules have been

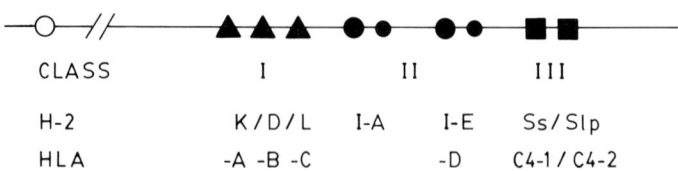

FIG. 1. Schematic view of the genetic structure of the MHS. The three major classes of MHS genes are depicted: Class I, Class II, and Class III. Below each type of gene are examples of the names given to them in the mouse (*H-2*) and human (HLA). Several other genes in the MHS have been identified, but they have been omitted for simplicity. The actual order of genes on the chromosome varies between species. The groupings shown here are for clarity.

described in the MHS of both human (Svejgaard et al., 1979) and mouse (Klein et al., 1978), and there is extensive evidence that other "Class I–like" genes exist in the MHS region (Margulies et al., 1982; Soloski et al., 1982). The number of Class II genes present in the MHS is not known. Three different Class II gene products have been characterized, but the exact numbers of genes that control the expression of these cellular products is still unclear (David, 1976, 1979; Klein and Figueroa, 1981).

Below each of the gene regions shown in Fig. 1 are the names that have been assigned to the principal MHS genes of human and mouse. The name *H-2* has been given to the MHS of the mouse, whereas the MHS of the human is called HLA. The abbreviation *H-2* stands for "histocompatibility locus-2," and HLA stands for "human lymphocyte antigen." The differences between species in the terminology for MHS loci and alleles are of historical origin. In general, the MHS genes of domestic animals have been named following the model used for the HLA system.

The principal Class I loci of mouse and human are called *H-2K*, *H-2D*, and *H-2L*, and HLA-A, HLA-B, and HLA-C, respectively. The Class II loci of the mouse code for at least three different products that are labeled A, E, and J. Analysis of the A and E gene products has shown that each consists of an α and a β polypeptide chain, which are expressed on the cell surface as a dimer. The Class II region of the mouse MHS should therefore contain an α and a β gene for both the A and E molecules. This appears to be true. However, the genes controlling the A and E molecules are not distributed as was originally expected. The genes that code for the A-α, A-β, and E-β proteins all map in the A region, whereas the E-α protein chain is controlled by an E-region gene (Uhr et al., 1979). The significance of this type of gene distribution is not known, but it may be of importance when an interaction between these different genes and/or their products is required. The J region of the *H-2* system is poorly understood, and homologous genes have not yet been identified in other species. Only one Class II region, called D or DR, has been well characterized in humans. However, there is mounting evidence that the region contains several genes coding for different products (Markert and Cresswell, 1980; Dick, 1982). The particular constellation of alleles on a single chromosome is called an MHS haplotype.

The Class III MHS genes code for components of the complement system. The relationship between the Class III molecules and the Class I and II molecules is not clear, and the Class III loci are not considered to be part of the MHS proper by some (Klein and Figueroa, 1981).

B. Molecular Structure and Tissue Distribution

The Class I and Class II MHS molecules have several points in common. They are both transmembrane glycoproteins that are expressed codominantly as cell surface antigens. Both classes of molecules exhibit considerable antigenic polymorphism, and both are involved in immune regulation. However, considerable information about the molecular biology of the Class I and II MHS molecules is available, and on this basis they can be distinguished (Table I).

The Class I MHS antigens are the classical transplantation antigens. They consist of two polypeptide chains: a large subunit of approximately 44,000 daltons and a small subunit of approximately 11,500 daltons, called β2 microglobulin. The two chains are noncovalently bound and expressed on the cell surface as a dimer. The larger subunit is coded for by an MHS gene and contains the polymorphic antigenic determinants. The gene for β2 microglobulin is not part of the MHS and is located on a separate chromosome (Strominger, 1981).

The large subunit can be divided into five regions or domains based on the overall three-dimensional structure that is generated by intrachain disulfide bonding. These domains include short intracellular and transmembrane portions, and three longer extracellular domains, each of approximately 10,000 daltons. These domains are called α-1, α-2, and α-3, of which α-3 is closest to the cell membrane (Strominger, 1981). It has structural homology with β2 microglobulin, an immunoglobulin domain, and the THY-1 molecule (Williams and Gagnon, 1982). The variable portions of the Class I molecule that characterize

TABLE I

Distinguishing Characteristics of Class I and Class II MHS Molecules

Characteristic	Class I	Class II
Approximate molecular weight	44,000	32,000 (α chain); 28,000 (β chain)
Membrane association with β2 microglobulin[a]	+	−
Tissue distribution	Wide: all nucleated cells	Narrow: restricted primarily to certain cell types of the lymphoreticular system
MHS Restriction	Cytotoxic lymphocytes	T-helper cell function; delayed-type hypersensitivity

[a] +, Association present; −, no association evident.

different alleles are located in the α-1 and α-2 domains (Strominger, 1981).

The structural homology between different Class I MHS allelic molecules is surprisingly high. Any two alleles at the *H-2K* locus have between 60 and 75% homology. However, a similar degree of homology exists between most *K*- and *D*-locus alleles and HLA-A and HLA-B locus alleles, or even between most human HLA and mouse *H-2* Class I antigens. The variation between Class I antigens occurs almost exclusively in the α-1 and α-2 domains, whereas the homology at other portions of the molecules is 90% or greater (Strominger, 1981). Earlier methods of determining homology by peptide mapping are gradually being replaced by amino acid sequencing (Coligan *et al.*, 1981), and this may change the early estimates. Techniques of DNA hybridization have already been applied to studies of the *H-2* system (Pease *et al.*, 1982), and further studies of this type will provide another view of the homology of MHS genes.

The Class I MHS antigens are present on virtually all tissues of the body. They are absent from mature erythrocytes of larger mammals such as humans and the domesticated species, but they are usually present on the erythrocytes of rodents, although at low density.

The Class II MHS molecules are dimers composed of two subunits: an α chain of 32,000 daltons and a smaller β chain of 28,000 daltons. Both of these subunits are transmembrane peptides and are expressed together on the cell surface. However, they are not covalently bound to one another (Owen and Crumpton, 1980).

The β subunits of the Class II molecules show considerable variation in peptide composition from allele to allele and therefore probably contain the polymorphic determinants. Overall, relatively little homology exists between the products of the A and E subregions (Cook *et al.*, 1978; Uhr *et al.*, 1979). Supporting data from studies in humans have also suggested that the β chain of the HLA-DR antigen expresses polymorphic differences (Walker *et al.*, 1980; Corte *et al.*, 1981). There also exists a high degree of homology between the murine Class II antigens from the E subregion and the best defined group of human DR antigens, suggesting their equivalence in the respective species (Allison *et al.*, 1978; Silver *et al.*, 1979). The human counterpart of the mouse Class II A-region antigen has been identified but is not yet well characterized (Goyert and Silver, 1981; Goyert *et al.*, 1982).

The three-dimensional structure of the polymorphic β chain is similar to that of the Class I antigen heavy chain (the 44,000-dalton unit). This includes the presence of two disulfied bond-created domains on the portion of the peptides that is on the cell surface as well as the

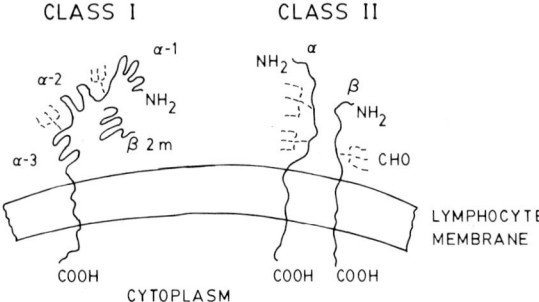

FIG. 2. Schematic diagram of Class I and Class II transmembrane glycoprotein molecules *in situ* at the cell surface. Both molecules have associated carbohydrate (CHO). The Class I molecule shows extracellular domains $\alpha-1$, $\alpha-2$, and $\alpha-3$. It is noncovalently associated with β2 microglobulin (β2m). Class II molecules are dimers with a larger α and a smaller β chain.

presence of intracellular and transmembrane portions. The domain that is closest to the cell membrane possesses a high degree of homology with the comparable Class I antigen domain (α-3) as well as with β2 microglobulin and an immunoglobulin domain. This homology suggests that the genes coding for all of these related proteins may have evolved from a single primordial gene (Larhammer *et al.*, 1981, 1982; Kaufman and Strominger, 1982). A schematic diagram of Class I and Class II MHS molecules *in situ* on the cell surface is shown in Fig. 2.

The Class II antigens have a narrow tissue distribution limited largely to cells of the lymphoreticular system. In peripheral blood these antigens are expressed most prominently on B lymphocytes, although some T lymphocytes and monocytes also express Class II antigens (Hammerling *et al.*, 1974, 1975; Winchester and Kunkel, 1979). The antigens of the J subregion of the *H-2* system are considered to be expressed only on T lymphocytes (Murphy *et al.*, 1976; Shreffler *et al.*, 1976). Expression of Class II antigens on B and T lymphocytes can also vary depending on disease states or the level of cell differentiation. For example, mature plasma cells or B lymphocytes that have been activated by pokeweed mitogen do not express Class II antigens (Halper *et al.*, 1978).

C. POPULATION STRUCTURE

The genetic variation in the genes of the MHS is one of its most remarkable features. Most genetic polymorphisms consist of a major allele that is very frequent and one or a few rare variant alleles that differ from the primary allele by only one or two amino acid substitutions. The genes of the MHS are very different. More than 20 alleles have been identified at the principal Class I MHS locus of the mouse, and it is estimated that more than 100 different alleles may exist in mouse populations worldwide (Klein and Figueroa, 1981). The polymorphism of Class II loci of the mouse is of the same order of magnitude, and the polymorphisms of the Class I and Class II HLA antigens of humans are equally extensive (Svejgaard et al., 1979). Additionally, any two Class I antigens are likely to differ from one another by several amino acid substitutions that are clustered in areas of the molecule distal to the cell surface (Strominger, 1981). Furthermore, as a consequence of the large number of MHS alleles in both human and mouse, few individuals in a population will carry identical MHS genes. As an example, individual wild mice heterozygous for the three principal Class I antigens and the two principal Class II antigens (A and E) would display 10 different MHS molecules on their cell surfaces. The functional significance of this tremendous genetic diversity has been a puzzle to immunologists for many years.

D. Immunological Function of MHS Molecules

Several important experiments have led to a partial elucidation of the functions of the Class I and Class II MHS molecules. Two types of experiments will be summarized.

1. Function of Class I Antigens

Zinkernagel and Doherty performed a series of experiments beginning in 1974 that have spawned thousands of variations and molded our current ideas about how T lymphocytes recognize antigens (Zinkernagel and Doherty, 1979). Using an *in vitro* system for measuring the cytotoxic reactivity of lymphocytes from mice that had been immunized with lymphocytic choriomeningitis virus, they demonstrated that immune T lymphocytes lyse virus-infected target cells under a particular set of conditions. This type of effector mechanism has immunological specificity: noninfected cells are not killed, nor are cells infected with non-cross-reacting viruses. However, the system also has genetic constraints: virus-infected target cells are not killed unless they carry the same Class I antigens as the immune T lymphocytes. Other genetic differences between the T lymphocytes and the target cells do not seem to influence the cytotoxic T-lymphocyte response. This phenomenon is called MHS-mediated restriction of T-lymphocyte function, because the Class I MHS antigen effectively restricts the way in which a conventional antigen is recognized by the T lymphocytes.

Doherty and Zinkernagel demonstrated in their experiments that the cellular target in virus-infected cells that is recognized by cytotoxic T lymphocytes consists of two parts. One part is viral antigen, and the second is a Class I antigen. The molecular basis of this dual recognition is yet to be elucidated.

2. Function of Class II Antigens

By similar kinds of experiments, it was shown that the antigen-specific proliferation by primed helper T lymphocytes is restricted by Class II antigens. Guinea pig T lymphocytes primed *in vivo* with soluble antigens such as tetanus toxoid or synthetic polypeptides such as poly-L-lysine can be induced to proliferate *in vitro* upon secondary challenge with the antigen. However, an antigen-presenting cell (macrophage-like) is required in this system in addition to the original antigen. These antigen-presenting cells must also carry the same Class II alleles as the primed T lymphocytes (Thomas et al., 1977; Shevach, 1978). This work demonstrated two points: (1) the T-lymphocyte receptor recognizes antigens only on cell surfaces and (2) part of the antigenic complex recognized by helper T lymphocytes consists of Class II antigens.

We now understand that T lymphocytes can be divided into several functionally distinct classes. Cytotoxic T lymphocytes, such as those that lyse virus-infected cells, are restricted by Class I antigens. The Class I antigens are present on virtually all cell types and therefore are distributed in a suitable fashion for this effector function. The T lymphocytes that help B lymphocytes produce antibody (helper T lymphocytes) and the T lymphocytes that produce delayed-type hypersensitivity (DTH) reactions are restricted by Class II antigens. These T lymphocytes are activated by antigen that is presented to the T-lymphocyte receptor by antigen-presenting cells of the lymphoreticular system. Class II antigens are expressed primarily by cells of the lymphoreticular system. Thus the specificity of receptors of the two principal classes of T lymphocytes (cytotoxic and helper/DTH) appears to be governed by the two principal classes of MHS molecules.

3. Immune Response Genes and Disease Associations

Observations linking the MHS and the genetic control of immune responsiveness have come from two sources. First, immune response (*Ir*) gene phenomena were identified in the inbred laboratory animal species. The first specific *Ir* gene was identified in guinea pigs by using the synthetic haptenated homopolymer dinitrophenyl-poly-L-lysine

(DNP-PLL). The ability to produce antibody to DNP-PLL was shown to be inherited as a simple Mendelian-dominant character. Further experimentation demonstrated that a particular strain of guinea pig (Strain 2) could respond to all PLL-hapten complexes, whereas Strain 13 could not. The gene determining this immune response was termed the PLL *Ir* gene. Subsequent to these observations, immune responses to a variety of synthetic polypeptides were studied in mice, and these experiments gave similar results to those obtained with guinea pigs (reviewed by Benacerraf, 1981; McDevitt, 1981).

The first evidence for linkage of *Ir* genes to the MHS was obtained in 1968 from the results of cell transfer experiments. The ability of mice to produce antibody against synthetic multichain polymers was transferred between responder and nonresponder strains by immune spleen and lymph node cells (McDevitt and Tyan, 1968). These cell transfer experiments and the results of a genetic analysis of backcrosses demonstrated that *Ir*-gene function was linked to the MHS.

The *Ir* genes of mice were mapped within the *H-2* complex between the *K* and *D* regions using recombinant strains in a cooperative effort involving several laboratories, thus defining the "*I* region" of the MHS (McDevitt *et al.*, 1972). The current usage of the term *I* region denotes the region between the *H-2K* and *H-2S* regions to which genes regulating immune responses to several antigens and the genes controlling the expression of Class II antigens are mapped (Klein *et al.*, 1974). The precise relationship between Class II antigens and *Ir* genes is still unclear. However, it has been suggested that the genetic defect in nonresponder strains lies at the level of the T-cell receptor (Nagy and Klein, 1981).

Epidemiological investigations in humans have identified "disease associations" between HLA and various pathological conditions (Dausset and Svejgaard, 1977). These associations simply mean that certain HLA antigens have a higher or lower frequency in individuals affected with certain diseases than they do in the population of unaffected individuals. Associations of HLA with disease have been shown with more than 50 conditions (Dausset and Svejgaard, 1977; Dick, 1978; Ryder *et al.*, 1979). Many of the conditions have inflammatory and/or immunological components, which suggests an autoimmune etiology. These include several arthropathies, acute anterior uveitis, psoriasis, and celiac disease. For some conditions the causes are unknown. Associations of HLA with allergic and infectious diseases are relatively rare (see following discussion).

The associations vary in the risk attributed to the inheritance of a particular HLA antigen and susceptibility to a given disease. Most of the associations are quite weak and raise the risk of developing a condition only two- to fourfold (Ryder et al., 1979). The fact that the associations are not absolute can be interpreted in several ways. The HLA gene may not be responsible for the disease association, but only linked to an *Ir* gene that is itself responsible. Linkage disequilibrium, the tendency for particular combinations of alleles of linked genes to occur together more often than expected on the basis of their respective gene frequencies in populations, is a characteristic feature of the HLA system (Alper et al., 1982). Alternatively, susceptibility may be a multigenic trait with the HLA gene controlling only a portion of the genetic basis of the disease. Finally, because the MHS is incompletely characterized and because diseases with different etiologies but similar manifestations may be grouped together, it follows that the ability to identify disease associations is also imperfect (Bodmer, 1980).

Although the pathophysiological basis of HLA disease associations is not known, several hypotheses have been put forward in explanation. First, it is possible that HLA antigens cross-react with antigens of pathogenic organisms, thus interfering with recognition by the immune system because of self-tolerance. The association of the HLA-antigenic specificity B27 and ankylosing spondylitis is believed to be related to a cross-reaction between the antigens of the HLA complex and the possible causative organism, *Klebsiella pneumoniae* (Ebringer et al., 1978). This hypothesis is supported by the results of *in vitro* leukocyte proliferation tests. The leukocytes from B27-positive individuals respond at a lower level against *K. pneumoniae* than do leukocytes from B27-negative individuals. Individuals who are B27 positive respond normally against other types of bacteria. That specific lack of responsiveness to *K. pneumoniae* may involve a self-tolerance is supported by reactivity patterns of antisera raised in rabbits against *K. pneumoniae*, which also react with lymphocytes carrying B27 (Seager et al., 1979). However, another report suggested that the *K. pneumoniae* organism may modify the B27 antigen and thus lead to autoimmune pathology (Geczy et al., 1980).

Second, a particular HLA antigen may act as a receptor for attachment or penetration to target cells by bacteria or viruses, thus causing an increased susceptibility to the infecting agent. There is only one example of HLA antigens serving as a receptor site for a pathogenic organism. The Semliki Forest virus has been demonstrated to bind to the Class I antigens (Helenius et al., 1978).

Finally, HLA disease associations may reflect the operation of human MHS-linked *Ir* genes. Human lymphocyte antigen–associated differences in the magnitude of antibody responses have been reported following infection with measles virus (Haverkorn *et al.*, 1975) and *Plasmodium falciparum* (Osoba *et al.*, 1979), as well as for poliomyelitis virus and diphtheria toxoid following vaccination (Haverkorn *et al.*, 1975). These differences in levels of specific antibody appear phenotypically similar to the variations in antibody levels attributed to MHS-linked *Ir* genes in rodents. In addition, several HLA-associated diseases and immune functions show stronger association with the human Class II antigens than with the Class I antigens (Keuning *et al.*, 1976; Sasazuki *et al.*, 1978). This lends support to the hypothesis that *Ir* genes are involved in at least some of the associations between the HLA system and the susceptibility to certain diseases.

4. Summary of Immunological Functions of the MHS

With the information just summarized, we can formulate hypotheses that attempt to answer the three questions posed at the beginning of this section.

Why are transplantation reactions to MHS antigens so violent? It is probably because of the nature of the T-lymphocyte receptor. Conventional antigens are normally recognized by T lymphocytes in association with their own MHS antigens. Foreign MHS antigens on grafted tissues may look to T lymphocytes like "self" MHS antigens coupled with foreign antigens, such as viruses. This could lead to abnormal triggering of large numbers of clones of T lymphocytes, resulting in the very strong immune responses mounted against MHS antigens associated with transplantation rejection (Lemmonier *et al.*, 1977).

How do immune response genes work? The repertoire of T-lymphocyte receptors must be able to recognize all conventional antigens in association with the MHS antigens of each species. In effect, two separate repertoires are required: one for cytotoxic T lymphocytes, which recognize antigen in association with Class I antigens, and one for helper T lymphocytes, which recognize antigens in association with Class II antigens. It is likely that "holes" exist in these repertoires. That is, receptors will be lacking for certain combinations of foreign antigens and MHS alleles (Schwartz, 1978). Animals carrying such alleles would be unable to make a response to those antigens. They would behave as "low responders" in *Ir*-gene terminology. The cellular mechanisms leading to a nonresponder state are not known, but they could involve specific clonal deletion or suppressor cell activity.

Why are there so many alleles at MHS loci? The answer may lie in a consideration of natural selection pressures in relation to *Ir* genes. If an animal cannot recognize a certain pathogen (i.e., lacks an *Ir* gene for a protective immune response), then it will succumb to infection when confronted with that pathogen. However, it is unlikely that the same *Ir*-gene deficit would occur with more than one MHS allele. Furthermore, deficits to different antigens would be expected to occur with different MHS alleles. With a large number of MHS alleles at the population level, it is likely that only a small percentage of individuals of any species would be susceptible to a given pathogen as a result of *Ir*-gene deficits. At the level of the individual animal, it would be advantageous to display as many different MHS alleles as possible in order to decrease the chance of being a nonresponder to an important pathogen. Thus MHS heterozygotes would be favored. Furthermore, duplication of MHS genes would also be favored, because this would increase the number of different Class I and Class II alleles that an individual could express. In support of this hypothesis is evidence that mice heterozygous for MHS antigens make stronger and broader responses to viral infections than do homozygous mice (Doherty and Zinkernagel, 1975).

E. Non-MHS–Linked Immune Response Genes

Although much emphasis has been placed on the role of MHS gene products in the regulation of immune responses, there is considerable evidence that other genes also contribute to immune reactions. Biozzi and colleagues (1979, 1981) have demonstrated through an extensive series of breeding experiments that between 10 and 15 genes influence the antibody response of mice to a number of natural antigens such as sheep red blood cells and bovine serum albumin. Two of these genes are linked to genes known to influence immune responses: *H-2* and a gene controlling immunoglobulin allotypes. Similar experiments revealed that selection of mice for high antibody production resulted in negative selection for cell-mediated immune responses, and vice versa. The effect of these genes on immune responses does not appear to be antigen specific, and thus differs from the MHS-linked *Ir* genes described previously.

An example of a specific *Ir* gene not linked to the MHS is the *Lsh* gene, which controls resistance to *Leishmania donovani* in mice (Plant et al., 1982). The *Lsh* gene is now thought to be identical to the *Ity* gene, which controls resistance to *Salmonella typhimurium* (Hormaeche, 1979). Resistance to most pathogenic organisms is likely to be influenced by many genes. In addition to the *Lsh* gene, a second gene or genes that map within or close to the *H-2* complex also appear to influence the course of *Leishmania* infections in mice (Blackwell *et al.*, 1980).

F. Nonimmunological Functions of the MHS

The majority of experiments designed to elucidate the functions of MHS molecules have concentrated on the role of the MHS in regulating immune responses. However, a substantial body of observations is accumulating that links the genetic control of a wide variety of nonimmunological traits to genes within or close to the MHS. Most of this information has been generated in the mouse *H-2* system mostly as a result of the availability of numbers of inbred strains that differ only at the MHS.

Many of these nonimmunological associations involve quantitative differences in physiological parameters (Ivanyi, 1978). Included are the genetic control of receptor levels for glucocorticoids (Gupta and Goldman, 1982) and total body weight (Simpson *et al.*, 1982). A fascinating study by Yamazaki and colleagues demonstrated that mice are capable of learning discrimination of MHS types, probably via chemosensory channels (Yamazaki *et al.*, 1979).

This introduction to the major histocompatibility system has been both selective and cursory. Large areas of MHS research have been barely mentioned, or omitted entirely, such as fetal–maternal interactions involving MHS genes. We refer interested readers to the many comprehensive reviews on this subject (Klein, 1975; Snell *et al.*, 1976; Götze, 1977).

G. Detection of MHS Polymorphisms

Polymorphisms at MHS loci may be detected in several ways: by skin graft rejection, serology, cell culture techniques, or biochemical characterization of alleles. For routine identification of MHS antigens (commonly called tissue typing), serology is used almost exclusively for the Class I antigen systems. Class II antigen polymorphisms are commonly defined either by serology or by cell culture. This section provides a short description of the most common methods of testing for Class I and Class II MHS alleles and the analysis of data that are generated using them. Detailed descriptions of these methods and others may be found in the *NIAID Manual of Tissue Typing Techniques* (Ray, 1979). Less frequently used methods will be described in the following sections as they arise. Most methods for histocompatibility testing in domestic animals have been adapted from methods used in HLA typing with little or no modification.

1. Serological Assays and Data Analysis

The serological assay used most extensively for detecting Class I MHS alleles of humans and other outbred species has been the microlymphocytotoxicity test. This test was developed by Terasaki and McClelland (1964) and has since undergone numerous minor modifications (Mittal et al., 1968; Ray, 1979). In this test 1–2 µl of an antiserum are incubated with 1000 to 3000 target cells in wells of specially designed microtest plates. The test is performed under an oil droplet to prevent evaporation of the reagents. The most widely used target cells are lymphocytes isolated from peripheral blood. The antiserum–lymphocyte mixture is incubated for 30 to 60 min to allow the antibodies to bind to the cell surface antigens, and then a complement source (usually rabbit serum) is added to effect cell lysis. The lytic reaction procedes for 1 to 2 hr. At the end of this stage the dead lymphocytes are stained by adding a vital stain such as eosin Y or trypan blue to the test mixture, and the reaction is then stopped and fixed by the addition of formaldehyde. The tests are scored visually using a tissue culture microscope, and the reactions are considered positive if a certain percentage (usually >50%) of the target cells have been killed.

A similar serological assay has been developed for the detection of Class II antigens. However, the more limited cellular expression of these antigens requires the use of different target cells. Generally, a B-lymphocyte–enriched target cell population is used. This enrichment can be achieved by various methods, including rosetting of T cells, "panning" on petri dishes coated with anti-Ig (Ray, 1979), and recovery of B cells from nylon wool columns (Julius et al., 1973). The rest of the microlymphocytotoxicity test is very similar to that used for Class I antigen typing (van Rood et al., 1975). The antisera used for Class I and Class II typing have been developed from a variety of sources and will be described for each domestic animal species in the appropriate sections.

The availability of inbred strains has facilitated histocompatibility research in laboratory rodents, because unlimited numbers of animals of known genotype are available for immunization and absorption experiments and experimental breeding. This has made analysis of serological data from these species relatively easy. For humans and the outbred animal species a variety of techniques for antiserum analysis have been developed to overcome the problems of genetic heterogeneity. A principal goal has been the identification of antisera from different sources that recognize the same MHS-antigenic specificities. Antisera to MHS antigens are generally complex, but it is possible to group sera that have antibodies in common. Researchers working with the HLA system have used statistical analysis based on a 2×2 chi square to compare lymphocytotoxicity patterns. Antisera that have high mutual correlation coefficients are grouped together or "clustered," because it is likely that they identify the same antigenic specificity (Albert and Götze, 1977). The use of computers has made this type of analysis feasible for the large volumes of data that are generated in MHS research (van Rood and van Leeuwen, 1963). The cluster analysis has been of enormous value and has been used extensively in the characterization of typing reagents in several outbred species.

2. Cell Culture Techniques

The mixed lymphocyte reaction (MLR) and cell-mediated lympholysis (CML) assays are *in vitro* tests of T-cell function. They have been widely used as models of the proliferative (MLR) and effector (CML) phases of graft rejection. The two assays are related. The MLR is a proliferative assay that measures genetic differences primarily, but not exclusively, at Class II MHS loci. Cytotoxic lymphocyte precursor cells in a mixed lymphocyte culture differentiate into cytotoxic T lymphocytes, which are the effector cells in the CML assay. When generated in an MLR, these cells are directed primarily against Class I MHS antigens.

These assays, in particular the MLR, can be used in the characterization of antigens of the MHS. In the MLR, mononuclear cells from different individuals are cultured together, and a subpopulation of cells, probably T-helper lymphocytes, is induced to proliferate if differences in the Class II antigens are present between the cell donors. This proliferation is usually measured by the specific uptake and incorporation of radioactive thymidine by the proliferating cell population. One-way reactions, in which the cells from only one of the donors are free to proliferate, are generated by blocking the cellular metabolism of the "stimulating" cell population by treatment with irradiation or mitomycin-C.

Homozygous typing cells (HTC) are stimulator lymphocytes from Class II antigen-homozygous individuals. These cells do not stimulate lymphocytes from an individual who carries the Class II-antigenic specificity of the HTCs. These cells can be used to type for allelic products of the Class II region on the basis of a lack of response in the MLR test.

In the CML test, cytotoxic T lymphocytes that are generated in extended MLR cultures are recovered and recultured with specific target cells. These target cells are generally blast cells from mitogen-stimulated cultures or leukemic cell lines that have been labeled with radioactive chromium (^{51}Cr). Target cells that express the same Class I antigen as the original MLR stimulator cell are specifically lysed. Lysis is measured by the release of ^{51}Cr into the culture supernatant. Details of the MLR and CML assays have been documented extensively (Klein, 1975; Snell *et al.*, 1976; Götze, 1977).

Polymorphisms at Class I and Class II loci can be detected using either the serological or lymphocyte culture assays just described. Although the two types of assays generally give similar results, they should be thought of as complementary tools for investigating antigens of the MHS. The serological and cellular assays represent, respectively, the B-lymphocyte and T-lymphocyte view of the MHS polymorphisms.

III. Histocompatibility Systems of Dogs

A. Introduction

Experimental studies of transplantation in dogs have led to two major advances in histocompatibility research. Morten Simonsen in 1953 rediscovered the graft-versus-host reaction during experimental studies of kidney allografts in dogs some 37 years after the phenomenon had first been described, misinterpreted, and forgotten (Murphy, 1916). Seven years later, again using the dog as a model for kidney transplantation, Govaerts (1960) identified cytotoxic lymphocytes in canine thoracic duct lymph which were generated as a result of sensitization to an allograft. This was the first description of the cytotoxic T lymphocyte. The importance of the dog to transplantation research has led to extensive characterization of histocompatibility systems in this species. At present the dog lymphocyte antigen (DLA) system represents the most extensively studied and best defined MHS of any of the domestic mammalian species.

B. DLA: Class I Antigens

1. Typing Reagents

The first work directed at the definition of the canine MHS centered on the production of typing reagents. Antisera were produced by planned immunizations with a variety of tissues, including lymph node cells, bone marrow cells, peripheral blood leukocytes, and tissue homogenates. Different immunization routes were also compared. Antisera were tested using hemagglutination, leukoagglutination, and complement-mediated lymphocytotoxicity assays. The resulting antisera reacted with antigens on leukocytes and occasionally against erythrocyte antigens (Kasakura et al., 1964; Puza et al., 1964; Cleton, 1965). The use of skin allografts as the immunization antigen source was also tested, giving similar results (Altman and Simonsen, 1964; Rubinstein and Ferrebee, 1964; Epstein et al., 1968; Cohen and Kozaki, 1969). Preliminary absorption studies of these antisera using leukocytes and erythrocytes suggested that several different antigenic specificities were being recognized (Rubinstein and Ferrebee, 1964).

The continued generation and characterization of antisera for use in identifying new antigen specificities has been an important aspect of work on the DLA system. Vriesendorp et al. (1971) compared the production of lymphocytotoxic antibodies following the rejection of intestine and skin grafts. Both types of grafts were capable of stimulating an antibody response: 8 of 18 dogs raised a high-titered antibody response following rejection of the intestinal grafts, and 21 of 26 responded in a similar manner to skin grafts. Antisera were also taken from postpartum dogs that had been immunized by transplacental passage of fetal antigens during pregnancy. This source of antisera can be very valuable, especially if large breeding colonies are available. However, the sera taken following graft rejection are considered a better source of DLA-typing reagents, because only about 15% of the parous dogs produced high-titered antibody responses (Vriesendorp et al., 1977).

Cross-immunization between family members, such as between parents and their offspring, has been widely used in the production of anti-DLA reagents. The principal benefit of this type of immunization is that it limits the DLA incompatibility to a single haplotype. In addition, it makes possible the generation of antiserum typing banks that can be used to type individuals of the same or related families and other colony members. This typing can in turn serve as the foundation for DLA functional studies (van der Does et al., 1973).

A final source of DLA antisera has been that made by immunization of rabbits with acetone-dried canine spleen powders. Preliminary results demonstrated that high-titered antibodies can be produced and that they recognize cell surface antigens on dog lymphocytes. The specificity of these reagents was increased by absorptions, also using powdered spleen tissue (Leon et al., 1975). This method has not been used extensively for DLA research.

2. Genetic Definition, Tissue Distribution, and Biochemical Analysis

Genetic analysis of the antigens recognized by the DLA antisera was accomplished using the same statistical techniques that had been used for HLA research. This included the use of computerized, chi-square–based cluster analysis of typing data on unrelated individuals to identify groups of antisera that recognize the same antigen. This was followed by genetic studies using full-sibling families. Six antigens were originally described. However, family studies showed that they were not all inherited independently, and it was suggested that two closely linked loci controlled the expression of these antigens (Vriesendorp et al., 1972). Subsequent experiments by other groups confirmed the existence of two DLA Class I loci, and the number of defined antigen specificities rose to eight at the first locus and seven at the second locus (Albert et al., 1973). The two DLA Class I antigen loci are very closely linked: only three recombinant offspring have been identified in 410 informative segregations (Vriesendorp et al., 1973). This recombination frequency is about 0.7%, which suggests a map distance of slightly less than 1 centimorgan. A third Class I locus has since been identified, and several of the antigens first thought to be part of the second locus have been reassigned to the third segregant series (Vriesendorp et al., 1977). These three loci are now commonly referred to as DLA-A, DLA-B, and DLA-C, following HLA terminology (Table II).

The phenotypic frequencies of the DLA Class I antigens vary greatly among different groups and breeds of dogs. This is most noticeable

TABLE II

GENE FREQUENCIES OF CURRENTLY RECOGNIZED DLA CLASS I ANTIGENS[a]

DLA-A		DLA-B		DLA-C	
1	0.013	4	0.163	11	0.172
2	0.058	5	0.163	12	0.130
3	0.296	6	0.106	R 15	0.146[b]
7	0.106	13	0.122	Blank	0.552
8	0.026	R 16	0.024[b]		
9	0.115	P 17	0.147[b]		
10	0.110	Blank	0.422		
Blank	0.276				

[a]Vriesendorp et al. (1977).
[b]New, provisionally defined specificity.

when comparing mongrel dogs to purebred beagles. The distribution of these antigens suggests that most of the alleles at the DLA-A and DLA-B loci are in Hardy–Weinberg equilibrium. However, several combinations of alleles from the three segregant series are present in the unrelated dog population and in families at higher frequencies than expected, suggesting linkage disequilibrium. This is especially true for certain products of the DLA-A and DLA-C loci (Vriesendorp et al., 1973, 1977).

The tissue distribution of the DLA Class I antigens has not been extensively investigated. The DLA antigens are present on lymphocytes, as these cells serve as targets for most of the Class I antigen-typing assays. The Class I antigens are also thought to be expressed by many other cell types such as skin cells and the tissues of most internal organs, because the rejection of these organs as grafts leads to the production of anti-Class I antibodies (Puza et al., 1964; Cohen and Kozaki, 1969; Vriesendorp et al., 1971; Westbroek et al., 1972). However, the stimulation for those antibodies could have come from passenger leukocytes in the grafted organs.

Preliminary biochemical analysis of the DLA Class I antigens has shown that they are composed of two subunits. The DLA-A2 antigen has been removed from the surface of spleen cells by papain digestion. The subunits have molecular weights of about 12,000 and 37,000. The smaller subunit is believed to be canine $\beta 2$ microglobulin. Purification of the solubilized DLA-A2 antigen was accomplished using lentil-lectin column chromatography, demonstrating that this antigen contains carbohydrate (van der Feltz et al., 1981).

C. DLA: Class II Antigens

1. Mixed Lymphocyte Reactivity (MLR)

The major direction of the research into the DLA Class II antigen system has involved the use of MLR assays. The culture conditions used for canine MLR have changed dramatically in the time span covering DLA research. Macroculture systems were used initially. These were done in test tubes with a total culture volume of 1 to 2 ml and 10^5 to 10^6 lymphocytes/ml (Rudolph et al., 1969). These assays have since been replaced by microculture systems that use 0.1–0.25 ml total culture volume and 96-well microtest culture plates. However, the number of cells per culture has not changed (Gluckman et al., 1973; Goldman and Flad, 1975). Cryopreserved lymphocytes have been used for both the stimulating and responding cell populations (Netzel et al.,

1975; Weaver *et al.*, 1975). The long culture period of 7 days (Rudolph *et al.*, 1969; Goldman *et al.*, 1975) has been partially replaced with shorter culture periods of 5 to 6 days (Goldman and Flad, 1975; Bijnen *et al.*, 1979). However, it has been suggested that the longer 7- to 8-day culture period may serve as a more definitive test when working with individuals that are likely to share haplotypes such as littermates or inbred dogs (Bijnen *et al.*, 1979). A peculiarity of canine lymphocyte culture systems is that they are incubated at 39°C, slightly higher than the 37.5°C used for most mammalian lymphocyte cultures.

Genetic control of MLR reactivity in dogs was demonstrated in the early days of DLA research. These genetic experiments took advantage of the large litter size of the dog. The distribution of MLR genotypes and their use in MLR analysis are shown in Fig. 3. In this type of test group, MLR-identical siblings are mutually nonstimulatory, and large families were found to consist of four such MLR-matched groups. Each group represents one of the four possible MLR genotypes, demonstrating that MLR proliferation was controlled by a single genetic system. Mutual lack of MLR stimulation was seldom observed in tests between unrelated dogs, which suggested the existence of multiple alleles (Rudolph *et al.*, 1969; Templeton and Thomas, 1971).

The typing of Class I antigens and MLR antigens in the same families demonstrated that the two antigen systems were associated: MLR responses were negative between DLA-identical, related dogs (Rudolph *et al.*, 1969; Albert *et al.*, 1973; Goldman *et al.*, 1975b). However, the results of MLR experiments using unrelated dogs could not be predicted reliably by Class I typing, demonstrating that the proliferative cellular response was not controlled by the same loci that controlled the expression of Class I antigens (Bachvaroff *et al.*, 1973). Using a more complete battery of typing reagents, van den Tweel *et al.* (1974) demonstrated that reactivity in the MLR test among unrelated dogs could usually be predicted using Class I antigen typing providing the typing was very complete. When unrelated dogs were matched for alleles at both the DLA-A and DLA-B loci, MLR test results were usually negative (10 of 14 pairs failed to respond). The proportion of nonreacting pairs dropped to 21 of 62 if only three alleles were shared between test dogs. Matching for only the DLA-A locus antigens led to intermediate results, with 17 of 38 negative tests, whereas only 4 of 24 tests were negative when dogs were matched only for DLA-B locus alleles. The higher frequency of negative responses associated with the matching of DLA-A locus alleles suggested that the genes involved in MLR control are more closely linked to DLA-A than to DLA-B.

The use of the MLR assay within families led to the identification of

HISTOCOMPATIBILITY POLYMORPHISMS OF DOMESTIC ANIMALS 23

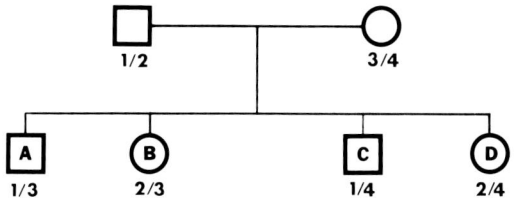

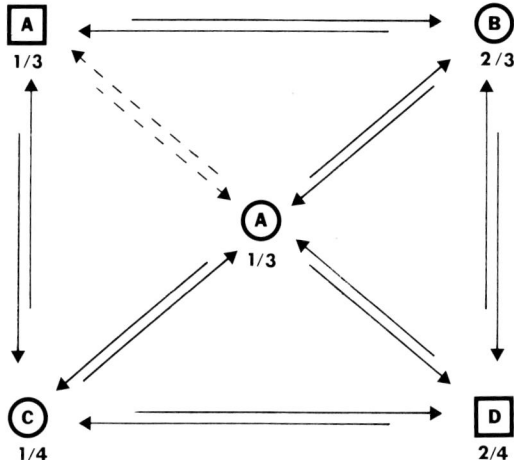

FIG. 3. Analysis of MLR data within full-sibling families. The top portion shows the four MLR genotypes that can occur in a family, assuming that alleles controlling the expression of MLR antigens belong to a single genetic system. The parents are both heterozygous for MLR alleles and carry 1 and 2 (sire), and 3 and 4 (dam), respectively. Four different MLR genotypes can be produced in the subsequent offspring (types A, B, C, and D), none of which are the same as the parents. The lower portion demonstrates the common MLR patterns found in tests between littermates (solid arrows, MLR stimulation; dashed arrows MLR nonstimulation). When more than four individuals are present in the family then some must be MLR identical, and subsequently they are mutually nonstimulatory in MLR assays.

dogs that were homozygous for their MLR antigens. These dogs were identified on the basis of the one-way reaction patterns obtained when they were tested against their heterozygous siblings with which they shared one haplotype (Grosse-Wilde et al., 1973; Schroeder et al., 1975a) (Fig. 4). These homozygous dogs could also be identified on the basis of their Class I DLA antigen genotypes (Gluckman et al., 1975). Lymphocytes from homozygous animals were used as stimulator cells

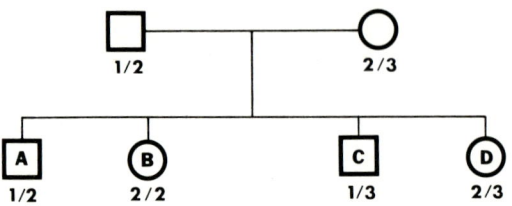

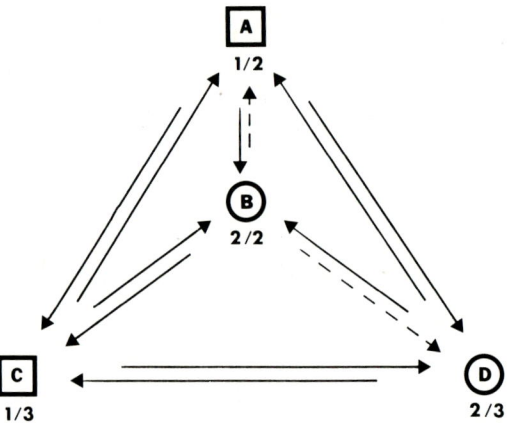

FIG. 4. Identification of MLR-homozygous individuals. The upper portion shows the MLR genotypes of a full-sibling family in which the parents share one MLR haploytpe. The four resulting genotypes of the offspring are represented as types A, B, C, and D. The lower portion depicts the MLR reactivity patterns expected from this family. Reciprocal MLR stimulation (solid arrows) is observed between individuals of types A and C, A and D, C and D, and C and B. The homozygous individual of type B does not stimulate (dashed arrows) family members that share MLR specificity 2, including the parents. The homozygous individual is stimulated by its nonidentical family members. This type of pairwise reaction is known as one-way MLR stimulation and is used to identify MLR-homozygous individuals.

(homozygous typing cells, HTC) to define MLR antigen specificities in unrelated dogs. Individuals that are not stimulated by an HTC are typed as "positive" for the MLR antigen expressed on the HTC. Grosse-Wilde et al. (1974) described four different MLR specificities using HTCs and suggested the existence of three others based on MLR reactions that could not be characterized with the available HTC panel. Nine DLA-MLR antigens have since been defined using HTCs (Vriesendorp et al., 1977). These MLR specificities have been given the internationally recognized designations DLA-50 to LDA-58 (Table III). The MLR antigens are frequently found in linkage disequilibrium with Class I antigens (Grosse-Wilde *et al.,* 1974; van den Tweel *et al.,* 1974; Vriesendorp *et al.,* 1977).

The inheritance of parental MLR antigens with Class I antigens in a haplotype suggests the presence of a single DLA-linked locus for MLR control. However, several one-way MLR reactions have been observed that could not be explained assuming MLR antigen homozygosity at a single locus. The existence of a second locus controlling MLR responses has been suggested (Goldman *et al.,* 1975a,b).

In another study, siblings that were totally matched for DLA antigens, including MLR antigens, were induced to respond to one another following a series of alloimmunizations. Skin grafts and blood were used for the immunizations. Peripheral blood lymphocytes taken from the immunized dogs became reactive in the *in vitro* MLR assay in 7 of 13 experiments when cells from the donor of the skin grafts and blood were used as the MLR stimulators. This response was specific: the immunized dogs failed to respond against other stimulator cells that had failed to stimulate in preimmunization tests (Gluckman, 1980). Similar results have been observed in the rhesus monkey and have been interpreted as evidence for a second, weaker MLR locus (van Es and Balner, 1979). This similarity of the dog MLR experiments with those of the rhesus monkey lend support to the hypothesis that a second MLR locus exists. However, it is also possible that the proliferative responses of these DLA-matched, immunized dogs were directed

TABLE III

WELL-DEFINED DLA–MLR ANTIGENS AND THEIR ASSOCIATION WITH DLA-A, DLA-B, AND DLA-C ANTIGEN SPECIFICITIES[a]

MLR Antigen	Frequently associated with
DLA-50	A2, B4, C11
DLA-51	A2, B5, C11
DLA-52	A9, B6, C12
DLA-53	A3
DLA-54	A10, B6
DLA-55	A3, C11
DLA-56	A1, B13
DLA-57	A8, B13, C11
DLA-58	A9, B4, C12

[a]Vriesendorp (1977).

against minor histocompatibility antigens and not against a DLA gene product.

The use of peripheral blood mononuclear cells (monocytes and lymphocytes) in the *in vitro* MLR assays demonstrates the presence of MLR antigens on some of these cells, but the possible differential expression of these antigens by subpopulations of canine mononuclear cells has not been studied. The use of nonlymphoid cells as stimulator cells in MLR assays can be considered as indirect evidence for the presence of MLR antigens on these cells. It has been shown that canine liver cells do not stimulate the MLR but that cells from the pancreatic islets of Langerhans do stimulate (Rabionvitch *et al.*, 1981). However, expression of MLR antigens on islet cells is difficult to prove because islet cells are very autostimulatory in MLR. It may be that tissue-specific antigens are also being recognized in these MLR tests (Miller *et al.*, 1981; Rabinovitch *et al.*, 1981).

2. B-Lymphocyte Antigens

Little work has been done with the serologically defined Class II antigens of the dog. In a preliminary experiment Vriesendorp *et al.* (1977) tested sera from parous dogs against target cell preparations that had been enriched for B lymphocytes and found no evidence for the presence of antibody to antigens expressed preferentially on B lymphocytes. Other results have since suggested that antibody to Class II antigens can be produced. Soulillou *et al.* (1980), by immunization with allogeneic spleen cells, successfully produced antisera that recognized antigens that were expressed on a portion of spleen cells, but that were not present on platelets. Further studies on the distribution of these antigens on blood cells and genetic studies have not been published, so it is not clear if these antisera do recognize DLA Class II antigens.

Monoclonal antibodies have been used to demonstrate Class II–like antigens in the dog. Deeg *et al.* (1982) used a monoclonal antibody that had been raised against HLA-DR antigens and found that it cross-reacted with antigens of canine tissues. The antibody recognized a cell surface protein that consisted of two subunits of molecular weights similar to the Class II antigens of other species: 29,000 and 34,000. Quantitative immunofluorescence studies have demonstrated that this antigen is expressed heavily by B lymphocytes and monocytes. However, this antigen is also present on all canine peripheral blood T lymphocytes, although the amount of antigen expressed appears to be less than that found on B lymphocytes and monocytes. The distribution of this antigen on lymphocytes of various lymphoid tissues is similar to that described for dog peripheral blood lymphocytes. This widespread tissue distribution of this Class II–like antigen is an apparent anomaly when compared to the distribution of Class II antigens in most other species. However, definitive proof that this monoclonal antibody is recognizing a Class II antigen product of the DLA system has not yet been provided. Such information will be required before conclusions can be drawn regarding the functional roles and significance of this antigen.

D. Immune Response Genes

A single preliminary study on *Ir* genes has been done in the dog. The random copolymers of L-glutamic acid with L-alanine (GA), L-lysine (GL), or L-tyrosine (GT) were chosen as the test antigens. Small doses of these antigens were used first to immunize a limited number of unrelated dogs. Specific antibody titers were measured 3 weeks after the primary immunization and 1 week after the booster. Preliminary results showed that responder and nonresponder dogs could be identified for each of the test antigens in the normal dog population. Subsequent experiments using families suggested that the ability of a dog to respond to these antigens was associated with the DLA system (Vriesendorp *et al.*, 1977). It was not possible to ascertain the exact DLA map position of the *Ir* genes in this study.

E. Functional Studies of the DLA System

1. Transplantation Biology and the DLA System

The earliest transplantation experiments that used DLA typing involved skin allografts. It was shown that the mean survival time of the grafts could be more than doubled if the selected donors and recipients were matched for all detectable DLA Class I specificities (Mollen *et al.*, 1968). Antibody production usually occurred in dogs that had rapidly rejected DLA-mismatched grafts, whereas matched grafts generally failed to evoke a detectable antibody response (Vriesendorp *et al.*, 1971). This association between prolonged survival of skin allografts and DLA antigen matching was important evidence in the identification of the DLA antigen system as the MHS of the dog.

Transplantation experiments with vascularized whole organs soon followed. Rapaport *et al.* (1970) demonstrated that mean survival time of renal allografts could be doubled in donor–recipient pairs that were DLA matched when compared to their mismatched counterparts. This extension of graft survival time was seen using both related donor–recipient pairs (littermates) and unrelated purebred beagles, and without the use of immunosuppression (Table IV). The degree of DLA matching was very important: good renal allograft survival was achieved only if all DLA Class I antigens were shared between the graft donor and recipient. The sharing of some DLA Class I antigens led to extended survival over totally mismatched pairs, but this ex-

TABLE IV

DLA Influence on Allograft Survival

Graft	DLA Status	Donor–recipient relationship	Mean survival time (days)[a]
Skin[b]	Matched	Littermates	29.8 ± 3.0 (SD)
	Mismatched	Beagles	13.7 ± 2.3 (SD)
Kidney[c]	Matched	Littermates	28.6 ± 8.2 (SD)
	Mismatched	Beagles	14.8 ± 3.0 (SD)
Kidney[c]	Matched	Nonlittermates	28.3 ± 8.7 (SD)
	Mismatched	Beagles	12.4 ± 2.1 (SD)
Heart[d]	Matched	Littermates	53.2 ± 30.8 (SD)
	Mismatched	Beagles	7.3 ± 1.8 (SD)
Heart[d]	Matched	Nonlittermates	26.3 ± 14.6 (SD)
	Mismatched	Beagles	6.3 ± 1.6 (SD)
Lung[e]	Matched	Related (not littermates)	98.1 ± 62.6 (SD)
	Mismatched	Beagles	10.5 ± 4.0 (SD)
Lung[e]	Matched	Unrelated	23.1 ± 15.6 (SD)
	Mismatched	Mongrels	8.8 ± 2.2 (SD)
Intestine[f]	Matched	Littermates	45.3 ± 19.9 (SD)
	Mismatched	Beagles	15.3 ± 13.2 (SD)
Intestine[f]	Matched	Nonlittermates	27.5 ± 16.2 (SD)
	Mismatched	Beagles	8.1 ± 1.0 (SD)
Liver[g]	Matched	Nonlittermates	43.9 ± 13.7 (SE)
	Mismatched	Beagles	8.7 ± 1.2 (SE)
Pancreas[h]	Matched	Littermates	42.0[i]
	Mismatched	Beagles	10.5[i]

[a]Mean survival time expressed as mean value ± the standard deviation (SD) or the standard error (SE) of the mean, as given by the authors of each cited reference or as calculated from their data.
[b]Mollen et al. (1968).
[c]Rapaport et al. (1970).
[d]Rapaport et al. (1971).
[e]Blumenstock et al. (1971).
[f]Westbroek et al. (1971).
[g]Chandler et al. (1972).
[h]de Gruyl et al. (1973).
[i]A measure of the variation was not given by the authors.

tended graft survival did not approach that attainable with totally matched pairs (Westbroek et al., 1972).

The lack of reactivity between donor–recipient pairs in the MLR test can also be used as a method of selection, although this test should be used only among littermates (Kisken and Malek, 1969). Experiments using unrelated mongrel dogs have confirmed and extended these findings for both the Class I and the Class II antigens. Westbroek et al. (1975) compared renal allograft survival in different groups of mongrel dogs that were matched either partially or totally for their Class I antigens or for their MLR antigens, or for both. The results demonstrated that the MLR antigens are the most important antigens in the DLA system with respect to renal allograft survival. However, the best renal allograft survival was achieved when donor–recipient pairs were matched for both the Class I and the MLR antigens.

Transplantation experiments using other organs also demonstrated the influence of the DLA system on allograft survival. Matching for DLA antigens increased the survival time of orthotopic heart (Rapaport et al., 1971), lung (Blumenstock et al., 1971), intestine (Westbroek et al., 1971), orthotopic liver (Chandler et al., 1972), isolated pancreas (de Gruyl et al., 1973), and intact nerve tissue allografts (Singh et al., 1977). Table IV summarizes these results.

The procedures involved in the allografting of live bone marrow cells differ from those used for other allografts. In most instances the allograft recipient is "conditioned," usually by whole-body irradiation, to ensure preliminary engraftment of the transplanted marrow cells. The long-term success or failure of bone marrow grafts is complicated further by the graft-versus-host (GvH) reaction. The earliest experiments with bone marrow allografts demonstrated the importance of DLA compatibility in survival of the graft and the recipient. A high degree of matching for both the Class I and the Class II DLA antigens was required for engraftment and long-term survival (Epstein et al., 1971; Storb et al., 1971a, 1973). However, a large proportion of dogs, usually greater than 50%, eventually died of GvH disease, even though the recipients had received bone marrow from DLA-identical littermates (Storb et al., 1971a). These results suggested that incompatibility at non-DLA histocompatibility genes could cause the GvH disease.

Vriesendorp et al. (1975b) found that DLA-mismatched donor–recipient pairs do occasionally survive and suggested that DLA-linked loci are probably also involved. Interaction between non-DLA histocompatibility genes and genes of the DLA system, or linkage of genes controlling GvH reactivity to the DLA system, have not been firmly established (Bachvaroff et al., 1978; Storb et al., 1976, 1978; Deeg et al., 1982).

The influence of the DLA system on allograft survival is important but not absolute. Most allografts are eventually rejected despite total DLA matching, probably as a result of minor histocompatibility antigen differences. Donor–recipient pairs were matched totally for DLA antigens to test for the influence of other antigen systems such as the Swisher erythrocyte antigens (Rapaport et al., 1971). Experiments involving different types of immunosuppression have also used matching or partial matching for DLA antigens in the donor–recipient pairs. Included were the use of antilymphocyte serum to extend the survival time of liver and pancreas allografts (Chandler et al., 1972; de Gruyl et al., 1973), the use of pretransplantation blood transfusions to increase kidney and bone marrow allograft survival (Storb et al., 1970, 1971b; Bijnen et al., 1982), and the use of immunosuppressive drugs (Storb et al., 1973; Blumenstock et al., 1981). Reviews covering these aspects of transplantation research in the dog are available (Rapaport and Bachvaroff, 1978; Vriesendorp, 1979).

2. Cell-mediated Lympholysis (CML) Assays

In vitro cell-mediated lympholysis (CML) assays have been used extensively in many species as models of the effector processes in organ graft rejection. Cytotoxic canine T cells were generated in bulk MLR cultures and tested for their effector capacity on ^{51}Cr-labeled PHA lymphoblast target cells from several donors. Specific release of label from target cells was seen only when the target cells carried the same DLA antigens as the stimulator cells used in the MLR cultures to generate the killer T cells (Flad et al., 1975; Schroeder et al., 1975b).

Using a similar assay system, the DLA antigens have been shown to restrict the cytotoxic lymphocyte response to virus-infected cells. Shek et al. (1980) demonstrated that canine distemper virus-specific cytotoxic lymphocytes could be produced by the inoculation of specific pathogen-free beagles with attenuated distemper virus. These specific cytotoxic lymphocytes killed virus-infected target cells (^{51}Cr-labeled canine testicular cells) but only when the effector and target cell populations shared DLA antigens. This restriction was not absolute, suggesting sharing of Class I alleles or cross-reactivity of antigens between the donors of the target cells.

3. Associations between DLA Antigens and Canine Diseases

The search for associations between the DLA system and canine disease has received little attention, with only four diseases having been investigated. These are leukosis or lymphoma, diabetes mellitus, hemolytic anemia, and the general susceptibility to allergies. Some weak positive associations were found for certain DLA antigens with diabetes mellitus and leukosis. Two alleles were present in the disease groups in slight excess. However, these associations were not statistically significant (Vriesendorp et al., 1973). Weak associations were also found between allergy and certain DLA antigen combinations, but a correlation between IgE levels and the same DLA antigens could not be demonstrated (Vriesendorp et al., 1975a).

F. Non-DLA Lymphocyte Alloantigens and Genes Linked to DLA

Antigens with cellular distributions that are similar to the DLA Class I antigens but are not controlled by genes within the DLA system have been identified. These antigens are present on peripheral blood lymphocytes and platelets and are identified by alloantisera. Alleles from two different antigen systems were identified and named DLB-1 and DLC-1 (Vriesendorp, 1973, 1976). Antisera that recognize a second allelic product in the DLB system have since been generated by alloimmunization with lymphocytes and platelets. The distribution of these two DLB antigens in families and in the dog population suggests that the DLB system is a closed, single-locus system controlling the expression of only two alleles (Krumbacher and Schnappauf, 1976). The biological roles and molecular constitution of the DLB and DLC antigens are not known.

A number of canine blood isoenzymes have also been studied, and several appear to be polymorphic, including phosphoglucomutase-3 (PGM-3) (Meera-Khan et al., 1973). Family analysis has shown that the locus controlling PGM-3 is linked to the DLA system (Vriesendorp, 1973, 1976). However, this linkage relationship is apparent only in the paternal haplotype, which suggests that a lower level of recombination occurs between the PGM-3 locus and the DLA system in males than in females. The exact map distance or map order of the DLA–PGM-3 complex has not been established (Vriesendorp et al., 1977).

G. International Workshops on Canine Immunogenetics

Investigators involved with DLA research have met in a combined effort to compare methods and antisera, and to analyze DLA-typing data at the international level (Vriesendorp, 1973, 1976). These workshops have led to confirmation of 13 DLA class I-antigenic specificities controlled by three separate loci. Data from MLR tests have also been analyzed at the workshop level and compared with Class I antigen typing to confirm the relationships reported by individual laboratories concerning these two antigen systems. Guidelines concerning the nomenclature of the DLA Class I and MLR antigens were also established during these workshops. A current list of established DLA antigens was published in 1977 by the IUIS committee on nomenclature (Vriesendorp, 1977).

Despite the efforts to standardize DLA typing, it still is not possible to compare the DLA-typing data from different laboratories directly. Both the one-stage and the two-stage lymphocytotoxicity assays have been used by different laboratories, and differences in test sensitivities have made the exchange of typing reagents difficult (Smid-Mercx et al., 1975). In addition, the suggested DLA nomenclature has not been totally accepted. One of the major DLA research groups prefers to report DLA antigen types by the letters b–o, as first described by Rubinstein and Ferrebee (1964). Genetic studies, functional studies, and transplantation experiments support the assumption that DLA typing performed in different laboratories is equivalent. However, a more widely accepted set of standard tests and nomenclature can only serve to simplify and promote the understanding of all future DLA research.

IV. Histocompatibility Systems of Swine

A. Introduction

Interest in the pig as a model for transplantation experiments stimulated the original studies of histocompatibility in this species. The experiments that provoked the most interest were those of Calne et al. (1969), which showed that livers exchanged as allografts between pigs could survive for extended periods without the use of immunosuppression or any cross-matching for histocompatibility antigens. Studies of the MHS of the pig soon followed.

B. SLA: Class I Antigen Definition, Serology, and Genetics

The earliest work on the MHS of the pig involved lymphocyte-typing assays and the use of antisera generated by alloimmunization, usually between related animals such as full siblings. Skin grafts, immunizations with lymphocytes, or combinations of these two techniques were used to generate antisera. The availability of large full-sibling litter families permitted comprehensive genetic studies to be performed. It was shown that all of the defined antigens were inherited as single units, probably as alleles at a single locus, and different from any of the known erythrocyte antigen systems (Vaiman *et al.*, 1970a, Simon and Hruban, 1971; White *et al.*, 1973).

Continued research led to the development of larger antisera-typing batteries and to the description of new antigenic specificities. Twenty-two Class I antigen specificities have been described thus far (Vaiman, 1979; Viaman *et al.*, 1979). The idea that more than a single locus was controlling these antigens was suggested to explain peculiar "cross-reactivities" that were found to exist between some of the newly defined antigens and those defined previously (Hruban *et al.*, 1977). This type of interpretation is based on the assumption that the alloantisera that were used probably recognized several antigens, all of which were present in a haplotype of the animal that donated the lymphocytes or the skin used in the immunization. When pigs from unrelated stock or from other breeds were used as lymphocyte donors, different combinations of alleles were probably being detected, assuming recombination at the population level between the genes under study. This means that "antihaplotype" antisera may recognize only parts of several of the new haplotypes and therefore give cytotoxicity reaction patterns that overlap or cross-react.

Formal proof for the existence of two Class I antigen loci came from large-scale genetic studies. Typing data from 268 families involving 2233 piglets identified two offspring that did not inherit their antigens in the expected parental haplotype but rather in combinations, which suggested that recombination had occurred between two Class I loci. A third Class I antigen locus in the SLA system has been tentatively identified by lysostrip analysis (Vaiman, 1979; Vaiman *et al.*, 1979).

The lysostripping technique takes advantage of the cell surface phenomenon of "antigen redistribution," whereby lymphocytes are induced to rearrange or "cap" surface antigens after these antigens have been cross-linked. In MHS research the cross-linking is achieved using specific anti-Class I antibodies. Lymphocytes that have been lysostripped are resistant to lysis in the microlymphocytotoxicity test when the same antiserum that was used for the lysostripping is also used as the cytotoxic test antiserum. If antisera against other gene products are used, cell lysis still is effected. The specific nature of this resistance to lysis means that it is possible to use different antiserum combinations for the lysostripping and the subsequent testing to ascertain the relationship between putatively different cell surface antigens. Class I antigens that are inherited together in a haplotype but that are distinct entities on the cell surface are likely to be products of different but closely linked MHS genes. The cell surface capping can also be monitored using immunofluorescence and antiimmunoglobulin reagents, which allow for direct visualization. The use of two different fluorochromes such as FITC and TRITC makes it possible to differentiate separate antigens: one antigen is capped whereas the other is left expressed in a more uniform or diffuse manner on the entire cell surface. The immunofluorescence variation of this technique is generally referred to as "co-capping" (Bernoco et al., 1972; Kourilsky et al., 1972). These techniques have proved to be very powerful tools and led to the identification of the third Class I antigen locus in both humans (HLA-C) and mice (H-$2L$) (Solheim et al., 1973; Demant and Neauport-Sautes, 1978).

The three loci of the SLA system that code for Class I antigens have been labeled SLA-A, SLA-B, and SLA-C. Twenty-six different SLA Class I–antigenic specificities have now been defined accurately using both family and population studies. However, the presence of linkage disequilibrium and serological cross-reactivity between both allelic products and antigens of different loci have made it impossible to assign all twenty-six specificities to particular SLA loci (Renard et al., 1982).

C. SLA: Class II Antigens

1. Mixed Lymphocyte Reactivity (MLR)

The use of MLR assays in pig families to study the MHS was done concurrently with Class I antigen serology. The presence of large full-sibling litters facilitated these studies. By using the one- and two-way MLR assays it was found that piglets of the same litter fell into four groups. Members of each group failed to respond to one another but responded to piglets from other groups. Piglets within each group were assumed to be identical to each other at loci coding for MLR antigens (Viza et al., 1970). These data were consistent with the hypothesis that one genetic region controls MLR in pigs. The rationale behind these experiments is the same as that described in the previous section on the dog (see Fig. 3).

Bradley and colleagues developed analytical methods for quantitating MLR reactions in pigs. They found that piglets could be characterized as totally matched, partially matched, or totally mismatched with their littermates based on the level of MLR test results. Totally mismatched pairs usually responded to the greatest extents whereas those that shared one antigen responded at a lower level (Bradley et al., 1972). A further extension of this finding made it possible to identify piglets within a litter that were homozygous for their MLR antigens. These pigs could then be used as a source for HTCs (Bradley et al., 1973). The use of serological typing for the Class I antigens in association with MLR assays showed that MLR test results could be predicted within litters based on Class I antigen-typing results, thus establishing an association between the antigens identified in the two test systems (Vaiman et al., 1970a, 1973). Recombinant animals found in family studies demonstrated that the Class I antigens and MLR antigens are controlled by separate loci that are closely linked (Vaiman et al., 1973). The genetic map distance between these different loci is about 0.4 centimorgans (Vaiman et al., 1979).

2. Class II Serology

Antisera against Class II SLA antigens were produced by alloimmunization between pigs that were matched for all known Class I-antigenic specificities but that differed in their MLR types. The antisera recognized polymorphic antigens, which are expressed primarily on B lymphocytes and a T-lymphocyte subpopulation, but not on platelets. Preliminary genetic studies demonstrated that the locus controlling these antigens was part of the SLA system and was linked closely to the locus controlling MLR antigens (Vaiman et al., 1975; Vaiman, 1979).

D. Miniature Pigs

A breed of miniature pigs has been used for transplantation research at the NIH Transplantation Biology Unit. These animals were selected because of their small adult size (150–250 pounds), short gestation period (4 months), and early onset of sexual maturity (4–6 months of age). They also have large litters. These miniature pigs have been inbred to a small degree to facilitate studies of the MHS and to help in assessing the role that the MHS plays in allograft survival.

Pigs were selected and bred to form MHS-homozygous lines. Selection was based on Class I antigen types, MLR studies, and the results of immunization studies carried out using sibling pairs. The immunization experiments were used in a fashion similar to the early swine MLR tests: pigs that did not respond to their littermates were assumed to share MHS antigens and were chosen for breeding to one another. This selection scheme led to the development of three miniature pig

MHS-homozygous lines, each of which has a different MHS type (Sachs *et al.*, 1976). The Class I antigens and MLR antigens are tightly linked: MLR-typing results can be predicted on the basis of Class I types (Sachs *et al.*, 1976; Leight *et al.*, 1977). The presence of serologically defined Class II antigens has been suggested by experiments using platelet-absorbed antisera (Lunney and Sachs, 1978). Genetic recombination between the Class I antigens and the MLR antigens has been documented. However, recombination between the MLR-stimulating antigens and Class II antigens defined by alloantisera has not been observed, suggesting that these antigens are the same, or at least that they map together in a region outside of the three Class I loci (Pennington *et al.*, 1981a).

E. Biochemical Characterization of SLA Antigens

Biochemical characterization of SLA antigens has shown that they are similar to those of other species. Class I antigens that have been removed from the surface of cells by papain digestion or detergent solubilization have a two-protein chain structure. The large unit has a molecular weight of 28,000 to 43,000, depending on the method of isolation, and the smaller unit is 11,000 to 12,000 (Arnoux *et al.*, 1974; Chardon *et al.*, 1978; Lunney and Sachs, 1978; Metzger *et al.*, 1981). The smaller subunit is homologous to a small protein present in pig urine, and it cross-reacts with human β2 microglobulin, suggesting that it is porcine β2 microglobulin (Chardon *et al.*, 1978). The partial amino acid sequence data for the N terminus of the heavy chain and of the β2 molecule demonstrated a high level of homology between these proteins and the analogous proteins in other species (Metzger *et al.*, 1982).

Class II antigens have also been isolated and characterized following detergent solubilization. These antigens are made up of two protein subunits, one with a molecular weight of 25,000 to 26,000 and the other with a molecular weight of 31,000 to 32,000 (Lunney and Sachs, 1979; Chardon *et al.*, 1981). At least one of the protein subunits of both the Class I and the Class II antigens are glycoproteins as demonstrated by their ability to bind to lentil lectin (Lunney and Sachs, 1978, 1979).

Biochemical studies using sequential immunoprecipitation techniques have demonstrated two Class II molecules that are expressed on pig lymphocytes (Lunney and Sachs, 1979; Chardon *et al.*, 1981). These molecules do not appear to be products of different alleles, suggesting the existence of two separate Class II loci.

Studies on the SLA Class I antigens have been expanded into the area of recombinant DNA technology. Singer et al. (1982) identified a sequence of pig genomic DNA that cross-reacts with a human HLA–DNA probe. The pig DNA that binds to the probe was purified, cloned, and inserted into the genome of a virus-transformed murine cell line (L cells). The L cells expressed the SLA Class I heavy chains on their cell surfaces, associated with murine $\beta 2$ microglobulin. The SLA-murine Class I antigen complex was recognized specifically by SLA-typing antisera.

This experiment demonstrates further the conservation of MHS genes between species in two ways. First, at the DNA level, human DNA was found to hybridize readily to pig DNA. Second, at the level of the protein products, pig Class I heavy chain was capable of associating with murine $\beta 2$ microglobulin to form an antigenically active cell surface product.

F. Histocompatibility Studies

Research in both the miniature pig lines and commercial pig breeds included experiments using skin allografts. Graft recipients that were matched for the Class I antigens of the skin donors rejected grafts in 8 to 12 days, whereas rejection occurred in 7 days or less in mismatched combinations. These results demonstrated that the serologically defined Class I antigens are part of the porcine MHS (Vaiman et al., 1970b; White et al., 1973; Hruban et al., 1974: Leight et al., 1978).

Similar results have been obtained using bone marrow and vascularized-whole-organ grafts such as kidney, intestine, and liver (Table V) (Vaiman et al., 1970a, 1972, 1981; Kirkman et al., 1979a; Fradelizi et al., 1981; Pazdera et al., 1981). Pigs that were totally mismatched for MLR antigens rejected grafts faster than those that shared one MLR antigen with the graft donor (Bradley et al., 1972).

Although the SLA system is known to play the major role in allograft survival, some characterization of minor histocompatibility antigens has also been achieved. Porcine erythrocyte antigens belong to a complex set of 15 systems (Rasmusen, 1975), several of which have been implicated in graft rejection. Leight et al. (1978) showed that split-thickness skin grafts were rejected in about 8 days if the graft donor and recipient were incompatible for the A-O erythrocyte antigens. This survival time is comparable to that found for A-O–compatible, SLA-incompatible pairs (Table VIA). The E-erythrocyte antigen system is also an important consideration when choosing transplantation donors and recipients. Matching for the E-system antigens in

TABLE V

SLA Influence on Allograft Survival

Graft type	SLA Status	Pig type[a]	Mean survival time (days)[b]
Skin[c]	Matched	Highly inbred	50.2 ± 29.2 (SD)
	Mismatched		9.1 ± 2.6 (SD)
Skin[c]	Matched	Partially inbred	9.8 ± 1.1 (SD)
	Mismatched		5.6 ± 1.1 (SD)
Skin[d]	Matched	Miniature pigs	11.8 ± 0.89 (SE)
	Mismatched		7.0 ± 0.36 (SE)
Kidney[e]	Matched	Commercial breeds	109.0 ± 22.1 (SE)
	Mismatched		11.5 ± 2.2 (SE)
Intestine[e]	Matched	Commercial breeds	49.5 ± 21.2 (SE)
	Mismatched		12.7 ± 4.8 (SE)
Liver[f]	Matched	Commercial breeds	63.5[g]
	Partial match		46.9[g]
	Total mismatch		32.8[g]

[a] Allografts were usually exchanged between full siblings. The term pig type refers to the source and genetic background of the experimental animals used.

[b] Mean survival time expressed as a mean value ± standard deviation (SD) or the standard error (SE) of the mean, as given by the authors of each cited reference.

[c] Pazdera et al. (1981).
[d] Leight et al. (1978).
[e] Vaiman et al. (1972).
[f] Vaiman et al. (1976).
[g] A measure of variation was not given by the authors.

SLA-compatible pigs increased skin graft survival time to about 11 days (Table VIB), and antibody to the E antigens was produced following transplantations with E-system incompatibilities (Hruban et al., 1974; Pazdera et al., 1981).

The involvement of other non-SLA systems in allograft survival has been suggested by inbreeding experiments. Survival times of skin allografts between full siblings increased from 10 days for outbred pigs to over 20 days for partially inbred pigs (Hruban et al., 1974; Pazdera et al., 1981). One explanation for this is that homozygosity for the erythrocyte antigens is increased within the inbred group, and this makes it more likely that erythrocyte compatibility can be achieved (Pazdera et al., 1981). However, other minor histocompatibility antigens may also be affected by this inbreeding.

Long-term graft survival also appears to be affected by minor histocompatibility systems. The rejection of renal or skin allografts leads to

TABLE VIA

INFLUENCE OF ERYTHROCYTE ANTIGENS ON SKIN ALLOGRAFT SURVIVAL: E-ERYTHROCYTE ANTIGENS IN HIGHLY INBRED PIGS[a]

Donor–recipient relationships		Number of experiments	Mean survival time (days ± SD)
SLA	E Blood groups		
Matched	Matched	36	54.4 ± 25.6
Matched	Mismatched	23	43.3 ± 28.0
Mismatched	Mismatched	13	9.1 ± 26.0

[a]Pazdera et al. (1981).

TABLE VIB

INFLUENCE OF ERYTHROCYTE ANTIGENS ON SKIN ALLOGRAFT SURVIVAL: A-O-ERYTHROCYTE ANTIGENS IN MINIATURE PIGS[a]

Donor–recipient relationships		Number of experiments	Mean survival time (days ± SE)
SLA	A-O Blood groups		
Matched	Matched	4	10.75 ± 0.25
Mismatched	Matched	6	7.00 ± 0.36
Matched	Mismatched	6	7.66 ± 0.54

[a]Leight et al. (1978).

the production of a potent and specific cell-mediated immune response that can be measured by an MLR assay with accelerated kinetics or by cell-mediated lympholysis assays. No antibody is produced in the presence of total SLA matching, but the cellular responses alone are sufficient to cause acute graft rejection (Kirkman et al., 1979b). It has also been suggested that the ability to respond to non-SLA histocompatibility antigens is under genetic control. Certain individuals can produce a more vigorous response than others. Most evidence suggests that both SLA-associated and non-SLA *Ir* genes are involved in graft rejection processes (Kirkman et al., 1979a; Pennington et al., 1981b).

G. TISSUE DISTRIBUTION OF SLA ANTIGENS

The Class I SLA antigens have been detected on cells from various tissues. Class I antigens are present on lymphocytes, platelets (Vaiman *et al.*, 1972), and granulocytes (Klaudy *et al.*, 1981). Soluble Class I antigens have been detected in serum by their ability to inhibit cytotoxic alloantisera (Schmid and Cwik, 1972; Cwik and Schmid, 1975), or by their ability to compete with papain-solubilized ^{125}I-labeled Class I antigen preparations in binding assays (Chardon *et al.*, 1977). It has been suggested that these soluble antigens may participate in the induction of tolerance toward foreign histocompatibility antigens. This theory is based on the observation that extended kidney and liver graft survival is achieved by the intravenous injection of graft donor blood, serum, or soluble cell membrane extracts prior to the implant of the graft (Calne *et al.*, 1970). Class I antigens are also expressed by kidney and liver cells. Cultured cell lines of liver and kidney parenchymal origin specifically absorbed antibody from cytotoxic antisera and were killed in an antibody-mediated cytotoxicity test (Davies *et al.*, 1976). Further studies have demonstrated that these antigens are also expressed by fresh cells in the kidney, particularly in the tubules and glomeruli. Expression on fresh liver parenchymal cells has also been established (Davies *et al.*, 1978). Finally, Class I antigens have been detected on spermatozoa by absorption using whole sperm (Jilek and Veselsky, 1972) and by direct cytotoxicity testing. It appears that these antigens may be expressed in a haploid fashion, reflecting the haploid nature of the germ line genome (Vaiman *et al.*, 1978c).

Class II SLA antigens appear to be expressed primarily on B lymphocytes and on a T-lymphocyte subpopulation, but not on platelets (Vaiman *et al.*, 1975). The presence of Class II antigens on cultured and fresh kidney cells has also been established. However, they do not appear to be expressed by liver parenchymal cells from either cultured lines or fresh liver isolates. This apparent lack of Class II antigen expression by liver parenchymal cells may explain the "privileged" status afforded to liver allografts by the immune system (Davies *et al.*, 1976, 1978). Class II antigens are also present on spermatozoa, but absorption studies suggest that they are expressed on sperm at much lower concentrations than on lymphocytes (Vaiman *et al.*, 1978c).

H. Antigens Shared by Erythrocytes and Lymphocytes

Experiments that used erythrocyte-typing reagents in lymphocytotoxicity tests have revealed three patterns of apparent shared antigen expression by these two cell types. First, specificities of the complex E system and at least one allele of the G system of erythrocyte antigens have been demonstrated to occur on lymphocytes. This was shown by typing a large panel of pigs with erythrocyte-typing reagents in both erythrocyte- and lymphocyte-typing assays. Reaction patterns in the erythrocyte-typing assay were highly correlated with those in the lymphocyte-typing assay for some of the E- and G-system antigens. That is, pigs positive for those erythrocyte antigens also had positive lymphocyte cytotoxicity reactions with the sera defining those antigens. The presence of these erythrocyte antigens on lymphocytes was confirmed by absorption studies (Hruban et al., 1972).

Second, antibodies specific for the erythrocyte antigens of the A-O system were found to be cytotoxic toward lymphocytes. Lymphocytotoxicity and positive erythrocyte-typing tests in individual pigs were highly correlated (Simon and Hruban, 1972). However, the expression of the A-O system antigens by lymphocytes has not been documented, and it has been suggested that these antigens are merely adsorbed to the surface of lymphocytes. These antigens are found in soluble form in many body fluids, including plasma, making this adsorption hypothesis a distinct possibility (Hojny and Glasnak, 1970).

Third, many other erythrocyte-typing reagents have been tested against lymphocytes, and most contain reactivity to lymphocyte antigens. However, none of these extra antilymphocyte reactivities is known to be associated with established erythrocyte antigen types. It is likely that the antilymphocyte reactivity in these reagents arose by contamination of erythrocyte immunogens with leukocytes, which would lead to active immunization against lymphocyte antigens not expressed by erythrocytes.

I. Non-MHS Lymphocyte Alloantigens

Two lymphocyte alloantigen polymorphisms that are not linked to the SLA system have been identified. Alloantisera that had been generated by lymphocyte immunization were used in identifying SLB. One detectable allele and a null allele have been described. These antigens are also present on thymocytes and are weakly expressed on kidney and liver cells. Attempts to generate antisera to the SLB antigens using skin graft techniques have been unsuccessful, suggesting that they are not present in skin (Hruban et al., 1978). The SLB antigen locus is apparently linked to an erythrocyte antigen system, the L system (Hruban et al., 1978). A similar lymphocyte alloantigenic system, called SLC, has been tentatively identified, but detailed reports have not yet been published (Pazdera et al., 1981).

J. Genes Linked to SLA

Analysis of litters using LOD scores (Morton, 1955) have shown that two of the erythrocyte antigen systems, J and C, are linked to the SLA system (Hruban et al., 1976, 1977). Breeding experiments using triple backcross matings have shown that the map order of this linkage group is SLA-J-C (Hradecky et al., 1982). Linkages between the SLA system and complement polymorphisms have not been documented. However, total hemolytic complement levels are associated with certain SLA haplotypes within families. Low complement levels are inherited as a recessive trait (Vaiman et al., 1978a).

The genetic control of the humoral immune response against hen egg-white lysozyme has been linked to the SLA system. The differences in response levels and the genetic control were first noticed using high doses of antigen (1 mg), but the differences were most prominent after secondary immunizations using lower antigen doses (10 μg). This pattern of control suggests that the response is under Ir-gene control (Vaiman et al., 1978b).

K. Association of Production Traits with SLA Antigens

The economic value of swine has led to a search for associations between detectable markers and production traits. Preliminary studies in three European breeds—the Large White, the French Landrace, and the Belgian Landrace—have shown that two important traits are associated with certain SLA antigen combinations. Lower growth performance is associated with the antigen combination of SLA 5, 20, 4 in the Large White breed, whereas higher carcass fatness is associated with the SLA 1, 15, 18 antigen group in the Landrace breeds (Capy et al., 1981). Similarly, neonatal weight gain rates have been associated with certain homozygous piglets (Kristensen et al., 1980). However, the generation of SLA-homozygous piglets may be detrimental in some instances. Vaiman and Renard (1980) have shown that certain homozygous SLA combinations are not present in the population at the frequencies that are expected, suggesting that selection against some homozygous antigen combinations may exist. Similarly, Kristensen et al. (1980) have shown that high mortality rates exist in certain homozygous SLA combinations. These preliminary results suggest that breeding and selection schemes based on SLA types may be of value to the future of the pig industry.

V. Histocompatibility Systems of Cattle

A. Introduction

The observations on red cell chimerism in cattle twins by Owen (1945) led to the classic studies on transplantation tolerance of Medawar and colleagues. These experiments, which were first carried out in cattle (Billingham et al., 1952), resulted in the formulation of the general theory of immunological tolerance in animals. After this early flush of success, the role of cattle as experimental animals in transplantation research declined dramatically. It was not until the 1970s that immunogeneticists again began to investigate histocompatibility systems of cattle. This work has led to the identification and partial characterization of the MHS of cattle, which is called BoLA, for bovine lymphocyte antigen.

B. Are Bovine Erythrocyte Antigens Expressed on Lymphocytes?

The bovine erythrocyte antigen and serum protein polymorphic systems represent one of the most comprehensively studied blood group systems of any domestic animal species. Currently, 11 erythrocyte antigen systems and several serum protein polymorphisms are used in standard cattle blood-typing services (Stormont, 1978). Several of these systems are very complex and polymorphic, and this high degree of antigenic complexity led to the idea that one of these systems might be the bovine MHS. This has turned out not to be true, but the experiments that demonstrated this are of historical interest.

Associations between bovine erythrocyte and lymphocyte antigen systems were sought by using antisera to known erythrocyte antigens in complement-mediated lymphocytotoxicity assays. Borovska and Demant (1967) tested typing antisera to 30 erythrocyte antigens against bovine lymph node lymphocytes. Varying degrees of antilymphocyte activity were detected in those antisera. Comparison of the lymphocytotoxicity patterns with the erythrocyte antigen types of the cell donors suggested that the lymphocyte antigens recognized were associated with the S-erythrocyte blood group system. The presence on peripheral blood lymphocytes of the erythrocyte and serum antigenic substance J (Hruban and Simon, 1973) and the B blood group system antigens E_3^- and Y^- (Schmid et al., 1978) were also demonstrated using lymphocytotoxicity testing with specific erythrocyte-typing reagents. In these reports a high degree of correlation was observed between the blood-typing results of the two cell types: only lymphocytes from those cows that expressed the test antigen on their erythrocytes were killed. Absorptions with either erythrocytes or lymphocytes were also specific and supported the cytotoxicity results. However, other reports have substantiated only the presence of lymphocytotoxic antibodies in erythrocyte-typing reagents. No correlations between lymphocytotoxicity patterns and erythrocyte types were found (Ostrand-Rosenberg and Stormont, 1974; Folger and Hines, 1976). Included in this study were the J and the B blood group antigens.

The reasons for these contradictions are unclear. However, it has been suggested that most of the antibody activity against lymphocyte antigens in antierythrocyte-typing sera is specific to those antigens and a by-product of the erythrocyte alloimmunizations, having been generated in response to a small number of contaminating leukocytes in the erythrocytes used as immunogen. Additionally, in the case of parous cattle, these antibodies may have been raised against fetal antigens of a previous pregnancy and therefore been present in the serum before any erythrocyte immunizations were performed (Folger and Hines, 1976). Subsequent research has shown that both of these hypotheses may explain the presence of lymphocytotoxic antibodies in erythrocyte-typing reagents. First, cattle do generate lymphocytotoxic antibody in response to pregnancy (Newman and Hines, 1979; Hines and Newman, 1981), and second, immunizations with small numbers of foreign lymphocytes (10^7) can generate a potent lymphocytotoxic antibody response (Newman and Brandon, 1981).

The presence of "extra" antibody reactivity in the antisera may explain the lymphocytotoxic nature of most blood-typing reagents, but it does not explain the specific cytotoxic and absorption reactivity seen against the J, E_3^-, and Y^- erythrocyte antigens. The J-antigen system differs from the other bovine erythrocyte antigen systems because the J-antigenic substance is present in the serum as well as on the erythrocyte surface in a J-positive individual. Actual expression of the J antigen by the cell is the result of specific adsorption of the J substance to the erythrocyte membrane (Stormont, 1978). It is feasible that a similar adsorption of the J substance may explain the expression of this antigen by lymphocytes. Differences in cell isolation techniques and washing steps could then account for the differences in the ability to detect the J antigen, because it may be removed by certain procedures. Adsorption of B blood group antigens has not been documented, and the specific expression or lack of expression of these antigens by lymphocytes has yet to be confirmed. In summary, erythrocyte antigens do not appear to be expressed on lymphocytes, with the possible exception of the adsorbed J antigen.

C. Class I Antigens

1. Source of Antisera

Most of the research effort into the bovine MHS has been directed at the identification and genetic characterization of the Class I antigens. The strategies employed follow those used in other outbred species, most notably those used in HLA research. These include the exclusive use of the complement-mediated microcytotoxicity assay, the use of large cell panels from unrelated individuals for preliminary characterization of typing antisera, a heavy reliance on statistical interpretation of the typing data, and the use of regional and international comparison tests and workshops to compare and disseminate pertinent data.

Antisera against Class I antigens have been obtained from two sources: (1) production by planned immunization with skin grafts, leukocytes, or purified lymphocytes and (2) the sera of parous cattle that have been immunized during pregnancy or at parturition with paternally inherited fetal antigens (Amorena and Stone, 1978; Caldwell and Cumberland, 1978; Spooner et al., 1978; Adams, 1980).

The antibody responses to lymphocyte alloantigens during bovine pregnancy have been followed in several experiments using cattle of different ages and involving different numbers of pregnancies. These studies have shown that a certain percentage (30–40%) of first-calf heifers can be expected to raise detectable antilymphocyte antibody either very late in the third trimester or following parturition. Very little antibody activity can be detected prior to the birth of the first calf (Newman and Hines, 1979, 1980). Antibody activity generated from a previous pregnancy may exist throughout subsequent pregnancies, and, as a consequence, sera from multiparous cows can be broadly reactive (Hines and Newman, 1981). The complex, polyspecific nature of the sera taken from older multiparous cows led to the suggestion that antisera for lymphocyte typing should be taken following the first or second pregnancies (Newman and Hines, 1979). However, subsequent studies have shown that sera from a large proportion of older cattle may also show restricted reaction patterns and therefore be valuable as typing sera (Table VII) (Hines and Newman, 1981).

Most parous sera, whether taken from first-calf heifers or multiparous cattle, are known to be polyspecific and generally have low

TABLE VII
Relationship of Serum Antilymphocyte Reactivity to Cow Age and Parity[a]

Age of cow (years)	Sera with reactivity (%)[b]	Sera with narrow reactivity (%)[c]	Number of pregnancies[d]	Number of sera tested
2	35	23	1	66
3	40	29	2	130
4	49	35	3	100
5	54	48	4	69
>5	60	40	>4	272

[a] Newman and Hines (1979, 1980); Hines and Newman (1981).
[b] The percentage of reactivity was determined using a panel of 36 selected test cattle.
[c] Narrow reactivity is defined as reactivity with lymphocytes of fewer than one-third of the panel animals. This level was chosen arbitrarily on the pretense that only sera of limited reactivity are likely to be valuable for use in tissue-typing research.
[d] The number of full-term pregnancies for the 2- and 3-year-old cattle were known. Parity of older cattle was estimated assuming the birth of one calf per year, the common reproduction rate in commercial herds.

titers, rarely exceeding 1:32. Because extensive absorptions may be required to produce monospecific antibody reagents, and the low titers of parous sera would preclude this, the value of these sera has been questioned (Spooner et al., 1979). However, the widespread use of antisera cluster groups that are formed by statistical analyses of the typing data means that monospecific antisera are not a prerequisite for accurate serological lymphocyte typing as they once were for the work with other bovine blood group systems. This ability to use polyspecific antisera and the widespread availability of parous sera, coupled with the lack of any required immunizations, has made this a most extensively used source of antisera for studies on the bovine MHS.

Despite the widespread use of parous sera, most laboratories have also generated specific antisera by other regimes. Two types of skin grafting have been used. Spooner et al. (1978) and Newman and Stear (1983) have described conventional methods using small full-thickness grafts that are placed in graft beds on the base of the tail or on the lower back. A novel skin implant technique has been described (Pringnitz et al., 1982). In this method a small full-thickness piece of skin is removed from the base of the ear of the donor and inserted into a small "pocket" that is cut in the loose skin of the recipient's neck.

Lymphocytotoxic antibody can be detected in serum 1–2 weeks following skin grafting. Peak titers are variable but are often very high

(1:128–1:2048), and they usually occur within the first 3 weeks after grafting. The early lymphocytotoxic response consists primarily of IgM; IgG is the predominant immunoglobulin later in the response. Antiserum of peak lymphocytotoxic titer is usually collected 2–4 weeks after grafting (Spooner et al., 1978; Newman and Stear, 1983). The antibody responses following skin implants appear to be similar, and it has been suggested that the best time to collect sera is 21 days after implanting the skin (Pringnitz et al., 1982).

Alloantisera generated by skin grafting tend to be multispecific (Spooner et al., 1978; Stone, 1981; Newman and Stear, 1983). In one study it was found that 12 of 12 sera taken at the time of peak titer (14–21 days postgrafting) reacted strongly with the lymphocytes from 73 to 100% of the cattle in a panel of 60 unrelated individuals from several breeds. This pattern of reactivity narrowed in subsequent weeks, but the titer also dropped significantly (Newman and Stear, 1983). Antisera such as these would need to be diluted or extensively absorbed to remove antibodies to all but the main specificities. Attempts to reduce the complexity of antisera generated by skin grafting, such as the exchange of grafts between siblings or dams and offspring, have been partially successful. However, absorptions were still required in most cases to make the antisera as specific as many parous sera (Spooner et al., 1978, 1979).

The final commonly used method to produce antisera to bovine lymphocyte alloantigens is by immunization with purified leukocytes or lymphocytes (Spooner et al., 1978; Amorena and Stone, 1980; Adams, 1980). The kinetics of the antibody responses following lymphocyte alloimmunizations is highly variable when compared to responses following skin grafting. In one study, 17 of 21 cattle produced detectable lymphocytotoxic antibody following one to four biweekly immunizations with 1 to 2×10^7 lymphocytes. Peak titers ranged from 1:2 to 1:1024. The immunoglobulin classes involved were the same as for skin grafting, primarily IgM early in the response followed by a predominance of IgG in later samples. The percentage reactivity of these sera in a panel of 60 cattle ranged from 3 to 100% after one or two immunizations. This percentage of reactivity increased as additional immunizations were given (Newman and Stear, 1983). The main advantage of immunizations with allogeneic leukocytes is that high-titered antisera of reduced specificity can be produced. The major disadvantage of this technique is that it is laborious, requiring isolation of the immunogen. Furthermore, two or more immunizations may be required to generate an antibody response (Amorena and Stone, 1982).

The antisera from these different sources all fit into the same cluster groups and therefore appear to recognize identical antigens (Spooner, 1979). It has been suggested that the most reliable method of MHS antigen definition may be to use antisera from all of these sources (Stone, 1981).

2. Serological, Genetic, and Biochemical Characterization

The Class I antigens of the bovine MHS have been described serologically. Amorena and Stone (1978) described 17 specificities using 70 typing sera; and the laboratory group at Texas A & M used 130 antisera to define 6 antigens (Caldwell and Cumberland, 1978; Caldwell, 1979). All of these defined antigens appeared to be products of a single polymorphic locus.

In 1978, nine different laboratories participated in the First International Bovine Lymphocyte Antigen Workshop. A total of 249 typing sera from the participating laboratories were tested against lymphocytes from 130 unrelated cattle of 21 breeds. The results of this comparison test demonstrated that the participating laboratories detected several antigens in common. Eleven antigens were designated "international workshop specificities." The locus controlling these antigens was termed BoLA for bovine lymphocyte antigens (Spooner, 1979). The results of regional workshops in 1979 in North America and Europe, and the Second International BoLA Workshop in 1980, have confirmed the identification of these 11 specificities and provided evidence for the existence of several others (Proceedings of the Second International Bovine Lymphocyte Antigen Workshop, 1982). The frequency distribution of these 11 specificities varies greatly among different cattle groups and breeds (Caldwell et al., 1979; Amorena and Stone, 1980; Oliver et al., 1981).

Absorption studies have been used to subdivide international workshop specificity BoLA-W6. It now appears as if BoLA-W6 represents a family of related antigens, similar to the subtypic–supertypic antigen families of the bovine erythrocyte antigen systems (Stormont, 1978; Spooner et al., 1980; Spooner and Morgan, 1981).

Unfortunately, many of the interlaboratory problems that exist among the DLA research groups are also present among the BoLA laboratories. Several slightly different microlymphocytotoxicity assays are used by various laboratories, and large differences in the sensitivities of these assays are thought to exist. This means that antisera characterized in one laboratory are not necessarily valuable to other BoLA workers and may require recharacterization upon exchange. Another problem exists with the distribution of the Class I-antigenic specificities. As mentioned previously, many of the alleles are present in different breeds with different frequencies. This difference in gene frequencies seems to extend to the geographic level: many of the international workshop-defined antigens have been detected only in European cattle, and they therefore cannot be easily studied by laboratories outside of Europe.

Preliminary biochemical characterization of one of the international BoLA antigens (W16) has shown that the bovine Class I antigen has a structure that is similar to that of other species. It is a glycoprotein with a molecular weight of about 44,000 that is associated with a second, smaller subunit with a molecular weight of about 12,000. It is assumed that this second subunit is bovine β2 microglobulin, but formal proof is lacking (Hoang-Xuan et al., 1982a).

The number of loci controlling the bovine Class I antigens is still unknown. Family studies have shown that at least 11 of the international workshop specificities behave as if controlled by alleles at a single locus with codominant expression (Caldwell, 1979; Amorena and Stone, 1980; Oliver et al., 1981). However, others have suggested that the data support the existence of a single genetic system that may consist of multiple linked loci (Adams, 1980; Stear et al., 1982b). In these studies antigens that have been defined by statistical analysis appear to be separate at the population level and yet are inherited together as a haplotype within families. These data have been interpreted to suggest the presence of separate but linked loci controlling the BoLA Class I antigens. Serological cross-reactivity between the antigens has also been suggested to explain these observations, but the statistical data do not support this idea. Additionally, co-capping experiments have demonstrated that at least two antigens that were inherited in one haplotype are expressed as separate antigens on the surface of lymphocytes, supporting the hypothesis that at least two loci are involved in controlling the BoLA Class I antigens (Stear et al., 1982b).

By analogy to other species, it is rather unexpected that a second or possibly a third Class I antigen locus has not yet been unambiguously identified. This may reflect several unique facets of the cattle population. First, genetic studies are usually done using paternal half-sibling families. In this situation a family consists of several offspring, all by a single sire, but out of several different dams. To collect segregation information on the antigens present in the sire requires a family of considerable size (more than five offspring plus their dams). This type of family provides information primarily about the bull's antigens;

little information is provided about maternal transmission of antigens. In addition, the widespread use of artificial insemination, segregation of cattle by breeds, and selection based on economic traits may be involved in maintaining strong linkage disequilibrium between different Class I loci, thus acting to keep certain antigen combinations intact within the population. The generation of more specific antisera and more extensive family studies, coupled with biochemical analyses and co-capping studies, will probably answer some of these questions about the number of genes involved in the BoLA system.

3. Histocompatibility Studies

Demonstration that the BoLA system is the bovine MHS has come from a series of simple transplantation experiments. Skin allografts were exchanged between groups of cattle that shared some, none, or all of their detectable Class I antigens. Experiments from two groups are in close agreement. Graft rejection could be detected in 10 to 12 days where Class I antigen mismatching was known to exist, whereas grafts exchanged between cattle that were matched for these antigens survived for about 16 days (Amorena and Stone, 1978, 1980; Adams, 1980).

D. Class II Antigens

1. Mixed Lymphocyte Reactivity (MLR)

A variety of cell culture parameters have been tested, and reproducible MLR assay protocols have been established for use with bovine peripheral blood lymphocytes (Emery and McCullagh, 1980; Splitter *et al.*, 1981). Usinger *et al.* (1977) first described the use of bovine MLR assays for genetic studies using paternal half-sibling families. This report demonstrated the existence of one- and two-way MLR responses between family members. By analysis of these one-way reactions it was possible to generate a hierarchy of responsiveness; by assuming that these responses were conforming to the mathematical law of transitivity, it was suggested that at least two loci control MLR in cattle.

The description of this MLR transitivity is unique to the cow, and it led to the suggestion that more than one locus controls MLR reactions. This differs markedly from the situations described in the dog and the pig, where genetic control of MLR responses appears to be under the control of a single locus. Details of the theory of MLR transitivity were described by Curie-Cohen *et al.* (1978), and an example is shown diagramatically in Fig. 5.

Subsequent studies of MLR reactions among full siblings generated

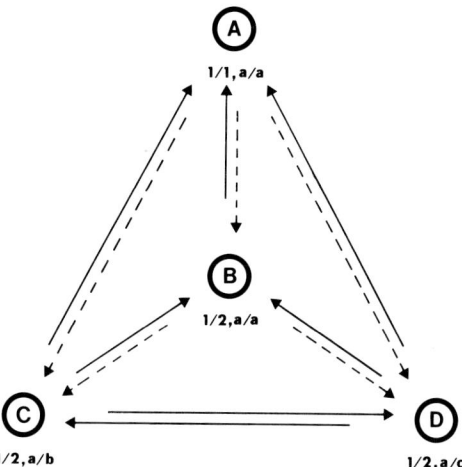

FIG. 5. Transitivity of bovine MLR. Individuals of type A are classified as homozygous and those of type B as heterozygous for a shared MLR specificity based on the one-way stimulation pattern (dashed arrows, MLR nonstimulation; solid arrows, MLR stimulation) between these types. However, MLR tests using types B, C, and D suggest that type B is also MLR homozygous, based on one-way stimulation patterns. This hierarchy of one-way MLR patterns is best explained by assuming that more than a single locus controls MLR responses. This theoretical example is diagrammed showing the involvement of two loci. The first locus is designated numerically and the second by lower case letters.

by embryo transfer were used to characterize further the genetic aspects of bovine MLR. These experiments demonstrated a significantly higher level of MLR response between BoLA-mismatched siblings than was observed between BoLA-matched siblings. However, a large portion of low responders from mismatched pairs was also observed, and this caused a large overlap between the two groups (Newman *et al.*, 1982b). Genetic linkage analysis of similar data revealed that the loci controlling MLR and the Class I antigens are linked, but it has not been possible to obtain an accurate estimate of the linkage distance using the available data (Usinger *et al.*, 1981).

The experiments using embryo transfer full siblings have neither supported nor refuted the two-locus MLR hypothesis suggested by the MLR transitivity data. Further analysis of larger families will be required to determine the number of loci that are stimulatory in bovine MLR cultures.

2. B-Lymphocyte Typing

Serological definition of bovine Class II antigens is still very much in its infancy. Newman *et al.* (1982a) have used alloantisera produced by immunization with lymphocytes and the two-color–fluorescence microcytotoxicity test (van Rood et al., 1976) to demonstrate the presence of B-lymphocyte alloantigens in cattle. The distribution of these antigens on blood cells suggests that they may be the bovine Class II antigens. These antigens are expressed primarily on B lymphocytes but not on platelets or erythrocytes. Their expression on monocytes and on a subpopulation of T lymphocytes was not investigated. Analysis of typing data on unrelated cattle using antisera that had been absorbed with platelets to remove antibody to Class I antigens demonstrated that these antigens are part of a complex, highly polymorphic system. Preliminary genetic studies indicated that the loci controlling Class I and Class II antigen expression are linked. However, an estimate of the linkage distance was not calculated. The number of loci coding for Class II antigens is not known. Family studies indicate that the antigens are probably controlled by a single genetic system. Absorption studies using lymphocytes and the reaction patterns of typing antisera suggest that two loci may be involved (Newman et al., 1982a).

A monoclonal antibody against human HLA-DR antigens and mouse alloantisera against both the A- and E-subregion antigens of the H-2 complex were found to react with antigens on the surface of some bovine lymphocytes. These cross-reactive antisera were used for partial biochemical characterization of the antigens. The antigens that were identified have a protein structure similar to the human and mouse Class II antigens. Subunits with molecular weights ranging from 27,000 to 34,000 were identified. Mouse antisera specific for A- or E-subregion antigens both exhibited this cross-reactivity, suggesting bovine counterparts for both of these antigens (Hoang-Xuan et al., 1982b). Formal proof that the molecules recognized by these cross-reacting antisera are the bovine Class II antigens was not provided. However, these results, coupled with the genetic data using bovine alloantisera and studies of MLR, support the hypothesis that an MHS-associated Class II antigen system is present in cattle.

E. Non-MHS Lymphocyte Alloantigens and Linkage of the BoLA Region to Other Genetic Markers

In addition to the BoLA system, a second locus controlling the expression of lymphocyte alloantigens has been described. Only a single antigenic specificity of this second system has been identified thus far. This antigen segregates from a blank or null allele in families, and the locus is apparently unlinked to BoLA. It was defined using antisera both from parous cows and from alloimmunizations, and it is expressed on all peripheral blood lymphocytes (Stear et al., 1982b).

Linkage analyses in large families using the LOD score method have failed to establish linkage between the BoLA system and any of the common erythrocyte antigen systems or polymorphic serum proteins. Included in these studies were the erythrocyte blood group systems of A, B, C, J, L. and Z, and the protein systems of transferrin, albumin, and hemoglobin (M. J. Stear and K. Bell, unpublished, 1982). Other studies have indicated that linkage may exist between the erythrocyte M system and the BoLA system (H. C. Hines, unpublished observations). However, the M antigens are expressed in an extremely low frequency in most of the common cattle breeds; therefore it may be difficult to determine accurately the exact linkage relationship. Linkage experiments using polymorphic isoenzymes or complement components have proved to be of limited value in cattle because of an apparent lack of polymorphism for many of these products (Stone, 1981). A similar lack of variation has been noted in preliminary experiments for total hemolytic complement levels (M. J. Stear, unpublished observations).

F. The BoLA System and Disease Associations

Speculations on associations between BoLA and cattle diseases (Adams et al., 1979) have led to preliminary experiments. Newman (1981) has shown that the BoLA system is associated with levels of resistance to the Australian cattle tick, *Boophilus microplus*. This association of the BoLA system with resistance to a complex ectoparasite is surprising when compared to the studies of *Ir* genes of the mouse *H-2* system, which have usually involved simple chemicals as antigens. However, studies on infestation by this tick have demonstrated that strong genetic (Wharton et al., 1970; Seifert, 1971) and immunological components (Roberts, 1968; Hewetson, 1971; Brossard, 1976; Schleger et al., 1976) are involved in resistance levels.

In another system, genetically restricted cell-mediated cytotoxicity against *Theileria parva* was demonstrated in peripheral blood lymphocyte populations from cattle immune to the parasite (Eugui and Emery, 1981). Although the experimental animals were not typed for MHS antigens, the patterns of responses observed were phenotypically similar to those seen in *H-2*–restricted cytotoxicity of virus-infected cells in mice (Zinkernagel and Doherty, 1979). The study was not designed to investigate genetically controlled resistance or susceptibility to *Theileria*, but its contribution to the understanding of immunological mechanisms operating in this important disease of cattle is significant.

G. BoLA AND HLA CROSS-REACTIVITY

An interesting aspect that has emerged from studies of the BoLA region is the antigenic cross-reactivity observed between the HLA and BoLA systems. This was first demonstrated by Iha *et al.* (1973), who showed that bovine alloantisera recognized alloantigens on human lymphocytes that were inherited in association with known HLA antigens. It was also found that HLA-typing antisera were cytotoxic against bovine lymphocytes. Monoclonal antibodies to HLA-A, HLA-B, HLA-C, and DR antigens, and human β2 microglobulin were tested against lymphocytes from numerous primate and nonprimate species, including the domestic farm animals. Cross-reactions with bovine lymphocytes were found much more frequently than for any of the other domestic species. In most instances the reactivity to bovine cells was similar in frequency to that seen using primate cells (Brodsky *et al.*, 1981; Brodsky and Parham, 1982; Teilland *et al.*, 1982). This high level of cross-reactivity between MHS antigens of two evolutionarily divergent species is extremely interesting and warrants continued investigation.

VI. Histocompatibility Systems of Horses

Compared to the homologous systems of dogs, swine, and cattle, relatively little is known about histocompatibility systems of the horse.

A. THE ELA REGION

The principal lymphocyte alloantigenic system of the horse is called ELA, for equine lymphocyte antigen. All evidence suggests that the ELA region is the MHS of the horse. However, critical transplantation experiments involving ELA-matched and ELA-mismatched donor–recipient pairs have not yet been reported.

1. Serology

The earliest description of ELA antigens used a ^{51}Cr-release assay to detect lymphocytotoxic antibodies in sera from pregnant mares and horses that had been immunized with allogeneic lymphocytes (Lazary *et al.*, 1975). Following this preliminary report, all subsequent descriptions of ELA antigens have used variations of the standard lymphocyte microcytotoxicity assay used in human tissue typing (Ray, 1979).

The ELA system has many similarities to the HLA and BoLA systems. Sera derived from pregnant or parturient mares have been the source of most of the alloantisera to ELA antigens (Bright *et al.*, 1978; DeWeck *et al.*, 1978; Mottironi *et al.*, 1981). However, some workers have also used alloimmunization with whole blood or lymphocytes as a source of reagents (Bailey, 1980). The ELA antigens have been shown to be expressed codominantly on peripheral blood lymphocytes by direct cytotoxicity testing (Bright *et al.*, 1978; Antczak *et al.*, 1982). On the basis of absorption experiments, they appear to occur on platelets (Bailey, 1980). Red blood cells lack ELA antigens (Bailey, 1980; Lazary *et al.*, 1980a).

Several groups have described ELA antigens that do not fit into a single allelic series (Bailey, 1980; Lazary *et al.*, 1980b; Antczak *et al.*, 1982). However, firm evidence for two or more linked loci in the ELA region, based on recombination in families or biochemical studies such as sequential immunoprecipitation of membrane molecules, is lacking. Evidence for 13 ELA antigens that behaved as alleles at a single locus was reported, with differences in the frequencies of particular antigens between breeds of horses (Antczak *et al.*, 1982). The 13 specificities in that study accounted for about 90% of the ELA alleles in both the Thoroughbred and Standardbred breeds of horses. Because unabsorbed pregnancy sera were the source of most of the reagents in that study, it is likely that the clusters of sera defining many of those ELA antigens contained antibodies against an entire haplotype of ELA antigens. Strong linkage disequilibrium and the population genetic structure of horse breeds, in which breeding males are rare relative to breeding females, could account for the difficulty in demonstrating a complex genetic structure for the ELA region.

A continuing series of international workshops foster collaboration on lymphocyte alloantigens of the horse. Twelve laboratories from four countries participated in the first antiserum exchange in 1981. These laboratories tested 200 antisera on lymphocytes from 1009 horses. The workshop discussions following computerized cluster analysis of the data resulted in the acceptance of six workshop clusters as international ELA specificities (manuscript in preparation). A similar serum exchange formed the basis of the 1982 workshop. Identification of the first six ELA specificities was confirmed at the 1982 workshop, and an additional five specificities were recognized (manuscript in preparation).

Of the 11 international workshop specificities, 10 behaved as alleles at a single locus, both at the workshop level and in individual laboratories. The gene frequencies of those 10 specificities in Standardbreds and Thoroughbreds are shown in Table VIII. The eleventh antiserum cluster accepted by the second workshop defined a lymphocyte alloantigen apparently not linked to the ELA region. The name proposed for the locus coding for this alloantigen was *Ely-2,* because it was considered to be different from the *Ely-1* gene described by Lazary and colleagues (1982). An important feature of the workshops on equine lymphocyte alloantigens has been a concerted attempt by participants to standardize reagents, procedures, and terminology.

2. Lymphocyte Culture

The genetic control of lymphocyte proliferation in mixed lymphocyte reaction (MLR) cultures was shown to parallel serological typing for ELA antigens in horse families (Lazary *et al.,* 1980b). Full siblings with identical ELA genotypes were mutually nonreactive in MLR cultures. In the same study, one offspring of a large horse clan was shown to be homozygous for both ELA antigens and MLR-stimulating determinants. These data suggest a genetic structure for the ELA region that is similar to that of the MHS of other species and therefore provides support for the hypothesis that the ELA region is the MHS of the horse. However, evidence for separate loci in the ELA region that determine serological and MLR-stimulating antigens has not been published.

3. Linked Loci

Bailey *et al.* (1979) have shown that the A blood group locus of the horse, which controls the expression of an erythrocyte membrane alloantigen, is linked to the ELA region. In the same study they found no evidence for linkage between the ELA region and genes coding for several other erythrocyte alloantigens, polymorphic serum enzymes, or coat color.

B. Non-ELA Lymphocyte Alloantigens

Reports of the possible existence of two or more linked loci determining ELA antigens (Bailey, 1980; Lazary *et al.,* 1980a,b) have not been substantiated at the level of the international workshops on equine lymphocyte alloantigens (1981 and 1982 reports in preparation). It is possible that cytotoxic antibodies to non-ELA lymphocyte alloantigens contaminating anti-ELA reagents could have caused serological reaction patterns that suggested two linked loci.

TABLE VIII

GENE FREQUENCIES OF INTERNATIONAL WORKSHOP SPECIFICITIES OF THE EQUINE LYMPHOCYTE ALLOANTIGEN SYSTEM[a,b]

	W1	W2	W3	W4	W5	W6	W7	W8	W9	W10	Total	Blank
Overall	0.13	0.08	0.12	0.05	0.10	0.05	0.03	0.04	0.07	0.11	0.78	0.22
Thoroughbred	0.00	0.16	0.18	0.00	0.18	0.01	0.01	0.00	0.19	0.04	0.77	0.23
Standardbred	0.25	0.01	0.05	0.11	0.07	0.06	0.05	0.10	0.00	0.25	0.95	0.05

[a] Data from the Second International Workshop on Lymphocyte Alloantigens of the Horse (1982, report in preparation).
[b] Gene frequencies (g) were determined from the phenotypic frequencies (f) by the formula: $g = 1 - \sqrt{1-f}$.

Lazary et al. (1982) have recently described a lymphocyte alloantigen that is inherited independently of the ELA antigens. Only one allele at the *Ely-1* locus has been identified by cytotoxic antisera, and because attempts to produce antibodies to other alleles by lymphocyte immunization have proved futile, it has been suggested that the *Ely-1*$^-$ allele may be a null mutant.

The *Ely-1* gene behaves as an autosomal dominant. The *Ely-1*$^+$ antigen is present on all lymphocytes and absent from red cells. Mixed lymphocyte reaction cultures between ELA-identical, *Ely-1*$^+$–disparate horses gave negative results. Sera from pregnant mares and antisera raised by alloimmunization with lymphocytes were used to define the *Ely-1*$^+$ antigen. The role of the *Ely-1* antigen in graft rejection is unknown.

The *Ely-1*$^+$ allele has a phenotypic frequency of about 50% in horse populations of several breeds. The *Ely-1* locus does not appear to be linked to loci determining erythrocyte alloantigens, polymorphic serum enzymes, or coat color. In a preliminary study of the distribution of the *Ely-1*$^+$ allele in diseased and normal horses, a statistically significant increase in *Ely-1*$^+$ horses was found in populations with chronic laminitis and navicular disease. The pathophysiological mechanisms causing these associations were not determined.

In an earlier study, Lazary and colleagues (1978) reported that certain of their antilymphocyte alloantisera reacted in differential fashion with lymphocytes from hyperimmunized horses making high-level (>2000 IU/ml) or low-level (<1000 IU/ml) antibody responses to tetanus toxoid. Positive cytotoxicity reactions with two antisera correlated well, but not absolutely, with high-level antibody responses. The antigen defined by those sera was not well defined in that study, but because the two antisera gave positive responses with about 50% of all horses, it is possible that they recognized the *Ely-1*$^+$ allele.

C. Histocompatibility and Pregnancy in Horses

The well-known hemolytic disease of newborn mules and foals is due to maternal immunization during pregnancy or at parturition with fetal red cells carrying histoincompatible, paternally inherited alloantigens. The initial descriptions of this condition represent some of the earliest investigations of untoward consequences of histoincompatibility and pregnancy in domestic animals (Caroli and Bessis, 1947; Bruner et al., 1948; Coombs et al., 1948). Maternal sensitization to fetal erythrocyte alloantigens is apparently rare, because only about 1 to 2%

of mares have serum antibody to erythrocyte antigens that was induced as a result of pregnancy (Bailey, 1982).

In contrast to this is the situation with respect to maternal sensitization to ELA antigens in the pregnant mare. Sera from stallions, geldings, and virgin mares are routinely found to be negative for alloantibody to ELA antigens (Bright et al., 1978). The reported frequency of antibody-positive sera from multiparous or primiparous mares has ranged from 85% (Bright et al., 1978) to 100% (DeWeck et al., 1978), respectively, in samples taken within 2 weeks after foaling. This is much higher than the frequency of pregnancy sera from cows (Newman and Hines, 1979), sheep (Ford and Elves, 1974), or humans (Ahrons, 1971) reported to contain cytotoxic antibody to MHS antigens.

Cytotoxic antibody to ELA antigens has been detected in colostrum with titers equivalent to those found in serum from the same animal (Lazary et al., 1980a). There is evidence that anti-ELA antibodies can be passively acquired by foals that ingest colostrum early in life. Of 32 serum samples from foals, 14 had antibody of the same specificity as that found in the serum of their dams, except for autoreactivity that had presumably been absorbed by the foals' tissues (Mottironi et al., 1981). Pathological effects on the foal of the ingestion and absorption of colostrum containing antibody to its own histocompatibility antigens have not been reported.

Independent evidence for a maternal immune response to fetal histocompatibility antigens has come from histological observations of the specialized tissues of the equine placenta called endometrial cups. The cups are small ulcer-like structures of the pregnant horn of the equine uterus. They develop from specialized trophoblast cells of the chorionic girdle that migrate into the endometrium of the mare at about day 35 of pregnancy. The endometrial cups secrete pregnant mare's serum gonadotropin. The so-called endometrial cup reaction is characterized by the accumulation of maternal leukocytes along the border of the cups. Leukocyte accumulations do not occur at other points along the endometrium–trophoblast border. It has been suggested that this leukocyte accumulation may represent a maternal cell-mediated immune response to fetal histocompatibility antigens (Allen, 1979). However, involvement of any particular alloantigenic system, such as ELA, has not been demonstrated for this cellular reaction.

Allen (1979) also reported that 9 of 10 primiparous Welsh pony mares produced cytotoxic antibody to paternal lymphocyte alloantigens, beginning as early as 44 days postconception. It was not determined if those antibodies recognized histocompatibility antigens of the

ELA system. The temporal relationship between the development of the endometrial cups and the maternal production of cytotoxic antibody suggests that the cup cells may have been the source of paternal histocompatibility antigens in this study.

In further investigations, Kydd et al. (1982) examined the sera from 69 equid pregnancies for the presence of cytotoxic alloantibodies to lymphocyte antigens. Normal and embryo transfer pregnancies were used in this study. Weekly serum samples from the mares were tested against lymphocytes from the stallion used for breeding or the sire and dam of the transferred embryos. In 16 intraspecies horse pregnancies, 94% of mares produced cytotoxic antibody that was first detectable between 44 and 70 days after ovulation. In all other types of pregnancies examined (19 intraspecies donkey, 6 interspecies mule, 2 interspecies hinny, 3 extraspecies horse-in-donkey, and 22 extraspecies donkey-in-horse), antibody production was observed less frequently, and sometimes with a more irregular onset. However, the dominant pattern of antibody response, which occurred in all types of pregnancy, was similar to that of intraspecies horse, with antibody first detectable between days 40 and 60 of pregnancy.

The cytotoxic antibody response of mares carrying extraspecies donkey conceptuses in the study of Kydd et al. (1982) was of particular interest for two reasons. First, the antibodies appeared to be directed primarily toward donkey alloantigens and not species-specific antigens, because some of the mares made antibodies that reacted only with cells from either the sire or the dam of the transferred donkey embryo they were carrying. This observation emphasizes the importance of maternal immunological recognition of paternally derived fetal histocompatibility antigens during normal equine pregnancy. Second, because endometrial cups apparently do not develop in that type of pregnancy, the stimulation of maternal cytotoxic antibody to fetal histocompatibility alloantigens in the absence of endometrial cup formation points to an alternative source of antigen that may also be immunogenic in normal horse pregnancy.

D. ELA AND COMBINED IMMUNODEFICIENCY DISEASE

Studies of the MHS of Arabian horses (Mottironi et al., 1981) were undertaken as part of a larger study of combined immunodeficiency disease (CID) in that breed (McGuire et al., 1974). No relationship between ELA and CID was demonstrated in that study (Mottironi et al., 1981). However, the availability of ELA typing in Arabians may make experimental immunological reconstitution of CID foals more feasible. Previous reconstitutions have been characterized by severe GvH disease (Perryman and Liu, 1980).

VII. Histocompatibility Systems of Sheep and Goats

A. HISTOCOMPATIBILITY SYSTEMS OF SHEEP

Early investigations of histocompatibility systems in sheep were used as a model for allograft rejection in humans. Schnickel and Ferguson (1953) observed that fetal sheep can reject maternal skin grafts as early as 80 days into gestation in a pregnancy of about 150 days. Using similar techniques, Silverstein et al. (1963) suggested that skin graft rejection by fetal sheep can occur in the absence of production of antibody to foreign histocompatibility antigens of the graft.

The description of lymphocyte alloantigen polymorphisms of sheep did not begin until the early 1970s. As for most other domestic species, the reported characteristics of the ovine lymphocyte antigen (OLA, also known as SH-LA) system are similar to those of the HLA system. Thus, Ford and Elves (1974) reported that 52.1% of sera from parous ewes contained antibody cytotoxic for sheep lymphocyte alloantigens. In the same study, sera from rams and lambs were found to be negative for antibody. The presence of cytotoxic antibody in ewes is evidence for maternal sensitization to paternally derived histocompatibility antigens. The effect of this sensitization on subsequent transplantation challenges is unclear, because a study of graft rejection between ewes and their offspring demonstrated no evidence for "second-set" rejection by mothers of skin of their offspring (Galton, 1965).

Studies by several investigators have used serological and genetic techniques to define lymphocyte alloantigens in a number of sheep breeds. Alloimmune sera raised by lymphocyte injections (Millot, 1978), skin grafts (Stear and Spooner, 1981), and osteoarticular grafts (Ford, 1974), as well as parous sera (Ford, 1974; Stear and Spooner, 1981; Cullen et al., 1982) have been used as a source of reagents. One group has used absorbed sera to define sheep lymphocyte antigens (Schmid et al., 1975).

The tissue distribution of sheep lymphocyte antigens has not been widely studied. However, it has been reported that absorption of sera with erythrocytes does not remove cytotoxic activity (Ford, 1974).

There have been few attempts to correlate and compare reagents and results among sheep researchers. One report provided little evidence for similarity between reagents from different laboratories (Stear and Spooner, 1981). However, breed differences could account for the lack of correlations, because some workers restricted their studies to a single breed (Millot, 1978), whereas others have reported differences in the frequencies of antigens between breeds (Ford, 1975).

Several investigators have provided evidence for a complex organization of the principal genetic region controlling the expression of sheep lymphocyte antigens (Ford, 1975; Millot, 1979; Stear and Spooner, 1981). This has been based primarily on serology conducted at the population level, but evidence for recombination in families also has been presented (Millot, 1979). It is difficult to estimate the extent of the OLA polymorphism at its present state of characterization. However, there is evidence that between 5 and 10 OLA specificities behave as alleles at a single locus (Millot, 1979; Stear and Spooner, 1981).

A method for cryopreservation of sheep lymphocytes has been reported (Stear *et al.*, 1982a). The use of frozen storage for lymphocytes should be of value to further studies of sheep lymphocyte alloantigens, as it can help overcome one of the disadvantages of working with sheep. Because sheep are usually raised for human consumption as lamb, individual sheep often have a short life span.

It has been assumed by most investigators of sheep lymphocyte alloantigens that they are studying the MHS of sheep, but evidence comparable to that provided in other species is lacking (linkage with genes determining MLR, biochemical characterization of MHS molecules, linkage with *Ir* genes, control of skin graft rejection, etc.). This lack of evidence is important because of the poor correlation between serological reagents from different laboratories (Stear and Spooner, 1981) and because one group has provided evidence for two additional loci coding for lymphocyte alloantigens: *Ol-X,* a locus probably on the same chromosome as OLA, and *Ol-Z,* a locus apparently unlinked to OLA (Millot, 1979). The existence of lymphocyte alloantigen polymorphisms that are not linked to the MHS can severely complicate the interpretation of serological data generated with unabsorbed, polyspecific sera.

B. Histocompatibility Systems of Goats

Only one group has reported investigations on histocompatibility systems of the goat (van Dam *et al.*, 1976, 1978, 1979). However, these studies have clearly defined the MHS of the goat, which has been termed GLA, for goat lymphocyte antigen (van Dam *et al.*, 1979). Alloantisera to lymphocyte antigens have been produced by immunization with lymphocytes, by skin grafting, and by screening sera from parous goats. Of 40 postpartum sera samples, 8 (20%) were found to contain cytotoxic alloantibody to lymphocyte antigens. As in other large domestic species, absorption of antilymphocyte antisera with erythrocytes did not remove cytotoxic activity (van Dam et al., 1976).

At least 10 serologically defined specificities have been identified (van Dam et al., 1976), and these antigens have been tentatively assigned to two linked loci (van Dam et al., 1979). Matching of donors and recipients for GLA antigens resulted in prolonged survival time of grafts (van Dam et al., 1976, 1978). In vitro culture techniques for the MLR have been developed (van Dam, et al., 1978), and these techniques are being applied to studies of the GLA region (van Dam et al., 1979).

VIII. Histocompatibility Systems of Cats

With regard to the characterization of its histocompatibility antigens, the cat has received less attention than any of the other common domestic species. However, a recent report is of considerable interest (Pollack et al., 1982). Pollack and co-workers have described their unsuccessful attempts to produce cytotoxic alloantisera to polymorphic cell surface molecules of cat lymphocytes by various immunization procedures. In addition, they reported their failure to observe strong mixed lymphocyte responses between unrelated cats. They have suggested that the cat may have a very restricted polymorphism at MHS loci, similar to the situation reported for the hamster (Duncan and Streilein, 1977). This is consistent with early reports of prolonged survival of kidney allografts between unrelated cats (Carrel, 1908). Such prolonged survival would be expected between animals differing at minor histocompatibility loci, but not the MHS. These observations could have relevance to the well-known susceptibility of cats to viral infections such as that caused by feline leukemia virus. Clearly, more research on this species is merited in the future.

IX. Conclusions

In this article we have attempted to summarize the most important biological aspects of the major histocompatibility system and to review

TABLE IX

Known Characteristics of the MHS of Domestic Species

Characteristic	Dog	Swine	Cattle	Horse	Sheep	Goat
Common name for MHS	DLA	SLA	BoLA	ELA	OLA	GLA
Class I loci	−A,−B,−C	−A,−B,−C	−A,−B?	−A	−A,−B	−A,−B?
Number of alleles per locus[a]	5–10	>7	10–15	10–15	5–10	5
Class II loci						
MLR	+	+	+	+	−	+
Serology	+	+	+	−	−	−
Number of alleles per locus[a]	10	?[b]	?	?	?	?
Ir-Gene function	+	+	−	−	−	−
Biochemical characterization of MHS antigens	+	+	+	−	−	−
MHS restriction of T-lymphocyte function	+	−	?	−	−	−
Identification of loci linked to MHS	+	+	?	+	−	−
MHS associations with production or disease	+	+	+	−	−	−

[a]Estimates made from published data.
[b]?, Only tentative evidence available, or numerical estimates not reported.

the current state of characterization of the MHS and other histocompatibility polymorphisms of the common domestic mammalian species. Table IX gives a synopsis of the traits of the MHS attributed to those species. Because so little is known about histocompatibility in the cat, it has been omitted from the table.

Students of histocompatibility eventually focused on the MHS because of its central role in the rejection of allografts. During the 1970s, the development of our understanding of the role of MHS genes in regulating immune responses shifted the emphasis of studies away from allograft transplantation and toward investigations of the true biological role of the MHS. Although the genes of the MHS are not the only genes that control immune responses, they do appear to play a central role in regulating several aspects of T-lymphocyte function.

Research on histocompatibility systems in domestic animals has increased dramatically during the past decade. There are several reasons for this. Some species, such as the pig and dog, have served as models of organ grafting in transplantation studies. As a result, the MHS of the dog and of the pig have received the most research attention and therefore are the best characterized of any of the domestic mammals (Table IX).

A second stimulus for histocompatibility studies of domestic species stems from the value of comparative investigations of homologous systems. The domestic species as a group have a unique genetic history. They have been highly selected for particular traits (e.g., milk, meat, or wool production, speed, or conformation), but a high degree of inbreeding has been avoided purposefully. Thus they occupy a niche separate from inbred laboratory animals and randomly bred wild species. They share the human environment to different extents, including many human diseases, such as tuberculosis, schistosomiasis, and Rift Valley fever.

Research on domestic species is likely to contribute to our overall understanding of the MHS in ways we cannot predict. Already, several aspects of histocompatibility research in domestic animals have been of particular interest. These include the peculiar control of mixed lymphocyte culture reactivity in cattle, the cross-reactivity between BoLA and HLA antigens, the privileged position of swine liver allografts, and the strong maternal antifetal histocompatibility antigen responses of pregnant mares. In addition, the lymphocyte alloantigens of dog, pigs, horses, and sheep that are not linked to the MHS of those species and that can be detected by cytotoxic alloantisera are fascinating and have no counterpart in rodents or primates. The new technologies of monoclonal antibody production, gene cloning, and embryo manipulation should permit rapid progress in future studies of histocompatibility systems of domestic species.

Finally, studies of the MHS of domestic animals are an important part of broader investigations of the genetic control of immune responses of domestic animals. The search for a genetic basis for disease resistance in domestic livestock has a long history (Hutt, 1958), but little progress has been made in mammalian species. Traditional schemes for vaccine development, vector control, and pharmacological therapeutics have all failed to control several important infectious diseases of both temperate and tropical zones. These include viral, bacterial, and parasitic diseases such as rabies, foot-and-mouth disease, rinderpest, bovine viral diarrhea, infectious bovine rhinotracheitis, brucellosis, trypanosomiasis, babesiosis, and anaplasmosis. Characterization of immune response genes might permit genetic selection for breeds of livestock with high levels of resistance to particular pathogens. Characterization of structural and functional features of the major histocompatibility system of domestic species will contribute to our understanding of important aspects of the genetic control of immune responses.

Acknowledgments

Support from USPHS grant HD–15799 and USDA-SEA grant 82–CRSR–2–1050 is gratefully acknowledged. The authors thank Ann Signore for typing the manuscript.

References

Adams, T. E., (1980). Ph.D. Thesis, Australian National University, Canberra.
Adams, T. E., Brandon, M. R., and Morris, B. (1979). *Anim. Blood Groups Biochem. Genet.* **10**, 155–163.
Ahrons, S. (1971). *Tissue Antigens* **1**, 178–183.
Albert, E. D., and Götze, D. (1977). *In* "The Major Histocompatibility System in Man and Animals" (D. Götze, ed.), pp. 7–78. Springer-Verlag, Berlin and New York.
Albert, E. D., Erickson, V. M., Graham, T. C., Parr, M., Templeton, J. W., Mickey, M. R., Thomas, E. D., and Storb, R. (1973). *Tissue Antigens* **3**, 417–430.
Allen, W. R. (1979). *Ciba Found. Symp. Ser.* **64** (new ser.), 323–352.
Allison, J. P., Walker, L. E., Russell, W. A., Pellegrino, M. A., Ferrone, S., Reisfeld, R. A., Frelinger, J. A., and Silver, J. (1978). *Proc. Natl. Acad. Sci. U.S.A.* **75**, 3953–3956.
Alper, C. A., Awdeh, Z. L., Raum, D. D., and Yunis, E. J. (1982). *Clin. Immunol. Immunopathol.* **24**, 276–285.
Altman, B., and Simonsen, M. (1964). *Ann. N.Y. Acad. Sci.* **120**, 28–34.
Amorena, B., and Stone, W. H. (1978). *Science* **201**, 159–160.
Amorena, B., and Stone, W. H. (1980). *Tissue Antigens* **16**, 212–225.
Amorena, B., and Stone, W. H. (1982). *Anim. Blood Groups Biochem. Genet.* **13**, 81–90.
Antczak, D. F., Bright, S. M., Remick, L. H., and Bauman, B. E. (1982). *Tissue Antigens* **20**, 172–187.
Arnoux, B., Chardon, P., Renard, C., Vaiman, M., and Haag, J. (1974). *C.R. Hebd. Seances Acad. Sci., Ser. D* **279**, 1817–1820.
Bachvaroff, R., Ozaki, A., Cannon, F. D., Mollen, N., Blumenstock, D. A., Ayvazian, J. H., Ferrebee, J. W., and Rapaport, F. T. (1973). *Transplant. Proc.* **5**, 1561–1565.
Bachvaroff, R., Cannon, F. D., Blumenstock, D. A., Ferrebee, J. W., and Rapaport, F. T. (1978). *Transplant. Proc.* **10**, 119–122.
Bailey, E. (1980). *Immunogenetics* **11**, 499–506.
Bailey, E. (1982). *Am. J. Vet. Res.* **43**, 1917–1921.
Bailey, E., Stormont, C., Suzuki, Y., and Trommershausen-Smith, A. (1979). *Science* **204**, 1317–1319.
Benacerraf, B. (1981). *Science* **212**, 1229–1238.
Bernoco, D., Cullen, S., Scudeller, G., Trinchieri, G., and Ceppellini, R. (1972). *In* "Histocompatibility Testing 1972" (J. Dausset and J. Colombani, eds.) pp. 527–537. Munksgaard, Copenhagen.
Bijnen, A. B., Dekkers-Bijma, A. M., Vriesendorp, H. M., and Westbroek, D. L. (1979). *Immunogenetics* **8**, 287–297.

Bijnen, A. B., Obertop, H., Niessen, G. J. C. M., Jeekel, J., and Westbroek, D. L. (1982). *Transplantation* **33**, 57–63.
Billingham, R. E., Lampkin, G. H., Medawar, P. B., and Williams, H. L. (1952). *Heredity* **6**, 201–212.
Binz, H., and Wigzell, H. (1975). *J. Exp. Med.* **142**, 1218–1230.
Biozzi, G., Mouton, D., Sant'Anna, O. A., Passos, H. C., Gennari, M., Reis, M. H., Ferreira, V. C. A., Heumann, A. M., Bouthillier, Y., Ibanéz, O. M., Stiffel, C., and Siqueira, M. (1979). *Curr. Top. Microbiol. Immunol.* **85**, 31–98.
Biozzi, G., Siqueira, M., Stiffel, C., Ibanéz, O. M., Mouton, D., and Ferreira, V. C. A. (1981). *In* "Immunology 80: Progress in Immunology IV" (M. Fougereau and J. Dausset, eds.), Vol. 2, Chapter 24, pp. 432–457. Academic Press, New York.
Blackwell, J., Freeman, J., and Bradley, D. (1980). *Nature(London)* **283**, 72–74.
Blumenstock, D., Wells, E., Sanford, C., and de Gillio, M. (1971). *Transplantation* **11**, 192–194.
Blumenstock, D. A., Cannon, F. D., Vlahovic, V. L., and Alpern, D. (1981). *Transplant. Proc.* **13**, 863–869.
Bodmer, W. F. (1972). *Nature (London)* **237**, 139–145.
Bodmer, W. F. (1978). *Br. Med. Bull.* **34**, 213–320.
Bodmer, W. F. (1980). *J. Exp. Med.* **152**, Suppl., 353S–357S.
Borovska, M., and Demant, P. (1967). *Folia Biol. (Prague)* **13**, 470–475.
Bradley, B. A., Edwards, J. M., Dunn, D. C., and Calne, R. Y. (1972). *Nature (London), New Biol.* **240**, 54–56.
Bradley, B. A., Edwards, J. M., and Franks, D. (1973). *Tissue Antigens* **3**, 340–347.
Bright, S., Antczak, D. F., and Ricketts, S. (1978). *J. Equine Med. Surg. Suppl.* **1**, 229–236.
Briles, W. E., and Briles, R. W. (1982). *Immunogenetics* **15**, 449–459.
Brodsky, F. M., and Parham, P. (1982). *Immunogenetics* **15**, 151–166.
Brodsky, F. M., Stone, W. H., and Parham, P. (1981). *Hum. Immunol.* **3**, 143–152.
Brossard, M. (1976). *Acta Trop.* **33**, 15–36.
Bruner, D. W., Edwards, P. R., and Doll, E. R. (1948). *Cornell Vet.* **38**, 363–366.
Caldwell, J. (1979). *Tissue Antigens* **13**, 319–326.
Caldwell, J., and Cumberland, P. A. (1978). *Transplant. Proc.* **10**, 889–892.
Caldwell, J., Cumberland, P. A., Weseli, D. F., and Williams, J. D. (1979). *Anim. Blood Groups Biochem. Genet.* **10**, 93–98.
Calne, R. Y., Sells, R. A., Pena, J. R., Davis, D. R., Millard, P. R., Herbertson, B. M., Binns, R. M., and Davies, D. A. L. (1969). *Nature (London)* **223**, 472–476.
Calne, R. Y., Davis, D. R., Hadjiyannakis, E., Sells, R. A., White, D., Herbertson, B. M., Millard, P. R., Joysey, V. C., Davies, D. A. L., Binns, R. M., and Festenstein, H. (1970). *Nature (London)* **227**, 903–906.
Capy, P., Renard, C., Sellier, P., and Vaiman, M. (1981). *Ann. Genet. Sel. Anim.* **13**, 441–446.
Caroli, H., and Bessis, M. (1947). *C. R. Hebd. Seances Acad. Sci. Ser. D* **224**, 969.
Carrel, A. (1908). *J. Exp. Med.* **10**, 98–104.
Chandler, J. G., Villar, H., Lee, S., Williams, R. J., Nakaji, N. T., Ferrebee, J. W., and Orloff, M. J. (1972). *Surgery* **71**, 807–816.
Chardon, P., Vaiman, M., Renard, C., and Arnoux, B. (1977). *Anim. Blood Groups Biochem. Genet.* **8**, 139–148.
Chardon, P., Vaiman, M., Renard, C., and Arnoux, B. (1978). *Transplantation* **26**, 107–112.
Chardon, P., Renard, C., and Vaiman, M. (1981). *Anim. Blood Groups Biochem. Genet.* **12**, 59–65.

Cleton, F. J. (1965). *In* "Histocompatibility Testing 1965" (H. Balner, F. J. Cleton, and J. G. Eernisse, eds.), pp. 263–264. Munksgaard, Copenhagen.
Cohen, I., and Kozaki, M. (1969). *Transplantation* **7**, 468–474.
Coligan, J. E., Kindt, T. J., Uehara, H., Martinko, J., and Natheson, S. G. (1981). *Nature (London)* **291**, 35–39.
Cook, R., Carroll, M. C., Uhr, J. W., Vitetta, E. S., and Capra, J. D. (1978). *Transplant. Proc.* **10**, 695–699.
Coombs, R. R. A., Crowhurst, R. C., Day, F. T., Heard, D. H., Hinde, I. T., Hoogstraten, J., and Parry, H. B. (1948). *J. Hyg.* **46**, 403–418.
Corte, G., Damiani, G., Calabi, F., Fabbi, M., and Bargellesi, A. (1981). *Proc. Natl. Acad. Sci. U.S.A.* **78**, 534–538.
Cullen, P., Bunch, C., Brownlie, J., and Morris, P. (1982). *Animal Blood Groups and Biochemical Genetics* **13**, 149–159.
Curie-Cohen, M., Usinger, W. R., and Stone, W. H. (1978). *Tissue Antigens* **12**, 170–178.
Cwik, S., and Schmid, D. O. (1975). *J. Immunogenet.* **2**, 27–30.
Dausset, J., and Svejgaard, A., eds. (1977). "HLA and Disease." Munksgaard, Copenhagen.
David, C. S. (1976). *Transplant. Rev.* **30**, 229–322.
David, C. S. (1979). *Transplant. Proc.* **11**, 677–682.
Davies, H. ff. S., Taylor, J. E., Daniel, M. R., and Wakerly, C. (1976). *J. Exp. Med.* **143**, 987–992.
Davies, H. ff. S., Taylor, J. E., White, D. J. G., and Binns, R. M. (1978). *Transplantation* **25**, 290–295.
Deeg, H. J., Storb, R., Raff, R. F., Weiden, P. L., de Rose, S., and Thomas, E. D. (1982). *Transplantation* **33**, 17–21.
Deeg, H. J., Wulff, J. C., de Rose, S., Sale, G. E., Braun, M., Brown, M. A., Springmeyer, S. C., Martin, P. J., and Storb, R. (1982). *Immunogenetics* **16**, 445–457.
de Gruyl, J., Westbroek, D. L., Dijkhuis, C. M., Vriesendorp, H. M., Mac Dicken, I., Elion-Gerritsen, W., Verschour, L., Hulsman, H. A. M., and Horchner, P. (1973). *Transplant. Proc.* **5**, 755–759.
Demant, P., and Neauport-Sautes, C. (1978). *Immunogenetics* **7**, 295–311.
deWeck, A. L., Lazary, S., Bullen, S., Gerber, H., and Meister, U. (1978). *J. Equine Med. Surg.* **2**, 221–227.
Dick, H. M. (1978). *Br. Med. Bull.* **34**, 271–274.
Dick, H. M. (1982). *Immunol. Today* **3**, 199–203.
Doherty, P. C., and Zinkernagel, R. M. (1975). *Lancet* **1**, 1406–1409.
Duncan, W. R., and Streilein, J. W. (1977). *J. Immunol.* **118**, 832–839.
Ebringer, R. W., Cawdell, D. R., Cowling, P., and Ebringer, A. (1978). *Ann. Rheum. Dis.* **37**, 146–151.
Emery, D., and McCullagh, P. (1980). *Transplantation* **29**, 17–22.
Epstein, R. B., Storb, R., Ragde, H., and Thomas, E. D. (1968). *Transplantation* **6**, 45–58.
Epstein, R. B., Storb, R., and Thomas, E. D. (1971). *Transplant. Proc.* **3**, 161–164.
Eugui, E. M., and Emery, D. L. (1981). *Nature (London)* **290**, 251–254.
Fischer-Lindahl, K., and Langhorne, J. (1981). *Scand. J. Immunol.* **14**, 643–654.
Flad, H. D., Goldmann, S. F., Krumbacher, K., Schnappauf, H., and Huget, R. P. (1975). *Transplant. Proc.* **7**, 407–410.
Folger, R. L., and Hines, H. C. (1976). *Anim. Blood Groups Biochem. Genet.* **7**, 137–145.
Ford, C. H. J. (1974). *J. Immunogenet.* **1**, 345–354.
Ford, C. H. J. (1975). *J. Immunogenet.* **2**, 31–40.
Ford, C. H. J., and Elves, M. W. (1974). *J. Immunogenet.* **1**, 259–264.
Ford, W. L., and Simonsen, M. (1971). *J. Exp. Med.* **133**, 938–949.

Ford, W. L., Simmonds, S. J., and Atkins, R. C. (1975). *J. Exp. Med.* **141**, 681–696.
Fradelizi, D., Mahouy, G., de Riberolles, C., Lecompte, Y., Alhomme, P., Douard, M. C., Chotin, G., Martelli, H., Daburow, F., and Vaiman, M. (1981). *Transplantation* **31**, 365–368.
Galton, M. (1965). *Transplantation* **3**, 39–43.
Geczy, A. F., Alexander, K., Bashir, H. V., and Edmonds, J. (1980). *Nature (London)* **283**, 782–784.
Gill, T. J., III, Cramer, D. V., and Kunz, H. W. (1978). *Am. J. Pathol.* **90**, 737–777.
Gluckman, E., Parr, M., Mickelson, E., Schroeder, M.-L., and Storb, R. (1973). *Transplantation* **15**, 642–645.
Gluckman, E., Schroeder, M. L., Storb, R., Goselink, H., Johnson, S., Graham, T. C., Pretorius, G., and Thomas, E. D. (1975). *Transplantation* **19**, 36–41.
Gluckman, J. C. (1980). *Eur. J. Immunol.* **10**, 693–697.
Goldman, S. F., and Flad, H. D. (1975). *Tissue Antigens* **5**, 145–154.
Goldman, S. F., Krumbacher, K., Schnappauf, H. P., Huget, R. P., and Flad, H. D. (1975a). *Tissue Antigens* **5**, 155–164.
Goldman, S. F., Krumbacher, K., Schnappauf, H., and Flad, H. D. (1975b). *Transplant. Proc.* **7**, 389–393.
Götze, D., ed. (1977). "The Major Histocompatibility System in Man and Animals." Springer-Verlag, Berlin and New York.
Govaerts, A. (1960). *J. Immunol.* **85**, 516–522.
Goyert, S. M., and Silver, J. (1981). *Nature (London)* **294**, 266–268.
Goyert, S. M., Shively, J. E., and Silver, J. (1982). *J. Exp. Med.* **156**, 550–566.
Grosse-Wilde, H., Baumann, P., Netzel, B., Kolb, H. J., Mempel, W., Wank, R., and Albert, E. D. (1973). *Transplant. Proc.* **5**, 1567–1571.
Grosse-Wilde, H., Vriesendorp, H. M., Wank, R., Mempel, W., de Champs, B., Honauer, U., Baumann, P., Netzel, B., Kolb, H. J., and Albert, E. D. (1974). *Tissue Antigens* **4**, 229–237.
Gupta, C., and Goldman, A. (1982). *Science* **216**, 994–996.
Halper, J., Fu, S. M., Wang, C. Y., Winchester, R., and Kunkel, H. G. (1978). *J. Immunol.* **120**, 1480–1484.
Hammerling, G. J., Deak, B. D., Mauve, G., Hammerling, U., and McDevitt, H. O. (1974). *Immunogenetics* **1**, 68–81.
Hammerling, G. J., Mauve, G., Goldberg, E., and McDevitt, H. O. (1975). *Immunogenetics* **1**, 428–437.
Haverkorn, M. J., Hofman, B., Masurel, N., and van Rood, J. J. (1975). *Transplant. Rev.* **22**, 120–124.
Helenius, A., Morein, B., Fries, E., Simons, K., Robinson, P., Schirrmacher, V., Terhorst, C., and Strominger, J. L. (1978). *Proc. Natl. Acad. Sci. U.S.A.* **75**, 3846–3850.
Hewetson, R. W. (1971). *Aust. J. Agric. Res.* **22**, 231–342.
Hines, H. C., and Newman, M. J. (1981). *Anim. Blood Groups Biochem. Genet.* **12**, 201–206.
Hoang-Xuan, M., Leveziel, H., Zilber, M. T., Parodi, A. L., and Levy, D. (1982a). *Immunogenetics* **15**, 207–211.
Hoang-Xuan, M., Charron, D., Zilber, M. T., and Levy, D. (1982b). *Immunogenetics* **15**, 621–624.
Hojny, J., and Glasnak, V. (1970). *Anim. Blood Groups Biochem. Genet.* **1**, 47–51.
Hormaeche, C. E. (1979). *Immunology* **37**, 319–327.
Hradecky, J., Hruban, V., Pazdera, J., and Klaudy, J. (1982). *Anim. Blood Groups Biochem. Genet.* **13**, 223–224.
Hruban, V., and Simon, M. (1973). *Anim. Blood Groups Biochem. Genet.* **4**, 183–184.

Hruban, V., Simon, M., and Hradecky, J. (1972). *Anim. Blood Groups Biochem. Genet.* **3,** 157–161.
Hruban, V., Simon, M., and Hradecky, J. (1974). *Anim. Blood Groups Biochem. Genet.* **5,** 171–176.
Hruban, V., Simon, M., Hradecky, J., and Jilek, F. (1976). *Tissue Antigens* **7,** 267–271.
Hruban, V., Simon, M., Hradecky, J., and Pazdera, J. (1977). *Anim. Blood Groups Biochem. Genet.* **8,** 85–92.
Hruban, V., Hradecky, J., Pazdera, J., Simon, M., and Veselsky, L. (1978). *J. Immunogenet.* **5,** 173–178.
Hutt, F. B., (1958). "Genetic Resistance to Disease in Domestic Animals." Cornell Univ. Press (Comstock), Ithaca, New York.
Iha, T. H., Gerbrandt, G., Bodmer, W. F., McGary, D., and Stone, W. H. (1973). *Tissue Antigens* **3,** 291–302.
Ivanyi, P., (1978). *Proc. R. Soc. London Ser. B* **202,** 117–158.
Jilek, F., and Veselsky, L. (1972). *J. Reprod. Fertil.* **31,** 295–298.
Julius, M., Simpson, E., and Herzenberg, L. (1973). *Eur. J. Immunol.* **3,** 645–649.
Kasakura, S., Thomas, E. D., and Ferrebee, J. W. (1964). *Transplantation* **2,** 274–280.
Kaufman, J. F., and Strominger, J. L. (1982). *Nature (London)* **297,** 694–697.
Keuning, J. J., Pena, A. S., van Hooff, J. P., van Leeuwen, A., and van Rood, J. J. (1976). *Lancet* **1,** 506–507.
Kirkman, R. L., Colvin, R. B., Flye, M. W., Leight, G. S., Rosenberg, S. A., Williams, G. M., and Sachs, D. H. (1979a). *Transplantation* **28,** 18–23.
Kirkman, R. L., Colvin, R. B., Flye, M. W., Williams, G. M., and Sachs, D. H. (1979b). *Transplantation* **28,** 24–30.
Kisken, W. A., and Malek, G. A. (1969). *Nature (London)* **224,** 1110–1111.
Klaudy, J., Hruban, V., Hradecky, J., Pazdera, J., and Pech, V. (1981). *Anim. Blood Groups Biochem Genet.* **12,** 67–74.
Klein, J. (1975). "Biology of the Mouse Histocompatibility-2 Complex." Springer-Verlag, Berlin and New York.
Klein, J. (1978). *Adv. Immunol.* **26,** 55–146.
Klein, J. (1979). *Science* **203,** 516–521, 516–521.
Klein, J., and Figueroa, F. (1981). *Immunol. Rev.* **60,** 23–57.
Klein, J., Bach, F. H., Festenstein, F., McDevitt, H. O., Shreffler, D. C., Snell, G. D., and Stimpfling, J. H. (1974). *Immunogenetics* **1,** 184–188.
Klein, J., Flaherty, L., VandeBerg, J. L., and Shreffler, D. C. (1978). *Immunogenetics* **6,** 489–512.
Kourlisky, F. M., Silvestre, D., Neauport-Sautes, C., Loosfelt, Y., and Dausset, J. (1972). *Eur. J. Immunol.* **2,** 249–257.
Kristensen, B., Wafler, P., and de Weck, A. L. (1980). *Anim. Blood Groups Biochem. Genet.* **11,** Suppl., 58–59.
Krumbacher, K., and Schnappauf, H. (1976). *Tissue Antigens* **7,** 181–182.
Kydd, J., Miller, J., Antczak, D. F., and Allen, W. R. (1982). *J. Reprod. Fertil., Suppl.* **32,** 361–369.
Larhammar, D., Wiman, K., Schenning, L., Claesson, L., Gustafsson, K., Peterson, P. A., and Rask, L. (1981). *Scand. J. Immunol.* **14,** 617–622.
Larhammar, D., Schenning, L., Gustafsson, K., Wiman, K., Claesson, L., Rask, L., and Peterson, P. A. (1982). *Proc. Natl. Acad. Sci. U.S.A.* **79,** 3687–3691.
Lazary, S., de Weck, A. L., Straub, R., and Gerber, H. (1975). In "Equine Hematology" (H. Kitchen and J. D. Krehbel, eds.), p. 132. Am. Assoc. Equine Practitioners, Golden, Colorado.

Lazary, S., Kuslys, A., Bullen, S., de Weck, A. L., and Gerber, H. (1978). *Equine Med. Surg.* **2**, 237–242.
Lazary, S., de Weck, A. L., Bullen, S., Straub, R., and Gerber, H. (1980a). *Transplantation* **30**, 203–209.
Lazary, S., Bullen, S., Müller, J., Kovacs, G., Bodo, I., Hockenjos, P., and de Weck, A. L. (1980b). *Transplantation* **30**, 210–215.
Lazary, S., Gerber, H., de Weck, A. L., and Arnold, P. (1982). *J. Immunogenetics* **9**, 327–334.
Lefkovits, I. (1974). *Curr. Top. Microbiol. Immunol.* **65**, 21–57.
Leight, G. S., Sachs, D. H., and Rosenberg, S. A. (1977). *Transplantation* **23**, 271–276.
Leight, G. S., Kirkman, R., Rasmusen, B. A., Rosenberg, S. A., Sachs, D. H., Terrill, R., and Williams, G. M. (1978). *Tissue Antigens* **12**, 65–74.
Lemmonier, F., Burakoff, S. J., Germain, R. J., and Benacerraf, B. (1977). *Proc. Natl. Acad. Sci. U.S.A.* **74**, 1229–1233.
Leon, S., Zweibaum, A., Vriesendorp, H. M., and Smid-Mercx, B. M. J. (1975). *Transplant. Proc.* **7**, 379–382.
Longenecker, B. M., and Mosmann, T. R. (1981). *Immunogenetics* **13**, 1–23.
Lunney, J. K., and Sachs, D. H. (1978). *J. Immunol.* **120**, 607–612.
Lunney, J. K., and Sachs, D. H. (1979). *J. Immunol.* **122**, 623–627.
McDevitt, H. O. (1981). *J. Immunogenet.* **8**, 287–295.
McDevitt, H. O., and Tyan, M. L. (1968). *J. Exp. Med.* **128**, 1–11.
McDevitt, H. O., Deak, B. D., Schreffler, D. C., Klein, J., Stimpfling, J. H., and Snell, G. D. (1972). *J. Exp. Med.* **135**, 1259–1278.
McGuire, T. C., Poppie, M. J., and Banks, K. L. (1974). *J. Am. Vet. Med. Assoc.* **164**, 70–76.
Margulies, D. H., Evans, G. A., Flaherty, L., and Seidman, J. G. (1982). *Nature (London)* **295**, 168–170.
Markert, M. L., and Cresswell, P. (1980). *Proc. Natl. Acad. Sci. U.S.A.* **77**, 6101–6104.
Meera-Kahn, P., Los, W. R. T., van der Does, J. A., and Epstein, R. B. (1973). *Transplantation* **15**, 624–628.
Metzger, J. J., Gilliland, G. L., Lunney, J. K., Osborne, B. A., Rudikoff, S., and Sachs, D. H. (1981). *J. Immunol.* **127**, 769–775.
Metzger, J. J., Lunney, J. K., Sachs, D. H., and Rudikoff, S. (1982). *J. Immunol.* **129**, 716–721.
Miller, J., Rabinovitch, A., Fuller, L., Kyriakides, G., Severyn, W., Noel, J., Flaa, C., and Mintz, D. (1981). *Transplant. Proc.* **13**, 807–809.
Millot, P. (1978). *Anim. Blood Groups Biochem. Genet.* **9**, 115–121.
Millot, P. (1979). *Immunogenetics* **9**, 509–534.
Mittal, K. K., Mickey, M. R., Singal, D. P., and Terasaki, P. I. (1968). *Transplantation* **6**, 913–927.
Mollen, N., St. John, D., Cannon, F. D., and Ferrebee, J. W. (1968). *Transplantation* **6**, 939–940.
Morton, N. E. (1955). *Am. J. Hum. Genet.* **7**, 277–318.
Mottironi, V. D., Perryman, L. E., Pollara, B., Mickey, M. R., Swift, R., and McGrath, P. (1981). *Transplantation* **31**, 290–294.
Murphy, D. B., Okumura, K., Herzenberg, L. A., Herzenberg, L. A., and McDevitt, H. O. (1976). *Cold Spring Harbor Symp. Quant. Biol.* **41**, 497–504.
Murphy, J. B. (1916). *J. Exp. Med.* **24**, 1–6.
Nagy, Z. A., and Klein, J. (1981). *Immunol. Today* **2**, 228–229.
Netzel, B., Grosse-Wilde, H., and Mempel, W. (1975). *Transplant. Proc.* **7**, 403–405.

Newman, M. J. (1981). Ph.D. Thesis, Australian National University, Canberra.
Newman, M. J., and Brandon, M. R. (1981). *Am. J. Vet. Res.* **42**, 923–926.
Newman, M. J., and Hines, H. C. (1979). *Anim. Blood Groups Biochem. Genet.* **10**, 87–92.
Newman, M. J., and Hines, H. C. (1980). *J. Reprod. Fertil.* **60**, 237–241.
Newman, M. J., and Stear, M. J. (1983). *Vet. Immunol. Immunopathol.* (in press).
Newman, M. J., Adams, T. E., and Brandon, M. R. (1982a). *Anim. Blood Groups Biochem. Genet.* **13**, 123–139.
Newman, M. J., Campion, J. E., and Stear, M. J. (1982b). *Tissue Antigens* **20**, 100–107.
Oliver, R. A., McCoubrey, C. M., Millar, P., Morgan, A. L. G., and Spooner, R. L. (1981). *Immunogenetics* **13**, 127–132.
Osoba, D., Dick, H. M., Voller, A., Goosen, T. J., Goosen, T., Draper, C. C., and de thé, G. (1979). *Immunogenetics* **8**, 323–338.
Ostrand-Rosenberg, S., and Stormont, C. (1974). *Anim. Blood Groups Biochem. Genet.* **5**, 231–237.
Owen, M. J., and Crumpton, M. J. (1980). *Immunol. Today* **1**, 117–122.
Owen, R. D. (1945). *Science* **102**, 400–401.
Pazdera, J., Hruban, V., Hradecky, J., Fortyn, K., Stanek, R., Pospisil, M., and Jilek, M. (1981). *Folia Biol. (Prague)* **27**, 96–106.
Pease, L. R., Nathenson, S. G., and Leinwand, L. A. (1982). *Nature(London)* 382–385.
Pennington, L. R., Lunney, J. K., and Sachs, D. H. (1981a). *Transplantation* **31**, 66–71.
Pennington, L. R., Flye, M. W., Kirkman, R. L., Thistlethwaite, J. R., Williams, G. M., and Sachs, D. H. (1981b). *Transplantation* **32**, 315–320.
Perryman, L. E., and Liu, I. K. M. (1980). *Am. J. Vet. Res.* **41**, 187–192.
Plant, J. E., Blackwell, J. M., O'Brien, A. D., Bradley, D. J., and Glynn, A. A. (1982). *Nature (London)* **297**, 510–511.
Pollack, M., Mastrota, F., Chin-Louie, J., Mooney, S., and Hayes, A. (1982). *Immunogenetics* **16**, 339–347.
Pringnitz, D. J., McLaughlin, K., Benforado, K., Strozinski, L., and Stone, W. H. (1982). *Anim. Blood Groups Biochem. Genet.* **13**, 91–96.
Proceedings of the Second International Bovine Lymphocyte Antigen (BoLA) Workshop (1982). *Anim. Blood Groups Biochem. Genet.* **13**, 33–53.
Puza, A., Rubinstein, P., Kasakura, S., Vlahovic, S., and Ferrebee, J. W. (1964). *Transplantation* **2**, 722–733.
Rabinovitch, A., Fuller, L., Mintz, D., Severyn, W., Noel, J. Flaa, C., and Dyriakides, G. (1981). *J. Clin. Invest.* **67**, 1507–1516.
Rapaport, F. T., and Bachvaroff, R. J. (1978). *Adv. Vet. Sci. Comp. Med.* **22**, 195–219.
Rapaport, F. T., Hanaoka, T., Shimada, T., Cannon, F. D., and Ferrebee, J. W. (1970). *J. Exp. Med.* **131**, 881–893.
Rapaport, F. T., Boyd, A. D., Spencer, F. C., Lower, R. R., Dausset, J., Cannon, F. D., and Ferrebee, J. W. (1971). *J. Exp. Med.* **133**, 261–274.
Rasmusen, B. A. (1975). In "Handbook of Genetics" (R. C. King, ed.), Vol. 4, pp. 447–458. Plenum, New York.
Ray, J. G., Jr., ed. (1979). "NIAID Manual of Tissue Typing Techniques,', NIH Publ. No. 80–545.
Renard, C., Chardon, P., and Vaiman, M. (1982). *Animal Blood Groups and Biochemical Genetics* **13**, 161–177.
Roberts, J. A. (1968). *J. Parasitol.* **54**, 657–662.
Rubinstein, R., and Ferrebee, J. W. (1964). *Transplantation* **2**, 734–742.
Rudolph, R. H., Hered, B., Epstein, R. B., and Thomas, E. D. (1969). *Transplantation* **8**, 141–146.

Ryder, L. P., Andersen, E., and Svejgaard, A. (1979). *Tissue Antigens,* Suppl.
Sachs, D. H., Leight, G., Cone, J., Schwarz, S., Stuart, L., and Rosenberg, S. (1976). *Transplantation* **22,** 559–567.
Sasazuki, T., Kohno, Y., Iwamoto, I., Tanimura, M., and Naito, S. (1978). *Nature (London)* **272,** 359–361.
Schinckel, P. G., and Ferguson, K. A. (1953). *Aust. J. Biol. Sci.* **6,** 533–546.
Schleger, A. V., Lincoln, D. T., McKenna, R. V., Kemp, D. H., and Roberts, J. A. (1976). *Aust. J. Biol. Sci.* **29,** 499–512.
Schmid, D. O., and Cwik, S. (1972). *Tissue Antigens* **2,** 255–261.
Schmid, D. O., Cwik, S., and Förschner, J. (1975). *Zentralbl. Veterinemed., Reihe B* **22,** 386–392.
Schmid, D. O., Rensmeyer, W., and Cwik, S. (1978). *Anim. Blood Groups Biochem. Genet.* **9,** 47–49.
Schroeder, M. L., Gluckman, E., Storb, R., and Thomas, E. D. (1975a). *Transplant. Proc.* **7,** 395–398.
Schroeder, M. L., Warren, R. P., Storb, R., Goselink, H., Johnson, S., and Brewer, M. (1975b). *Transplant. Proc.* **7,** 411–413.
Schwartz, R. (1978). *Scad. J. Immunol.* **7,** 3–10.
Seager, K., Bashir, H. V., Geczy, A. F., Edmonds, J., and de Vere-Tyndall, A. (1979). *Nature (London)* **277,** 68–70.
Seifert, G. W. (1971). *Aust. J. Agric. Res.* **22,** 159–168.
Shek, W. R., Schultz, R. D., and Appel, M. J. G. (1980). *Infect. Immun.* **28,** 724–734.
Shevach, E. M. (1978). *Springer Semin. Immunopathol.* **1,** 207–234.
Shreffler, D. C., David, C. S., Cullen, S. E., Frelinger, J. A., and Niederhuber, J. E. (1976). *Cold Spring Harbor Symp. Quant. Biol.* **41,** 477–487.
Silver, J., Walker, L. E., Reisfeld, R. A., Pellegrino, M. A., and Ferrone, S. (1979). *Mol. Immunol.* **16,** 37–42.
Silverstein, A. M., Prendergast, R. A., and Kraner, K. L. (1963). *Science* **142,** 1172–1173.
Simon, M., and Hruban, V. (1971). *Anim. Blood Groups Biochem. Genet.* **2,** 95–100.
Simon, M., and Hruban, V. (1972). *Vox Sang.* **23,** 208–211.
Simonsen, M. (1953). *Acta Pathol. Microbiol Scand.* **32,** 36–84.
Simpson, E., Bulfield, G., Brenan, M., Fitzpatric, W., Hetherington, C., and Blann, A. (1982). *Immunogenetics* **15,** 63–70.
Singer, D. S., Camerini-Otero, R. D., Satz, M. L., Osborne, B., Sachs, D., and Rudikoff, S. (1982). *Proc. Natl. Acad. Sci. U.S.A.* **79,** 1403–1407.
Singh, R., Mechelse, K., and Stefanko, S. (1977). *J. Neurol., Neurosurg. Psychiatry* **40,** 865–871.
Smid-Mercx, B. M. J., Duyzer-den Hartog, B., Visser, T. P., and Vriesendorp, H. M. (1975). *Transplant. Proc.* **7,** 361–364.
Snell, G. D., Dausset, J., and Nathenson, S. (1976). "Histocompatibility." Academic Press, New York.
Solheim, B. G., Bratlie, A., Sandberg, L., Staub-Nielsen, L., and Thorsby, E. (1973). *Tissue Antigens* **3,** 439–453.
Soloski, M. J., Uhr, J. W., and Vitetta, E. S. (1982). *Nature (London)* **296,** 759–761.
Soulillou, J. P., Keribin, D., Lecoguic, G., and Robine-Leon, S. (1980). *Transplantation* **29,** 314–319.
Splitter, G. A., Everlith, K. M., and Usinger, W. R. (1981). *Vet. Immunol. Immunopathol.* **2,** 215–232.
Spooner, R. L. (1979). *Anim. Blood Groups Biochem. Genet.* **10,** 63–86.
Spooner, R. L., and Morgan, A. L. G. (1981). *Tissue Antigens* **17,** 178–188.

Spooner, R. L., Leveziel, H., Grosclaude, F., Oliver, R. A., and Vaiman, M. (1978). *J. Immunogenet.* **5,** 335–346.
Spooner, R. L., Millar, P., and Oliver, R. A. (1979). *Anim. Blood Groups Biochem. Genet.* **10,** 99–105.
Spooner, R. L., Morgan, A. L. G., and Oliver, R. A. (1980). *Tissue Antigens* **15,** 289–296.
Stear, M. J., and Spooner, R. L. (1981). *Anim. Blood Groups Biochem. Genet.* **12,** 265–276.
Stear, M. J., Allen, D., and Spooner, R. L. (1982a). *Tissue Antigens* **19,** 134–139.
Stear, M. J., Newman, M. J., and Nicholas, F. W. (1982b). *Tissue Antigens* **20,** 289–299.
Stone, W. H. (1981). *Adv. Exp. Med. Biol.* **137,** 433–540.
Storb, R., Epstein, R. B., Rudolph, R. H., and Thomas, E. D. (1970). *J. Immunol.* **105,** 627–633.
Storb, R., Rudolph, R. H., and Thomas, E. D. (1971a). *J. Clin. Invest.* **50,** 1272–1275.
Storb, R., Rudolph, R. H., Graham, T. C., and Thomas, E. D. (1971b). *J. Immunol.* **107,** 409–413.
Storb, R., Rudolph, R. H., Kolb, H. J., Graham, T. C., Mickelson, E., Erickson, V., Lerner, K. G., Kolb, H., and Thomas, E. D. (1973). *Transplantation* **15,** 92–100.
Storb, R., Weiden, P. L., Schroeder, M. L., Graham, T. C., Lerner, K. G., and Thomas, E. D. (1976). *Transplantation* **21,** 299–306.
Storb, R., Weiden, P. L., Graham, T. C., and Thomas, E. D. (1978). *Transplant. Proc.* **10,** 113–118.
Stormont, C. (1978). *Immunogenetics* **6,** 1–15.
Strominger, J. L. (1981). *In* "Immunology 80: Progress in Immunology IV" (M. Fougereau and J. Dausset, eds.), Vol. 2, Chapter 30, pp. 541–554. Academic Press, New York.
Svejgaard, A., Hauge, M., Jersild, C., Platz, P., Ryder, L. P., Staub-Nielsen, L. and Thomsen, M. (1979). *Monogr. Hum. Genet.* **7,** 1–111.
Teillaud, J. L., Crevat, D., Chardon, P., Kalil, J., Goujet-Zalc, C., Mahouy, G., Vaiman, M., Fellous, M., and Pious, D. (1982). *Immunogenetics* **15,** 377–384.
Templeton, J. W., and Thomas, E. D. (1971). *Transplantation* **11,** 429–431.
Terasaki, P. I., and McClelland, D. (1964). *Nature (London)* **204,** 998–1000.
Thomas, D. W., Yamashita U., and Shevach, E. M. (1977). *Immunol. Rev.* **35,** 97–120.
Uhr, J. W., Capra, J. D., Vitetta, E. S., and Cook, R. G. (1979). *Science* **206,** 292–297.
Usinger, W. R., Curie-Cohen, M., and Stone, W. H. (1977). *Science* **196,** 1017–1018.
Usinger, W. R., Curie-Cohen, M., Benforado, K., Pringnitz, D., Rowe, R., Splitter, G. A., and Stone, W. H. (1981). *Immunogenetics* **14,** 423–428.
Vaiman, M. (1979). *Anim. Blood Groups Biochem. Genet.* **10,** 125–126.
Vaiman, M., and Renard, C. (1980). *Anim. Blood Groups Biochem. Genet.* **11,** *(Suppl.),* 57.
Vaiman, M., Arnoux, A., Filleul, X., and Nizza, P. (1970a). *C. R. Hebd. Seances Acad. Sci. Ser. D* **271,** 1724–1727.
Vaiman, M., Renard, C., LaFage, P., Ameteau, J., and Nizza, P. (1970b). *Transplantation* **10,** 155–164.
Vaiman, M., Garnier, H., Kunlin, A., Hay, J. M., Parc, R., Bacour, F., Fagniez, P. H., Villiers, P. A., Lecointre, J., Bara, M. F., and Nizza, P. (1972). *Transplantation* **14,** 541–550.
Vaiman, M., Haag, J., Arnoux, A., and Nizza, P. (1973). *Tissue Antigens* **3,** 204–211.
Vaiman, M., Renard, C., Ponceau, M., Lecointre, J., and Villiers, P. A. (1975). *C. R. Hebd. Seances Acad. Sci., Ser. D* **280,** 2809–2812.
Vaiman, M., Bacourt, F., Villiers, P. A., and Garnier, H. (1976). *Transplantation* **22,** 402–404.

Vaiman, M., Hauptmann, G., and Mayer, S. (1978a). *J. Immunogenet.* **5**, 59–65.
Vaiman, M., Metzger, J. J., Renard, C., and Vila, J. P. (1978b). *Immunogenetics* **7**, 231–238.
Vaiman, M., Fellous, M., Wiels, J., Renard, C., Lecointre, J., De Mesnil du Buisson, F., and Dausset, J. (1978c). *J. Immunogenet.* **5**, 135–142.
Vaiman, M., Chardon, P., and Renard, C. (1979). *Immunogenetics* **9**, 353–361.
Vaiman, M., Daburon, F., Remy, J., Villiers, P. A., de Riberolles, C., Lecompte, Y., Mahouy, G., and Fradelizi, D. (1981). *Transplantation* **31**, 358–364.
van Dam, R. H., Borst-van Werkhoven, C., van der Donk, J. A., and Goudswaard, J. (1976). *J. Immunogenet.* **3**, 237–244.
van Dam, R. H., Boot, R., van der Donk, J. A., and Goudswaard, J. (1977). *Am. J. Vet. Res.* **39**, 1359–1362.
van Dam, R. H., van Kooten, P. J. S., and van der Donk, J. A. (1978). *J. Immunol. Methods* **21**, 217–228.
van Dam, R. H., d'Amaro, J., van Kooten, P. J. S., van der Donk, J. A., and Goudswaard, J. (1979). *Anim. Blood Groups Biochem. Genet.* **10**, 121–124.
van den Tweel, J. G., Vriesendorp, H. M., Termijtelen, A., Westbroek, D. L., Bach, M. L., and van Rood, J. J. (1974). *J. Exp. Med.* **140**, 825–836.
van der Does, J. A., van Rood, J. J., Walker, W. S., and Epstein, R. B. (1973). *J. Exp. Med.* **137**, 494–503.
van der Feltz, M. J. M., van der Korput, J. A. G. M., Giphart, M. J., and Westbroek, D. L. (1981). *Transplantation* **32**, 253–255.
van Es, A. A., and Balner, H. (1979). *Tissue Antigens* **13**, 239–254.
van Rood, J. J., and van Leeuwen, A. (1963). *J. Clin. Invest.* **42**, 1382–1390.
van Rood, J. J., van Leeuwen, A., Keuning, J. J., and Blusse van Oud Alblas, A. (1975). *Tissue Antigens* **5**, 73–79.
van Rood, J. J., van Leeuwen, A., and Ploem, J. S. (1976). *Nature (London)* **262**, 795–797.
Viza, D., Sugar, J. R., and Binns, R. M. (1970). *Nature (London)* **227**, 949–950.
Vriesendorp, H. M. (1973). *Tissue Antigens* **3**, 145–163.
Vriesendorp, H. M. (1976). *Transplant. Proc.* **8**, 289–314.
Vriesendorp, H. M. (1977). *Transplant. Proc.* **9**, 1909–1910.
Vriesendorp, H. M. (1979). *Adv. Vet. Sci. Comp. Med.* **23**, 229–265.
Vriesendorp, H. M., Rothengatter, C., Bos, E., Westbroek, D. L., and van Rood, J. J. (1971). *Transplantation* **11**, 440–445.
Vriesendorp, H. M., Epstein, R. B., d'Amaro, J., Westbroek, D. L., and van Rood, J. J. (1972). *Transplantation* **14**, 229–307.
Vriesendorp, H. M., d'Amaro, J., van der Does, J. A., Westbroek, D. L., and Epstein, R. B. (1973). *Transplant. Proc.* **5**, 311–315.
Vriesendorp, H. M., Smid-Mercx, B. M. J., Visser, T. P., Halliwell, R. E. W., and Schwartzman, R. M. (1975a). *Transplant. Proc.* **7**, 375–377.
Vriesendorp, H. M., Zurcher, C., and van Bekkum, D. W. (1975b). *Transplant. Proc.* **7**, 465–468.
Vriesendorp, H. M., Grosse-Wilde, H., and Dorf, M. E. (1977). *In* "The Major Histocompatibility System in Man and Animals" (D. Götze, ed.), pp. 129–164. Springer-Verlag, Berlin and New York.
Walker, L. E., Ferrone, S., Pellegrino, M. E., and Reisfeld, R. A. (1980). *Mol. Immunol.* **17**, 1443–1448.
Weaver, W. J., Weber, F. S., Holmes, K., Jacob, S. W., and Templeton, J. W. (1975). *Transplant. Proc.* **7**, 399–401.
Westbroek, D. L., Rothengatter, C., Vriesendorp, H. M., van Rood, J. J., Willighagen, R. G. J., and de Vries, M. J. (1971). *Transplant. Proc.* **3**, 157–160.

Westbroek, D. L., Silberbusch, J., Vriesendorp, H. M., van Urk, H., Roemeling, H. W., Schonherr-Scholtes, Y., and de Vries, M. J. (1972). *Transplantation* **14,** 582–589.
Westbroek, D. L., Vriesendorp, H. M., van den Tweel, J. G., de Gruyl, J., and van Urk, H. (1975). *Transplant. Proc.* **7,** 427–429.
Wharton, R. H., Utech, K. B. W., and Turner, H. G. (1970). *Aust. J. Agric. Res.* **21,** 163–181.
White, D. J. G., Bradley, B., Calne, R. Y., and Binns, R. M. (1973). *Transplant. Proc.* **5,** 317–320.
Williams, A. F., and Gagnon, J. (1982). *Science* **216,** 696–703.
Wilson, B. D., Blyth, J. L., and Nowell, P. C. (1968). *J. Exp. Med.* **128,** 1157–1181.
Winchester, R. J., and Kunkel, H. G. (1979). *Adv. Immunol.* **28,** 221–292.
Yamazaki, K., Yamaguchi, M., Baranoski, L., Bard, J., Boyse, E. A., and Thomas, L. (1979). *J. Exp. Med.* **150,** 755–760.
Zinkernagel, R. M., and Doherty, P. C. (1979). *Adv. Immunol.* **27,** 221–292.

Sickled Red Cells in the Cervidae

W. JAPE TAYLOR

Department of Medicine, University of Florida College of Medicine, Gainesville, Florida

I.	Introduction	77
II.	Production and Behavior of Sickled Cells	80
	A. Sickling in Deer	80
	B. Sickling in Other Species.......................................	81
III.	Molecular Mechanisms of Sickling	83
IV.	Primary Structure and Genetics of the Hemoglobins...................	90
	A. α-Chain Duplication	90
	B. β-Chain Variability...	92
V.	Summary	94
	References...	95

I. Introduction

The sickling of deer erythrocytes is not associated with a disease and would probably have remained an obscure biological phenomenon were it not for its close resemblance to the distortion of red cells found in the serious human disease, sickle cell anemia (Fig. 1). Gulliver (1840a,b) first described the sickling of deer cells, and subsequent studies of numerous species of deer have demonstrated that the sickling phenomenon is virtually universal in members of the family Cervidae from both the Old and the New Worlds (Table I) (Undritz 1946; Untritz *et al.*, 1960; Kitchen *et al.*, 1966; Maughan and Williams, 1967; Butcher and Hawkey, 1977). Among the species that have been examined, only in the Chinese water deer (*Hydropotes inermis*), reindeer (*Rangifer tarandus*), and moose (*Alces alces*) is sickling not seen, whereas in the wapiti (*Cervus canadensis*) it is induced only with overnight storage.

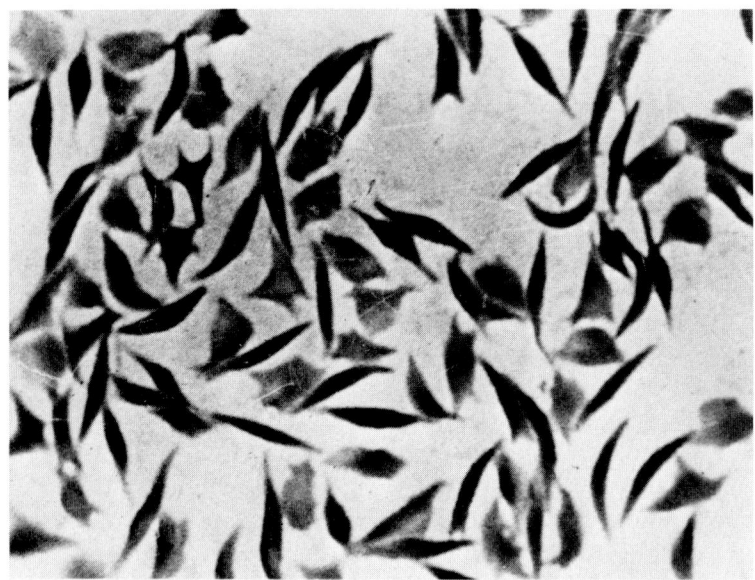

Fig. 1. Although hemoglobin polymerization causes the typically sickled cell of the deer to assume a variety of shapes, needle-like protrusions of varying lengths characterize all of them.

The biological significance of the widespread occurrence of sickling in deer is not known, for it has not been shown to be related to any evolutionary advantage such as the disease resistance that has been postulated for human sickle cell disease relative to malaria. The red blood cell survival in deer is approximately 125 days and is the same in both sickling and nonsickling animals (Noyes et al., 1966). The average adult values for hemoglobin, hematocrit, and red blood cell count are also identical regardless of the sickling state in white-tailed deer, *Odocoileus virginianus;* 18 gm/100 ml, 54%, and 18 m/cm, respectively, with the red cells being smaller than human erythrocytes (Kitchen et al., 1964).

Although sickling has been identified in many species of deer, the most extensive studies have involved the white-tailed deer, and this article will focus on that species. The production and behavior of sickled deer cells will be contrasted with those of human cells, and sickling in other species will be reviewed briefly. Hemoglobin polymerization is the critical requirement for sickling, and the relationship of this to specific β chains will be outlined. Finally, the primary structure of the hemoglobin chains and the unusual features of their genetic control will be examined.

TABLE I

Incidence and Distribution of the Sickling Phenomenon and Polymorphic Hemoglobins in the Family Cervidae

Common name (genus/species)	Geographical origin	Sickling[a]	Multiple hemoglobins[a]
Elk (*Alces alces*)	Europe and Asia	−	n.d.
Moose (*Alces americana*)	North America	−	n.d.
Axis deer (*Axis axis*)	Asia	+	+
Hog deer (*Axis porcinus*)	Asia	+	−
Roe deer (*Capreolus capreolus*)	Europe	+	−
Rocky Mountain wapiti (*Cervus canadensis nelsoni*)	North America	+	+
Tule wapiti (*Cervus canadensis nannodes*)	North America	+	+
Barasingha (*Cervus duvauceli*)	Asia	+	−
Red deer (*Cervus elaphus*)	Europe	+	−
Sika deer (*Cervus nippon*)	Asia	+; −	+
Dybowski's sika (*Cervus nippon hortulorum*)	Asia	+	n.d.
Timor deer (*Cervus timoriensis*)	Indonesia	+	+
Sambar (*Cervus unicolor*)	Asia	+	n.d.
Fallow deer (*Dama dama*)	Europe and East Asia	+	+
Père David deer (*Elaphurus davidianus*)	Asia	+	−
Chinese water deer (*Hydropotes inermis*)	Asia	−	+
Reeves muntjac (*Muntiacus muntjac reevesii*)	Asia	+	+
Panama deer (*Odocoileus chiriquensis*)	Central America	+	−
Black-tailed deer (*Odocoileus hemionus columbianus*)	North America	+	+
Mule deer (*Odocoileus hemionus hemionus*)	North America	+	+
Mexican deer (*Odocoileus mexicanus*)	North America	+	n.d.
White-tailed deer (*Odocoileus virginianus*)	North America	+; −	+
Reindeer (*Rangifer tarandus*)	Arctic	−	−

[a] +, Present; −, not present; n.d., no data.

II. Production and Behavior of Sickled Cells

A. Sickling in Deer

The reversible shifting of deer red cells from biconcave disks to bizarrely distorted cells with long needle-like protrusions and irregularities along the margins is a truly remarkable phenomenon. This event is primarily an *in vitro* occurrence, with sickling requiring an oxygenated cell in an environment with an elevated pH—optimally in the range of 7.6 to 7.8, although sickling begins at a pH of 7.4 in the white-tailed deer (Kitchen *et al.*, 1964). Undritz (1946), Undritz *et al.* (1960), and Butcher and Hawkey (1977) have emphasized the importance of high pH in the production of sickled deer erythrocytes from European and Asiatic deer. It is possible that alkalosis alone is suficient to induce sickling in some species; however, this has not been proven, and it appears clear that both high pH and high pO_2 are the optimal circumstances. *In vitro* sickling can also be induced by incubation with carbon monoxide and is accelerated by hypertonic media and other circumstances that concentrate the hemoglobin. Reducing agents inhibit the distortion of deer cells, in contrast to human sickling.

It is of note that requirements for the sickling of deer cells are the inverse of those that induce human sickling; they are also beyond the usual *in vivo* physiological parameters. Despite an occasional report to the contrary (Whitten, 1967), when precautions are taken to fix the red cells in their *in vivo* morphology, few sickled cells are found (Kitchen and Taylor, 1973: Parshall *et al.*, 1975). With drastic intravenous alkalinization, augmented by forced ventilation with 100% oxygen, Parshall *et al.* (1975) induced transient *in vivo* sickling in the sika deer, *Cervus nippon*. The procedure resulted in a high mortality, and the investigators were unable to produce chronic sicklemia. The evidence seems overwhelming that, in contrast to the human situation, a significant number of sickled cells is not present for any appreciable period of time in deer, thereby accounting for the absence of an associated disease.

In human sickle cell anemia, the classical concept of pathogenesis has been that the bizarre shapes and large, protruding spicules of the sickled cells increase their mechanical fragility and viscosity, thereby promoting intravascular hemolysis and stagnation (Ham and Castle, 1940). Lesser degrees of polymerization of human deoxyhemoglobin S precede the end product of overt sickling, and it has been postulated that the deformability of cells containing this partially gelled hemoglobin is limited, thereby impeding flow at the arterioles and capillaries even in the absence of overt sickling (Noguchi and Schecter, 1981). It is also known that the kinetics of oxygen uptake and release are abnormal in sickled cells, thereby contributing to a low arterial oxygen saturation (Jensen *et al.*, 1957; Sproule *et al.*, 1958; Harrington *et al.*, 1977).

In studies of the mechanical fragility and viscosity of sickled deer cells, Taylor *et al.* (1962) demonstrated both parameters to be increased, and Whitten (1967) also reported an increase in viscosity related to sickling but did not confirm the change in mechanical fragility. It is of interest, although not related to pathogenetic mechanisms, that increased ultrasonic absorption is a feature of sickled cells from both humans and deer (Shung *et al.*, 1981). In view of the marked similarity of the hemoglobin polymerization, that produces sickling in both species, the morphological identity of the cells, and the comparable behavior of sickled cells in humans and deer, the absence of a major disease in the deer relates primarily to the different requirements for the induction of polymerization and to the smaller size of their cells, which facilitates capillary transit.

Theoretically, the vascular area in which sickled erythrocytes or lesser degrees of intracellular hemoglobin aggregation would be most likely to occur in deer is the pulmonary capillary bed, where the pH and pO_2 are relatively high. In this regard, it is notable that an occasional deer that has been hyperventilating from either anxiety or the chase will die abruptly with congestive atelectasis of the lungs. Sickle cells are present in the pathological specimens, but it is not known if these were formed antemortem. Furthermore, the exact significance of this congestive atelectasis is unknown, because in other species that do not have sickling erythrocytes, the same phenomenon may be observed, although rarely. One other pathological peculiarity in such cases suggests the possibility of increased intravascular resistance. The deer heart has a striking increase in thickness of the free wall of both ventricles, which is illustrated in Fig. 2. However, if this cardiac finding is due to the sickling phenomenon, the relationship is a subtle one, because resting cardiac output and pulmonary artery pressure are not high in deer (Good *et al.*, 1961), and the hearts of sickling and nonsickling deer are comparable.

B. Sickling in Other Species

In the same survey of animals in the London Zoo that led to the description of sickling in deer in 1840, Gulliver (1840a) noted similar

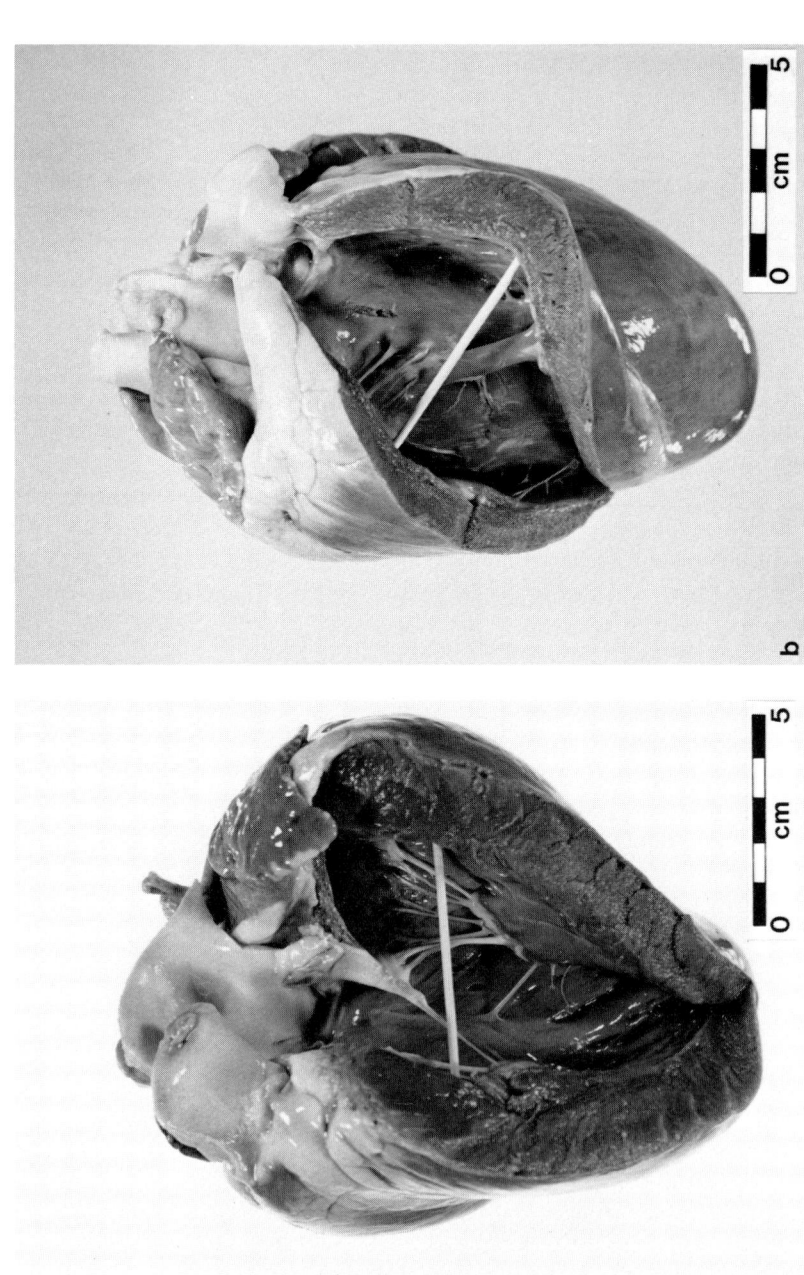

FIG. 2. Photograph of heart from a 9-year-old, 160-pound buck. (a) The thickness of the free wall of the left ventricle measures over 2 cm. (b) The wall of the right ventricle is over 1 cm thick, considerably greater than that of a sheep of comparable size.

cells in the genet. This observation has been confirmed by Ball *et al.* (1976), who induced sickling in erythrocytes from two species of genets, *Genetta genetta genetta* and *G. genetta tigrina,* under conditions similar to those that sickle deer red cells. It is probable that hemoglobin polymerization induces the sickling in genets, but this has not been demonstrated, and the mechanism of sickling in genets remains unknown. Deoxygenated erythrocytes of cats, whose hemoglobin is known to be relatively insoluble, will also assume a holly leaf configuration (Mauk *et al.,* 1974).

From time to time, reports of sickling of erythrocytes from a variety of other animals have appeared. Usually these have been various artiodactyls such as sheep (Evans, 1968) or goats (Holman and Dew, 1964), but some of the published pictures have not been convincing, and hemoglobin polymerization, the sine qua non for true sickling, has generally not been demonstrated. By electron microscopy, Jain and Kono (1977) did show that aggregated hemoglobin fibers induce a form of sickling in some angora goats. Interestingly, no difference between nonsickling and sickling goats in hemoglobin type was demonstrated by electrophoresis, but induction of a new adult hemoglobin C by bleeding did decrease the fusiform sickling (Jain *et al.,* 1980), suggesting a relationship to a specific hemoglobin.

The only nonmammalian species in which sickling polymerization of hemoglobin has been described are two iguana lizards of the Caribbean (Simpson *et al.,* 1983). Although gross distortion of the erythrocytes of the iguana is apparently prevented by the dense cell membranes and nuclei, the electron micrographic appearance of the polymerized hemoglobin in both cytoplasm and nuclei is strikingly similar to that of sickled cells from humans and deer. The hemoglobin of the iguana also shares the relative insolubility of other sickling hemoglobins.

III. Molecular Mechanisms of Sickling

As in other mammals, the adult hemoglobin of deer consists of two identical α chains and two identical β chains, each of which has approximately 145 amino acid residues. In the white-tailed deer, three α-chain variants have been identified, as well as seven β-chain types, so that a remarkable degree of hemoglobin polymorphism is found in this species. After the disappearance of the fetal γ chains in early life, the adult chains of any individual deer remain constant throughout life, in contrast to the situation in sheep and goats in which hemoglobin C is induced by acute anemia (Huisman *et al.,* 1969).

The sickling propensity is related to specific β chains in the white-tailed deer and is not influenced by α-chain type. The majority of these β chains are readily separated by standard electrophoretic techniques, and the more common ones have been designated $β^2$, $β^3$, $β^{4d}$, $β^{4e}$, $β^5$, and $β^7$; the seventh β chain has been found only in a single animal. The sickling $β^2$ and $β^3$ chains are most prevalent, being found in approximately 85% of deer, but regional differences in incidence may occur (Kitchen et al., 1966; Harris et al., 1973). Two of the α-chain variants have major charge differences producing altered electrophoretic migrations of the entire hemoglobin. For example, the $β^3$ chain produces hemoglobin I in combination with one α chain and hemoglobin III when present with another α chain. The less common $β^5$ and $β^7$ chains and the γ chain of fetal hemoglobin inhibit sickling, even when in heterozygous combination with either of the sickling chains. The two $β^4$ chains do not permit sickling, but instead an atypical burr cell (Taylor and Easley, 1974). Only limited numbers of animals of other species have been examined, but from the report of Butcher and Hawkey (1977), it appears that there are both sickling and nonsickling hemoglobins in other deer species as well.

Two major forms of reversibly sickling deer cells have been recognized and correlated with specific β chains. Both are characterized by elongated projections from the cells; in typical sickle cells, these protrude at a variety of angles, giving crescent, comma-shaped, or holly leaf types of deformation, whereas in the "matchstick" cell the entire cell becomes a long rod from which spicules may extend at either or both ends (Fig. 3). The in vitro conditions under which both of these sickled forms are induced appear to be identical, but typical sickling depends on the presence of the $β^3$ chain whereas the $β^2$ chain dictates the formation of matchsticks. As mentioned before, both the crescent and matchstick forms are found in white-tailed deer, and both have also been described in the hog deer (Axis porcinus), timor deer (Cervus timoirensis), barasingha (C. duvauceli), and Père David deer (Elaphurus davidianus). In these latter species, it is not known if the two forms are associated with different β chains as they are in the white-tailed deer.

The internal architecture of sickled cells is as spectacular as the external morphology. Transmission electron microscopy reveals fibers of polymerized hemoglobin that distort the cell membranes, thereby producing bizarre shapes. In the typically sickled cells, the aggregates appear as linear densities that are relatively short and interspersed at many angles except in the projecting spicules where they are more nearly parallel in the long axis of the protrusions. At high magnifica-

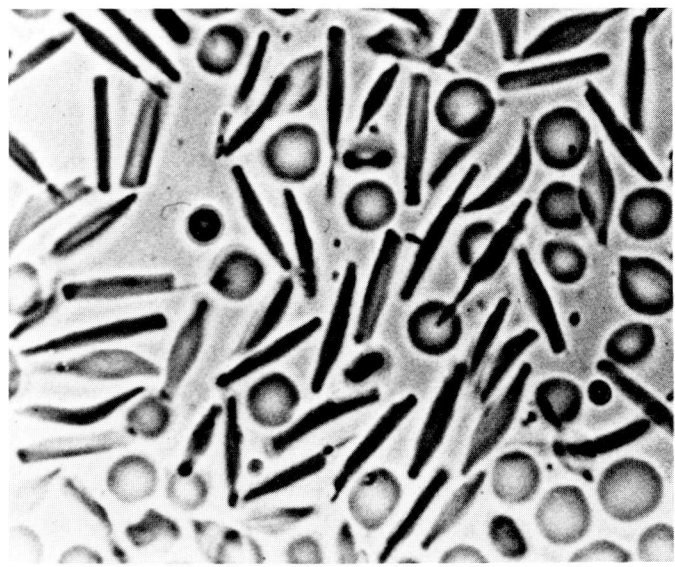

FIG. 3. The matchstick sickle cell has been seen only in deer and is induced by the same *in vitro* conditions of high pH and pO_2 that yield the typical sickle cell.

tions, the linear electron-dense aggregates are seen to consist of multi-sided tubules, 160–190 Å in diameter. Most of the fibers appear to be hexagonal and are virtually identical to those that are seen in human sickle cells, in which hemoglobin molecules align as stacked layers in a helical fashion (Finch et al., 1973; Simpson and Taylor, 1974a; Josephs et al., 1976). It is known that the β chains move approximately 6 Å closer together with oxygenation, and it is probable that this movement exposes or brings together contact areas of the hemoglobin chains so that intermolecular bonding can then produce polymerization of the hemoglobin.

The matchstick form of sickle cell contains polymerized hemoglobin that is aligned quite differently from the microtubules of the typically sickled cells (Taylor and Simpson, 1974). In the matchstick sickled cells one sees long linear aggregates that are not randomly dispersed but are always parallel. These produce long filaments that vary from 75 to 85 Å in diameter with center to center spacing of 120 to 125 Å, so that a very regular pattern resembling the trees in an orchard is produced in cross section. Spicules that contain only a few of these filaments may project from the ends of the matchsticks. In individual deer that have both hemoglobins II and III, because of heterozygosity for $β^2$

and β^3 chains, both the microtubular formation of typical sickle cells and the long filaments of the matchstick cell are found (Simpson and Taylor, 1974b). A comparable but not entirely identical alignment of polymerized hemoglobin is seen in previously unpublished electron micrographs (Figs. 4, 5, and 6) of the late C. A. Stetson, who was one of the first investigators to recognize the intracellular structure of the human sickle cell (Stetson, 1966). These electron micrographs of red cells of the Père David deer demonstrate a very orderly array of polymerized hemoglobin in long linear filaments that are very similar to those seen in the matchstick cell. Electron micrographs have not been published for other species, but it is probable that minor variations in the type of hemoglobin polymerization will be seen in the cells from different deer species relating to the different primary structures of their hemoglobins.

Interest in the structure of the hemoglobin polymers that occur in human sickle cell anemia has been intense because of the theoretical possibility of developing chemicals to block the intermolecular bonding that produces these polymers and their associated sickling. It has long been agreed that fibers of polymerized hemoglobin develop in human sickle cells and in gels of concentrated deoxyhemoglobin S, and that the solubility of that deoxyhemoglobin S is much less than that of deoxyhemoglobin A (Perutz and Mitchison, 1950; Stetson, 1966; Edelstein et al., 1973; Finch et al., 1973). However, a variety of models have been proposed to explain the intermolecular bonding that produces these fibers, and the precise mechanism of this linkage remains unknown. It has been demonstrated that strands of hemoglobin molecules may fuse into fibers that may, in turn, by appropriate manipulations be induced to crystallize (Josephs et al., 1976; Wellems and Josephs, 1979). This has led to the suggestion that the hemoglobin fibers of human sickle cells are composed of eight double strands; like previous models, the known single amino acid substitution of valine for glutamic acid at the β^6 position is emphasized as a point of abnormal contact.

The primary structure of the β chains of the deer hemoglobins are quite variable in contrast to the single amino acid difference between human hemoglobins A and S. It seems likely that the unifying feature between the hemoglobin polymers of the typical deer sickle cell and the matchstick form is the formation of strands of hemoglobin molecules, which then align into either tubular fibers or the more regular pattern of the matchstick cell or that seen in the Père David deer. This interpretation is consistent with the crystallographic data from deer hemoglobins II and III, which have demonstrated quite different forms of

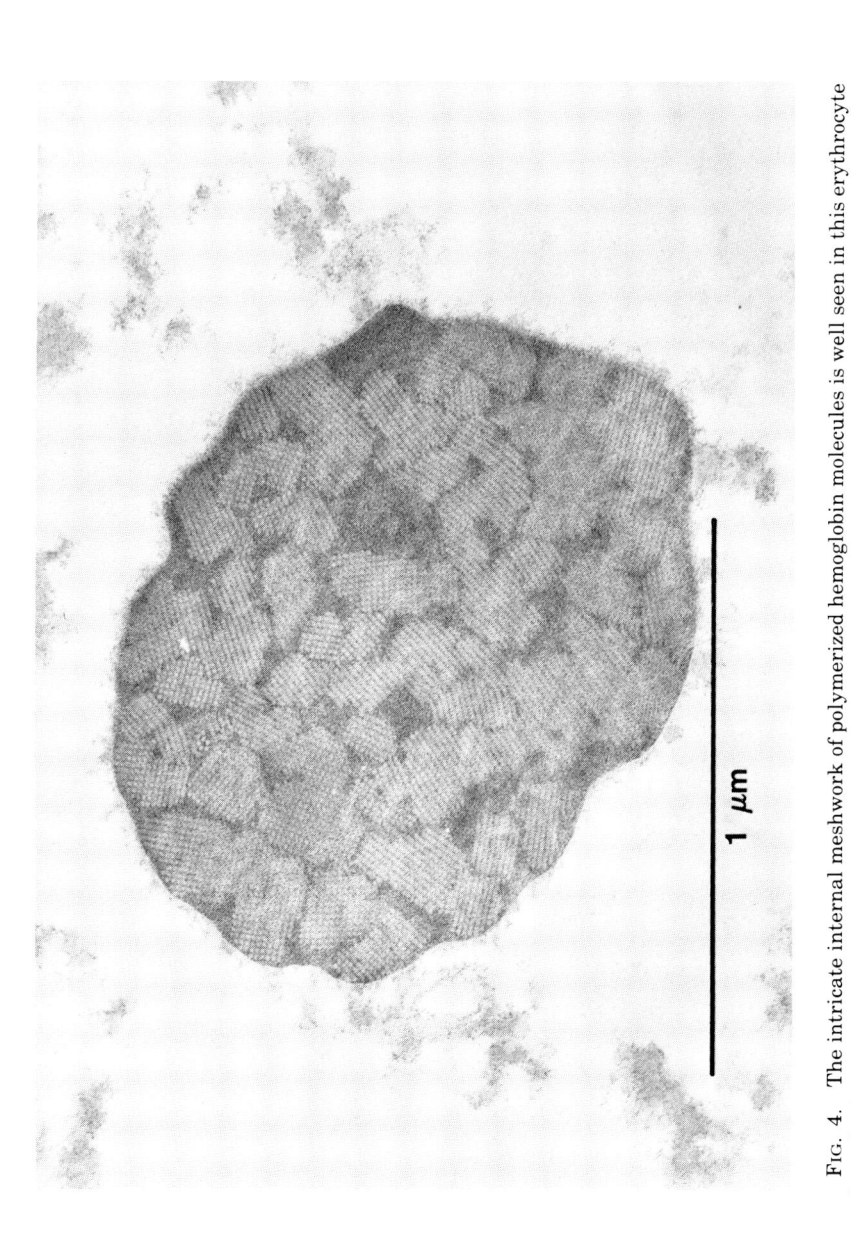

FIG. 4. The intricate internal meshwork of polymerized hemoglobin molecules is well seen in this erythrocyte from the Père David deer. Fixed in glutaraldehyde (×120,000).

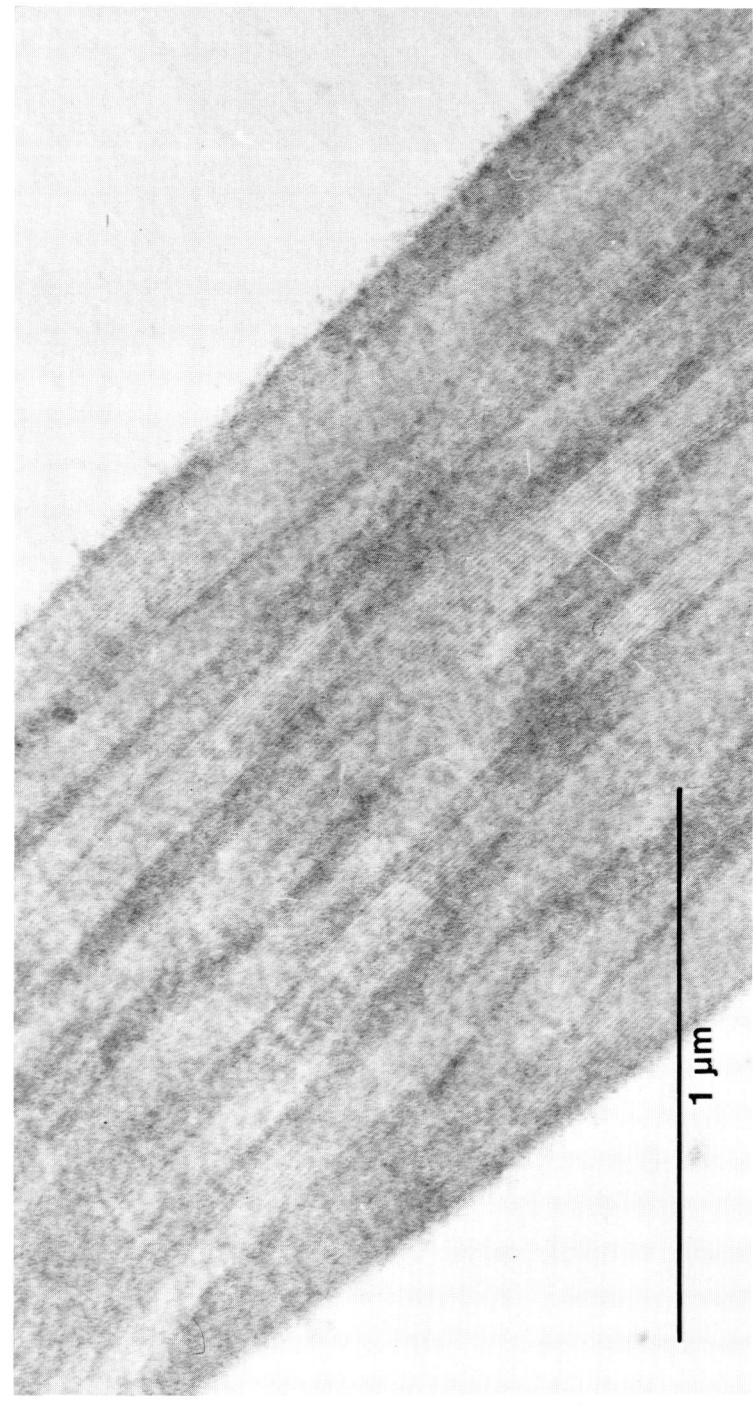

FIG. 5. The long linear strands of hemoglobin that produce matchstick cells are seen in the Père David deer. Fixed in glutaraldehyde (×120,000).

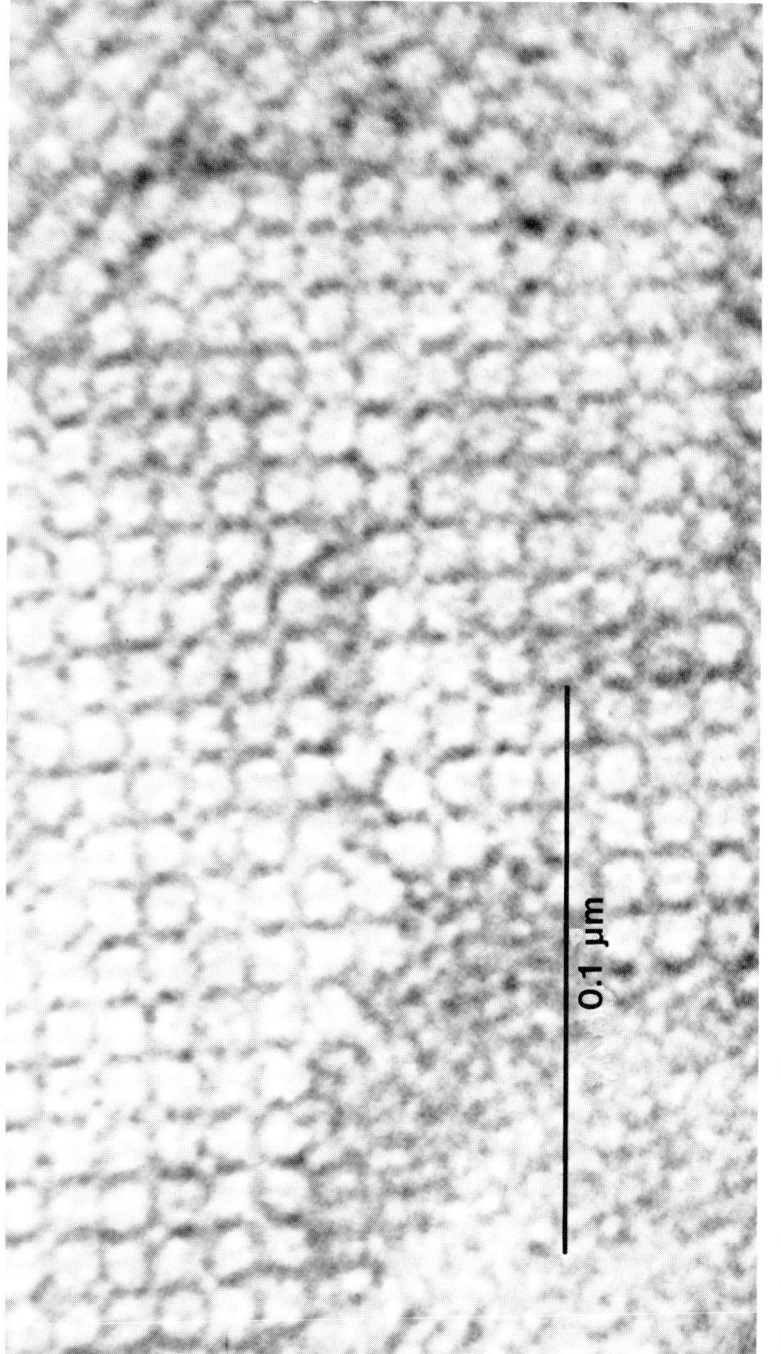

FIG. 6. At extreme magnification, a honeycomb appearance is produced by a latticework in which eight or more hemoglobin molecules surround central cavities with diameters of approximately 100 Å. Fixed in glutaraldehyde (×1,200,000).

molecular packing in crystals of these two hemoglobins (Houston *et al.*, 1978; Girling *et al.*, 1979).

IV. Primary Structure and Genetics of the Hemoglobins

Even if they did not possess the sickling propensity, the deer hemoglobins would be set apart as an unusual biological series by their extreme polymorphism. The usual genetic mechanism for mammalian hemoglobin production includes structural gene pairs at individual loci that dictate the structure of the individual hemoglobin chains. Accordingly, for adult hemoglobins one pair of genes controls the β chains and another pair the α chains; however, in many species two pairs of genes govern α-chain synthesis. If a minor hemoglobin component such as A_2 of humans is present, a separate gene pair at another locus is needed. The same requirement exists for the γ chains of fetal life, which, when combined with α chains, produce fetal hemoglobin and the even earlier embryonic hemoglobin chains.

Most of the common human hemoglobin variants are due to single-point mutations such as the one that produces the valine for glutamic acid substitution at the $β^6$ position of hemoglobin S. However, a variety of other genetic alterations such as deletions, chain elongation, and translocations occur (Lang and Lorkin, 1976; Weatherall and Clegg, 1979). The developmental sequences in which hemoglobins appear and the rates of individual chain synthesis are also under genetic control.

Duplication of α-chain gene loci in a number of species, including many primates, has been recognized with increasing frequency in recent years (Nute, 1974). Deer of at least two species are excellent examples of this phenomenon. In addition, the β chains of the white-tailed deer demonstrate deletions and a remarkable variability in primary structure despite being the products of allelic genes. Both the α-chain gene duplication and the β-chain variability will be outlined.

A. α-Chain Duplication

In the white-tailed deer, electrophoretic separation of dissociated α and β chains led to the identification of at least two α-chain variants. Selective breeding of apparently heterozygous animals produced deer that were homozygous for one of the α chains, but the other was never seen in the homozygous state. This prompted isolation and chemical study of the α chains, which revealed that some animals had three distinct α chains, two of which had the same electrophoretic mobility so that they had not been identified by that technique. Other animals had only a single α chain, whereas, another group had two α chains, so that an individual deer could have from one to three different α chains. Clearly, the presence of three α chains in a single animal could not be explained by alleles at a single gene locus, and required the presence of at least two α-gene loci.

Structural studies revealed two major sites of variation between the three chains. The $^I\alpha^3$ and $^I\alpha^{3'}$ chains contain tyrosine and phenylalanine at position 24, respectively, but are otherwise identical. The $^{II}\alpha^1$ chain contains lysine at position 20, where the $^I\alpha^3$ and $^I\alpha^{3'}$ chains have aspartic acid, but otherwise $^{II}\alpha^1$ is identical to $^I\alpha^{3'}$. This charge difference between aspartic acid and lysine not only had permitted the easy differentiation of the $^{II}\alpha^1$ chain from the other $^I\alpha$ chains, but is responsible for electrophoretic distinction between whole hemoglobins I and III. In combination with the common sickling β^3 chain, the $^{II}\alpha^1$ chain makes hemoglobin I whereas the hemoglobin III consists of the β^3 chain and either of the $^I\alpha^3$ chains. It is also of significance that the $^{II}\alpha^1$ is never seen in isolation but always in association with the $^I\alpha^{3'}$. Either of the $^I\alpha$ chains may exist alone. These data, which are similar to those of Harris *et al.* (1972), were considered to indicate that the gene for the $^I\alpha^{3'}$ chain was the original structural gene that had undergone a simple mutation at position 24 to produce the $^I\alpha^3$ gene, but also a duplication and subsequent mutation at position 20 to produce the $^{II}\alpha^1$ gene (Taylor *et al.*, 1972). It is fascinating that the nonduplicated gene has persisted for millions of years since the duplication occurred, suggesting that the duplicated gene has not had any major survival benefit. However, it is of note that it has, by its mutation, introduced a much less conservative change—the lysine–aspartic acid substitution—than is present in the tyrosine–phenylalanine variant at the twenty-fourth residue. In the overall evolutionary scheme, gene duplication is an obvious necessity, but its impact on the deer hemoglobins is by no means clear, although it has resulted in apparent heterogeneity of α-chain gene loci, with some deer having one locus and others two.

The only other deer species for which the primary structure of the α chain has been investigated in detail is the sika deer (*Cervus nippon*), in which a surprising array of α chains was found, even though electrophoresis of these chains revealed only a single band (Taylor and Easley, 1977). At least five, and possibly seven, α chains were identified in the sika deer by Taylor and Easley, with the points of substitution in the same general area as is found in the white-tailed deer, namely α-chain residues 15, 20, and 22. Although gene duplication was not unequivocally proven to be the cause of the multiple sika α chains, it appears most likely that this is true, and comparison of the sika chains with those of the white-tailed deer also suggests that the original lineage that evolved into the present sika deer branched from the stock that became white-tailed deer after the duplication of the α-chain gene. The incidence of α-chain duplication in other artiodactyls is not known, but it is present in domestic sheep and goats as well as the Barbary sheep (*Ammotragus lervia*), and appears to be high considering the limited number of species that has been investigated (Adams *et al.*, 1969; Wilson *et al.*, 1970; Vestri *et al.*, 1980).

Classic genetic data have indicated duplication of human α-chain genes for several years, but recent mapping of the genes has confirmed this fact (Orkin, 1978). Knowledge of the existence of α-chain gene duplication and its exploration at a molecular level has greatly expanded understanding of the α-thalassemias, a group of human diseases with varying degrees of diminished α-chain synthesis. In many populations, it is clear that variants of this disorder are due to gene deletions at one or the other of the α-chain gene loci, but other mechanisms exist as well (Kan *et al.*, 1977; Weatherall and Clegg, 1979). Accordingly, the heterogeneity of α-chain gene loci in deer is of interest relative to the very common thalassemia syndromes, just as the cell morphology is relative to sickle cell anemia.

B. β-Chain Variability

In one sense, the genetics of the deer β chains is not as complex as that of the α chain, but in another it is even more puzzling. Long-term multigenerational breeding experiments have never revealed evidence of more than a single gene locus controlling β-chain synthesis. However, the six common β chains that have been studied have an incredible degree of variation in their primary structure. With the exception of the $β^{4d}$ and $β^{4e}$ chains, which appear to be distinguished by only a single amino acid substitution, all of the other chains differ at multiple sites.

Amino acid variations have been identified in at least 11 sites of the deer β chain, and the structures of the entire chains have not been elucidated as yet (Table II). Aside from deletions at the beginning of the $β^5$ chain, it is possible that the other substitutions represent only single-point mutations. If this is so, it would appear that the genes have been extremely vulnerable to mutation and that the substitutions have had no major evolutionary impact but have been neutral,

TABLE II

STRUCTURAL VARIATION IN THE DEER β CHAINS

Position	2	3	12	61	66	69	70	73	135	143	144
β²	Met	Leu	Thr	Lys	Lys	Glx	Ser	Glx	Thr	Leu	Gly
β³	Met	Leu	Val	Lys	Arg	Asx	Ala	Glx	Ala	His	Arg
β⁴ᵈ	Met	Leu	Thr	Val	Arg	Asx	Ala	Asx	Thr	His	Arg
β⁴ᵉ	Met	Leu	Thr	Val	Arg	Asx	Ala	Glx	Thr	His	Arg
β⁵	—	—	Thr	Leu	Arg	Asx	Ala	Asx	Thr	His	Arg

thereby allowing the accumulation of a large number of hemoglobin variants. However, some as yet unidentified genetic mechanism may have produced the extreme diversity of the β chains.

Other ruminants share this characteristic of marked β-chain variability (Kitchen et al., 1968). Although only the sheep has a comparable degree of structural variability between the β chains (Boyer et al., 1967), the cow also has more than a single substitution (Schroeder et al., 1972). In contrast, the α chains of these species are very similar, with those of the sheep and the deer being almost identical. It is not clear why the intraspecies differences in hemoglobin structure in the ruminants is greater than the interspecies variations between many primates.

After the γ chains of fetal hemoglobin have been replaced by the particular adult β chain or chains at approximately 2 months of age, the β-chain type does not change. This contrasts to the situation in a number of other ruminants, particularly sheep and goats, in which a new hemoglobin C can be induced by anemia (Tucker and Clarke, 1980). Sequential studies of fetal erythropoietic stem cells demonstrates that this fascinating hemoglobin switch is not modulated by the same mechanism as is the fetal–adult hemoglobin switch (Barker et al., 1980).

V. Summary

Hemoglobin polymerizes within the red cells from most species of deer when exposed to oxygen and an elevated pH. This hemoglobin aggregation is related to specific β chains, which also dictate the precise alignment of the molecules and the type of cellular distortion. The typical sickle cell is virtually identical in shape, mechanical fragility, and viscosity to the human sickle cell, whereas the matchstick cell shares the latter properties but is an elongate cell from which spicules protrude in only one direction. The conditions of pH and pO_2 that are required are beyond the usual physiological ranges; therefore, neither *in vivo* sickling nor disease is seen in deer.

The genetic makeup of deer hemoglobin is of interest because of duplication of the α-chain gene loci and because of an extreme variability of the primary structure of the β chains, at least in the white-tailed deer.

Many facets of the deer hemoglobins remain fascinating objects for speculation. The evolutionary significance, if any, of the almost universal presence of sickling in the Cervidae is unknown. The meaning of the extreme polymorphism of the deer hemoglobins and the mechanisms by which they occurred are also obscure. It may be, however, that they may provide a tool by which one can elucidate the contact points and bonds that lead to the polymerization that produces the picturesque sickle cell.

Acknowledgments

Much of the original research on the white-tailed deer was done in satisfying collaboration with Hyram Kitchen, Caroline W. Easley, and Charles F. Simpson. Bottle-feeding of numerous fawns by my wife, Audrey Dennison Taylor, was critical to many of the long-term genetic studies. Skilled technical assistance was provided by Beatrice P. Godwin, John L. Neal, Jr., and J. W. Carlisle. Typing and assistance in preparation of the manuscript was given by Deborah Hodges. Financial support was provided by grants from the National Institutes of Health, chapters of the Florida Affiliate of the American Heart Association, and the W. Jape Taylor Medical Research and Teaching Foundation.

References

Adams, H. R., Wrightstone, R. N., Miller, A., and Huisman, T. H. J. (1969). Quantitation of hemoglobin α-chains in adult and fetal goats: Gene duplication and the production of polypeptide chains. *Arch. Biochem. Biophys.* **132**, 223–236.

Ball, S., Hawkey, C. M., Hime, J. M., Keymer, I. F., and Brambell, M. R. (1976). Red cell sickling in genets. *Comp. Biochem. Physiol. A* **54A**, 49–54.

Barker, J. E., Pierce, J. E., and Nienhuis, A. W. (1980). Hemoglobin switching in sheep: A comparison of the erythropoietin-induced switch to HbC and the fetal to adult hemoglobin switch. *Blood* **56**, 488–493.

Boyer, S. H., Hathaway, P., Pascasio, F., Bordley, J., Orton, C., and Naughton, M. A. (1967). Differences in the amino acid sequences of tryptic peptides from three sheep hemoglobin β-chains. *J. Biol. Chem.* **242**, 2211–2231.

Butcher, P. D., and Hawkey, C. M. (1977). Haemoglobins and erythrocyte sickling in the Artiodactyla: A survey. *Comp. Biochem. Physiol. A* **57A**, 391–398.

Edelstein, S. J., Telford, J. N., and Crepeau, R. H. (1973). Structure of fibers of sickle cell hemoglobin. *Proc. Natl. Acad. Sci. U.S.A.* **70**, 1104–1107.

Evans, E. T. R. (1968). Sickling phenomenon in sheep. *Nature (London)* **217**, 74–75.

Finch, J. T., Perutz, M. F., Bertles, J. B., and Dobler, J. (1973). Structure of sickled erythrocytes and sickle-cell hemoglobin fibers. *Proc. Natl. Acad. Sci. U.S.A.* **70**, 718–722.

Girling, R. L., Schmidt, W. C., Jr., Houston, T. E., Amma, E. L., and Huisman, T. H. J. (1979). The molecular packing and intermolecular contacts of sickling deer type III hemoglobin. *J. Mol. Biol.* **131**, 417–433.

Good, A. L., Stowe, C. M., and Blankenship, L. (1961). Cardiac output and related values in anesthetized deer. *Am. J. Vet. Res.* **22**, 156–158.

Gulliver, G. (1840a). Observations on certain peculiarities of form in the blood corpuscles of the mammiferous animals. *Philos. Mag.* [3] **17**, 325–327.

Gulliver, G. (1840b). Observations on the blood corpuscles of certain species of the genus Cervus. *Philos. Mag.* [3] **17**, 327–331.

Ham, T. H., and Castle, W. B. (1940). Relation of increased hypotonic fragility and of erythrostasis to the mechanism of hemolysis in certain anemias. *Trans. Assoc. Am. Physicians* **55**, 127–132.

Harrington, J. P., Elbaum, D., Bookchin, R. M., Wittenberg, J. B., and Nagel, R. L. (1977). Ligand kinetics of hemoglobin S containing erythrocytes. *Proc. Natl. Acad. Sci. U.S.A.* **74**, 203–206.

Harris, M. H., Wilson, J. B., and Huisman, T. H. J. (1972). Structural studies of hemoglobin α-chains from Virginia white-tailed deer. *Arch. Biochem. Biophys.* **151**, 540–548.

Harris, M. J., Huisman, T. H. J., and Hayes, F. A. (1973). Geographic distribution of hemoglobin variants in the white-tailed deer. *J. Mammal.* **54**, 270–274.

Holman, H. H., and Dew, S. M. (1964). The blood picture of the goat. II. Changes in erythrocyte shape, size, and number associated with age. *Res. Vet. Sci.* **5**, 274–285.

Houston, T. E., Plese, C. F., Girling, R. L., Amma, E. L., and Huisman, T. H. J. (1978). Crystallography and oriented single crystal electron microscopy of hemoglobin deer. II. A hemoglobin that exhibits match-stick-shaped erythrocytes. *Biochim. Biophys. Acta* **535**, 413–417.

Huisman, T. H. J., Lewis, J. P., Blunt, M. H., Adams, N. R., Miller, A., Dozy, A. M., and Boyd, E. M. (1969). Hemoglobin C in newborn sheep and goats: A possible explanation for its function and biosynthesis. *Pediatr. Res.* **3**, 189–198.

Jain, N. C., and Kono, C. S. (1977). Fusiform erythrocytes resembling sickle cells in angora goats: Light and electron microscopic observations. *Res. Vet. Sci.* **22**, 169–180.

Jain, N. C., Kono, C. S., Myers, A., and Bottomly, K. (1980). Fusiform erythrocytes resembling sickle cells in angora goats: Observations on osmotic and mechanical fragility and reversal of cell shape during anemia. *Res. Vet. Sci.* **28**, 25–35.

Jensen, W. N., Rucknagel, D. C., and Taylor, W. J. (1957). Arterial oxygen unsaturation and possible mechanism of production in sickle cell anemia. *J. Clin. Invest.* **37**, 905–906.

Josephs, R., Jarosch, H. S., and Edelstein, S. J. (1976). Polymorphism of sickle cell hemoglobin fibers. *J. Mol. Biol.* **102**, 409–426.

Kan, Y. W., Dozy, A. M., Trecartin, R., and Todd, D. (1977). Identification of a nondeletion defect in α thalassemia. *N. Engl. J. Med.* **297**, 1081–1083.

Kitchen, H., and Taylor, W. J. (1973). The sickling phenomenon of deer erythrocytes. In "Hemoglobin and Red Cell Structure and Function" (G. J. Brewer, ed.), pp. 325–336. Plenum, New York.

Kitchen, H., Putnam, F. W., and Taylor, W. J. (1964). Hemoglobin polymorphism: Its relation to sickling of erythrocytes in white-tailed deer. *Science* **144**, 1237–1239.

Kitchen, H., Putnam, F. W., and Taylor, W. J. (1966). The structural basis for the polymorphic hemoglobins of white-tailed deer (*Odocoileus virginianus*): A comparison of the hemoglobins associated with sickled and nonsickled erythrocytes. *Proc. Int. Symp. Comp. Hemoglobin Struct.* pp. 73–82.

Kitchen, H., Easley, C. W., Putnam, F. W., and Taylor, W. J. (1968). Structural comparison of polymorphic hemoglobins of deer with those of sheep and other species. *J. Biol. Chem.* **243**, 1204–1211.

Lang, A., and Lorkin, P. A. (1976). Genetics of human haemoglobins. *Br. Med. Bull.* **32**, 239–245.

Maughan, E., and Williams, J. R. B. (1967). Haemoglobin types in deer. *Nature (London)* **215**, 404–405.

Mauk, A. G., Whelan, H. T., and Taketa, F. (1974). "Holly wreath" morphology of feline erythrocytes—The effects of cyanate and 4,4′-dipyridyldisulfide (37855). *Proc. Soc. Exp. Biol. Med.* **145**, 578–585.

Noguchi, C. T., and Schecter, A. N. (1981). The intracellular polymerization of sickle hemoglobin and its relevance to sickle cell disease. *Blood* **58**, 1057–1068.

Noyes, W. D., Kitchen, H., and Taylor, W. J. (1966). Red cell life span of white-tailed deer, *Odocoileus virginianus*. *Comp. Biochem. Physiol.* **19**, 471–473.

Nute, P. E. (1974). Multiple hemoglobin α-chain loci in monkeys, apes and man. *Ann. N.Y. Acad. Sci.* **241**, 39–60.

Orkin, S. H. (1978). The duplicated human alpha globin genes lie close together in cellular DNA. *Proc. Natl. Acad. Sci. U.S.A.* **75**, 5950–5954.

Parshall, C. J., Vainisi, S. J., Goldberg, M. F., and Wolf, E. D. (1975). In vivo erythrocyte sickling in the Japanese Sika deer (*Cervus nippon*): Methodology. *Am. J. Vet. Res.* **36**, 749–752.

Perutz, M. F., and Mitchison, J. M. (1950). State of haemoglobin in sickle-cell anaemia. *Nature (London)* **166**, 677–679.

Schroeder, W. A., Shelton, J. R., Shelton, J. B., Apell, G., Huisman, T. H. S., Smith, L. L., and Carr, W. R. (1972). Amino acid sequences in the β-chains of adult bovine hemoglobins C-Rhodesia and D-Zambia. *Arch. Biochem. Biophys.* **152**, 222–232.

Shung, K. K., Rocco, M., and Ballard, J. O. III. (1981). Ultrasonic absorption in deer blood. *J. Acoust. Soc. Am.* **70**, 664–668.

Simpson, C. F., and Taylor, W. J. (1974a). Ultrastructure of sickled deer erythrocytes. I. The typical crescent and holly leaf forms. *Blood* **43**, 899–906.

Simpson, C. F., and Taylor, W. J. (1974b). Morphological and submicroscopic comparison of sickle erythrocytes of humans and deer. *Ann. N.Y. Acad. Sci.* **241**, 614–622.

Simpson, C. F., Taylor, W. J., and Jacobson, E. R. (1982). Sickling hemoglobin polymerization in iguana erythrocytes. *Comp. Biochem. Physiol.* **73A**, 703–708.

Sproule, B. J., Halden, E. R., and Miller, N. F. (1958). A study of cardiopulmonary alterations in patients with sickle cell disease and its variants. *J. Clin. Invest.* **37**, 486–495.

Stetson, C. A. (1966). The state of hemoglobin in sickled erythrocytes. *J. Exp. Med.* **123**, 341–346.

Taylor, W. J., and Easley, C. W. (1974). Sickling phenomena of deer. *Ann. N.Y. Acad. Sci.* **241**, 594–604.

Taylor, W. J., and Easley, C. W. (1977). Multiple hemoglobin α-chains in the sika deer (*Cervus nippon*). *Biochim. Biophys. Acta* **492**, 126–135.

Taylor, W. J., Childress, R. C., and Kitchen, H. (1962). The production and behavior of sockled erythrocytes in deer blood. *Clin. Res.* **10**, 208.

Taylor, W. J., Easley, C. W., and Kitchen, H. (1972). Structural evidence for heterogeneity of two hemoglobin α-chain gene loci in white-tailed deer. *J. Biol. Chem.* **247**, 7320–7324.

Tucker, E. M., and Clarke, S. W. (1980). Comparative aspects of biochemical polymorphism in the blood of Caprinae species and their hybrids. *Anim. Blood Groups Biochem. Genet.* **11**, 163–183.

Undritz, E. (1946). Über das vorkommen von sichelzell-erythrozyten und anderer Blutzellen-varianten unter normalen verkältnissen und als anomalie bie meusch und tier. *Arch. Julius Klaus-Stift. Vererbungsforsch., Sozialanthropol. Rassenhyg.* **21**, 288–295.

Undritz, E., Betke, K., and Lehmann, H. (1960). Sickling phenomenon in deer. *Nature (London)* **187**, 333–334.

Vestri, R., Crema, C., Marinucci, M., Giordano, P. C., and Bernini, L. F. (1980). Possible duplication of the hemoglobin α chain locus in sheep. *Biochim. Biophys. Acta* **625**, 328, 336.

Weatherall, D. J., and Clegg, J. B. (1979). Recent developments in the molecular genetics of human hemoglobin. *Cell* **16,** 467–479.

Wellems, T. E., and Josephs, R. (1979). Crystallization of deoxyhemoglobin S by fiber alignment and fusion. *J. Mol. Biol.* **135,** 651–674.

Whitten, C. F. (1967). Innocuous nature of the sickling (pseudosickling) phenomenon in deer. *Br. J. Haematol.* **13,** 650–655.

Wilson, J. B., Wrightstone, R. N., and Huisman, T. H. J. (1970). Haemoglobin α chain duplication in Barbary sheep, *Ammotragus lervia, Pallas,* 1777. *Nature (London)* **226,** 354–355.

Corticosteroid Teratogenicity

J. M. ROWLAND AND A. G. HENDRICKX

California Primate Research Center, University of California, Davis, California

I. Introduction 99
II. Interspecies Comparison of Corticosteroid Teratogenicity 100
    A. Mice 100
    B. Rats 103
    C. Nonhuman Primates 105
    D. Hamsters 106
    E. Others 107
    F. Summary 109
III. Factors Determining Corticosteroid-Induced Cleft Palate 111
    A. Exposure to the Teratogenic Agent 111
    B. Molecular Mechanisms 114
    C. Embryological Characteristics 117
IV. Conclusion 123
    References 124

I. Introduction

Corticosteroids have been extensively studied as teratogenic agents since the initial report by Baxter and Fraser (1950) that administration of cortisone to pregnant mice resulted in cleft palates in the offspring. Since that time, corticosteroids have become a widely used tool for the study of cleft palate (Green and Kochhar, 1975; Salomon and Pratt, 1979). It has not been as well recognized that corticosteroid effects are not confined to the developing palate but encompass a wide variety of organ systems and developmental events. This is not an unexpected finding given the diverse physiological and pharmacological effects displayed by these compounds in the adult animal. They are known to influence protein, carbohydrate, fat, and purine metabolism and to alter the function of a variety of organ systems including the cardiovascular system, nervous system, immune system, kidneys, muscle, and bone.

The demonstrated teratogenicity of corticosteroids in laboratory animals raises the question of possible human teratogenicity. Several authors have concluded that corticosteriods probably do not have an adverse effect on human intrauterine development (Bongiovanni and McPadden, 1960; Popert, 1962; Wilson, 1977), although cleft palate (Doig and Coltman, 1956: Harris and Ross, 1956; Popert, 1962; Schatz *et al.*, 1975) and a number of other malformations (Guilbeau, 1953; Wells, 1953; Rees and Williams, 1962; Malpas, 1965; Williams, 1967; Kraus, 1975; Schatz *et al.*, 1975) have been reported in offspring exposed to corticosteroids during development. A number of deficiencies exist in the human studies, such as inadequate documentation of dosage, time of treatment, and end points evaluated. In light of the equivocal results and inadequacies of the data base, the possibility that corticosteroids may be teratogenic in humans cannot be eliminated.

The purpose of this article is to review the teratogenic effects of corticosteroids in mammalian species, giving special emphasis to the multisystemic effects reported, and to examine some of the critical factors responsible for interstrain and interspecies differences in corticosteroid-induced cleft palate.

II. Interspecies Comparison of Corticosteroid Teratogenicity

A. Mice

The teratogenicity of corticosteroids was first reported in mice by Fraser and associates (Baxter and Fraser, 1950; Fraser and Fainstat, 1951). These initial studies determined that a dose of 2.5 mg/day of cortisone acetate administered to the pregnant female on Days 11–14 of gestation was the optimal teratogenic regimen in A/J mice, resulting in 100% cleft palate and a low incidence of resorption. Cortisol was also found to be teratogenic in mice (Kalter and Fraser, 1952), although further studies have indicated that it is not as potent as cortisone in inducing cleft palate in Strain A mice. Pinsky and DiGeorge (1965) reported an incidence of 18% cleft palate in offspring of A/J mice when 4 mg of cortisol were administered intramuscularly on Days 11–14 of gestation, whereas Lahti *et al.* (1972) found 56% cleft palate in A/J mice with the same dose and treatment period but using intraperitoneal injection. Heiberg et al. (1959) provided evidence that the maternal adrenals were capable of secreting teratogenic levels of corticosteroid with the finding that the administration of ACTH to the pregnant female produced cleft palate in the offspring. Further support for this conclusion came with the reports by Blaustein et al. (1971) and Hackman and Brown (1972) that corticosterone, the primary adrenocorticosteroid in mice, was teratogenic. Subcutaneous (sc) administration of 2.5 mg/day of corticosterone to pregnant A/J mice on Days 11–14 of gestation resulted in 31% cleft palate (Hackman and Brown, 1972). Thus all of the major naturally occurring corticosteroids, corticosterone, cortisol, and cortisone, as well as adrenocorticotropic hormone (ACTH), have been demonstrated to be deleterious to normal development in mice when administered at appropriate doses and stages of gestation.

A number of synthetic corticosteroids—triamcinolone acetonide (TAC), dexamethasone, and prednisolone—have also been demonstrated to be teratogenic in A/J mice (Pinsky and DiGeorge, 1965; Walker, 1965), although there are wide variations in the relative teratogenic potencies of these compounds. From a comparative standpoint, based on the dosage required to induce a similar incidence of defects, triamcinolone acetonide is the most potent teratogen, followed by dexamethasone, prednisolone, cortisone, cortisol, and corticosterone. Deoxycorticosterone, a mineralocorticoid, failed to induce cleft palate at doses up to 2000 times the human therapeutic dose. Triamcinolone acetonide was approximately 12 times more potent than dexamethasone and 200 times more potent than cortisone in inducing cleft palate in 100% of the treated fetuses.

Different strains of inbred mice exhibit different degrees of susceptibility to corticosteroid-induced cleft palate (Fraser et al., 1954). For example, 2.5 mg of cortisone acetate administered on Days 11–14 of gestation produce 100% cleft palate in A/J mice but only 20–25% in C57BL/6J. Reciprocal crosses of sensitive and resistant strains result in intermediate cleft palate sensitivity in the offspring. The offspring of interstrain crosses using A/J (sensitive) mothers and C57BL/6J (resistant) fathers are more sensitive than those from a cross of A/J fathers and C57BL/6J mothers, indicating a maternal effect in addition to the altered embryo genotype (Kalter, 1954). However, patrilinial sensitivity has been found in offspring of analogous crosses between the C3H (moderate sensitivity) and A/J or A/St (sensitive) strains (Loevy, 1962, 1963; Kalter, 1965). Backcrosses of reciprocal F_1 hybrid males to inbred females have been used to test the hypothesis that sex-linked genes affect embryonic sensitivity to cortisone-induced cleft palate. Francis (1973) has reported that sex-linked genes contribute to the embryonic reactivity to cortisone-induced cleft palate whereas Biddle and Fraser (1976,1977) found no evidence to support this hypothesis.

The sensitivity to corticosteroid-induced cleft palate appears to be a multigenic trait (Kalter, 1954, 1965; Walker and Fraser, 1957; Loevy, 1963; Dostal and Jelinek, 1973; Biddle and Fraser, 1977). At least one of the loci contributing to cleft palate sensitivity appears to be closely associated with the major histocompatibility locus in the mouse (Biddle and Fraser, 1977). Several laboratories have reported an association of certain H-2 haplotypes with susceptibility to corticosteroid-induced cleft palate (Bonner and Slavkin, 1975; Tyan and Miller, 1978), although conflicting data have been reported by Jirsakova and Valhova (1971). Mice with the H-2^a haplotype, A/J and B10.A, are highly susceptible to corticosteroid-induced cleft palate, whereas those with H-2^b haplotypes, C57BL/6J and C57BL/10ScSn, are resistant. The frequency of cleft palate in hybrid animals bearing a maternally derived H-2^a haplotype is much higher than in hybrids with a paternally derived H-2^a. Similarly, the frequency of cleft palate was lowered more significantly if the H-2^b haplotype was maternally rather than paternally derived. It is clear that despite the positive associations between certain H-2 haplotypes and cleft palate sensitivity, the H-2 locus is not the sole determinant of susceptibility to corticosteroid-induced cleft palate. For example, C57 and bm/bm mice have the same H-2 haplotype, H-2^b, but very different cleft palate frequencies after corticosteroid administration (Pratt et al., 1980a). Similarly, C3H/HeJ and CBA/J mice both contain the H-2^K haplotype but different sensitivity to cortisone-induced cleft palate (Goldman et al., 1977). These results indicate that additional, non-H-2–associated genetic differences must contribute to susceptibility to corticosteroid-induced cleft palate.

Studies involving corticosteroid teratogenicity in mice have focused primarily on cleft palate as the primary defect. However, a number of other defects have been reported and should be considered before making conclusions regarding the specificity of corticosteroids toward the developing palate. The initial report of cleft palate induction by cortisone also contained evidence of several other defects that occurred sporadically, such as spina bifida and shortening of the head and mandible (Fraser and Fainstat, 1951). Jurand (1968) reported that 25 mg/kg of cortisol on Days 10–12 (sc) caused micromelia (10.3%) and abnormal digits (5.8%), as well as cleft palate (52.7%). When embryos were evaluated on Day 14 of gestation, 26% showed some form of abnormality. The most frequent abnormalities detected were dilation of the marginal venous sinus (14.5%), distal limb bud necrosis (7.9%), or hemorrhage (10.7%) and subepidermal blisters. The decrease in frequency of embryos with abnormal digits on Day 18 compared to Day 14 suggests that many of the embryos with hemorrhage or necrosis of the foot plates do not survive until Day 18. It is important to note that no limb abnormalities have ever been detected at term by any other investigators.

Abnormal ovarian position was reported in offspring of CD-1 mice treated with prednisolone or dexamethasone (ocular administration) on Days 10–13 of gestation (Ballard et al., 1977). These anomalies were unilateral and consisted of the ovary being located at various locations on the ventral surface of the kidney whereas the contralateral gonad appeared in its normal position. The frequency of ovarian abnormalities was less than that found for cleft palate. An increase in the anogenital distance of female offspring (measured on postnatal Day 60) and reduced body weight were reported following the subcutaneous administration of prednisolone to pregnant mice from Day 13 to Day 18 of gestation at dosages of 50–400 µg/day (Gandelman and Rosenthal, 1981). Delays in attainment of eye opening, lifting, walking, and gripping were also noted. All of these effects were found at doses below that required to cause cleft palate.

Abnormalities of the eye as well as the palate were detected following subcutaneous administration of cortisol at varying periods during organogenesis (Rogoyski and Trzcinska-Dabrowska, 1960). Histological examination of the fetal lens (Day 18 of gestation) showed a high incidence of cataracts in the treated groups. The effects on the eye were most marked in the group treated on Day 8 and 9 of gestation, whereas cleft palate was most common in animals treated on Days 11–14 of gestation.

B. Rats

Numerous investigators have reported no increased cleft palate incidence following administration of either cortisol or cortisone to pregnant rats (Gunberg, 1957; Mercier-Parot, 1957; Curry and Beaton, 1958; Csaba et al., 1967; Walker, 1971). However, intraamniotic injections of cortisol do cause cleft palate in rat embryos (Dostal and Jelinek, 1971), and data obtained in our laboratory have demonstrated that maternally administered cortisol can, at very high dosages (500 mg/kg), induce a small but significant increase in cleft palates in the fetuses (Rowland and Hendrickx, 1982).

Similarly, prednisolone treatment has not been reported to cause cleft palate in rats (Kalter, 1962; Walker, 1971) but has been demonstrated to cause morphological changes in the placenta (Blackburn et al., 1965). Prednisone treatment on Days 11–20 of gestation causes adrenal and thymic atrophy and fetal growth retardation but no cleft palates or other malformations (Angervall and Lundin, 1964).

In contrast to the refractoriness of rats to cleft palate induction by cortisol, cortisone, prednisolone, and prednisone, the more potent synthetic corticosteroids have been demonstrated to cause malformations. Vannier et al. (1969) demonstrated that administration of dexamethasone to the pregnant female resulted in cleft palate and umbilical hernia in the offspring. Cleft palate induction by administration of dexamethasone during midgestation was confirmed by Nanda et al. (1970) and Chamberlain and Kasahara (1971). Furthermore, intraamniotic injection of dexamethasone (40–120 μg) resulted in 88–98% cleft palate in the embryos (Chamberlain and Kasahara, 1971), suggesting that the teratogenic effects result from a direct effect on the embryo. Walker (1971) reported that dexamethasone, triamcinolone acetonide, and betamethasone all produced cleft palate in the rat but methylprednisolone, prednisolone, and cortisone did not.

Rowland and Hendrickx (1983) have confirmed the observation that triamcinolone acetonide induces cleft palate in the rat and demonstrated that decreased fetal viability, fetal growth retardation, umbilical hernias, undescended testes, and decreased ossification of the skeleton are also produced by TAC treatment. These effects were all produced at doses causing no maternal lethality. In addition, fetal growth retardation was produced at doses lower than those required to produce malformations and during periods of gestation where no malformations are produced, supporting the use of this parameter as a sensitive indicator of embryotoxicity. Furthermore, an increased incidence of fetuses with a hypoplastic thymus was detected following treatment on Days 15–17 of gestation. This is in agreement with earlier reports of reduced thymus weights in offspring of rats treated with cortisone (Angervall and Lundin, 1964, 1965) or prednisone (Angervall and Lundin, 1965) during the second half of gestation. Russel et al. (1972) examined the effects of cortisone on thymolymphatic differentiation in the rat and found that the thymus was the most severely affected organ, exhibiting marked hypoplasia primarily due to cortical thinning, and gross lymphocytic depletion of both medullary and cortical portions. Similarly, the spleen and adrenals were reduced in size relative to the control organs, and the thymic-derived zones of the spleen and lymph nodes were depleted of lymphocytes.

Mosier et al. (1981) reported that dexamethasone and betamethasone reduced ossification of the axial skeleton in rats but enhanced ossification of some bones of the appendicular skeleton at low doses. Rowland and Hendrickx (1983) reported only a reduction of ossification with no enhanced ossification in any part of the skeleton at any dose of triamcinolone acetonide (0.125–0.5 mg/kg/day for 3 days) studied. This difference between the different corticosteroids may reflect actual pharmacodynamic differences between the drugs or may simply be the result of the considerable variation in the number of centers of ossification in Day-20 rat fetuses (Aliverti *et al.*, 1979).

C. Nonhuman Primates

Triamcinolone acetonide (TAC) is the only corticosteroid that has been studied during the embryonic period in nonhuman primates. Hendrickx *et al.* (1980) have reported the effects of various dosages of TAC (5–20 mg/kg) administered on single or multiple days between Days 21 and 43 of gestation in rhesus monkeys, bonnet monkeys, and baboons. The pattern of malformations is essentially the same in all three species and was similar following single- and multiple-day treatments, with the principal difference being an increased severity of the defects following multiple-dose treatment. The central nervous system and cranium were the most commonly malformed areas in all three species.

Cranium bifidum, associated with encephalocele, meningocele, and less frequently, hydrocephalus, was a commonly observed skeletal defect in the multiple-dose treatment groups. Cranium bifidum occultum in association with aplasia cutis congenita or in the absence of any exterior gross lesions was more frequently observed in single-day–treated cases. The calvarial defects were characterized by an underossification of the frontal, parietal, and occipital bones, with a thin membranous tissue (dense fibrous connective tissue) covering the unossified areas. The underossification was most apparent at the midline and involved the metopic, sagittal, coronal, and lamboid sutures. This underossification was still apparent at 2 to $2\frac{1}{2}$ years of age in several bonnet monkeys; although some compensatory growth had occurred to reduce the size of the original defect. Abnormalities of the cranial base were also observed, mainly affecting the occipital, frontal, and sphenoid bones.

A variety of facial abnormalities, described collectively as craniofacial dysmorphia, were seen in all three species. These were frequently accompanied by cleft or arched palate, with arched palate being much more frequent. In addition to the encephaloceles and hydrocephalus discussed earlier, a number of cerebellar and midbrain defects were described. Minor malformations of the skeleton and viscera were also observed, including cutaneous syndactyly, hypoplastic spleen, and hypoplastic thymus. Growth retardation was observed in all three species, with a combined percentage of 39.5% of all macaques and baboons, receiving multiple-day treatments being growth retarded.

The effects of TAC (3–28 mg/kg) administered for 1 to 4 consecutive days during later periods of development included resorption, intrauterine death, and malformaion (Hendrickx et al., 1975). Defects were seen in the orofacial region (including one cleft palate), thorax, hindlimbs, thymus, adrenal, and kidney. A large proportion of bonnet and rhesus monkeys had alterations of craniofacial development, such as protrusion of the forehead, widening of the head, and expansion of the cranial sutures, which were similar to the craniofacial dysmorphia reported by Hendrickx et al. (1980).

Malformations of the viscera, with the exception of the thymus, were infrequent and showed no specific pattern. The thymus was the most severely affected organ. It was grossly hypoplastic in all 5 bonnet monkeys and in 13 of 17 rhesus monkeys, although grossly normal in 4 baboon fetuses. Histologically, the lobular structure of the thymus is still present, but there are almost total depletion of thymic lymphocytes and a reduction in the epithelial component. Lymphocyte studies on three surviving baboon infants revealed a persistent lymphopenia with a marked decrease in peripheral blood lymphocytes forming spontaneous nonimmune rosettes with sheep erythrocytes. There was also an increased percentage of the peripheral blood lymphocytes with detectable surface immunoglobulin.

Sawyer et al. (1977) extended these observations by studying the effects of 10 to 14 mg/kg TAC administered for 4 consecutive days between Days 45 and 83 of gestation to seven pregnant rhesus monkeys. Treated animals lacked a distinct thymus but did have thymic rudiments present. Although some degree of lobulation was retained, the separation of the thymus into cortical and medullary zones was not evident, and there was a dramatic depletion of lymphoid elements, especially the cortical lymphocytes. All but one specimen showed large cystic Hassell's bodies containing cellular debris. In two fetuses exposed at Days 80–83 of gestation, the Hassell's bodies contained polymorphonuclear lymphocytes.

D. Hamsters

A large number of corticosteroids have been evaluated for teratogenicity in hamsters. Single intramuscular doses of cortisol (25–75 mg) can produce 100% cleft palate (Shah and Chaudhry, 1973). Day 11 of gestation was found to be the most sensitive day for production of cleft palate (Chaudhry and Shah, 1973). The effects of administration of different doses of cortisone, corticosterone, dexamethasone, triamcinolone, and prednisolone were reported by Shah and Kilistoff (1976). All of these compounds, with the exception of cortisone, produced cleft palate in the fetuses. However, the relative teratogenic potencies varied considerably with the ED50 for cleft palate induction, ranging from 0.484 mg for triamcinolone to 9.349 mg for corticosterone. The total incidence of cleft palate, the morphological type of cleft palate, and the degree of fetal growth retardation were all related to the dose of corticosteroid administered. It would be valuable to know whether higher doses of cortisone would cause an increased incidence of cleft palate. The small number of treated litters examined by Shah and Kilistoff (1976) make the lack of effect of cortisone treatment tentative at present. It is particularly surprising in relation to the high efficacy of cortisol in producing cleft palate in the hamster. If the refractoriness of the hamster to cortisone is confirmed as absolute, it would imply a deficiency of 11β-hydroxysteroid reductase activity.

Administration of long-acting ACTH (Synacthen-Depot®) also results in an increased incidence of cleft palate in the offspring (Shah, 1977). These clefts were all partial clefts of the anterior portion of the secondary palate and were found in only 9 of 32 treated fetuses, indicating that ACTH is only mildly teratogenic in this species. The teratogenic action of ACTH is presumably mediated through stimulation of the maternal adrenal glands to secrete teratogenic amounts of endogenous corticosteroid.

The only other report of corticosteroid-induced malformations in hamsters is that of Kelly (1981). Triamcinolone acetonide was found to cause the highest incidence of malformations on Days 9–11 of gestation. A dosage of 1.0 mg/kg on Day 9, 10, or 11 resulted in an 80–100% incidence of malformed embryos. No increase in either malformations or resorptions was detected at 0.1 mg/kg, indicating the presence of a threshold. Cranium bifidum was the most common defect. This was usually located over the mesencephalon, which protruded through the cleft in the presumptive skull, resulting in encephalocele.

E. OTHERS

1. Rabbits

Rabbits were first determined to be sensitive to corticosteroid-induced cleft palate by Fainstat (1954). Administration of cortisone at dosages of 10 to 30 mg/day for 4 days in the period just prior to palate closure resulted in cleft palate in several strains of rabbits. Clavert *et al.* (1961) demonstrated that a variety of malformations could be produced by the injection of dexamethasone on Days 11–14 of gestation. The most frequent malformations were umbilical hernias and omphaloceles, cleft palates, and cardiac malformations. In addition, one case each of spina bifida, exencephaly, and anencephaly was seen.

The effects of dexamethasone on cardiac development were further investigated by Clavert *et al.* (1965). Dosages of 2 mg/day on Days 11–14 of gestation resulted in approximately 41% of the embryos being abnormal. Interventricular septal defect was the most common cardiac malformation, followed by atrial septal defect and one case of total agenesis of the atrial septum. These malformations showed a dose–response effect with dosages of 1 mg/day or less causing only small ventricular septal defects in the membranous portion of the ventricular septum. The optimal sensitive period for the production of cardiac malformations was found to be Days 11–14. Treatment on Days 14–17 with 2 mg/day resulted in only an 8% malformation rate, which consisted of small ventricular septal defects. Single injections of 8 gm on either Day 11 or Day 14 resulted in defects similar to those found after multiple treatment with 2 mg/day from Day 11 to Day 14.

Other vascular anomalies that were produced consisted of irregularities of vessel diameter, with both dilations and irregular constrictions reported. Histologically, there was a net diminution of elastic tissue in the aorta of these animals.

Walker (1967) compared the effects of triamcinolone acetonide, dexamethasone, methylprednisolone, prednisolone, betamethasone, and cortisone administered on gestational Days 13–16 in New Zealand white rabbits. There was a high incidence of resorption at the upper dose levels with all the drugs. It is difficult to compare the teratogenic potencies of these drugs quantitatively because of the small number of animals and considerable variation in response at different dose levels. Triamcinolone acetonide and dexamethasone both caused some cleft palates at dosages of less than 1 mg. Betamethasone treatment (1–4 mg/day) resulted in resorption of 21 of 24 litters. In the remaining litters there were 9 cleft palate fetuses, all from the same litter. Methylprednisolone caused resorption of 6 of 7 litters, with 3 normal fetuses in the remaining litter at 1 to 4 mg/day and no cleft palates in fetuses from 11 surviving litters treated with lower dosages. Cortisone also caused a low incidence of cleft palate (affecting 3 of 7 litters), with several litters being totally resorbed.

Cortisol, cortisone, and dexamethasone are all teratogenic when administered via the conjunctival sac to New Zealand white rabbits (Kasirsky and Lombardi, 1970). The spectrum of malformations was similar for each of the drugs, with hypoplastic kidneys, herniated abdominal viscera, absence of the intestinal tract, asymmetric cerebral hemispheres, and partial anencephaly being the most frequently reported malformations.

2. Guinea Pigs

Guinea pigs were demonstrated to be sensitive to corticosteroid teratogenicity by Hoar (1962). Subcutaneous injections of hydrocortisone resulted in a variety of malformations, including open eyelid, abdominal eventration, umbilical hernia, edema, cleft palate, syringomyelomeningocele, syndactyly, and limb torsion. The frequency of malformation was highest in animals treated on Days 16–17 of gestation. No dose–response relationship was demonstrated, as a doubling of the dosage (administered twice daily) from 3 mg/kg to 6 mg/kg did not result in an increase in the malformation rate. No other corticosteroids have been evaluated for teratogenicity in guinea pigs.

F. SUMMARY

A variety of abnormalities have been reported following corticosteroid treatment in a variety of species (Table I). The most prevalent malformation in most of the species studied is cleft palate. However, in the nonhuman primate species studied (Hendrickx et al., 1980), this was less common than the cranial and central nervous system defects. It is important to remember that the treatment period used by

TABLE I

ABNORMALITIES INDUCED BY CORTICOSTEROIDS IN MAMMALIAN SPECIES

Abnormality	Species
Cleft palate	Mice, rats, nonhuman primates, rabbits, hamsters, guinea pigs
Umbilical hernias	Rats, guinea pigs, rabbits
Cranium bifidum with associated abnormalities	Nonhuman primates—rhesus monkeys, bonnet monkeys, baboons, hamsters
Genital defects	
Male	Rats
Female	Mice
Cardiovascular defects	Rabbits
Limb anomalies	Mice
Cataract	Mice

Hendrickx et al. (1980) is earlier than that normally associated with sensitivity to cleft palate. No definitive studies have been reported in nonhuman primates that specifically address the sensitivity of these species to corticosteroid-induced cleft palate. Preliminary studies in our laboratory (J. M. Rowland and A. G. Hendrickx, unpublished data) suggest that rhesus monkeys are less susceptible to triamcinolone acetonide-induced cleft palate than the lower laboratory animals. No cleft palates have been detected in nine animals treated with as much as 4.0 mg/kg/day on Days 35–43 of gestation. Further work is needed to determine if these preliminary results are indicative of a quantitatively different response in rhesus monkeys than in other laboratory animals.

None of the other abnormalities have been reported in more than three species, and many have only been detected in one species. These data should not be interpreted to mean that these abnormalities are necessarily more species specific than cleft palate. In many cases, the method of evaluation was not appropriate to detect some of the defects. In addition, the widespread use of corticosteroids as cleft palate-inducing agents has narrowed the focus of many investigations of these compounds to stages of development relevant to palate formation and has restricted examinations to the secondary palate. It is important to determine in future studies whether there are substantial interspecies differences in the teratogenicity of these compounds. At the present time we are unable to determine whether there are any qualitative interspecies differences in response to this class of compounds.

Another area of interest is whether there are any qualitative or quantitative differences in response to the various individual corticosteroids. There are widespread potency differences between the different corticosteroids that have at times resulted in apparently qualitative differences in response. For example, triamcinolone acetonide is a very potent teratogen in all of the species tested, inducing significant frequencies of abnormality at relatively low dosages. In contrast, cortisol and cortisone are much less potent corticosteroids. Whereas these compounds are capable of inducing 100% cleft palate in sensitive strains of mice, they are very mild teratogens in rats even when administered at maximal doses. In fact, for many years the rat was considered refractory to the cleft palate-inducing effects of corticosteroids because of this difference. It has, however, now become apparent that this was at least partially a result of differential embryonal exposure. This will be discussed in detail in the following section.

The available data, at present, indicate that all of the corticosteroids are basically similar in terms of the abnormalities they produce. Differences in potency result in certain alterations in response between different compounds or a given compound in different species. These anomalies in the general pattern should be useful in suggesting certain factors that are responsible for mediating the teratogenic effects of these compounds. It also illustrates the importance of testing several corticosteroids (as suggested by Walker, 1971) and several species before making any conclusions regarding the teratogenic potential of the compounds. It is also important to evaluate a sufficiently wide dose range and determine dose–response characteristics of each compound studied. This provides a more valuable source of comparison than the effects of a drug at a single dose level.

III. Factors Determining Corticosteroid-Induced Cleft Palate

At this time it is not possible to determine whether there are any true qualitative differences in response between different species. However, it is very clear (and has been recognized from the early days of corticosteroid teratogenicity studies) that significant intra- and interspecies differences in sensitivity to various corticosteroids do exist. In this section we will examine a number of factors that have been proposed as contributing to these differences. These will be examined under the basic subdivisions: exposure to the teratogenic agent, molecular mechanisms, and embryological characteristics. The largest body of available literature concerns interspecies differences in sensitivity to corticosteroid-induced cleft palate, and therefore this will be a major focus of the discussion.

A. Exposure to the Teratogenic Agent

A fundamental parameter in assessing dose–response characteristics of any pharmacological agent is the concentration of drug at the site of action. In Section III,B we review the evidence implicating glucocorticoid receptor proteins as the ultimate molecular site of action. Differences in the concentration of corticosteroid that reaches the appropriate site of action in the embryo could be a factor in inter- and intraspecies variations in teratogenic sensitivity.

A number of drug distribution studies have been conducted in mice in an attempt to explain the significant interstrain variation in teratogenic sensitivity seen in that species. Levine et al. (1968) injected pregnant mice with [^{14}C]cortisol on Day 11 of gestation and found a higher concentration of total radioactivity in A/J (more sensitive) embryos than in CBA (less sensitive) embryos. No separation of parent compound and metabolites was attempted, thus no comparison of exposure to the active agent is possible.

Waddell (1971, 1972) used autoradiography to investigate the possibility of differential localization of drug within the pregnant mouse. No difference in localization was seen between teratogenic (cortisone, hydrocortisone, and corticosterone) and nonteratogenic (deoxycorticosterone) corticosteroids. Autoradiographic techniques are unable to distinguish between the parent compound and metabolites, therefore no definitive answers regarding localization of the active agent can be found from these data.

Zimmerman and Bowen (1972a) administered [^{3}H]triamcinolone acetonide to pregnant A/J mice on Day 11 of gestation and examined maternal and embryonic tissue at selected periods after drug administration. Although triamcinolone acetonide was extensively metabolized by the maternal system, only unmetabolized drug was found in the embryo at the earliest time measured (30 min). After that time, the concentration of unmetabolized triamcinolone acetonide in the embryo fell markedly, and the percentage of metabolites increased. The distribution and metabolism of triamcinolone acetonide was compared in these strains of mice with different degrees of susceptibility to corticosteroid-induced cleft palate (Zimmerman and Bowen, 1972b). There was a lower concentration of unchanged triamcinolone acetonide in embryos of CBA (low-sensitivity) mice than in embryos of C3H (intermediate-sensitivity) or A/J (high-sensitivity) mice. This was attributed to a more rapid metabolism of triamcinolone acetonide by the CBA females.

Embryonic exposure was similar in C3H and A/J mice despite the differences in sensitivity. The greater sensitivity of A/J than C3H may be due to embryological differences or receptor characteristics of the embryo. The palate shelves elevate slightly later in A/J mice than in C3H, and the period of optimal sensitivity to TAC-induced cleft palate is on Day 11.5 in C3H but Day 12.5 for A/J (Andrew et al., 1973). Goldman et al. (1977) found that A/J embryos had several times as much cytosolic cortisol-binding protein as C3H mice, although Hackney (1980) has reported similar levels of glucocorticoid receptors in the two strains.

Spain et al. (1975) administered [^{3}H]cortisol in a solution of unlabeled cortisone to A/J mice on Day 12 of gestation and analyzed several tissues for parent cortisol and metabolites. The highest concentration of total radioactivity was found at 30 min after injection for all tissues (embryonic jaws, yolk sac, placenta, and maternal liver). Unchanged cortisol was the predominant compound detected in embryonic jaws at all time points, and its percentage composition of the total radioactivity was unchanged over the 3-hr course of the experiment. The percentage of cortisone decreased steadily with time. The use of cortisone acetate as the cold carrier for [^{3}H]cortisol makes interpretation of the metabolic conversions speculative. If a high concentration of unchanged cortisone was present in the various tissues, it could hinder the conversion of cortisol to cortisone by 11β-hydroxysteroid dehydrogenase. It would be valuable to know whether [^{3}H]cortisol metabolism and distribution are the same when cortisol is used as the cold carrier. It would also be valuable to know the concentration of [^{3}H]cortisol achieved in the embryo when a teratogenic dose of [^{3}H]cortisone is administered to the pregnant female. Without this additional data it is not possible to assess the contribution of embryonal exposure to cortisol in determining teratogenic sensitivity of the mouse to cortisol and cortisone. Administration of [^{14}C]cortisone to pregnant A/J and C57BL mice on Day 12 of gestation resulted in a significantly higher concentration of radioactivity firmly bound to embryonic tissue in A/J than in C57BL mice. This "bound" material represents methanol-insoluble radioactivity. No further characterization of this material was conducted, so it is not known whether this represents parent compound or a metabolite. More extensive organic extractions would be necessary before one could conclude that this material was covalently bound (Siekevitz, 1952; Jollow et al., 1973). The extractable radioactivity was partially separated by differential extraction into conjugated and unconjugated fractions, but no further separation to obtain the concentration of cortisol was attempted.

Pharmacokinetic data will also be important in attempting to explain interspecies variations in teratogenic response and performing interspecies extrapolations. Triamcinolone acetonide metabolism and distribution in the pregnant rat during the sensitive period for cleft palate induction have been studied using high-performance liquid chromatography techniques (Rowland et al., 1983). The pharmacokinetics of triamcinolone acetonide were found to be dose independent over the teratogenic dosage range of 0.125 to 0.5 mg/kg. There were no marked alterations in maternal or embryonal metabolism following multiple-dose administration (once daily or Day 12, 13, and 14), although a transient elevation in the embryonal concentration of TAC at 1 hr following the second or third injection was detected. The majority of TAC-derived radioactivity found in the embryo at the earliest time points represents unchanged TAC, which is in agreement with results in mice (Zimmerman and Bowen, 1972a). However, it appears that the embryonal concentration of TAC and the duration of exposure are greater in A/J mice than in rats. This correlates with the greater sensitivity of A/J mice to TAC-induced cleft palate. A dosage of 2.0 mg/kg of TAC administered to A/J mice on Day 11.5 of gestation resulted in 92% cleft palate (Zimmerman and Bowen, 1972b), whereas a dosage of 5.0 mg/kg administered on Day 13 of gestation was required to induce 92% cleft palate in the rat (Rowland and Hendrickx, 1982).

Pharmacokinetic differences can also be used to evaluate differences in teratogenic potency between various corticosteroids. The rat has been demonstrated to be much more resistant to cortisol induction of cleft palate than to triamcinolone acetonide (Rowland and Hendrickx, 1982; Section II,B). The demonstration that a relatively high incidence of cleft palate can be induced in rat embryos when cortisol is injected into the amniotic sac (Dostal and Jelinek, 1971) indicates that this resistance is not due to an inability of the rat embryo to respond to cortisol but may be due to a relative lack of transfer of the drug into the embryo when compared to potent teratogens like triamcinolone acetonide. When [^{3}H]TAC and [^{14}C]cortisol were administered to pregnant rats on Day 12 of gestation, there was significantly greater embryonal exposure to TAC than to cortisol (Rowland *et al.,* 1980). This was found to be partially due to rapid maternal metabolism of cortisol but also to differences in placental transfer and metabolism. No direct comparisons of embryonal exposure to cortisol in rats and mice are possible because of differences in experimental design. However, the significant proportion of unchanged cortisol still present in A/J embryos 3 hr after injection (Spain *et al.,* 1975) suggests that embryonal exposure to a teratogenic dose of cortisol would be much greater in mice than in rats.

Studies on exposure of the embryo to different corticosteroids have yielded important data regarding intra- and interspecies differences in teratogenicity. Further work is needed with other corticosteroids in several species to clarify the role of pharmacokinetics in corticosteroid teratogenicity.

B. Molecular Mechanisms

Corticosteroids are thought to exert most, if not all, their diverse physiological and pharmacological effects through interaction of the steroid with specific intracellular receptor proteins in the cytoplasm of sensitive cells (Thompson and Lippman, 1974; Cake and Litwack, 1975). The steroid receptor complex undergoes a conformational change, becomes activated, and translocates into the nucleus where it interacts with chromatin. The cellular response evoked by this interaction is dependent on the target tissue.

Corticosteroids have been recognized as important factors in the morphological and biochemical development of a variety of tissues (Jost and Picon, 1970; Greengard, 1975; Sugimoto et al., 1976). The presence of a specific glucocorticoid receptor in these tissues is often associated with the onset of responsiveness of the tissue to corticosteroids (Cake and Litwack, 1975). High-affinity receptor proteins for glucocorticoids have been detected in mouse facial mesenchymal cells (Salomon and Pratt, 1976), mouse palatal mesenchyme (Salomon and Pratt, 1976, 1978), mouse embryonic jaws (Goldman et al., 1977), mouse embryonic heads (Hackney, 1980), whole mouse embryos (Salomon et al., 1978), rat maxillary processes (Salomon and Pratt, 1979), and human fetal palatal mesenchymal cells (Goldman et al., 1978). The most definitive biochemical characterization of these receptors has been conducted on receptors isolated from homogenates of whole mouse embryos (Salomon et al., 1978). The physicochemical properties of these receptors are similar to those described for cytoplasmic glucocorticoid receptors in adult target tissue (Baxter and Tomkins, 1971; Rousseau et al., 1972), although some subtle differences may exist with regard to specificity of the receptor for various steroids (Salomon et al., 1978). The glucocorticoid receptor proteins can be distinguished from corticosteroid-binding globulin (CBG) by a number of characteristics including heat sensitivity, sedimentation coefficients, gel filtration properties, and sensitivity to sulfhydryl reagents. The receptor proteins are present in mouse embryonic cytosol as early as Day 12 of gestation, and their concentration increases (expressed on a per embryo basis) on Days 13 and 14 of gestation (Salomon et al., 1978). The presence of specific glucocorticoid receptors in structures involved in formation of the secondary palate during the time of palate development suggests a role for corticosteroids in normal palate growth and differentiation. The interactions of physiological levels of corticosteroids and other hormones and growth factors in relation to secondary palate development have been reviewed (Salomon and Pratt, 1979; Pratt et al., 1980b).

Interaction of teratogenic levels of corticosteroids with these receptors may provide a molecular mechanism leading to corticosteroid-induced cleft palate. The relationship of glucocorticoid receptor levels in midgestation mouse embryos to cleft palate sensitivity has not yet been clearly defined. Embryonic facial mesenchymal cells obtained on Day 14 of gestation from A/J mice have two to three times more cytoplasmic receptors than those from C57 mice (Salomon and Pratt, 1976). A similar correlation between receptor level and cleft palate sensitivity has been reported for DBA/IJ, CBA/J, SWR/FR, and SWR/NIH mice (Salomon and Pratt, 1978, 1979). The level of cytosolic cortisol-binding proteins in maternal palates and embryonic jaw regions on Day 11 of gestation have been found to correlate with cleft palate susceptibility for seven strains of mice (Goldman et al., 1977). One specific protein with a microelectrofocusing pI of 6.9 to 7.0 was also correlated with cleft palate sensitivity and was proposed as a candidate for the glucocorticoid receptor. However, no definitive binding evidence was reported for this protein, such as affinity constants or competition by other steroids. The use of cortisol as the ligand for the binding studies also raises the question of binding to serum proteins, such as CBG (Westphal, 1969). A dexamethasone-binding protein that has a pI similar to that reported for the murine cortisol-binding protein has been detected in palate mesenchyme of human fetuses obtained after the period of palate closure, indicating that the cortisol-binding protein may in fact be a specific glucocorticoid receptor (Goldman et al., 1978). Salomon et al. (1978) found that A/J mice had a higher concentration of receptor sites in whole-embryo cytosols on Day 12 of gestation than C57BL mice, which was attributed to a high level of nonspecific binding in the A/J strain. There was no difference in receptor concentration on Day 13 or 14 of gestation. Hackney (1980) reported that there was no correlation between binding of triamcinolone acetonide to glucocorticoid receptors from embryonic heads on Day 13 of gestation, and teratogenic sensitivity. In face, heads from A/J embryos bound less glucocorticoid than either C3H or C57 embryos. Similar results were obtained when the oropalatal region was examined and when embryos were obtained on Day 11 of gestation.

The variations in the results of these studies may be due to the different sources of tissue examined. The concentration of receptors appears to be higher in the orofacial region than in other embryonic tissues (Salomon and Pratt, 1979). The use of preparations from whole embryos or embryonic heads could possibly mask strain differences in the palate region, although Hackney (1980) found differences in receptor levels in oropalatal regions similar to those in whole heads. Variations in biochemical techniques, source of tissue, and age of tissue could all be factors in the conflicting results. Further work is needed to clarify the relationship between strain differences in receptor levels and cleft palate sensitivity.

Despite the uncertainty as to the importance of receptor concentration, there is evidence implicating the receptor as a factor in corticosteroid-induced cleft palate. Specific binding of dexamethasone to the mouse embryonic cytosol receptor was most effectively inhibited by other active corticosteroids (Salomon and Pratt, 1978; Salomon et al., 1978; Hackney, 1980) and less affected by inactive corticosteroids such as cortisone or sex steroids. The ability of these compounds to compete for the glucocorticoid receptor is correlated with their teratogenic potency (Hackney, 1980).

Once a glucocorticoid has bound to the receptor, a number of other steps must occur before a cellular response is elicited. Interaction of the receptor–steroid complex with the genetic material is a critical event in this process. Bekhor et al. (1978) have reported that chromatin isolated from triamcinolone acetonide-treated embryos had reduced template activity as compared to comparably obtained controls. These changes were associated with binding of triamcinolone acetonide– receptor complexes to specific chromosomal proteins, which may function as the acceptor sites on the chromatin. Further studies show that although administration of triamcinolone acetonide to A/J mice caused an increase in RNA snythesis and RNA polymerases A and B in nuclei of maternal liver, it caused a decrease in transcription in nuclei from embryonic maxillary processes and no increase in either polymerase A or B (Anne and Bekhor, 1978). These studies provide a more specific mechanism for the inhibition of RNA synthesis reported by Zimmerman and associates (Zimmerman et al., 1970; Andrew et al., 1973). Zimmerman et al. (1970) originally suggested that all species of RNA (mRNA, rRNA, tRNA) were inhibited by corticosteroids, but no effect on tRNA or polymerase C (which is specific for tRNA synthesis) was detected by Anne and Bekhor (1978).

More definitive data are required to assess the role of glucocorticoid receptors in determining sensitivity to corticosteroid-induced cleft palate. Interspecies comparisons of receptor levels in relation to teratogenic sensitivity are particularly lacking. Technical limitations have limited studies of receptor proteins in the target tissues at the time of peak sensitivity. It is hoped that advances will soon allow an accurate assessment of the ontogeny of glucocorticoid receptors and their relation to corticosteroid sensitivity.

C. Embryological Characteristics

This section will integrate, whenever possible, information on the normal process of palate development with data on effects of corticosteroids on various aspects of this process. This discussion will focus primarily on data derived from studies in rate and mice. It should be noted that although the overall process of palate formation is generally similar among the various species studied, there are species differences in the pattern of shelf elevation and fusion that may be important in analyzing corticosteroid-induced cleft palate (Shah and Travill, 1976a). More extensive studies of normal palate embryology in a number of mammalian species and its relationship to teratogen-induced cleft palate will further our understanding of mechanisms of normal and abnormal development.

Development of the secondary palate involves an integrated series of events that combine to accomplish palatal shelf elevation, contact, and fusion (Greene and Pratt, 1976; Diewert, 1980). The relative roles of various intrinsic and extrinsic factors in accomplishing normal palate development are still under active investigation.

The first phase of normal palate development is the elevation of the palatal shelves from a vertical to a horizontal position. Corticosteroids have been demonstrated to delay palatal shelf elevation in various strains of mice (Fraser et al., 1954; Walker and Fraser, 1957; Ross and Walker, 1967; Greene and Kochhar, 1973; Vekemans and Fraser, 1979; Pratt et al., 1980a; Diewert and Pratt, 1981). The specific mechanisms by which corticosteroids cause this delay in shelf elevation are still not established (see reviews by Greene and Kochhar, 1975; Salomon and Pratt, 1979). In order to examine this problem a better understanding of normal palate development is required.

Analyses of three-dimensional craniofacial growth and palate development in the rat have shown an intimate association between a variety of changing spatial relations in the oronasal cavity and palatal shelf elevation (Deiwert, 1980). Forward growth of the lower face is more rapid than that of the upper face (Sicher, 1915; Zeiler et al., 1964; Babula et al., 1970: Wragg et al., 1970; Hart et al., 1972; Diewert, 1974, 1976). The mandible becomes more prominent in relation to the primary palate (Burdi and Silvey, 1969; Diewert, 1974, 1976), and the vertical dimension of the face increases (Hart et al., 1972; Diewert, 1974, 1976). During this time the width of the maxilla decreases in rats (Wragg et al., 1972) but remains unchanged in mice (Smiley et al., 1971). There is a rapid growth of Meckel's cartilage resulting in a doubling of its length during this period, which contributes to the downward and forward displacement of the tongue (Diewert, 1976). Coincident with these changes there is an increase in the volume of the palatomaxillary processes, which in conjunction with the displacement of the tongue and the lack of increase of maxillary width results in the palatal shelves bulging medially over the tongue (Diewert, 1978).

Differences in craniofacial growth help explain the delayed shelf elevation in A/J compared to C57BL mice (Diewert, 1979, 1980). It was found that A/J mice had longer palatal shelves, smaller tongues and mandibles, and smaller vertical dimensions in the oronasal cavity, which combined to delay palatal shelf elevation in this strain.

The tongue represents an obstacle to the elevating palatal shelves. Surgical removal of the tongue has been demonstrated to facilitate shelf elevation in mice *in vivo* (Walker and Quarles, 1976; Walker and Patterson, 1978) and *in vitro* (Brinkley et al., 1978). In addition to the influence of craniofacial growth on tongue position, there is the possibility that active muscular contraction may help to remove the tongue as an impediment to shelf elevation. The tongue appears to be capable of responding to neural stimulation at the time of palatal shelf elevation and fusion (Wragg et al., 1972; Holt, 1975). Other embryonic movements such as neck flexion and swallowing may play a role in allowing the shelves to elevate (Humphrey, 1969; Walker, 1969).

Walker and Quarles (1975) have reported that teratogenic doses of cortisone and triamcinolone acetonide decrease the number of spontaneous muscular movements in mouse embryos and suggest that these muscular movements are necessary to move the tongue from its position between the shelves. Surgical removal of the tongue decreased the incidence of cleft palate in cortisone-treated CD-1 mice (Walker and Patterson, 1978). A less traumatic mechanical displacement of the tongue has also been shown to decrease the incidence of cortisone-induced cleft palate (Walker, 1982). Although palate closure is more readily accomplished when the tongue is removed, this does not necessarily mean that contraction of the tongue is the primary motive force for its removal or that cortisone exerts its primary effect on the musculature of the tongue.

Although some studies have shown involvement of the cranial base in shelf elevation (Harris, 1967; Verusio, 1970; Wragg et al., 1970; Hart et al., 1972; Long et al., 1973), it cannot play a primary role, because isolated palatal shelves are capable of elevating *in vitro* (Brinkley et al., 1975: Wee et al., 1976). Diewert (1974) found that no significant change in cranial base angulation occurred during shelf elevation in the rat, although straightening of the cranial base was observed as the nasomaxillary complex lifted. Furthermore, the cranial base of the A/J mouse is more developed and straighter than that of the C57BL mouse prior to shelf elevation (Diewert, 1979), despite the fact that the A/J strain is more delayed in time of palate elevation. Neither of these two studies supports a direct role for the cranial base in palatal shelf elevation.

Aside from the contribution of various extrinsic factors in palatal shelf elevation, there is considerable evidence of a contribution by the palatal shelves. Walker and Fraser (1956) proposed the development of an intrinsic shelf force in mice that provided an inherent ability of the palatal shelves to elevate. It was suggested that the intrinsic shelf force resided in elastic fibers within the palatal shelves (Clark, 1956; Walker and Fraser, 1956). However, no evidence has been found for the presence of these fibers in the palatal shelf at the time of elevation (Stark and Ehrmann, 1958; Walker, 1961; Isaacson and Chaudhry, 1962; Frommer, 1968; Frommer and Monroe, 1969).

Investigators have since focused on the possibility that actin and myosin may play a role in generating the shelf force. These proteins are present in palatal mesenchymal cells just prior to shelf elevation (Lessard et al., 1974; Krawczyk and Gillon, 1976) and appear to be arranged in cytoplasmic fibrils of microfilaments (Babiarz et al., 1975; Innes, 1978; Shah, 1979). These fibers may function as nonmuscle contractile systems and have been shown to contract and rotate the palatal shelves *in vitro* when incubated with ATP (Wee and Zimmerman, 1980).

The palatal shelves increase in volume during the time of shelf elevation and fusion (Lazzaro, 1940; Diewert, 1978). This increase in volume is probably important in promoting elevation of the shelves as well as providing adequate shelf contact for fusion once elevation is accomplished. The possibility that a rapid increase in the proliferation rate of mesenchymal cells in appropriate areas of the palate could contribute to this increase in volume has been investigated. There is no evidence for an exceptionally high mitotic rate in the palate mesenchyme during shelf elevation (Walker and Fraser, 1956; Hughes et al., 1967). In fact, the peak period for proliferation of these cells precedes shelf elevation by 24 to 48 hr (Mott et al., 1969; Jelinek and Dostal, 1973, 1975; Hassell et al., 1974; Nanda and Romeo, 1975; Cleaton-Jones, 1976; Diewert, 1980). This does not preclude the possibility that corticosteroid-induced cleft palate may be at least partially due to inhibition of mesenchymal cell proliferation (Jelinek and Dostal, 1975; Mott et al., 1969; Nanda and Romeo, 1978). Corticosteroids have been shown to cause a reduction in cell number and a decrease in [^{3}H]thymidine incorporation into DNA in both A/J and C57 facial mesenchymal cells in culture. The A/J cells are more sensitive to corticosteroid-induced growth inhibition than C57 cells. Similar effects have been noted in palatal shelves cultured *in vitro* in the presence of cortisol or dexamethasone (Saxen, 1973; Pratt et al., 1979). This growth inhibition helps create a reduced shelf size, which decreases the amount of the shelves in contact and ultimately decreases the degree of fusion that can occur.

Diewert (1978, 1980) has demonstrated that as shelf volume increases, cell density decreases, suggesting that accumulation of extracellular matrix components contribute a major portion of the increase in palatal shelf volume. The formation and accumulation of glycosaminoglycan (GAG) before and during shelf elevation has been linked with palatal shelf elevation (Larsson et al., 1959; Larsson, 1962b; Walker, 1961; Jacobs, 1964a; Anderson and Matthiessen, 1967; Pratt et al., 1973; Ferguson, 1978). Collagen may also play a role in shelf elevation in that a significant increase in palatal collagen is found at the time of shelf elevation (Pratt and King, 1971). In the rat these collagen fibers are found throughout the mesenchyme but are particularly abundant adjacent to the basal lamina of the presumptive oral epithelium. The fibers are oriented uniformly along the anteroposterior axis of the shelf in this area (Hassell and Orkin, 1976).

Corticosteriods are known to affect the extracellular matrix (Nacht and Garzon, 1974; Moscatelli and Rubin, 1977; Newman and Cutroneo, 1977). However, a direct link between effects on extracellular matrix components and cleft palate has not been established. Jacobs (1964a) reported a decreased accumulation of GAG (measured histochemically) in palatal mesenchyme of cortisone-treated mice at the time of shelf elevation. In contrast, several other investigators have reported no difference in histochemical staining intensity of palatal shelves between control and treated mice (Larsson, 1962a; Loevy, 1962). A delay in the peak of accumulation of sulfated GAG in palatal mesenchyme of cortisone-treated mice has been detected using autoradiographic (Larsson, 1962a) and liquid scintillation counting techniques (Jacobs, 1964b). However, Larsson (1962a) could not detect a difference in [^{35}S]sulfate incorporation between two strains of mice differing in sensitivity, and Andrew and Zimmerman (1971) found that although triamcinolone acetonide (10 mg/kg) and cortisol (320 mg/kg) induced similar frequencies of cleft palate in C3H mice, there were substantial differences in the degree of inhibition of [^{25}S]sulfate incorporation. In addition, a nonteratogenic dose of cortisol acetate decreased sulfated GAG synthesis to an extent that was similar to a teratogenic dose of triamcinolone acetonide. These negative results based on ^{35}S uptake should be interpreted with caution, because they only measure the accumulation of sulfated GAG. Hyaluronate, a nonsulfated GAG, represents approximately 60–65% of total GAG in the palate at the time of elevation (Pratt et al., 1973) and appears to play an important role in hydration of embryonic tissues and associated morphogenetic movements (Toole et al., 1980). Further studies using more definitive biochemical techniques are needed to determine whether corticosteroids decrease the accumulation of hyaluronate in palatal shelves. Until such studies become available, no definitive answer regarding the role of glycosaminoglycans in general, and hyaluronate in particular, in corticosteroid-induced cleft palate can be derived.

Shapiro and Shoshan (1972) have demonstrated that administration of cortisone to pregnant mice causes a reduced synthesis of collagen in the embryonic palates. Similar results have been obtained *in vitro* with A/J and C57 maxillary mesenchymal cell cultures (Salomon and Pratt, 1979). There was a greater reduction in collagen synthesis in A/J cells than in comparably exposed C57 cells indicating another possible source of the interstrain sensitivity differences. However, Uitto and Thesleff (1979) found that cortisol increased the production of collagen in palatal explants of two strains of mice differing in sensitivity to corticosteroid-induced cleft palate and reported that there was no difference between the two strains in the degree of response. The discrepancy between these results may be due to the different *in vitro* culture systems used. Uitto and Thesleff (1979) cultured palatal explants that included the cranial base and septal cartilage. It is possible that changes in collagen synthesis in these nonpalatal tissues masked the changes occurring in the palatal shelves. Alternatively, the differences in the corticosteroids tested, age of the embryos from which the palate tissue was obtained, and strains of mice used could all have contributed to the contradictory results. Again, further work is needed to determine the nature of corticosteroid effects on palatal collagen synthesis before a definitive assessment can be made of this as a factor in corticosteroid-induced cleft palate.

The second phase of normal palate development involves adhesion and subsequent fusion of the palatal shelves. Initial adhesion of the opposing palatal shelves is probably made thorugh an extracellular carbohydrate-rich surface coat on the medial-edge epithelial cells. The presence of this surface coat has been demonstrated ultrastructurally by the binding of concanavalin A (Pratt et al., 1973; Pratt and Hassell, 1975) and by staining with ruthenium red (Greene and Kochhar, 1974). The exact chemical nature of the surface coat is not known, but it appears to contain a large amount of glycoprotein. The progression from palatal shelf adhesion to the actual fusion of mesenchyme from opposing palatal shelves requires the breakdown of the midline epithelial seam. The palatal medial edge epithelial cells undergo a programmed cell death at a specific stage of development (Mato et al., 1966; Smiley, 1970; Smiley and Koch, 1971; Matthiessen and Anderson, 1972; Chaudhry and Shah, 1973). The first sign of the programmed cell death is a cessation of DNA synthesis in the medial-edge cells, which occurs as early as 36 hr prior to shelf contact (Hudson and

Shapiro, 1973; Pratt and Martin, 1975). A lysosomal-mediated autolysis is presumed to cause the death of the midline epithelial cells (Mato et al., 1967). As the basal lamina of the opposing shelves break down, phagocytosis of the degenerating epithelial cells is accomplished by macrophages that migrate into the region (Koziol and Steffek, 1969; Matthiessen and Anderson, 1972; Shah and Chaudhry, 1974).

The suggestion that cortisone may interfere with the process of shelf fusion was made by Greene and Kochhar (1973) following the observation that palatal shelves of cortisone-treated ICR/DUB mice sometimes do make contact with each other and with the nasal septum. Similar observations have recently been made in A/J mice by Diewert and Pratt (1981). Shah and Travill (1976a) reported that there was no effect of cortisol on the early stages of palate formation (shelf elevation) in the hamster but an inhibition of fusion. Further study in the hamster showed necrotic changes in some of the basal epithelial cells of the palatal shelf, alterations of the basal lamina, and absence of lysosomes (Shah and Travill, 1976b). The superficial epithelial cells that normally undergo programmed cell death never underwent necrosis but became keratinized instead. An inhibition of breakdown of the medial-edge epithelium of the palatal shelf *in vitro* has also been reported (Herold and Futran, 1980). These results conflict with those of Lahti and Saxen (1967) and Lahti et al. (1972), who found that cortisol delayed palate closure *in vitro* but never prevented fusion from taking place. Treatment of CF1 mice with triamcinolone acetonide delayed but did not prevent breakdown of medial epithelial cells (Kurisu et al., 1977, 1981). It is possible that some of these conflicting results are due to the different species and corticosteroids studied, differences in response of the palatal epithelium *in vivo* and *in vitro,* or differences in the *in vitro* culture system used. Although some shelf contact has been reported in corticosteroid-treated embryos, the degree of contact is much less extensive than in control palates (Greene and Kochhar, 1973; Shah and Travill, 1976a; Diewert and Pratt, 1981). This suggests that the major effect of corticosteroids in producing cleft palate must be exerted on either shelf elevation or shelf size, and any possible effect on shelf fusion would primarily affect the size of the cleft.

IV. Conclusion

Despite the extensive studies of corticosteroid teratogenicity conducted, there still remain a number of unresolved issues. It is clear that corticosteroids are teratogenic in all of the mammalian species that have been adequately tested. A wide spectrum of abnormalities can be produced depending on such factors as developmental age, dosage, and embryological characteristics. Progress has been made in determining some of the critical factors determining teratogenic sensitivity and possible mechanisms of action. Continued research on these topics promises to yield a significant increase in our understanding of corticosteroid teratogenicity in the years to come.

REFERENCES

Aliverti, V., Bonanomi, L., Giavini, E., Leone, V. G., and Mariani, L. (1979). *Teratology* **20,** 237–242.
Anderson, H., and Mathiessen, M. E. (1967). *Acta Anat.* **68,** 473–508.
Andrew, F. D., Bowen, D., and Zimmerman, E. F. (1973). *Teratology* **7,** 167–176.
Andrew, R. D., and Zimmerman, E. F. (1971). *Teratology* **4,** 31–38.
Angervall, L., and Lundin, P. M. (1964). *Endocrinology* **74,** 986–989.
Angervall, L., and Lundin, P. M. (1965). *Acta Endocrinol.* **50,** 104–114.
Anne, L., and Bekhor, I. (1978). *Teratology* **18,** 343–352.
Babiarz, B., Allenspach, A. L., and Zimmerman, E. F. (1975). *Dev. Biol.* **47,** 32–44.
Babula, W. J., Smiley, G. R., and Dixon, A. D. (1970). *Am. J. Orthod.* **58,** 250–263.
Ballard, P. D., Hearney, E. F., and Smith, M. B. (1977). *Teratology* **16,** 175–180.
Baxter, H., and Fraser, F. C. (1950). *McGill Med. J.* **19,** 245–248.
Baxter, J. D., and Tomkins, G. M. (1971). *Proc. Natl. Acad. Sci. U.S.A.* **68,** 932–937.
Bekhor, I., Mirell, C., and Anne, L. (1978). *Cleft Palate J.* **15,** 220–232.
Biddle, F. G., and Fraser, F. C. (1976). *Genetics* **84,** 743–754.
Biddle, F. G., and Fraser, F. C. (1977). *Genetics* **85,** 289–302.
Blackburn, W. R., Kaplan, H. S., and McKay, D. G. (1965). *Am. J. Obstet. Gynecol.* **92,** 234–246.
Blaustein, F. M., Feller, R., and Rosenzweig, S. (1971). *J. Dent. Res.* **50,** 609–612.
Bongiovanni, A. M., and McPadden, A. J. (1960). *Fertil. Steril.* **11,** 181–186.
Bonner, J. J., and Slavkin, H. C. (1975). *Immunogenetics* **2,** 213–218.
Brinkley, L., Basehoar, G., Branch, A., and Avery, J. (1975). *J. Embryol. Exp. Morphol.* **34,** 485–495.
Brinkley, L., Basehoar, G., and Avery, J. (1978). *J. Dent. Res.* **57,** 402–411.
Burdi, A., and Silvey, R. G. (1969). *Teratology* **2,** 297–304.
Cake, M. H., and Litwack, G. (1975). *In* "Biochemical Actions of Hormones" (G. Litwack, ed.), Vol. 3, pp. 317–390. Academic Press, New York.
Chamberlain, J. G., and Kasahara, M. (1971). *Proc. Soc. Exp. Biol. Med.* **138,** 290–293.
Chaudhry, A. P., and Shah, R. M. (1973). *Teratology* **8,** 139–142.
Clark, K. H. (1956). *Genetics* **41,** 637–648.
Clavert, J., Buck, P., and Rumpler, Y. (1961). *C. R. Seances Soc. Biol. Ses Fil.* **155,** 1569–1571.
Clavert, J., Buck, P., Rumpler, Y., and Ruch, J. V. (1965). *Therapie* **20,** 1579–1584.
Cleaton-Jones, P. (1976). *J. Dent Res.* **55,** 437–441.
Csaba, G., Toro, I., and Fischer, J. (1967). *Acta Paediatr. Acad. Sci. Hung.* **8,** 217–223.
Curry, D. M., and Beaton, G. H. (1958). *Endocrinology* **63,** 155–161.
Diewert, V. M. (1974). *Arch. Oral Biol.* **19,** 303–315.
Diewert, V. M. (1976). *Teratology* **14,** 291–314.

Diewert, V. M. (1978). *Arch. Oral Biol.* **23,** 607–629.
Diewert, V. M. (1979). *Anat. Rec.* **193,** 523 (abstr.).
Diewert, V. M. (1980). *In* "Current Research Trends in Prenatal Craniofacial Development" (R. M. Pratt and R. L. Christiansen, eds.), pp. 165–186. Elsevier/North-Holland, New York.
Diewert, V. M., and Pratt, R. M. (1981). *Teratology* **24,** 149–162.
Doig, R. K., and Coltman, O. McK. (1956). *Lancet* **2,** 730–731.
Dostal, M., and Jelinek, R. (1971). *Nature (London)* **230,** 464.
Dostal, M., and Jelinek, R. (1973). *Teratology* **8,** 245–252.
Fainstat, T. (1954). *Endocrinology* **55,** 502–508.
Ferguson, M. W. J. (1978). *J. Anat.* **125,** 555–577.
Francis, B. M. (1973). *Teratology* **7,** 119–126.
Fraser, F. C., and Fainstat, T. (1951). *Pediatrics* **8,** 527–533.
Fraser, F. C., Kalter, H., Walker, B. E., and Fainstat, T. D. (1954). *J. Cell. Comp. Physiol.* **43,** Suppl. 1, 237–259.
Frommer, J. (1968). *Anat. Rec.* **160,** 471.
Frommer, J., and Monroe, C. W. (1969). *J. Dent. Res.* **48,** 155–156.
Gandelman, R., and Rosenthal, C. (1981). *Teratology* **24,** 293–301.
Goldman, A. S., Katsumata, M., Yaffe, S. J., and Gasser, D. L. (1977). *Nature (London)* **265,** 643–645.
Goldman, A. S., Shapiro, B. H., and Katsumata, M. (1978). *Nature (London)* **272,** 464–466.
Greene, R. M., and Kochhar, D. M. (1973). *Am. J. Anat.* **137,** 477–482.
Greene, R. M., and Kochhar, D. M. (1974). *J. Embryol. Exp. Morphol.* **31,** 683–692.
Greene, R. M., and Kochhar, D. M. (1975). *Teratology* **11,** 47–56.
Greene, R. M., and Pratt, R. M. (1976). *J. Embryol. Exp. Morphol.* **36,** 225–245.
Greengard, O. (1975). *J. Steroid Biochem.* **6,** 639–642.
Guilbeau, J. A. (1953). *Am. J. Obstet. Gynecol.* **65,** 227.
Gunberg, D. L. (1957). *Anat. Rec.* **129,** 133–153.
Hackman, R. M., and Brown, K. S. (1972). *Teratology* **6,** 313–316.
Hackney, J. F. (1980). *Teratology* **21,** 39–51.
Harris, J. W. S. (1967). *Sci. Basis Med.* pp. 356–370.
Harris, J. W. S., and Ross, I. P. (1956). *Lancet* **1,** 1045–1047.
Hart, J. C., Smiley, G. R., and Dixon, A. D. (1972). *Teratology* **6,** 43–50.
Hassell, J. R., and Orkin, R. W. (1976). *Dev. Biol.* **49,** 80–88.
Hassell, J. R., Pratt, R. M., and King, C. T. G. (1974). *Teratology* **9,** 19 (abstract).
Heiberg, K., Kalter, H., and Fraser, F. C. (1959). *Biol. Neonat.* **1,** 33–37.
Hendrickx, A. G., Sawyer, R. H., Terrell, T. G., Osburn, B. I., Henrickson, R. V., and Steffek, A. J. (1975). *Fed. Proc., Fed. Am. Soc. Exp. Biol.* **34,** 1661–1665.
Hendrickx, A. G., Pellegrini, M., Tarara, R., Parker, R., Silverman, S., and Steffek, A. J. (1980). *Teratology* **22,** 103–114.
Herold, R. C., and Futran, N. (1980). *Arch. Oral Biol.* **25,** 423–429.
Hoar, R. M. (1962). *Anat. Rec.* **144,** 155–163.
Holt, T. M. (1975). *Am. J. Anat.* **144,** 169–196.
Hudson, C. D., and Shapiro, B. L. (1973). *Arch. Oral Biol.* **18,** 77–84.
Hughes, L. V., Furstman, L., and Berdick, S. (1967). *J. Dent. Res.* **46,** 373–379.
Humphrey, T. (1969). *Am. J. Anat.* **125,** 317–344.
Innes, R. B. (1978). *J. Embryol. Exp. Morphol.* **43,** 185–194.
Isaacson, R. J., and Chaudhry, A. P. (1962). *Anat. Rec.* **142,** 479–484.
Jacobs, R. M. (1964a). *Anat. Rec.* **149,** 691–697.

Jacobs, R. M. (1964b). *Anat. Rec.* **150**, 271–277.
Jelinek, R., and Dostal, M. (1973). *Acta Chir. Plast.* **15**, 216–222.
Jelinek, R., and Dostal, M. (1975). *Teratology* **11**, 193–198.
Jirsakova, A., and Valhova, I. (1971). *Folia Biol. (Prague)* **17**, 286–289.
Jollow, D. J., Mitchell, J. R., Potter, W. Z., Davis, D. C., Gillette, J. R., and Brodie, B. B. (1973). *J. Pharmacol. Exp. Ther.* **187**, 195–202.
Jost, A., and Picon, L. (1970). *Adv. Metab. Disord.* **4**, 123–184.
Jurand, A. (1968). *J. Embryol. Exp. Morphol.* **20**, 355–366.
Kalter, H. (1954). *Genetics* **39**, 185–196.
Kalter, H. (1962). *Anat. Rec.* **142**, 311 (abstr.).
Kalter, H. (1965). *Ann. N. Y. Acad. Sci.* **123**, 287–294.
Kalter, H., and Fraser, F. C. (1952). *Nature (London)* **169**, 665.
Kasirsky, G., and Lombardi, L. (1970). *Toxicol. Appl. Pharmacol.* **16**, 773–778.
Kelly, A. (1981). Ph.D. Dissertation, University of Texas, San Antonio.
Koziol, C. A., and Steffek, A. K. (1969). *Arch. Oral Biol.* **14**, 317–321.
Kraus, A. M. (1975). *J. Pediatr. Ophthalmol.* **12**, 107–108.
Krawczyk, W., and Gillon, D. (1976). *Arch. Oral Biol.* **21**, 503–508.
Kurisu, K., Shimizu, K., and Wada, K. (1977). *Jpn. J. Oral Biol.* **19**, 288–299.
Kurisu, K., Sasaki, S., Shimazaki, K., Ohsaki, Y., and Wada, R. (1981). *J. Craniofacial Genet. Dev. Biol.* **1**, 273.
Lahti, A., and Saxen, L. (1967). *Nature (London)* **216**, 1217–1218.
Lahti, A., Antila, E., and Saxen, L. (1972). *Teratology* **6**, 37–42.
Larsson, K. S. (1962a). *Acta Odontol. Scand.* **20**, Suppl. 31, 1–35.
Larsson, K. S. (1962b). *Acta Morphol. Neerl. Scand.* **4**, 349–367.
Larsson, K. S., Boström, H., and Carlsöö, S. (1959). *Exp. Cell Res.* **16**, 379–383.
Lazzaro, C. (1940). *Monit. Zool. Ital.* **51**, 249–265.
Lessard, J. L., Wee, E. L., and Zimmerman, D. F. (1974). *Teratology* **9**, 113–126.
Levine, A., Yaffe, S. J., and Back, N. (1968). *Proc. Soc. Exp. Biol. Med.* **129**, 86–88.
Loevy, H. (1962). *Anat. Rec.* **142**, 375–389.
Loevy, H. (1963). *Anat. Rec.* **145**, 117–122.
Long, S. Y., Larsson, K. S., and Lohmander, S. (1973). *Teratology* **8**, 137–138.
Malpas, P. ((1965). *Br. Med. J.* **1**, 795.
Mato, M., Aikawa, E., and Katahira, M. (1966). *Gunma J. Med. Sci.* **15**, 46–56.
Mato, M., Aikawa, E., and Katahira, M. (1967). *Gunma J. Med. Sci.* **16**, 79–99.
Matthiessen, M., and Anderson, H. (1972). *Z. Anat. Entwicklungsgesch.* **137**, 153–169.
Mercier-Parot, L. (1957). *Biol. Med. (Paris)* **46**, 672–680.
Moscatteli, D., and Rubin, H. (1977). *J. Cell. Physiol.* **91**, 79–88.
Mosier, H. D., Jr., Dearden, L. C., Roberts, R. C., Jansons, R. A., and Biggs, C. S. (1981). *Teratology* **23**, 15–24.
Mott, W., Toto, P., and Hilgers, D. (1969). *J. Dent. Res.* **48**, 263–269.
Nacht, S., and Garzon, P. (1974). *Adv. Steroid Biochem. Pharmacol.* **4**, 157–187.
Nanda, R., and Romeo, D. (1975). *Cleft Palate J.* **12**, 436–442.
Nanda, R., and Romeo, D. (1978). *Cleft Palate J.* **15**, 176–181.
Nanda, R., Van Der Linden, F. P. G. M., and Jansen, H. W. B. (1970). *Experientia* **26**, 1111–1112.
Newman, R. A., and Cutroneo, K. R. (1977). *Mol. Pharmacol.* **14**, 189–198.
Pinsky, L., and DiGeorge, A. M. (1965). *Science* **147**, 402–403.
Popert, A. J. (1962). *Br. Med. J.* **1**, 967–971.
Pratt, R. M., and Hassell, J. R. (1975). *Dev. Biol.* **45**, 192–198.
Pratt, R. M., and King, C. T. G. (1971). *Arch. Oral Biol.* **16**, 1181–1185.

Pratt, R. M., and Martin, G. R. (1975). *Proc. Natl. Acad. Sci. U.S.A.* **72,** 874–877.
Pratt, R. M., Goggins, J. R., Wilk, A. L., and King, C. T. G. (1973). *Dev. Biol.* **32,** 230–237.
Pratt, R. M., Figueroa, A. A., Greene, R. M., Wilk, A. L., and Salomon, D. S. (1979). *In* "Advances in the study of Birth Defects and Abnormal Embryogenesis: Cellular and Molecular Aspects" (T. V. N. Persaud, ed.), Vol. 4, pp. 161–176. MTP Press, Ltd., London.
Pratt, R. M., Salomon, D. S., Diewert, V. M., Erickson, R. P., Burns, R., and Brown, K. S. (1980a). *Teratog., Carcinog., Mutagen.* **1,** 15–23.
Pratt, R. M., Yoneda, T., Silver, M. H., and Salomon, D. S. (1980b). *In* "Current Research Trends in Prenatal Craniofacial Development (R. M. Pratt and R. L. Christiansen, eds.), pp. 235–252. Elsevier/North-Holland, New York.
Rees, H. A., and Williams, D. A. (1962). *Br. Med. J.* **1,** 1575–1579.
Rogoyski, A., and Trzcinska-Dabrowska, Z. (1969). *Am. J. Ophthalmol.* **69,** 128–133.
Ross, L. M., and Walker, B. E. (1967). *Am. J. Anat.* **121,** 509–521.
Rousseau, G. G., Baxter, J. D., and Tomkins, G. M. (1972). *J. Mol. Biol.* **67,** 99–115.
Rowland, J. M., and Hendrickx, A. G. (1982). *Teratology* **25,** 72 (abstr.).
Rowland, J. M., and Hendrickx, A. G. (1983). *Teratology* **27,** 13–18.
Rowland, J. M., Althaus, Z. R., Slikker, J. W., Jr., and Hendrickx, A. G. (1980). *Teratology* **21,** 65–66 (abstr.).
Rowland, J. M., Althaus, Z. R., Slikker, W., and Hendrickx, A. G. (1983). *Toxicol. Appl. Pharmacol.* **67,** 70–77.
Russell, A., Ornoy, A., Ritchie, J., Golenser, J., Fein, A., and Nebel, L. (1972). *Adv. Exp. Med. Biol.* **27,** 257–271.
Salomon, D. S., and Pratt, R. M. (1976). *Nature (London)* **264,** 174–177.
Salomon, D. S., and Pratt, R. M. (1978). *J. Cell. Physiol.* **97,** 315–327.
Salomon, D. S., and Pratt, R. M. (1979). *Differentiation* **13,** 141–154.
Salomon, D. S., Zubairi, Y., and Thompson, E. B. (1978). *J. Steroid Biochem.* **9,** 95–107.
Sawyer, R., Hendrickx, A., Osburn, B., Terrell, T., and Anderson, J. (1977). *J. Med. Primatol.* **6,** 145–150.
Saxen, I. (1973). *Arch. Oral Biol.* **18,** 1469–1479.
Schatz, M., Patterson, R., Zeitz, S., O'Rourke, J., and Melam, H. (1975). *JAMA, J. Am. Med. Assoc.* **233,** 804–807.
Shah, R. M. (1977). *Toxicol. Appl. Pharmacol.* **42,** 229–231.
Shah, R. M. (1979). *J. Anat.* **129,** 531–539.
Shah, R. M., and Chaudhry, A. P. (1973). *Teratology* **7,** 191–194.
Shah, R. M., and Chaudhry, A. P. (1974). *Teratology* **10,** 17–30.
Shah, R. M., and Kilistoff, A. (1976). *J. Embryol. Exp. Morphol.* **36,** 101–108.
Shah, R. M., and Travill, A. A. (1976a). *Teratology* **13,** 71–83.
Shah, R. M., and Travill, A. A. (1976b). *Am. J. Anat.* **145,** 149–165.
Shapira, Y., and Shoshan, S. (1972). *Arch. Oral Biol.* **17,** 1699–1703.
Sicher, H. (1915). *Anat. Anz.* **47,** 513–523, 545–562.
Siekevitz, P. (1952). *J. Biol. Chem.* **195,** 549–565.
Smiley, G. R. (1970). *Arch. Oral Biol.* **15,** 287–296.
Smiley, G. R., and Koch, W. E. (1971). *J. Dent. Res.* **59,** 1671–1677.
Smiley, G. R., Hart, J. D., and Dixon, A. D. (1971). *J. Dent. Res.* **50,** 1506–1507.
Spain, K. M., Kisieleski, W., and Wood, N. K. (1975). *J. Dent. Res.* **54,** 1069–1077.
Stark, R. B. M., and Ehrmann, N. A. (1958). *Plast. Reconstr. Surg.* **21,** 177–184.
Sugimoto, M., Kojima, M., and Endo, H. (1976). *Dev., Growth Differ.* **18,** 319–327.
Thompson, E. B., and Lippman, M. E. (1974). *Metab., Clin. Exp.* **23,** 159–202.

Toole, B. P., Underhill, C. B., Mikumi-Takagaki, Y., and Orkin, R. W. (1980). In "Current Research Trends in Craniofacial Development" (R. M. Pratt and R. L. Christiansen, eds.), pp. 263–275. Elsevier/North-Holland, New York.
Tyan, M. L., and Miller, K. K. (1978). Proc. Soc. Exp. Biol. Med. **158**, 618–621.
Uitto, V. J., and Thesleff, I. (1979). Arch. Oral Biol. **24**, 575–583.
Vannier, B., Jequier, R., and Jude, A. (1969). C. R. Seances Soc. Biol. Ses Fil. **163**, 1269–1272.
Vekemans, M., and Fraser, F. C. (1979). Am. J. Med. Genet. **4**, 95–102.
Verrusio, A. C. (1970). Teratology **3**, 17–20.
Waddell, W. J. (1971). Teratology **4**, 355–366.
Waddell, W. J. (1972). Teratology **5**, 219–221.
Walker, B. E. (1961). J. Embryol. Exp. Morphol. **9**, 22–31.
Walker, B. E. (1965). Science **149**, 862–863.
Walker, B. E. (1967). Proc. Soc. Exp. Biol. Med. **125**, 1281–1284.
Walker, B. E. (1969). Teratology **2**, 191–198.
Walker, B. E. (1971). Teratology **4**, 39–42.
Walker, B. E. (1982). Arch. Oral Biol. **27**, 175–176.
Walker, B. E., and Fraser, F. C. (1956). J. Embryol. Exp. Morphol. **4**, 176–189.
Walker, B. E., and Fraser, F. C. (1957). J. Embryol. Exp. Morphol. **5**, 201–209.
Walker, B. E., and Patterson, A. (1978). Teratology **17**, 51–56.
Walker, B. E., and Quarles, J. (1975). J. Dent. Res. **54**, 1200–1206.
Walker, B. E., and Quarles, J. (1976). Arch. Oral Biol. **21**, 405–412.
Wee, E. L., and Zimmerman, E. F. (1980). Teratology **21**, 15–27.
Wee, E. L., Wolfson, L. G., and Zimmerman, E. F. (1976). Dev. Biol. **48**, 91–103.
Wells, C. N. (1953). Am. J. Obstet. Gynecol. **66**, 598–601.
Westphal, U. (1969). In "Methods in Enzymology" (R. B. Clayton, ed.), Vol. 15, pp. 761–796. Academic Press, New York.
Williams, D. A. (1967). Acta Allergol. **22**, 311–323.
Wilson, J. G. (1977). In "Handbook of Teratology" (J. G. Wilson and F. C. Fraser, eds.), Vol. 1, pp. 309–355. Plenum, New York.
Wragg, L. E., Klein, M., Steinvorth, G., and Warpeha, R. (1970). Arch. Oral Biol. **15**, 705–719.
Wragg, L. E., Diewert, V. M., and Klein, M. (1972). Arch. Oral Biol. **17**, 683–690.
Zeiler, K. B., Weinstein, S., and Gibson, R. D. (1964). Arch. Oral Biol. **9**, 545–554.
Zimmerman, E. F., and Bowen, D. (1972a). Teratology **5**, 57–69.
Zimmerman, E. F., and Bowen, D. (1972b). Teratology **5**, 335–344.
Zimmerman, E. F., Andrew, F., and Kalter, H. (1970). Proc. Natl. Aad. Sci. U.S.A. **67**, 779–785.

Embryo Transfer in Domestic Animals

GARY B. ANDERSON

Department of Animal Science, University of California, Davis, California

I. Introduction 129
II. History.. 130
III. Applications of Embryo Transfer to Large Animals..................... 132
    A. Enhanced Reproductive Rate of Donor Females 132
    B. Production of Offspring from Infertile Females.................... 134
    C. Importation and Exportation of Embryos 135
    D. Induction of Twins in Cattle 136
    E. Research 137
    F. Detection of Undesirable Recessives.............................. 137
IV. Current Embryo Transfer Technology 138
    A. Cattle.. 138
    B. Horses 147
    C. Sheep 150
    D. Goats 151
    E. Swine.. 152
    F. Other Species... 153
V. Future Developments in Embryo Transfer 154
    References... 156

I. Introduction

Embryo transfer is the removal and transfer of a developing embryo from the reproductive tract of one female to that of another, where the pregnancy may continue. The term embryo transfer is often used to describe collectively a variety of techniques such as superovulation of the donor, synchronization of estrus in the donor and recipient, and various manipulations of the embryo *in vitro*, in addition to the physical transfer of an embryo. Embryo transfer technology has developed exceedingly fast, more rapidly than most investigators in the field could have predicted. A great deal is known today about embryo transfer, particularly in cattle; in fact, it is one physiological process where more is known about a farm animal species than about the laboratory rat. Information learned from work with cattle is now being applied to other domestic species.

Several excellent reviews of embryo transfer technology are available. As with any rapidly changing field, new information must be continually incorporated as dogma is disproven, breakthroughs are made, and new questions are raised. The purpose of this article is to draw together up-to-date information dealing with embryo transfer in domestic animals. Emphasis has been placed on recent reports in the scientific literature. Older reviews that contain information from earlier work that was important in developing this new field are cited where appropriate.

II. History

Historically, the development of embryo transfer technology has had two phases, one fairly long and slow moving, the other very recent and rapidly changing. The first phase relates to the intellectual and academic elaboration of embryo transfer techniques, whereas the second involves commercialization of embryo transfer. Betteridge (1981) has reviewed the evolution of concepts held today regarding the production of ova by the mammalian female and has reported on the application of embryo transfer to a range of species.

The first successful embryo transfer was performed with rabbits by Walter Heape (1891, 1897). His often-cited work was not carried out to be "a first," nor was it intended to capitalize on commercial or other practical considerations; rather, it was designed to make use of the tremendous potential of embryo transfer as a research tool to separate fetal and maternal influences. Offspring produced by embryo transfer in farm animal species were reported for the sheep and goat in 1934 (Warwick et al., 1934), cow and pig in 1951 (Kvasnickii, 1951; Willet et al., 1951), and horse in 1974 (Oguri and Tsutsumi, 1974). Except for the report of successes with the horse, these early achievements remained fairly isolated events, and few intensive research efforts were initiated to improve and perfect technology per se. In fact, as with much of mammalian embryology, embryo transfer techniques were developed and utilized widely in research before they were applied to any great extent to domestic animal production. Much of the credit for rekindling interest in large-animal embryo transfer, which later led to commercial application, is given to the researchers at Cambridge University. A series of articles from Cambridge demonstrated that high pregnancy rates could be achieved in cattle using methods of surgical embryo collection and transfer (Rowson et al., 1969, 1971, 1972). Such early investigations utilized only small numbers of animals and did not take advantage of the flexibility realized today in such areas as synchronization of estrus in donors and recipients. They did, however, stimulate research in countries around the world to refine and apply transfer techniques. Likewise, interest in possible commercial application was initiated, which lead to rapid development of the embryo transfer industry.

The history of the commercial embryo transfer industry is short but includes the major portion of what is known about the technique. Application on a commerical scale began while procedures were as yet imperfect and results were extremely variable. A demand for reliable embryo transfer services provided the stimulus and financial backing for expansion of the industry. Seidel and Seidel (1982) have emphasized the unique nature of the evolution of embryo transfer techniques. Rather than development and promotion by scientists and extension, financial backing from the private sector was primarily responsible for establishment of the commercial industry and its support during the early years of rapidly changing technology. The primary impetus has been attributed to the so-called exotic boom (Carmichael, 1980; Schultz, 1980). Inflated cattle prices resulting from introduction of European breeds of cattle during the early 1970s provided incentives to utilize embryo transfer as a method of reproducing more rapidly the few imported purebred "exotics" and to hasten upgrading of crossbreds from artificial insemination of North American cattle with imported semen. Most of the early commercial embryo transfers were carried out on exotics using surgical collection and transfer, which limited the procedures to well-equipped facilities built exclusively for embryo transfer. Unpredictability of the results meant that only high-priced cattle whose offspring were potentially valuable would be commercially feasible candidates for embryo transfer. As the demand for exotics lessened and beef cattle markets entered a slump during the mid-1970s, the demand for embryo transfer services fell, and a number of commercial units folded. The commercial industry itself suffered and could have been reduced to an insignificant force in large-animal reproduction, but development of nonsurgical embryo collection techniques during this time was giving the industry wider potential for applying embryo transfer to lactating, high-producing dairy cattle. Improvements in nonsurgical techniques resulting in pregnancy rates similar to those achieved with surgical transfer have further taken embryo transfer from commercial facilities to the farm. Lower investments in facilities and greater confidence in achieving positive results have opened the field to private individuals, such as veterinarians wishing to provide the service to their clients without necessarily excluding other aspects of a clinical practice. A limited but growing industry is developing in equine embryo transfer, and on an even smaller but perhaps equally significant scale, commercial embryo transfer is being applied to sheep, goats, and pigs. Economic value rather than genetic merit is the primary criterion for selection of donors in these other farm animal species, as it is in the case with bovine embryo transfer.

III. Applications of Embryo Transfer to Large Animals

A. Enhanced Reproductive Rate of Donor Females

Together, superovulation and embryo transfer offer the opportunity to produce substantially more offspring from a donor female than she is capable of producing naturally. Single embryos may be collected from nonsuperovulated donors during recurring estrous cycles and transferred to recipients. Seidel (1981a) has calculated that even with repeated embryo collections of nonsuperovulated cows, fewer than half as many calves could be expected than if the dams were superovulated an optimal three times during the year.

The mare, unlike females of the other farm animal species, is resistant to superovulation attempts, and currently, collection of only singly ovulated embryos is possible. Single-embryo recoveries coupled with the seasonal nature of the equine reproductive cycle limit the potential number of offspring that can be produced with embryo transfer. Restrictions imposed by equine breed registries on the number of offspring that may be produced per breeding season currently make the potential number of foals that may be generated of academic interest only.

Only for the cow do adequate data exist on the number of offspring produced through embryo transfer. Reports in popular magazines of individual donors producing large litters of calves have often left the impression that this is the rule rather than the exception. Analysis of data from large numbers of donors from commercial embryo transfer units indicates that, on the average, 3.5 pregnancies per superovulation treatment may be expected from normal, healthy cows (Schneider et al., 1980; Seidel, 1981a). This average is based on a mean of 10 embryos collected per superovulation, approximately 8 of which are fertilized, 6 of which are judged to have sufficiently normal morphology for transfer, and 2–3 of which will either not implant or will miscarry, resulting in approximately 3.5 pregnancies. Seidel (1981a) has indicated that, on the average, half of the total pregnancies are produced by embryos from only a quarter of the donors. Furthermore, of 64 superovulated donors, 10% did not show estrus, 22% produced no pregnancies after transfer, 25% produced 1–2 pregnancies, 25% had 3–4 pregnancies, and 18% had 5–12 pregnancies. From this latter 18%, much of the publicity related to embryo transfer is generated. Although reports exist of cows that have produced over 50 calves in a single year (Seidel, 1981a), the data just presented would suggest that 10 calves is a more reasonable expectation. It should be remembered that this is a mean value, and considerable variation may be expected between donors and between superovulation treatments of individual donors.

It would appear that embryo transfer offers tremendous potential for genetic improvement through enhanced reproduction of genetically superior females. Because artificial insemination provides a means of augmenting the numbers of offspring from genetically superior males, and dramatic increases in production have occurred as a result (e.g., development of today's high-producing dairy cows), it may seem natural to equate embryo transfer with artificial insemination. Animal breeders who have estimated the genetic progress possible with embryo transfer, however, have unanimously concluded that the addition of embryo transfer to a breeding scheme already using artificial insemination will result in substantially less additional genetic progress than would be obtained with artificial insemination alone. Even with superovulation, the reproductive potential of the female in terms of the number of offspring she can produce is many times less than that of the male. In addition, the true genetic merit of a female is often difficult to determine because of a limited number of records on any cow and her progeny. Nevertheless, embryo transfer can contribute to genetic improvement, for example, at the herd level by allowing dairy farmers to produce all of their replacement heifers from the top 10% rather than the entire herd. With current costs, the value of the additional product would be less than the cost of the procedure (Wilmut and Hume, 1978; Bradford and Kennedy, 1980: Van Velck, 1982). However, in view of the tremendous advances that have been made during the past decade, it would be very short-sighted not to conclude that technology will develop sufficiently for practical application at a reduced cost to hasten genetic progress through embryo transfer.

As mentioned earlier, market value rather than genetic superiority has been the primary criterion for selecting females as donors for embryo transfer programs. Because a number of factors contribute to market value, some of which are unrelated to genetic merit, it cannot be assumed that a female in an embryo transfer program will produce genetically superior offspring, only that she is likely to produce economically valuable offspring. It is encouraging that an analysis by Seidel (1981a) of milk production by embryo transfer donors revealed that dairy cattle used as donors to date have been in the top twenty-fifth percentile for genetic value in milk production. However, the sires used to produce progeny by embryo transfer have been at approximately the second percentile in genetic value for milk production of all bulls born (Seidel, 1981a), further demonstrating the greater selection pressure that can be exerted through the male with artificial insemination.

B. Production of Offspring from Infertile Females

Failure of a female to produce offspring may occur in spite of production of fertile ova, normal fertilization, and early preimplantation development. Various conditions of the female reproductive tract, particularly in older animals, preclude normal maintenance of pregnancy. Offspring can often be produced from these females by flushing the embryo from the reproductive tract during the first week of development and transferring it to the uterus of a fertile recipient. Commercial embryo transfer has been used for this purpose in cattle and, because of restrictions imposed by breed registries, it is the primary commercial application of embryo transfer in horses. Generally, lower rates of success are achieved with infertile than with normal fertile animals. Elsden *et al.* (1979) compared superovulation response, number of fertilized ova recovered, and pregnancy rates of fertile and infertile cows. All three variables were significantly lower in the infertile than in the fertile cows. In the same study, attempts to collect embryos from nonsuperovulated infertile cows were less successful than with fertile cows. Similar results were reported for the mare where fewer embryos were collected from infertile than fertile mares, but normal embryos resulted in similar pregnancy rates for the two groups (Imel *et al.*, 1981a).

Adequate data have yet to be collected to determine the ultimate effect and desirability of reproducing infertile females. Over the short term it is economically acceptable when the market value of the offspring justifies the cost of the procedure. Because some types of infertility have a genetic component, the wisdom of reproducing these females artificially may be open to some question. An intelligent recommendation will require further characterization of the causes of infertility and analysis by animal geneticists.

C. Importation and Exportation of Embryos

Importation and exportation of breeding animals between countries have certain inherent problems, some of which may be at least partially overcome by using embryo transfer. Embryos may be transported at ambient or body temperature (Bedirian et al., 1979), refrigerated (BonDurant et al., 1982), or frozen (de los Santos-Valadez et al., 1981). Importation of embryos may facilitate introduction of bloodlines into countries where animal agriculture is developing. If the embryos are shipped rather than carried by an individual capable of doing the transfers, sufficient technical knowledge and expertise are required to successfully carry out synchronization of estrus in the recipients, the transfer itself, and posttransfer maintenance of the recipients.

Importation of embryos and transfer to indigenous recipients appear to have several practical advantages over importation of animals after birth. First, transporting an embryo can be done more cheaply than transporting an animal, although the long time period until the imported embryo is capable of reproducing should be considered. Second, the risk of transmitting a disease, which is an important consideration when animals are moved between countries, is probably reduced by importing embryos. It is known that certain pathogens may infect mammalian embryos and be transmitted via transfer of these embryos (Waters, 1981). However, many pathogens appear unable to penetrate the zona pellucida, and disease transmission is less likely to occur by embryo importation than if an animal is imported after birth. Tight restrictions exist on importation of embryos into some countries. Although there is an active market for export of embryos from the United States, embryos may not currently be imported. These restrictions are expected to be lifted once disease transmission is more fully understood.

Finally, it has been suggested that an animal born into a new environment has a better chance of adjusting than if it were imported after birth. No clear evidence exists to support this contention, but it is known that animals suffer serious health problems and significantly reduced production when sent to environments for which they are not adapted, for example, exportation of Canadian or U.S. Holstein cattle to countries in tropical zones. In addition to an early opportunity to build active immunities and adjust to other environmental conditions, passive immunity may be conferred upon the imported offspring by transfer of antibodies across the placenta or in the colostrum from a recipient that is well adapted to the particular environment. Each of the advantages of importing embryos rather than livestock may in most cases still be accomplished satisfactorily by importation of semen from genetically superior males.

D. Induction of Twins in Cattle

Multiple ovulation and pregnancy are characteristics of sheep, goats, and pigs; consequently, induction of twins is likely to be of greatest application in cattle, specifically beef cattle. It has been demonstrated that embryo transfer can be used successfully to induce twin pregnancies in cattle (Rowson et al., 1971; Anderson, 1978a). Conflicting results exist (Newcomb et al., 1980), but induction of twins is likely to be most successful if an embryo is transferred to each uterine horn, rather than two embryos to one uterine horn. Twin pregnancy will result either from transfer of two embryos to a nonbred recipient or transfer of a single embryo to the uterine horn contralateral to the corpus luteum of a bred recipient. High rates of twin pregnancy may be achieved with either surgical (Anderson et al., 1978, 1979, 1982) or nonsurgical transfer (Gordon and Boland, 1979).

Producers of breeding stock are hesitant to use twin pregnancy because half of the heifer calves are likely to be freemartins (Horton et al., 1980). Results from experiments designed to study the phenomenon of twinning in cattle have provided data for evaluating the economics of producing twins for the commercial market. The experiments have demonstrated that when cows are managed for the production of twins, including adjustment of prepartum and postpartum nutrition, many other complications that are usually reported to occur with twins are avoided (Price et al., 1981; Anderson et al., 1982; Wheeler et al., 1982).

Because the primary cost of producing a calf is associated not with the requirements for pregnancy but with the cost of maintaining the cow, production of two calves rather than one should result in increased production per cow. However, the cost of inducing the twin pregnancy cannot be greater than the value of the calf and still be economically feasible. At present, the cost of embryo transfer is greater than the value of a calf to be used for meat. There are currently two trends likely to make embryo transfer to produce twins more useful. On-the-farm collections and transfers are becoming more widespread as the producer provides labor for superovulation of donors and synchronization of estrus in the recipients, as well as providing the recipients themselves. The cost of embryo transfer may now be as low as several hundred dollars per pregnancy rather than several thousand. At the same time, advances are being made in the ability to sex embryos prior to transfer (White *et al.*, 1982), which may make production of twins more attractive to producers of purebred stock.

E. Research

As discussed earlier, embryo transfer techniques were used in research, extensively in laboratory animals and to a lesser extent in large animals, before commercial embryo transfer was established. Embryo transfer provides the ultimate separation of genetic effects of the fetus from genetic effects of the dam. For example, reciprocal transfer of embryos between two breeds of sheep that differ in gestation period proved that it is primarily the genotype of the fetus that determines length of gestation (Bradford *et al.*, 1972). Transfer of one embryo of each breed resulted in an intermediate gestation (Anderson *et al.*, 1981), providing a unique model for studying the initiation of parturition that would not have been possible without embryo transfer.

F. Detection of Undesirable Recessives

Superovulation of known carriers of undesirable recessives and insemination with semen from potential carriers can rapidly provide sufficient offspring to demonstrate, on a statistical basis, the presence or absence of recessive genes. Such a method was used to test young bulls as carriers of mulefoot prior to release of their semen for widespread use in artificial insemination (Johnson *et al.*, 1980). Some recessives (e.g., dwarf gene) are often lethal in the homozygous state, and others (e.g., mulefoot) are debilitating when expressed, which restricts testing to heterozygous females. This requires production of a larger number of offspring to give high confidence levels when testing males. With superovulation of homozygous or heterozygous females, large numbers of embryos may be transferred to normal females, reducing the number of carriers of the mutant genes that must be kept. For some genes, including both dwarf and mulefoot genes, fetuses may be recovered at slaughter of recipients and the phenotype determined, reducing the time required to test a male. It is likely that this type of testing will be employed more in the future to screen bulls to be used in artificial insemination.

IV. Current Embryo Transfer Technology

A. CATTLE

In spite of growing interest in use of embryo transfer for other farm animals, cattle still represent the most widely used species. The rapid development of embryo transfer technology, which has been applied even to humans (Steptoe and Edwards, 1978; Trounson *et al.*, 1980), has centered around techniques used in the cow. Accurate and current data on volume of transfers are difficult to obtain, but Seidel (1981a) determined that in 1979 approximately 17,000 pregnancies were established by commercial embryo transfer in North America, the center of the industry. This figure represents an approximate 80% increase in volume over the previous year, which Seidel ascribes in part to acceptance of improved technologies by animal breeders. The effect of improved technology on volume of transfers is difficult to quantitate but was demonstrated by a dramatic increase in use of embryo transfer by dairy farmers when nonsurgical embryo collection replaced surgical collection. After 1979 a shift also took place from surgical to nonsurgical methods of transferring embryos to recipients, resulting in a wave of on-the-farm transfers. The volume of commercial embryo transfer for 1982 is likely to be several times that determined for 1979. Description of current bovine embryo transfer technology is provided in the following section. Several extensive literature reviews are also available (Betteridge, 1977; Seidel, 1981a; Seidel and Seidel, 1982).

1. *Superovulation*

The major variable affecting the number of calves produced by embryo transfer is the unpredictability of the superovulation response. It is widely accepted that with a large population of superovulated donors, an average of 10 ovulations may be expected at each superovulation attempt (Elsden *et al.*, 1978; Schneider *et al.*, 1980). However, this mean is calculated from a large range in superovulation response and is not useful in predicting the response of an individual animal, because two donors receiving the same superovulation treatment may respond quite differently. Furthermore, the repeatability of response from one superovulation to the next within a donor is low (Seidel, 1981a). Age and breed of the donor, stage of the estrous cycle at which treatment is initiated, previous superovulation treatment, lactation, nutrition, and season may all affect superovulation and account for the large differences in response. Although conflicting data exist (Newcomb et al., 1979; Lubbadeh et al., 1980), cows may be repeatedly superovulated without a significant reduction in response (Nelson et al., 1979; Seidel, 1981a). It is important that sufficient time be allowed between successive treatments, however. The subject of bovine superovulation has been extensively reviewed by Gordon (1975) and Betteridge (1977).

Various treatments using several different gonadotropins have been devised to induce superovulation. Pregnant mare serum gonadotropin (PMSG) was the primary hormone used until the 1980s. Dosages of approximately 2000 IU were given at the time of normal luteal regression, Day 16 of the estrous cycle. At the ensuing estrus, which occurred at the normal time, multiple ovulation generally resulted. The long biological half-life of PMSG (Cole et al., 1967) allowed superovulation with a single injection. Sensitivity to exogenous PMSG tends to be greatest when it is injected between Days 8 and 12 of the estrous cycle (Greve, 1976; Sreenan and Gosling, 1977). The availability of prostaglandin $F_{2\alpha}$ and its analogs, two forms of which are currently marketed in the United States, allowed superovulation to be accomplished at selected times throughout the estrous cycle. This provided not only greater convenience, but probably slightly greater superovulatory response (Elsden et al., 1974). The typical regime involved a single injection of PMSG followed in 48 hr by a luteolytic dose of $PGF_{2\alpha}$. Estrus occurs in superovulated donors approximately 48–60 hr after $PGF_{2\alpha}$, slightly sooner after $PGF_{2\alpha}$ than in nonsuperovulated cattle (e.g., synchronized recipients) (Tervit et al., 1973).

Variation in response to PMSG continues to be studied. It is believed by some researchers that the long biological half-life of PMSG may contribute to variability in superovulatory response and recovery of normal embryos by continued ovarian stimulation after ovulation. However, attempts to neutralize PMSG with PMSG antiserum administered at estrus have not improved superovulation response (Jensen and Greve, 1980; Saumande and Chupin, 1981). Another possible source of variation is the FSH:LH ratio of the PMSG used. Stewart et al. (1976) reported a relatively constant FSH:LH ratio in PMSG collected from six mares between Days 40 and 80 of gestation. Humphrey et al. (1979), in contrast, reported significant differences in the FSH:LH ratio between PMSG collected at 60 and 90 days relative to that collected at 45 and 120 days. Furthermore, PMSG with high FSH:LH ratio appeared to superovulate more effectively than PMSG with low FSH:LH ratio. Newcomb *et al.* (1979) reported differences in FSH:LH ratio among commercial batches of PMSG. It is worth noting that even if the activity of PMSG is held constant, other sources of variation mentioned earlier will still contribute to the unpredictable nature of superovulation. When it is available, PMSG will continue to be used for superovulation.

A combination of FSH and LH, injected twice a day for 5 days in decreasing doses, has also been used for superovulation. When compared with PMSG, this regime yielded slightly more corpora lutea, recovered ova, and pregnancies per superovulated donor in some experiments (Elsden *et al.*, 1978) and was equivalent in others (Hasler, 1978). It is now generally accepted that addition of LH is unnecessary. Furthermore, FSH alone, administered for 3 or 4 days, is as efficacious as the 5-day treatment (Garcia *et al.*, 1982). Once-a-day rather than twice-a-day treatment with FSH also shows promise for superovulation (Looney *et al.*, 1981, 1982).

Another gonadotropin treatment that may be used successfully to induce superovulation is crude equine pituitary extract. Like PMSG, it has the advantage of being used as a single injection (Boland *et al.*, 1981; Danner and Oxender, 1980). Progesterone-releasing intravaginal devices (Kunkel, 1979), intravaginal pessaries containing progesterone (Sreenan and Beehan, 1976), and subcutaneous gestagen implants (Holtz *et al.*, 1979) have also been used rather than prostaglandin to synchronize estrus in superovulated donors and recipients.

2. Embryo Collection and Transfer

Early procedures for embryo collection in cattle were carried out surgically with the donor under general anesthesia (Rowson *et al.*, 1969; Newcomb and Rowson, 1975; Elsden, 1977a). Recovery of embryos with surgical collection, based on the number of corpora lutea on the ovaries, ranged from slightly over 75% 3 days after estrus to slightly under 50% at 8 days following estrus (Sreenan and Beehan, 1976). Although used almost exclusively for at least 5 years in commercial embryo transfer, surgical collection had numerous disadvantages. In addition to the risk of losing a high-priced donor under general anesthesia, resulting adhesions of the reproductive tract often made subsequent collections difficult and sometimes caused permanent impaired fertility. Dairy farmers were reluctant to subject high-producing dairy cows to surgery that would likely affect lactation and require the animal to spend peak lactation time at an embryo transfer facility. The extensive facilities required for surgery also precluded reduction of costs to the client through on-the-farm collection. Successful nonsurgical collection of bovine embryos was reported early in the era of commercial transfer (Sugie et al., 1972), but not until 1976 were methods described from which today's techniques were developed (Drost et al., 1976; Elsden et al., 1976; Rowe et al., 1976). Individual investigators and commercial groups have modified basic procedures to fit their needs, facilities, and personnel. In addition, further modifications in technique and equipment aimed at facilitating embryo collection have been reported (Ozil et al., 1979; Rowe et al., 1980a). It is generally accepted that recovery of embryos by nonsurgical means is at least equivalent to that of the surgical approach. Recovery rates of 60 to 80%, based on estimates of the number of corpora lutea obtained by palpation of the ovary per rectum, have been reported (Nelson et al., 1978; Rowe et al., 1980a). Recovery rates of Day-7 to Day-9 embryos tend to be higher than for Day-5 to Day-6.5 embryos (Nelson et al., 1978). Bovine embryo collection is now almost exclusively nonsurgical. The technique can be used repeatedly without serious complications. Shelton et al. (1979) reported as many as 11 collections per donor.

Elsden (1977b) has described the procedures most commonly used for surgical transfer of embryos to recipients. One procedure involves a midventral incision with the recipient under general anesthesia, similar to that used in surgical collection of embryos from the donor. The other involves a flank incision with the recipient in a standing position under local anesthesia. Under many conditions slightly lower pregnancy rates were obtained with the flank than with the midventral approach (Newcomb, 1979), although other authors have reported similar results for the two (Shelton et al., 1980). Evans et al. (1979) reported a 79% pregnancy rate with the flank method, which is probably higher than can be expected consistently with the midventral procedure. The improved speed, economy, and convenience of the flank approach, plus the greater application for on-the-farm transfers, made it the method of choice for some commercial units. Because of the high value of the calves resulting from a successful pregnancy, other units relied on midventral transfer because of its presumed slightly higher pregnancy rate.

The debate over which surgical approach yields the best results has nearly become academic, as pregnancy rates resulting from nonsurgical transfer steadily improve and, in some cases, equal those of surgical transfer (Rowe et al., 1979, 1980b; Tervit et al., 1980). The standard technique for nonsurgical embryo transfer requires a cassou insemination gun with a 0.25-cm^3 straw and sheath, equipment commonly used for artificial insemination. The tip of the cassou gun is introduced through the cervix into the uterine horn, where the embryo is deposited. Pregnancy rates with nonsurgical embryo transfer continue to improve, even without major modifications in technique. Technical expertise has been shown to be very important to high pregnancy rates (Rowe et al., 1980b; Curtis et al., 1981), and those individuals who do the greatest number of transfers tend to report the highest rates of success (Wright, 1981). As more individuals become competent with nonsurgical transfer, there is likely to be a complete replacement of surgical transfer with nonsurgical transfer as has already occurred at some insitutions. At the same time, an increasing proportion of superovulation, embryo collection, and embryo transfer procedures will be performed entirely at the ranch or farm, with the owner's own recipients (Greve and Lehn-Jensen, 1979). This should reduce the costs of embryo transfer and make it more available to the average producer. Additional information may be obtained from reviews of development and problems of nonsurgical embryo transfer (Sreenan, 1978; Newcomb and Rowson, 1980; Wright, 1981).

Transfer of a single embryo to an unmated recipient is usually made to the uterine horn ipsilateral to the corpus luteum as determined by palpation per rectum of the ovaries. Seidel (1981b) reviewed experiments comparing transfer of embryos to the uterine horn ipsilateral versus contralateral to the corpus luteum, and survival was consistently lower in the contralateral horn. Maintenance of the corpus luteum is apparently affected by the presence of a viable embryo in the ipsilateral uterine horn. With transfer of one embryo to each uterine horn of a recipient, survival of the embryo in the contralateral horn is somewhat dependent on survival of the embryo in the ipsilateral horn. If that embryo fails to develop, the chances are reduced that the pregnancy will be maintained. Under normal conditions, migration of an embryo from one uterine horn to the other occurs infrequently (Gordon et al., 1962). This local effect of the embryo on maintenance of the corpus luteum seems to be inherent in bovine reproduction, and until a mechanism is devised for preventing luteolysis, survival of a single embryo in the contralateral horn is likely to be reduced. Christie et al. (1979) attempted to assist the embryo in the contralateral horn by giving human chorionic gonadotropin (hCG) or progesterone to recipients on Days 13–23 or 13–35 of pregnancy. Compared to controls there seemed to be little benefit from the treatment. Interestingly, in a few recipients receiving progesterone, the pregnancy but not the corpus luteum was maintained until slaughter. Other workers have attempted to improve pregnancy rates with embryo transfer by giving hCG to recipients on Day 15 after estrus, shortly before luteolysis occurs (de los Santos-Valadez et al., 1982), or every other day from Day 13 to Day 35 of pregnancy (Greve and Lehn-Jensen, 1982). In general, the treatments stimulated accessory corpora lutea, which were sometimes maintained to parturition, and tended to increase peripheral progesterone levels, but had no significant effect on pregnancy rate at 60 days of gestation.

There is some indication that even after the corpus luteum has been maintained and the recipient fails to return to estrus and may be presumed pregnant, high embryonic loss occurs between Days 35 and 40 of pregnancy in nonsurgical recipients. The weighted average, calculated from data of six separate reports (Hahn and Hahn, 1976; Brand et al., 1978: Jillella and Baker, 1978; Tervit et al., 1980: Curtis et al., 1981; de los Santos-Valadez et al., 1981), is approximately 20% for embryonic loss between Days 35 and 40 of pregnancy following nonsurgical embryo transfer. Comparable figures were 9% between Days 25 and 60 with surgical transfer (Markette et al., 1980) and 7–12% between Days 25 and 75 with artificial insemination (Kummerfeld et al., 1978; Bulman and Lamming, 1979). Further study is needed to verify that higher than normal embryo loss indeed occurs with nonsurgical embryo transfer and to identify and correct the cause.

Evaluation of the embryo for viability after it has been collected is important in determining whether its transfer is likely to result in a calf. Subjective evaluation of morphology remains the primary means of assessing viability. Criteria included in evaluation are stage of development of the embryo for its postovulatory age, uniformity of blastomere size, and texture and symmetry of the blastomeres. The first of these, stage of development for age, appears to be the best indicator of viability (Shea, 1981). A range in stage of development may be expected at times, yet be normal, because ovulation in superovulated cows may occur over a period of at least 24 hr (Maxwell et al., 1978). Likewise, certain abnormalities of the zona pellucida and failure of some blastomeres to divide often have little effect on viability (Shea, 1981). With experience, an individual is able to classify embryos into categories that reflect the potential for development after transfer to recipients (e.g., Schneider et al., 1980; Shea, 1981; Wright, 1981). Unfortunately, not all embryos classified as excellent will develop after transfer, and not all embryos classified as poor or degenerated fail to develop. The latter are particularly intriguing, because they clearly demonstrate that embryos are capable of overcoming conditions that seem, with our current knowledge, highly abnormal.

Attempts to make embryo evaluation less subjective include the use of fluorescent dyes that stain either living or dead cells (Schilling et al., 1979a,b; Renard et al., 1982), uptake of glucose in vitro (Renard et al., 1980c), and release of enzymes from the embryo into the surrounding medium in vitro (Renard et al., 1982). Unfortunately, these criteria do little to improve predictions of viability.

In order for an embryo to continue development after it is transferred to a recipient it is necessary that the estrous cycle of the recipient be synchronized with that of the donor. The degree of synchrony required is still a matter of some debate. The earliest study of synchronization requirements indicated that exact synchrony was ideal, and variation of estrus in the recipient of even 1 day before or after estrus in the donor would result in a dramatic decline in pregnancy rate (Rowson et al., 1972). This study was conducted with embryos collected and transferred surgically as early as 3 days after estrus. Subsequent studies with later stage embryos collected nonsurgically on Days 6–8 after estrus affirm that close synchrony is ideal; however, pregnancy rate drops slowly rather than rapidly with the degree of asynchrony (Schneider et al., 1980). Furthermore, Wright (1981) reported that with transfer of over 2000 embryos, no reduction in pregnancy rate was observed when the recipient was in estrus 12, 24, or 36 hr before the donor compared with exact synchrony. There was no reduction in pregnancy when the recipient was observed in estrus 12 or 24 hr after the donor, but pregnancy rate fell with 36-hr asynchrony. It appears that with nonsurgical collection and transfer of Day-7 to Day-9 late morulae and blastocysts, synchrony requirements are not as exacting as for earlier stage embryos. Two other interesting observations regarding donor and recipient synchrony are that embryos classified as excellent based on morphology tend to tolerate greater asynchrony than embryos judged to have abnormalities (Nelson et al., 1982), and stage of development of the embryo rather than estrus in the donor may be a better criterion for determining the optimum luteal stage of the recipient (Kunkel and Stricklin, 1978).

3. Storage of Embryos

After the embryos have been flushed from the reproductive tract of the donor and until they have been transferred to recipients, they must be maintained in vitro under conditions that will ensure that viability will be maintained. Initially, the interval from collection to transfer was only a matter of hours, but to provide additional flexibility for embryo transfer procedures, methods have been sought that will allow successful extension of in vitro storage periods. Bovine embryos may now be kept viable in vitro for up to several days at body, room, or refrigeration temperatures. A recent development has been successful freezing of embryos in liquid nitrogen, which allows for long-term storage for months and probably years. Embryos may also be stored in the rabbit oviduct for 1 to 2 days, but because simpler *in vitro* techniques provide equal success, the rabbit oviduct is used more in research than for practical storage of embryos (Lawson et al., 1972a).

A large number of systems have been tested for culturing embryos at near body temperature (37°C). Conditions have differed according to the culture medium, additives to the culture medium, vessels in which cultures are carried out, and gaseous atmosphere. Reviews and descriptions of the various approaches are available (Seidel, 1977, 1981b; Anderson, 1978b; Wright and Bondioli, 1981). Generally, development to the blastocyst stage is considered the end point for most culture systems; development beyond the blastocyst stage requires conditions that have been identified only for laboratory species. Embryos in early cleavage stages, such as those collected with surgical techniques on Days 3–5 after estrus, are much more difficult to culture to the blastocyst stage than are Day-7 to Day-8 embryos collected nonsurgically. This is partly because of the time required to reach the blastocyst stage. A bovine embryo collected on Day 8 is likely to be a blastocyst and in culture will hatch from the zona pellucida; an eight-cell embryo collected on Day 3 will require at least 5 days and perhaps even longer to reach the blastocyst stage. Beyond the fact that early embryos must develop for longer periods *in vitro*, for as yet unexplained reasons early cleavages do not proceed *in vitro* as readily as the cell divisions and morphological transition from the morula to blastocyst stage. The development and acceptance of nonsurgical transfer, and consequent collection of blastocyst-stage embryos, have reduced the interest in culturing bovine embryos for more than a day or so. Modified phosphate-buffered saline (PBS) with heat-treated fetal calf serum is adequate for these short culture periods (Trounson et al., 1976c), allowing blastocysts to survive even at ambient temperatures (Trounson et al., 1976a). It should be remembered, however, that the requirements for maintaining viability for a day may be quite different from those for supporting continued development for a longer period of time. Thus, more sophisticated systems have been used for earlier stage embryos to be cultured for several days. Such culture systems generally employ bicarbonate-buffered media, energy substrates, serum or bovine serum albumin, and often vitamins and amino acids. An advantage has also been demonstrated for culturing bovine embryos under an atmosphere of 5% CO_2, 5% O_2, and 90% N_2. In such complex culture systems, bovine embryos have been shown to develop from early cleavage stages to hatched blastocysts (Wright *et al.*, 1976b,c). Although the blastocysts that developed in these systems appeared to be morphologically normal, viability was not tested by transferring the cultured embryos back to recipients. It is well known that viability of embryos from laboratory species tends to decrease with length of time in culture, even though apparently normal cleavage and morphology continue. Normal rates of pregnancy have been achieved with transfer of embryos cultured for 24 hr (Peters *et al.*, 1978; Schneider *et al.*, 1980; and others). Pregnancies have resulted from transfer of embryos cultured for longer periods (Tervit *et al.*, 1972; McKenzie and Kenney, 1973: Shea *et al.*, 1974), but further research is needed before it may be assumed that normal viability is maintained as long as normal morphology. A disturbing trend has recently been reported; in embryos cultured for 24 hr at 37°C, higher than usual embryonic losses occur between Days 21 and 60 of pregnancy (Renard *et al.*, 1980a,b). This, too, requires additional research to determine if the apparent trend is real.

Temperatures higher than approximately 20°C foster development in mammalian embryos. At lower temperatures, however, mitosis is halted, and embryos remain suspended at the stage of development at which they were cooled. Storage at refrigeration temperatures is effective for short periods, up to several days, whereas freezing in liquid nitrogen will maintain viability for an indefinite period of time. Premorula-stage bovine embryos do not survive refrigeration as well as later stage embryos (Trounson *et al.*, 1976b; Lindner *et al.*, 1982). Bovine blastocysts may be stored for 48 hr at 4°C in PBS supplemented with fetal calf serum without a significant loss in viability (BonDurant *et al.*, 1982). Survival is reduced to zero by 5 days at 4°C (Lindner *et al.*, 1983). It is interesting that embryos that have been refrigerated for 3 to 5 days tend to develop in culture at 37°C but not after transfer to recipients. Cells of the inner cell mass, from which the fetus will develop, are apparently more sensitive to low temperature than are trophoblast cells, which form placental membranes (Lindner *et al.*, 1982). Longer storage periods are probably possible with modifications of storage conditions. Successful short-term storage of embryos would be useful when the number of embryos collected exceeds the number of synchronized recipients available, but for this purpose viability after more than 2 days of storage is desirable.

The first successful freezing and thawing of mammalian embryos was achieved with mouse embryos (Whittingham, 1971). The first calf born from a frozen–thawed bovine embryo was reported shortly thereafter (Wilmut and Rowson, 1973). Improvements in survival after freezing have come about by altering cooling and rewarming rates, by altering the cryoprotectants used, and by making other modifications of earlier work (Trounson et al., 1978; Willadsen et al., 1978; Renard et al., 1981b; Smorag et al., 1981). A number of cryoprotectants have been demonstrated effective for bovine embryos, such as dimethyl sulfoxide, ethylene glycol, glycerol (Elsden et al., 1982), and propanediol (Renard et al., 1981a). Survival rates equivalent to those achieved with embryos frozen in glass ampules and tubes have been recently reported for plastic semen straws (Massip et al., 1979; Bouyssou and Chupin, 1982). This may facilitate the direct transfer of a frozen–thawed embryo without the intermediate step of transferring it from the freezing vessel to a straw for transfer to a recipient.

Despite the very encouraging results achieved to date, optimum survival of frozen–thawed bovine embryos has not yet been achieved. An embryo is capable of recovering from loss of some blastomeres, which will inevitably occur at times as a result of intracellular crystal formation. If a majority of the cells are damaged, the embryo may be unable to recover and viability will be lost. Often embryos are cultured at 37°C for a short time after thawing, and only those that develop *in vitro* or appear to be viable are transferred to recipients. Pregnancy rates after careful selection of frozen–thawed embryos are often as high as those of nonfrozen embryos, but are inflated compared to pregnancy rates based on all embryos frozen (Lehn-Jensen and Greve, 1982). Schneider et al. (1980) reported that of 68 frozen embryos, 34 were adjudged viable upon thawing. Of these 34 embryos, 23 resulted in pregnancy when transferred to recipients, or approximately one-third of the embryos frozen were capable of developing into calves. Both slightly higher and slightly lower survival rates have also been reported (Tervit and Elsden, 1981; Elsden et al., 1982). Improvements in methodology can be expected to continue, but at this time, freezing and thawing of bovine embryos result in the loss of some potential calves. Reviews of the development of embryo-freezing technology are available (Whittingham, 1977; Maurer, 1978).

B. Horses

The first pregnancy established by embryo transfer in horses was reported by Oguri and Tsutsumi (1974). Technical difficulties are not a major limitation of the technique; the large size and ease of dilatation of the mare's cervix make nonsurgical collection and transfer in some ways easier in the horse than in the cow. However, breed registries are reluctant to accept embryo transfer in horses, and therefore the incentives for development of a commercial industry have not been as great as for cattle. Registries that do allow registration of foals produced by embryo transfer have imposed restrictions as to which mares may be used as donors (e.g., only mares over a certain age and only those that have not produced a foal for several years in spite of repeated breedings) and on the number of foals (one) per breeding season that may be registered. Nevertheless, several commercial companies and research groups are actively working to improve embryo transfer technology for use in the horse.

1. Superovulation

Why superovulation is less effective in the mare than in females of the other domestic species is unknown. It may be related to the large size of the ovulating follicle relative to the ovulation fossa, a limitation difficult to overcome. There is also evidence that equine gonadotropins are different and have different actions than those of other species. For example, Irvine (1981) stated that instead of the FSH-like activity that is observed when used in other domestic animals, PMSG has LH-like activity in the mare. It may be that a satisfactory exogenous gonadotropin treatment for superovulation needs to be identified. Attempts to superovulate and synchronize ovulation in mares have been reviewed by Douglas (1979), Irvine (1981), and Woods *et al.* (1982). The use of crude and partially purified equine pituitary extracts has provided some success during both the anestrous (Douglas *et al.*, 1974) and the estrous seasons (Lapin and Ginther, 1977), inducing ovulation in more than 80% of the mares and multiple ovulations in over half of these. Whether these successes will improve the supply of equine embryos is still subject to some debate, however, following the report of preliminary data by Douglas (1979), in which rates of embryo recovery based on the number of ovulations were significantly lower in gonadotropin-treated mares than in controls. At this time, embryo transfer in horses is based primarily on collection and transfer of singly ovulated ova.

2. Embryo Collection and Transfer

Techniques for collecting and transferring equine embryos are based on modifications of procedures developed for cattle. Surgical and nonsurgical collection and transfer have been described by several researchers (Allen and Rowson, 1975; Douglas, 1979; Imel *et al.*, 1981b; Squires *et al.*, 1982). Nonsurgical collections are usually carried out 6–8 days after ovulation using a larger volume of medium (3 liters of PBS) than is used in cattle. Nonsurgical collections prior to Day 6 tend to be unsuccessful because the embryo has not yet moved into the uterus (Steffenhagen et al., 1972). By Day 8, equine embryos are macroscopic, and flushing of the uterus is discontinued when the embryo appears in the recovered medium. Nonsurgical recovery rates of singly ovulated ova as high as 90% have been reported (Oguri and Tsutsumi, 1974), although rates of 50 to 60% seem to be more common (Allen and Rowson, 1975; Castleberry et al., 1980; Griffin et al., 1981a; Squires et al., 1982). Because unfertilized ova are retained in the oviduct of the mare, recovery rates of embryos may be affected by the stallion used to breed the donor (Douglas, 1979). Squires et al. (1982) did not observe such an effect, but it would be expected to occur only if stallions of different fertility were used. As in cattle, a lower recovery rate of embryos occurs from infertile than fertile donors (Imel et al., 1981a).

To circumvent the problems of a limited supply of embryos due to difficulty of superovulation and the seasonal nature of their reproductive cycles, mares are often subjected to a schedule of intensive embryo collection. Single embryos may be collected during each estrous cycle. Griffin et al. (1981a) described a schedule in which embryos were collected every 2 weeks by initiating a new estrous cycle with prostaglandin immediately after collection. With this scheme, one mare was reported to have produced three embryos in 35 days. There are several reports that nonsurgical collection of embryos has no effect on subsequent fertility of the donor (Vogelsang et al., 1979; Tischner and Bielanski, 1980), but studies of fertility after repeated manipulation of the estrous cycle and embryo collection have not been reported.

Transfer of embryos by surgical means usually produces a higher pregnancy rate than nonsurgical transfer (50–60% versus approximately 25% or less) (Imel et al., 1981b; Castleberry et al., 1980). Squires et al. (1982) recently reported four of five recipients pregnant after surgical transfer via a flank approach. They also reported a significant effect of the technician on pregnancy after nonsurgical transfer; for one technician 46% of the attempted nonsurgical transfers resulted in pregnancy. An effect on pregnancy rate of the timing of embryo transfer has also been reported, but requires further study (Squires et al., 1982).

3. Storage of Embryos

Very little is known about the requirements for maintaining equine embryos *in vitro*, thus transfer to a recipient is usually accomplished as soon as possible. Phosphate-buffered saline is reported to be a satisfactory medium for short-term storage of embryos prior to transfer (Squires et al., 1982). Attempts to hold equine embryos *in vitro* for 24 hr in PBS have been largely unsuccessful (Imel et al., 1981c), although

Allen et al. (1976) were able to store equine embryos in the oviduct of the rabbit for approximately 48 hr. Griffin et al. (1981b) obtained one pregnancy from 19 frozen embryos, but the pregnancy was lost between Days 60 and 85 of gestation.

C. SHEEP

Embryo transfer in sheep has been used extensively in research for over 20 years (reviewed by Lawson, 1977). Purebred sheep have been successfully reproduced by embryo transfer (Tervit et al., 1976), but on a small scale commerically. Limited use of embryo transfer has been made to import new breeds and bloodlines (Hunter et al., 1962; Baker et al., 1971). The small size of the ewe makes nonsurgical techniques impractical, and therefore surgical collection and transfer, with their higher costs, are required. Currently, embryo transfer in sheep is only economically feasible in exceptional cases.

1. Superovulation

A variety of approaches have been used for superovulation and synchronization of estrus in sheep. Although various hormone treatments have been compared, the optimum has not been determined, and acceptable superovulation can be achieved with several combinations of gonadotropins and either progestogens (Anderson et al., 1981) or prostaglandins (Trounson et al., 1976a). Superovulation in sheep has been reviewed by Betteridge and Moore (1977). Most commonly used is PMSG, because a single injection is adequate to induce superovulation, but FSH or FSH plus LH (Bondioli and Wright, 1980) and HAP (Crosby et al., 1980) have also been used successfully. Lack of a standardized superovulation treatment among experiments makes a prediction of ovulation rate difficult, but a typical response may be 6–12 ovulations per ewe. Premature regression of corpora lutea resulting from superovulation has been reported (Tervit et al., 1976; Betteridge and Moore, 1977), which may affect recovery of embryos.

2. Embryo Collection and Transfer

Embryos are collected and transferred surgically while the donor and recipient are under general anesthesia. Flushing of the oviduct and tip of the uterine horn on Day 3 or 4 after estrus typically results in high embryo recovery rates. Two to six embryos per recipient have been transferred (Anderson et al., 1981). In general, the more embryos transferred the higher the percentage of recipients that become pregnant, but the lower the proportion of embryos that survive. Ovine embryos appear to tolerate asynchrony in donor and recipient estrous cycles as well as, or perhaps even better than, bovine embryos. This conclusion is based on a small number of transfers in sheep as compared to cattle (Rowson and Moor, 1966).

3. Storage of Embryos

Between collection from the donor and transfer to the recipient, ovine embryos may be stored at body temperature, at refrigeration temperatures (0–10°C), or in liquid nitrogen (−196°C). Sheep embryos will develop in culture at 37°C from early cleavage stages to the blastocyst stage in a relatively simple, defined, bicarbonate-buffered medium (Tervit and Rowson, 1974; Wright et al., 1976a; Peters et al., 1977; Wright and Bondioli, 1981). Lambs have been produced after transfer of embryos cultured for as long as 4 days (Tervit and Rowson, 1974). Ovine embryos will also survive in the ligated oviduct of the pseudopregnant rabbit. Retransfer of embryos to a sheep after 3 days in the rabbit resulted in high survival to birth: survival was reduced after 5 days in the rabbit (Lawson et al., 1972b). Sheep embryos will also survive at refrigeration temperatures (Moore and Bilton, 1973), as long as 10 days in one report (Kardymowicz, 1972), and develop to lambs after transfer to recipient ewes. Lambs have also been born from embryos frozen at −196°C and stored for a month or more (Willadsen et al., 1976).

D. GOATS

Embryo transfer has been used less in goats than in sheep, even though procedures and results are similar for the two species. Growing interest in enhanced reproduction of both high-producing dairy does and Angora does may result in substantially greater use of embryo transfer in the future.

1. Superovulation

Superovulation and synchronization of estrus have been accomplished with PMSG, FSH (Armstrong et al., 1982), FSH and LH (Bondioli and Wright, 1981), and HAP (Moore, 1974), in combination with prostaglandin or intravaginal progestogen sponges (Armstrong et al., 1982). As has been observed in ewes, does tend to display a higher superovulation response during the breeding season than during anestrus. Premature regression of corpora lutea in superovulated does may also affect embryo recovery rates (Armstrong et al., 1982). Depending on the superovulation treatment used, an average of five to eight kids per doe has been reported (Armstrong *et al.*, 1982). Moore and Eppleston (1979) reported only three kids per doe.

2. *Embryo Collection and Transfer*

Collection and transfer procedures in goats are similar to those used in sheep. Reluctance to subject lactating does to surgical collection may provide the impetus for developing an acceptable technique for nonsurgical embryo collection.

3. *Storage of Embryos*

Morulae and blastocysts have been cultured for 2 days at 37°C, stored at 5°C for 2 days, and frozen to −196°C for as long as a month (Bilton and Moore, 1976). In each case, survival was verified by the birth of kids after transfer to recipient does. Early cleavage-stage embryos do not develop in culture as readily as morulae and blastocysts (Wright and Bondioli, 1981).

E. SWINE

Embryo transfer is used in swine for both research (Dziuk, 1975; Dziuk and Day, 1977) and practical swine production (James and Reeser, 1979; Day, 1979). In addition to enhanced reproduction in valuable sows and international transport of genetic material, embryo transfer may also be important for introducing new animals into a closed swine herd. With greater emphasis on confinement systems of production, introduction of disease with new breeding animals is a serious consideration. Introducing new breeding stock as embryos transferable to sows in the existing herd may reduce the risks of disease outbreaks (Day, 1979).

1. *Superovulation*

Injection of 1200 to 1500 IU PMSG on Day 15 of the estrous cycle is successful in inducing approximately 30 ovulations (Guthrie *et al.*, 1974; Hunter, 1964, 1966). Embryos may also be collected from prepuberal gilts following injection of PMSG to stimulate follicular development and hCG to induce ovulation (Baker, 1979). These two gonadotropins may also be used to stimulate ovulation in lactating sows (James and Reeser, 1979). Even without superovulation, the high normal ovulation rate in swine allows collection of a large number of embryos.

2. Embryo Collection and Transfer

Both collection and transfer procedures are carried out surgically; attempts to use nonsurgical collection have been unsuccessful because of the tortuous nature of the cervix (Altenhof et al., 1982). Descriptions of the surgical collection and transfer procedures are given by Dziuk (1971) and Day (1979).

Even without nonsurgical embryo collection procedures available for swine, intensive collections have been carried out. James and Reeser (1979) described repeated collection at 3- to 6-week intervals on a group of gilts and sows. Embryos were collected as many as seven times per donor with no apparent effects on subsequent fertility. With the intensive schedule used, five surgical recoveries could be carried out over a 90-day period.

3. Storage of Embryos

Swine embryos may be successfully cultured *in vitro* at 37°C (Wright and Bondioli, 1981; Menino and Wright, 1982) or transferred to the rabbit oviduct (Polge et al., 1972). Attempts to store embryos at low temperatures have not yet been successful (Wilmut, 1972).

F. OTHER SPECIES

Information on embryo transfer in other species is limited. The technology described throughout this article is available for application to other species and has been recently reported for both the dog (Kinney et al., 1979) and the cat (Schriver and Kraemer, 1978). Kraemer et al. (1979) have provided a review of embryo transfer in nonhuman primates, which to date has been used primarily as a research tool. Durrant and Benirschke (1981) have reviewed the literature on interspecies embryo transfer; their special interest was in possibilities for preserving endangered species. It is hoped that superovulation of endangered females and transfer of their embryos to females of a related, more plentiful species may be a useful approach to revitalizing species facing extinction. Some individuals interested in interspecies tranfers are concerned that the phenotype of the embryo be unaffected by developing in a foreign species, that is, that the characteristics of the endangered species remain intact. Our knowledge of interspecies embryo transfer is increasing through research with nonendangered species. Examples include the transfer of African eland embryos to cattle (Dresser et al., 1982) and reciprocal transfers between horses and donkeys (Allen and Rowson, 1972) and between sheep and goats (Hancock and McGovern, 1963).

V. Future Developments in Embryo Transfer

Not long ago, without the tremendous advances in mammalian embryology, the following discussion would have seemed more appropriate for science fiction. The highly successful techniques currently used in cattle will continue to be extended to other species until equally high rates of success are achieved. Potential for improvements in existing technology still exists. High variability in the number of calves produced per donor is due primarily to the unpredictable response to superovulation. As understanding of the control of follicular development and ovulation is increased, we will be better able to collect a uniformly high number of embryos. Improvements are also needed in embryo storage systems, so that viability is not lost during freezing and thawing, or while the embryos are held for several days at body or refrigeration temperature. Major breakthroughs in superovulation and embryo storage have occurred; minor improvements that remain are likely to be made at a slow rate.

There are other areas where major achievements may be expected in embryo transfer technology. It is not currently possible to determine with a high degree of success the sex of an embryo prior to transfer. Sex chromosome analysis of cells from the chorion of Day 12–15 bovine embryos is reasonably successful; approximately 68% of the embryos can be sexed, but the large size of such embryos makes transfer difficult, and resulting pregnancy rates are unacceptable (Betteridge et al., 1982). Day-6 bovine morulae survive well after transfer, but determination of sex is difficult and less successful than with older embryos (Singh and Hare, 1980). Antibodies to H-Y antigen have recently been shown to be 86% effective in correctly identifying the sex of eight-cell mouse embryos (White et al., 1982). Betteridge et al. (1982) have reviewed methods of selecting the sex of an embryo to be transferred, including the possibility of altering the sex ratio by treatment of the semen.

The possibility also exists for harvesting a larger number of oocytes from the ovary than can be obtained with superovulation. Most females have many times more oocytes than will be ovulated naturally. Freed from the follicle, resting oocytes resume meiosis *in vitro* and may be capable of being fertilized, although few young of any species have been produced from oocytes matured *in vitro*. Such oocytes may be fertilized by transfer to the oviduct of a female of the same species (Trounson et al., 1977) or of another species (xenogenous fertilization) (Hirst et al., 1981), or in vitro. Most current efforts to fertilize in vitro (reviewed by Brackett, 1981a,b) deal with oocytes collected shortly before or shortly after ovulation, after oocyte maturation has occurred in vivo. Viable young born from in vitro–fertilized ova from domestic animals have been limited to laboratory species, except for one report of the birth of a calf (Brackett et al., 1982). The success being achieved with fertilization of human ova in vitro surpasses what is currently possible in large domestic animals (Steptoe and Edwards, 1978; Trounson et al., 1980).

The production of clones in domestic animals may also soon be reality (Markert and Seidel, 1982). Production of identical twins by splitting embryos is highly successful in both sheep and cattle (Willadsen, 1979; Willadsen et al., 1981; Williams et al., 1982). In fact, split ovine embryos have been frozen for later transfer, resulting in the birth of identical offspring several months apart (Willadsen, 1980). Clones of desirable animals may also be produced by nuclear transplantation; successful transfer of nuclei from embryonic tissue has been carried out in mice by Illmensee and Hoppe (1981). Offspring produced by nuclear transplants were previously limited to non-mammalian species (McKinnell, 1982).

Homozygous diploid mice have been produced by removal of either the male or the female pronucleus from a fertilized zygote (Hoppe and Illmensee, 1977; Markert and Petters, 1977). The micromanipulation techniques required for such a feat may well be applied to embryos of large domestic animals. Homozygous offspring have yet to be produced in mammals by induced parthenogenesis. The practical advantages for producing single-parent homozygous offspring from genetically superior males and females are unknown.

Exciting possibilities exist for use of gene transfer in domestic animals, which will depend on use of embryo transfer technology. The first successful gene transfer in mammals was recently reported by Wagner et al. (1981). Use of gene transfer in food-producing animals for the benefit of humanity is likely to be some years away. Few major genes affecting production traits in domestic animals have as yet been identified. The physiological effects of genes that have been isolated and are under investigation (e.g., the gene for growth hormone) have not been studied adequately to determine whether transfer of such genes will have beneficial effects. Their potential may rest with production of gene products in the laboratory. The achievements made in embryo transfer to date are phenomenal, and progress continues to be made in the field, providing us with useful tools in the understanding and cultivation of food animals and beneficial animal products.

ACKNOWLEDGEMENTS

The assistance of S. E. Donahue, M. B. Horton, and S. Winkler in preparation of this manuscript is gratefully acknowledged. The large volume of scientific literature dealing with various phases of embryo transfer precludes reference to all relevant articles in this review. Apologies are extended to investigators whose important contributions to development of today's embryo transfer technology have been omitted.

REFERENCES

Allen, W. R., and Rowson, L. E. A. (1972). *Proc. Int. Congr. Anim. Reprod. Artif. Insemin., 7th, 1972* Vol 1, pp. 483–488.
Allen, W. R., and Rowson, L. E. A. (1975). *J. Reprod. Fertil., Suppl.* **23,** 525–530.
Allen, W. R., Francesca, S., Trounson, A. L., Tischner, M., and Bielanski, W. (1976). *J. Reprod. Fertil.* **47,** 387–390.
Altenhof, R. L., Tanksley, T. D., Jr., Knabe, D. A., Harms, P. G., Bowen, M. J., and Kraemer, D. L. (1982). *Theriogenology* **17,** 75.
Anderson, G. B. (1978a). *Theriogenology* **9,** 3–16.
Anderson, G. B. (1978b). *In* "Methods in Mammalian Reproduction" (J. C. Daniel, Jr., ed.), pp. 273–283. Academic Press, New York.
Anderson, G. B., Cupps, P. T., Drost, M., Horton, M. B., and Wright, R. W., Jr. (1978). *J. Anim. Sci.* **46,** 449–452.
Anderson, G. B., Cupps, P. T., and Drost, M. (1979). *J. Anim. Sci.* **49,** 1037–1042.
Anderson, G. B., Bradford, G. E., and Cupps, P. T. (1981). *Theriogenology* **16,** 119–129.
Anderson, G. B., BonDurant, R. H., and Cupps, P. T. (1982). *J. Anim. Sci.* **54,** 485–490.
Armstrong, D. T., Pfitzner, A. P., and Seamark, R. F. (1982). *Theriogenology* **17,** 76.
Baker, R. D. (1979). *Theriogenology* **11,** 91.
Baker, R. D., Webel, S., Ellicott, A., and Dzuik, P. J. (1971). *Can. J. Anim. Sci.* **51,** 542–543.
Bedirian, K. N., Mills, M. S., Bligh, P. J., Geroldi, R., and Kilmer, B. A. (1979). *Theriogenology* **11,** 3–4.
Betteridge, K. J. (1977). "Embryo Transfer in Farm Animals," Monogr. 16. Canada Department of Agriculture, Ottawa.
Betteridge, K. J. (1981). *J. Reprod. Fertil.* **62,** 1–13.
Betteridge, K. J., and Moore, N. W. (1977). *In* "Embryo Transfer in Farm Animals" (K. J. Betteridge, ed.), Monogr. 16, pp. 37–38. Canada Department of Agriculture, Ottawa.
Betteridge, K. J., Hare, W. C. D., and Singh, E. L. (1982). *In* "New Technologies in Animal Breeding" (B. G. Brackett, G. E. Seidel, Jr., and S. M. Seidel, eds.), pp. 109–125. Academic Press, New York.
Bilton, R. J., and Moore, N. W. (1976). *Aust. J. Biol. Sci.* **29,** 125–129.
Boland, M. P., Kennedy, L. G., Crosby, T. F., and Gordon, I. (1981). *Theriogenology* **15,** 110.
Bondioli, K. R., and Wright, R. W., Jr. (1980). *Theriogenology* **13,** 89.
Bondioli, K. R., and Wright, R. W., Jr. (1981). *Theriogenology* **15,** 118.
BonDurant, R. H., Anderson, G. B., Boland, M. P., Cupps, P. T., and Hughes, M. A. (1982). *Theriogenology* **17,** 223–230.

Bouyssou, B., and Chupin, D. (1982). *Theriogenology* **17**, 80.
Brackett, B. G. (1981). *In* "Fertilization and Embryonic Development *in Vitro*" (L. Mastroianni, Jr. and J. Biggers, eds.), pp. 61–79. Plenum. New York.
Brackett, B. G. (1982). *In* "New Technologies in Animal Breeding" (B. G. Brackett, G. E. Seidel, Jr., and S. M. Seidel, eds.), pp. 141–161. Academic Press, New York.
Brackett, B. G., Bousquet, D., Boice, M. L., Donawick, W. J., Evans, J. F., and Dressel, M. A. (1982). *Biol. Reprod.* **27**, 147–158.
Bradford, G. E., and Kennedy, B. W. (1980). *Theriogenology* **13**, 13–26.
Bradford, G. E., Hart, R., Quirke, J. F., and Land, R. B. (1972). *J. Reprod. Fertil.* **30**, 459–463.
Brand, A., Aarts, M. H., Zaayer, D., and Oxender, W. D. (1978). *In* "Control of Reproduction in the Cow" (J. M. Sreenan, ed.) pp. 281–291. Nijhoff, The Hague.
Bulman, D. C., and Lamming, G. E. (1979). *Br. Vet. J.* **135**, 559–567.
Carmichael, R. A. (1980). *Theriogenology* **13**, 3–6.
Castleberry, R. S., Schneider, H. J., Jr., and Griffin, J. L. (1980). *Theriogenology* **13**, 90.
Christie, W. B., Newcomb, R., and Rowson, L. E. A. (1979). *J. Reprod. Fertil.* **56**, 701–706.
Cole, H. H., Bigelow, M., Finkel, J., and Rupp, G. R. (1967). *Endocrinology* **81**, 927–930.
Crosby, T. F., Boland, M. P., El-Kamali, A. A., and Gordon, I. (1980). *Theriogenology* **13**, 92.
Curtis, J. L., Elsden, R. P., and Seidel, G. E., Jr. (1981). *Theriogenology* **15**, 124.
Danner, M. L., and Oxender, W. D. (1980). *Theriogenology* **13**, 94.
Day, B. N. (1979). *Theriogenology* **11**, 27–31.
de los Santos-Valadez, S., Tervit, H. R., Elsden, R. P., and Seidel, G. E., Jr. (1981). *Theriogenology* **15**, 123.
de los Santos-Valadez, S., Seidel, G. E., Jr., and Elsden, R. P. (1982). *Theriogenology* **17**, 85.
Douglas, R. H. (1979). *Theriogenology* **11**, 33–46.
Douglas, R. H., Nuti, L., and Ginther, O. J. (1974). *Theriogenology* **2**, 133–142.
Dresser, B. L., Kramer, L., Pope, C. E., Dahlhausen, R. D., and Blauser, C. (1982). *Theriogenology* **17**, 86.
Drost, M., Brand, A., and Aarts, M. H. (1976). *Theriogenology* **6**, 503–507.
Durrant, B., and Benirschke, K. (1981). *Theriogenology* **15**, 77–83.
Dziuk, P. J. (1971). *In* "Methods in Mammalian Embryology" (J. C. Daniel, Jr., ed.), pp. 76–85. Freeman, San Francisco, California.
Dziuk, P. J. (1975). *BioScience* **25**, 102–104.
Dziuk, P. J., and Day, D. N. (1977). *In* "Embryo Transfer in Farm Animals" (K. J. Betteridge, ed.), Monogr. 16, pp. 78–79. Canada Department of Agriculture, Ottawa.
Elsden, R. P. (1977a). *In* "Embryo Transfer in Farm Animals" (K. J. Betteridge, ed.), Monogr. 16. pp. 10–13. Canada Department of Agriculture, Ottawa.
Elsden, R. P. (1977b). *In* "Embryo Transfer in Farm Animals" (K. J. Betteridge, ed.), Monogr. 16. pp. 27–28. Canada Department of Agriculture, Ottawa.
Elsden, R. P., Lewis, S., Cumming, I. A., and Lawson, R. A. S. (1974). *J. Reprod. Fertil.* **36**, 455–456.
Elsden, R. P., Hasler, J. F., and Seidel, G. E., Jr. (1976). *Theriogenology* **6**, 523–532.
Elsden, R. P., Nelson, L. D., and Seidel, G. E., Jr. (1978). *Theriogenology* **9**, 17–26.
Elsden, R. P., Nelson, L. D., and Seidel, G. E., Jr. (1979). *Theriogenology* **11**, 17–25.
Elsden, R. P., Seidel, G. E., Jr., Takeda, T., and Farrand, G. D. (1982). *Theriogenology* **17**, 1–10.
Evans, J. F., Hesseltive, G. R., and Kenney, R. M. (1979). *Theriogenology* **11**, 97.

Garcia, G. J. K., Seidel, G. E., Jr., and Elsden, R. P. (1982). *Theriogenology* **17**, 90.
Gordon, I. (1975). *Ir. Vet. J.* **29**, 21–30, 39–62.
Gordon, I., and Boland, M. P. (1979). *Vet. Sci. Commun.* **3**, 177–186.
Gordon, I., Williams, G., and Edwards, J. (1962). *J. Agric. Sci.* **59**, 143–197.
Greve, T. (1976). *Theriogenology* **5**, 15–19.
Greve, T., and Lehn-Jensen, H. (1979). *Acta Vet Scand.* **20**, 135–144.
Greve, T., and Lehn-Jensen, H. (1982). *Theriogenology* **17**, 91.
Griffin, J. L., Castleberry, R. S., and Schneider, H. S., Jr. (1981a). *Theriogenology* **15**, 105.
Griffin, J. L., Castleberry, R. S., and Schneider, H. S., Jr. (1981b). *Theriogenology* **15**, 106.
Guthrie, H. D., Henricks, D. M., and Handlin, D. L. (1974). *J. Reprod. Fertil.* **41**, 361–370.
Hahn, J., and Hahn, R. (1976). *In* "Egg Transfer in Cattle" (L. E. A. Rowson, ed.), EEC Publ. EUR5491, pp. 199–204. Comm. Eur. Commun., Luxembourg.
Hancock, J. L., and McGovern, P. T. (1963). *Res. Vet. Sci.* **9**, 411–415.
Hasler, J. F. (1978). *Theriogenology* **9**, 94.
Heape, W. (1891). *Proc. R. Soc. London* **48**, 457–458.
Heape, W. (1897). *Proc. R. London* **62**, 178–183.
Hirst, P. J., DeMayo, F. J., and Dukelow, W. R. (1981). *Theriogenology* **15**, 67–75.
Holtz, W., Herrmann, H. H., and Voss, H. J. (1979). *Theriogenology* **12**, 197–205.
Hoppe, P. C., and Illmensee, K. (1977). *Proc. Natl. Acad. Sci. U.S.A.* **74**, 5657–5661.
Horton, M. B., Anderson, G. B., BonDurant, R. H., and Cupps, P. T. (1980). *Theriogenology* **14**, 443–451.
Humphrey, W. D., Murphy, B. D., Rieger, D., Mapletoft, R. J., Manns, J. G., and Fretz, P. B. (1979). *Theriogenology* **11**, 101.
Hunter, G. L., Bishop, G. P., Adams, C. E., and Rowson, L. E. A. (1962). *J. Reprod. Fertil.* **3**, 33–40.
Hunter, R. H. F. (1964). *Anim. Prod.* **6**, 189–194.
Hunter, R. H. F. (1966). *Anim. Prod.* **8**, 457–465.
Illmensee, K., and Hoppe, P. C. (1981). *Cell* **23**, 9–18.
Imel, K. J., Squires, E. L., and Shideler, R. K. (1981a). *Theriogenology* **15**, 107.
Imel, K. J., Squires, E. L., Elsden, R. P., and Schdeler, R. K. (1981b). *J. Am. Vet. Med. Assoc.* **179**, 987–991.
Imel, K. J., Squires, E. L., Elsden, R. P., and Shideler, R. K. (1981c). *Proc. 73rd Annu. Meet. Am. Soc. Anim. Sci.* Abstract 508.
Irvine, C. H. G. (1981). *Theriogenology* **15**, 85–104.
James, J. E., and Reeser, P. O. (1979). *Theriogenology* **11**, 47–50.
Jensen, A. M., and Greve, T. (1980). *Theriogenology* **13**, 98.
Jillella, D., and Baker, A. A. (1978). *Vet. Rec.* **103**, 574–576.
Johnson, J. L., Leipold, H. W., Snider, G. W., and Baker, R. D. (1980). *J. Am. Vet. Med. Assoc.* **176**, 549–550.
Kardymowicz, O. (1972). *Proc. Int. Congr. Anim. Reprod. Artif. Insemin., 7th, 1972* Vol. 1, pp. 499–502.
Kinney, G. M., Pennycook, J. W., Schriver, M. D., Templeton, J. W., and Kraemer, D. C. (1979). *Biol. Reprod.* **20**, Suppl. 1, 96.
Kraemer, D. C., Flow, B. L., Schriver, M. D., Kinney, G. M., and Pennycook, J. W. (1979). *Theriogenology* **11**, 51–62.
Kummerfeld, H. L., Oltenacu, E. A. B., and Foote, R. H. (1978). *J. Dairy Sci.* **51**, 1773–1777.
Kunkel, R. N. (1979). *Theriogenology* **11**, 102.

Kunkel, R. N., and Stricklin, W. R. (1978). *Theriogenology* **9**, 96.
Kvasnickii, A. V. (1951). *Anim. Breed. Abstr.* **19**, 224.
Lapin, D. R., and Ginther, O. J. (1977). *J. Anim. Sci.* **44**, 834–842.
Lawson, R. A. S. (1977). *In* "Embryo Transfer in Farm Animals" (K. J. Betteridge, ed.), Monogr. 16, pp. 72–78. Canada Department of Agriculture, Ottawa.
Lawson, R. A. S., Rowson, L. E. A., and Adams, C. E. (1972a). *J. Reprod. Fertil.* **28**, 313–315.
Lawson, R. A. S., Adams, C. E., and Rowson, L. E. A. (1972b). *J. Reprod. Fertil.* **29**, 105–116.
Lehn-Jensen, H., and Greve, T. (1982). *Theriogenology* **17**, 95.
Lindner, G. M., Anderson, G. B., BonDurant, R. H., and Cupps, P. T. (1983). Theriogenology (in press).
Looney, C. R., Boutte, B. W., Archbald, L. F., and Godke, R. A. (1981). *Theriogenology* **15**, 13–22.
Looney, C. R., Hill, K. G., Thompson, D. L., Jr., Archbald, L. F., and Godke, R. A. (1982). *Theriogenology* **17**, 97.
Lubbadeh, W. F., Graves, C. N., and Spahr, S. L. (1980). *J. Anim. Sci.* **50**, 124–127.
McKenzie, B. E., and Kenney, R. M. (1973). *Am. J. Vet. Res.* **34**, 1271–1275.
McKinnell, R. G. (1982). *In* "New Technologies in Animal Breeding" (B. G. Brackett, G. E. Seidel, Jr., and S. M. Seidel, eds.) pp. 163–180. Academic Press, New York.
Markert, C. L., and Petters, R. M. (1977). *J. Exp. Zool.* **201**, 295–302.
Markert, C. L., and Seidel, G. E., Jr. (1982). *In* "New Technologies in Animal Breeding" (B. G. Brackett, G. E. Seidel, Jr., and S. M. Seidel, eds.), pp. 181–200. Academic Press, New York.
Markette, K. L., Seidel, G. E., Jr., and Elsden, R. P. (1980). *Theriogenology* **13**, 105.
Massip, A., Van der Zwalmen, P., Ectors, F., De Coster, R., D'Ieteren, G., and Hanzen, C. (1979). *Theriogenology* **12**, 79–84.
Maurer, R. R. (1978). *Theriogenology* **9**, 45–68.
Maxwell, D. P., Massey, J. M., and Kraemer, D. C. (1978). *Theriogenology* **9**, 97.
Menino, A. R., Jr., and Wright, R. W., Jr. (1982). *J. Anim. Sci.* **54**, 583–588.
Moore, N. W. (1974). *Proc. Aust. Soc. Anim. Prod.* **10**, 246–249.
Moore, N. W., and Bilton, R. J. (1973). *Aust. J. Biol. Sci.* **26**, 1421–1427.
Moore, N. W., and Eppleston, J. (1979). *Aust. J. Agric. Res.* **30**, 973–981.
Nelson, L. D., Elsden, R. P., Case, L. G., and Homan, N. R. (1978). *Theriogenology* **9**, 98.
Nelson, L. D., Seidel, G. E., Jr., and Elsden, R. P. (1979). *Theriogenology* **11**, 104.
Nelson, L. D., Elsden, R. P., and Seidel, G. E., Jr. (1982). *Theriogenology* **17**, 101.
Newcomb, R. (1979). *Vet. Rec.* **105**, 432–434.
Newcomb, R., and Rowson, L. E. A. (1975). *Vet. Rec.* **96**, 468–469.
Newcomb, R., and Rowson, L. E. A. (1980). *Theriogenology* **13**, 41–49.
Newcomb, R., Christie, W. B., Rowson, L. E. A., Walters, D. E., and Bousfield, W. E. D. (1979). *J. Reprod. Fertil.* **56**, 113–118.
Newcomb, R., Christie, W. B., and Rowson, L. E. A. (1980). *J. Reprod. Fertil.* **59**, 31–36.
Oguri, N., and Tsutsumi, Y. (1974). *J. Reprod. Fertil.* **41**, 313–320.
Ozil, J. P., Heyman, Y., and Renard, J. P. (1979). *Theriogenology* **11**, 173–183.
Peters, D. F., Anderson, G. B., and Cupps, P. T. (1977). *J. Anim. Sci.* **45**, 350–354.
Peters, D. F., Anderson, G. B., BonDurant, R., Cupps, P. T., and Drost, M. (1978). *Theriogenology* **10**, 337–342.
Polge, C., Adams, C. E., and Baker, R. D. (1972). *Proc. Int. Congr. Anim. Reprod. Artif. Insemin., 7th, 1972* Vol. 1, pp. 513–517.
Price, E. O., Thos, J., and Anderson, G. B. (1981). *J. Anim. Sci.* **53**, 934–939.
Renard, J.-P., Heyman, Y., and Ozil, J.-P. (1980a). *Vet. Rec.* **107**, 152–153.

Renard, J.-P., Heyman, Y. and Ozil, J.-P. (1980b). *Theriogenology* **13**, 109.
Renard, J.-P., Philippon, A., and Menezo, Y. (1980c). *J. Reprod. Fertil.* **58**, 161–164.
Renard, J.-P., Heyman, Y., and Ozil, J.-P. (1981a). *Theriogenology* **15**, 113.
Renard, J.-P., Ozil, J.-P., and Heyman, Y. (1981b). *Theriogenology* **15**, 311–320.
Renard, J.-P., Menezo, Y., and Heyman, Y. (1982). *Theriogenology* **17**, 106.
Rowe, R. F., Del Campo, M. R., Eilts, C. L., French, L. R., Winch, R. P., and Ginther, O. J. (1976). *Theriogenology* **6**, 471–483.
Rowe, R. F., Critser, J. K., and Ginther, O. J. (1979). *Theriogenology* **11**, 107.
Rowe, R. F., Del Campo, M. R., Critser, J. K., and Ginther, O. J. (1980a). *Am. J. Vet. Res.* **41**, 106–108.
Rowe, R. F., Del Campo, M. R., Critser, J. K., and Ginther, O. J. (1980b). *Am. J. Vet. Res.* **41**, 1024–1028.
Rowson, L. E. A., and Moor, R. M. (1966). *J. Reprod. Fertil.* **11**, 207–212.
Rowson, L. E. A., Moor, R. M., and Lawson, R. A. S. (1969). *J. Reprod. Fertil.* **18**, 517–523.
Rowson, L. E. A., Lawson, R. A. S., and Moor, R. M. (1971). *J. Reprod. Fertil.* **25**, 261–268.
Rowson, L. E. A., Lawson, R. A. S., Moor, R. M., and Baker, A. A. (1972). *J. Reprod. Fertil.* **28**, 427–431.
Saumande, J., and Chupin, D. (1981). *Theriogenology* **15**, 108.
Schilling, E., Niemann, H., Cheng, S. P., and Doepke, H. H. (1979a). *Zuechthyg.* **14**, 170–172.
Schilling, E., Smidt, D., Sacher, B., Petac, D., and El Kaschab, S. (1979b). *Ann. Biol. Anim., Biochim., Biophys.* **19**, 1625–1629.
Schneider, H. J., Jr., Castleberry, R. S., and Griffin, J. L. (1980). *Theriogenology* **13**, 73–85.
Schriver, M. D., and Kraemer, D. C. (1978). *Am. Assoc. Lab. Anim. Sci. Publ.* **78–4**, 12.
Schultz, R. H. (1980). *Theriogenology* **13**, 7–11.
Seidel, G. E., Jr. (1977). *In* "Embryo Transfer in Farm Animals" (K. J. Betteridge, ed.), Monogr. 16, pp. 20–24. Canada Department of Agriculture, Ottawa.
Seidel, G. E., Jr. (1981a). *Science* **211**, 351–358.
Seidel, G. E., Jr. (1981b). *In* "Fertilization and Embryonic Development *in Vitro*" (L. Mastroianni, Jr. and J. D. Biggers, eds), pp. 323–353. Plenum, New York.
Seidel, G. E., Jr., and Seidel, S. M. (1982). *In* "New Technology in Animal Breeding" (B. G. Brackett, G. E. Seidel, Jr., and S. M. Seidel, eds.), pp. 41–80. Academic Press, New York.
Shea, B. F. (1981). *Theriogenology* **15**, 31–42.
Shea, B. F., Church, R. B., and Tervit, R. (1974). *Proc. 7th Ann. Meeting Soc. Study Reprod.* Abstract 147.
Shelton, J. N., Heath, T. D., Old, K. G., and Turnbull, G. E. (1979). *Theriogenology* **11**, 149–152.
Shelton, J. N., Heath, T. D., Turnbull, G. E., and Old, K. G. (1980). *Vet. Rec.* **106**, 514.
Singh, E. L., and Hare, W. C. D. (1980). *Theriogenology* **13**, 421–427.
Smorag, K., Katska, L., and Wierzchos, E. (1981). *Anim. Reprod. Sci.* **4**, 65–72.
Squires, E. L., Iuliano, M. F., and Shideler, R. K. (1982). *Theriogenology* **17**, 35–41.
Sreenan, J. M. (1978). *Theriogenology* **9**, 69–83.
Sreenan, J. M., and Beehan, D. (1976). *In* "Egg Transfer in Cattle" (L. E. A. Rowson, ed.), EEC Publ. EUR5491, pp. 19–34. Comm. Eur. Commun., Luxembourg.
Sreenan, J. M., and Gosling, J. P. (1977). *J. Reprod. Fertil.* **50**, 367–369.
Steffenhagen, W. P., Pineda, M. H., and Ginther, O. J. (1972). *Am. J. Vet. Res.* **33**, 2391–2398.

Steptoe, P. C., and Edwards, R. G. (1978). *Lancet* **1**, 366.
Stewart, F., Allen, W. R., and Moor, R. M. (1976). *J. Endocrinol.* **71**, 371–382.
Sugie, T., Soma, T., Fukumitsu, S., and Otsuki, K. (1972). *Natl. Inst. Anim. Ind. Bull.* **25**, 27–34.
Tervit, H. R., and Elsden, R. P. (1981). *Theriogenology* **15**, 395–403.
Tervit, H. R., and Rowson, L. E. A. (1974). *J. Reprod. Fertil.* **38**, 177–179.
Tervit, H. R., Whittingham, D. G., and Rowson, L. E. A. (1972). *J. Reprod. Fertil.* **30**, 493–497.
Tervit, H. R., Rowson, L. E. A., and Brand, A. (1973). *J. Reprod. Fertil.* **34**, 179–181.
Tervit, H. R., Allison, A. J., Smith, J. F., Harvey, T. M., and Havik, P. G. (1976). *Proc. N. Z. Soc. Anim. Prod.* **36**, 67–75.
Tervit, H. R., Cooper, M. W., Goold, P. G., and Haszard, G. M. (1980). *Theriogenology* **13**, 63–72.
Tischner, M., and Bielanski, A. (1980). *J. Reprod. Fertil.* **58**, 357–361.
Trounson, A. O., Willadsen, S. M., and Moor, R. M. (1976a). *J. Agric. Sci.* **86**, 609–611.
Trounson, A. O., Willadsen, S. M., Rowson, L. E. A., and Newcomb, R. (1976b). *J. Reprod. Fertil.* **46**, 173–178.
Trounson, A. O., Willadsen, S. M., and Rowson, L. E. A. (1976c). *J. Reprod. Fertil.* **47**, 367–370.
Trounson, A. O., Willadsen, S. M., and Rowson, L. E. A. (1977). *J. Reprod. Fertil.* **51**, 321–327.
Trounson, A. O., Shea, B. F., Ollis, G. W., and Jacobson, M. E. (1978). *J. Anim. Sci.* **47**, 677–681.
Trounson, A. O., Leeton, J. F., Wood, C., Webb, J., and Wood, J. (1980). *Science* **221**, 681–682.
Van Vleck, L. D. (1982). *In* "New Technologies in Animal Breeding" (B. G. Brackett, G. E. Seidel, Jr., and S. M. Seidel, eds.), pp. 221–242. Academic Press, New York.
Vogelsang, S. G., Sorensen, A. M., Jr., Potter, G. D., Burns, S. J., and Kraemer, D. C. (1979). *J. Reprod. Fertil. Suppl.* **27**, 383–386.
Wagner, T. E., Hoppe, P. C., Jollick, J. D., Scholl, D. R., Hodinka, R. L., and Gault, J. B. (1981). *Proc. Natl. Acad. Sci. U.S.A.* **78**, 6376–6380.
Warwick, B. L., Berry, R. O., and Horlacher, W. R. (1934). *Proc. Am. Soc. Anim. Prod.* **27**, 225–227.
Waters, H. A. (1981). *Theriogenology* **15**, 57–66.
Wheeler, M. B., Anderson, G. B., BonDurant, R. H., and Stabenfeldt, G. H. (1982). *J. Anim. Sci.* **54**, 589–593.
White, K. L., Lindner, G. M., Anderson, G. B., and BonDurant, R. H. (1982). *Theriogenology* **18**, 655–662.
Whittingham, D. G. (1971). *Nature (London)* **233**, 125–126.
Whittingham, D. G. (1977). *In* "Embryo Transfer in Farm Animals" (K. G. Betteridge, ed.), Monogr. 16, pp. 50–53. Canada Department of Agriculture, Ottawa.
Willadsen, S. M. (1979). *Nature (London)* **277**, 298–300.
Willadsen, S. M. (1980). *J. Reprod. Fertil.* **59**, 357–362.
Willadsen, S. M., Polge, C., Rowson, L. E. A., and Moor, R. M. (1976). *J. Reprod. Fertil.* **46**, 151–154.
Willadsen, S. M., Polge, C., and Rowson, L. E. A. (1978). *J. Reprod. Fertil.* **52**, 391–393.
Willadsen, S. M., Lehn-Jensen, H., Fehilly, C. B., and Newcomb, R. (1981). *Theriogenology* **15**, 23–29.
Willett, E. L., Black, W. G., Casida, L. E., Stone, W. H., and Buckner, P. J. (1951). *Science* **113**, 247.
Williams, T. J., Elsden, R. P., and Seidel, G. E., Jr. (1982). *Theriogenology* **17**, 114.

Wilmut, I. (1972). *J. Reprod. Fertil.* **31,** 513–514.
Wilmut, I., and Hume, A. (1978). *Vet. Rec.* **103,** 107–110.
Wilmut, I., and Rowson, L. E. A. (1973). *J. Reprod. Fertil.* **33,** 352–353.
Woods, G. L., Scraba, S. T., and Ginther, O. J. (1982). *Theriogenology* **17,** 61–72.
Wright, J. M. (1981). *Theriogenology* **15,** 43–56.
Wright, R. W., Jr., and Bondioli, K. R. (1981). *J. Anim. Sci.* **53,** 702–729.
Wright, R. W., Jr., Anderson, G. B., Cupps, P. T., Drost, M., and Bradford, G. E. (1976a). *J. Anim. Sci.* **42,** 912–917.
Wright, R. W., Jr., Anderson, G. B., Cupps, P. T., and Drost, M. (1976b). *Biol. Reprod.* **14,** 157–162.
Wright, R. W., Jr., Anderson, G. B., Cupps, P. T., and Drost, M. (1976c). *J. Anim. Sci.* **43,** 170–174.

Immune-Mediated Diseases of the Blood

W. JEAN DODDS

Division of Laboratories and Research, New York State Department of Health, Albany, New York

I. Introduction ... 163
II. Clinical Signs ... 165
III. Diagnosis ... 166
    A. History ... 166
    B. Clinicopathological Tests ... 167
    C. Serial Monitoring ... 173
IV. Findings ... 173
    A. Family and Breed Histories ... 173
    B. Case Histories ... 178
V. Predisposing Factors ... 178
    A. Increased Frequency ... 180
    B. Sex Predisposition ... 181
    C. Breed Predisposition ... 181
    D. Genetic Influences ... 181
    E. Relationship to Viral Infections and Vaccinations ... 182
    F. Hormonal Influences ... 187
    G. Drug Reactions ... 188
    H. Stress and Underlying Disease ... 189
VI. Management and Treatment ... 190
    A. Red Cell Disorders ... 190
    B. Platelet Disorders ... 192
VII. Prevention ... 194
    References ... 195

I. Introduction

The immune-mediated and true autoimmune diseases of humans and animals comprise a group of poorly understood disorders in which antibodies are produced against tissues of the body, thus violating the premise of immune self-tolerance (Dacie, 1967; Dacie and Worlledge, 1968; Schalm et al., 1975; Dodds, 1977; Tizard, 1977; Halliwell, 1978). In true autoimmune disease, a rare entity, the host's immune system goes awry and reacts against its own body. The mechanism for this failure to recognize self is unclear, so that the prognosis for survival on a long-term basis is frequently guarded or unfavorable. In the immune-mediated situation, in contrast, the chances for recovery are much better if the causative agent or trigger of the immune reaction can be identified and removed. In common usage, the term autoimmune disease is loosely applied to most types of immunological disorders of the blood and tissues, although this is technically incorrect as most cases are, in fact, immune mediated. For purposes of this article, therefore, the term immune mediated is preferred.

One of the oldest recognized immune-mediated diseases of both humans and dogs is called autoimmune hemolytic anemia (Dacie, 1967; Schalm, 1975). The clinical entity was known long before the immunological basis of the pathogenesis was understood (Bielschowsky et al., 1959; Videbaek, 1962; Fialkow, 1964; Dobbs, 1965; Robbins et al., 1969). In autoimmune hemolytic disease (AIHD) the antibodies formed are directed against the red blood cell and are best demonstrated by the direct Coombs' antiglobulin test (Dacie, 1967; Williams et al., 1972; Schalm, 1975; Schultz, 1976; Dodds, 1977; Tizard, 1977, 1978; Halliwell, 1978; Slappendel, 1979). Diagnosis is based on a positive Coombs' test, the finding of a responsive bone marrow, and a history that rules out other underlying causes of hemolysis, such as transfusion and sepsis, as well as intrinsic red cell abnormalities such as pyruvate kinase deficiency.

In addition to producing antibodies targeted against red cells, immune-mediated diseases frequently elicit antiplatelet antibodies with resultant thrombocytopenia (Oski and Naiman, 1966; Bachand et al., 1967; Williams et al., 1972; Wilkins et al., 1973; Karpatkin, 1980). The most commonly affected animal species are the dog, horse, and cat (Dodds and Wilkins, 1977; Halliwell, 1978; Byars and Greene, 1982). On average, about two-thirds of the chronic, recurrent thrombocytopenias of humans and animals have an immunological basis (Williams et al., 1972; Wilkins et al., 1973; Schalm et al., 1975; Dodds and Wilkins, 1977; Halliwell, 1978; Karpatkin, 1980; Wilkins and Hurvitz, 1981; Dodds, 1982). Antiplatelet antibodies and/or thrombocytopenia may be associated with antierythrocyte antibodies and/or anemia, or can occur in the absence of red blood cell involvement. Generally, about two-thirds of cases with red cell destruction show a concomitant involvement of platelets.

There has been a significant increase in the number of dogs recognized to have immune-mediated diseases (Dodds, 1982; R. J. Wilkins and A. I. Hurvitz, 1981, K. Young, 1981, and C. Pertz, 1981, personal communications). These include a number of specific immunological diseases that can affect tissues or organs as well as the blood. The conditions have been both autoimmune, in which the body's immune system forms antibodies against self-antigens, or immune mediated, in which foreign antigenic materials such as viruses and drugs act as haptens and adhere to or alter the surface or body tissues and cells, forming antibodies against the hapten–cellular complex. Both types of immunological disease produce similar clinical signs in the affected individual, because the resultant antibodies destroy the target organs or cells. The target tissues can be the kidneys as occurs in systemic lupus erythematosus (Lewis et al., 1965, 1973; Osborne et al., 1973; Schwartz, 1975), the joints as with rheumatoid arthritis (Newton et al., 1976; Pedersen et al., 1976), the skin as in pemphigus (Slappendel et al., 1970; Halliwell, 1978), the muscles as in myasthenia gravis and eosinophilic myositis (Tizard, 1977), and the thyroid gland as in Hashimoto's disease (Halliwell, 1978). In some cases, other tissues such as the bone, intestinal tract, brain, or nervous system can be involved in destructive processes, and specific names have been given to each type of disorder. When several tissues are affected, the resulting disease is more serious.

II. Clinical Signs

If the immune-mediated disease is destroying red blood cells, the affected animal can become suddenly or gradually anemic and weak. The gums and eye membranes may be icteric, and the urine may be dark brown or dark red in color. Diagnosis is confirmed by blood tests and especially the direct Coombs' test, which is positive at some time during the course of the disease. It is important to perform this test before the animal is treated with corticosteroids, because false negative results can occur once treatment has been initiated. If the immune-mediated disease is destroying platelets, the animal will usually show a bleeding tendency from the skin and mucosal surfaces. Typical signs are small pinpoint bruises (petechiae) in the skin, gums, and eye membranes, nosebleeds, large patchy bruises (ecchymoses) in the skin, and bleeding from the gastrointestinal tract (melena) or into the urine (hematuria). The platelet count is usually less than 150,000 per mm^3, and prognosis depends on the severity of the platelet reduction. Very low counts (less than 30,000 per mm^3) are quite dangerous, because internal bleeding can be fatal. Curiously, a number of severely thrombocytopenic patients do not show clinical signs of a bleeding tendency unless provoked by stress, trauma, or surgery, despite platelet counts of less than 50,000 (Karpatkin, 1980; Dodds, 1982). Why some individuals fail to bleed whereas others with similar histories and laboratory findings have recurrent problems is not understood. Perhaps the function of those few circulating platelets is enhanced in the former cases, which affords a measure of protection. Diagnosis is confirmed by laboratory tests to detect the presence of antiplatelet antibody in the blood. Again, this test should be done before corticosteroid therapy is given.

III. Diagnosis

A. History

The typical history of affected animals will depend on two factors: whether the onset is gradual or sudden, and whether or not both red cells and platelets are involved. The classical acute case of AIHD is presented with a sudden collapse of a previously healthy animal. The gums are usually blanched and frequently are icteric. When platelets are concomitantly depleted, there may be petechiae spread over the ventral abdomen, gums, and sclera. In isolated cases of thrombocytopenia, the disease is less dramatic. The owner may notice small bruises when grooming the dog, or the veterinarian may observe such bruises as the animal is being examined for a routine checkup or vaccination procedure. Chronic cases of AIHD progress slowly to a nonspecific general weakness, lethargy, and inappetence. Episodes of overt illness are usually preceded by environmental or physiological stresses such as extremes of hot or cold weather, hormonal changes (estrus, pseudocyesis), and other disease processes (especially viral infections). The affected animal is frequently a young to middle-aged adult female with a previous history of reproductive irregularities including heat cycles of varying lengths and intervals of anestrus, silent heats, prolonged estrual bleeding, and pseudopregnancy. The owner may also mention that other family members have had similar problems or a series of undiagnosed chronic or acute and fatal illnesses. Some cases have a family history of chronic allergies, which includes various types of seasonal, chronic dermatitis. The history of other illnesses among relatives may reflect "tumors" of the liver and spleen as well as anemia. Questioning the veterinarian involved frequently reveals that this was nonspecific hepatosplenomegaly of unknown cause. Typically there has been an incomplete workup of the case from a clinical pathological or histopathological standpoint.

A second form of immune-mediated anemia is associated with the presence of cold erythrocyte agglutinins. These are more rare than the usual warm-reactive antibodies that produce the classical AIHD syndrome. Cold antibodies are most active below 20°C and produce microcirculatory failure at the extremities rather than hemolytic anemia. Thus the nose, feet, tail, and tips of the ears are affected with dry gangrene-like lesions caused by intravascular erythrocyte agglutination.

In addition to the nonspecific signs of regenerative anemia, affected animals will have hemoglobinuria and may have hemoglobinemia if intravascular hemolysis is sufficient to exceed clearance of erythrocyte breakdown products by the reticuloendothelial system. There may also be anorexia, pyrexia, polydipsia, peripheral lymphadenopathy, and hepatosplenomegaly in chronic cases. Most animals respond well if they are treated aggressively after the initial onset of signs. In some cases the course of the disease is unpredictable, and in others there is a spontaneous remission.

If the dog with AIHD also has systemic lupus erythematosus (SLE), it will show a variety of other clinical signs at some point (Lewis *et al.*, 1965, 1973). About two-thirds of the cases have concomitant thrombocytopenia, and there is progressive renal failure from immune-complex glomerulonephritis. Additional signs include polyarthritis, polymyositis, skin lesions that blanket the muzzle, pleurisy, and pericarditis. Diagnosis is confirmed by clinicopathological tests.

B. Clinicopathological Tests

1. Red Cell Tests

The diagnosis of immune-mediated blood diseases is confirmed by clinicopathological testing (Schultz, 1976). When the red cells are involved, the resulting disease can be classified according to the type of erythrocyte antibody produced (Dodds, 1977). This classification has been described in detail by Halliwell (1978). Basically the antibodies are divided into the warm- and cold-acting types, the former being much more common. A classification scheme is shown in Table I.

Warm-reacting antibodies give a positive Coombs' antiglobulin test at 37°C, whereas cold-reacting antibodies are Coombs' positive at 4°C

TABLE I
Classification of Immune-Mediated Antierythrocyte Agglutinins[a]

Type	Characteristics
Warm Antibodies	
Spontaneous agglutinins	Visible in freshly collected blood; probably is occurring *in vivo;* differentiated from rouleaux by persistence upon dilution with isotonic saline; Coombs' test unnecessary; prognosis guarded to poor
In vivo hemolysins	Massive red cell destruction with hemoglobinuria and hemoglobinemia; sudden onset of serious illness with icterus is common; Coombs' test needed to confirm
Incomplete antibody type	Most common form; Coombs' test important; intravascular hemolysis uncommon; splenomegaly common; hemoglobinuria but not hemoglobinemia present; chronic course with gradual onset
Cold Antibodies	
Cold agglutinins	Optimum effect below 20°C; cold weather-induced anemia and hemoglobulinuria; dry gangrene of extremities common; intravascular hemolysis uncommon; Coombs' test negative at 37°C but strongly positive at 4°C; can occur in warm weather
Nonagglutinating cold antibodies	Coombs' test positive at 4°C only; icterus and hemoglobinuria common especially in cold weather; rare

[a] After Halliwell (1978).

and negative at 37°C. In fact, warming of cold-agglutinated blood will usually reverse the process. The preferred form of the Coombs' assay is the direct test, which uses the patient's washed red cells tested against species-specific antiglobulin serum (Dodds, 1977; Tizard, 1977; Halliwell, 1978; Slappendel, 1979). The indirect form of the test, which uses the patient's serum and normal washed red cells, precludes diagnosis if the antibody titer is too low to elicit a positive reaction. Because these antibodies are most destructive at the cell surface, the direct test is more meaningful and reliable.

The red cell agglutinins can be directed at IgG (15–50% incidence), at complement components, especially C3 and/or C4 (30–50% incidence), at a combination of these two (25% incidence), and at other antibody types such as IgM or IgA, which are rare (Dodds, 1977). In a recent analysis of 371 anemic dogs (Slappendel, 1979), 134 cases or 36% had positive direct Coombs' tests, and of these 11% had IgG antibodies, 31% had IgG + complement antibodies, 55% had complement antibodies, and about 2% had IgM + complement antibodies. In two Coombs'-positive dogs the type of reaction was unclear, and occasionally IgM and/or IgA reactions occurred along with strong IgG and complement antibodies. Eighty-four of the Coombs'-positive dogs had one or more symptoms of hemolysis including hemoglobinemia, indirect hyperbilirubinemia, increased red cell osmotic fragility, and increased fecal excretion of urobilinogen. Most dogs with the IgG + complement-type agglutinins had severe hemolysis, and primary or secondary diseases were present in only half of these. Thus overt anemia was usually associated with dogs having either the IgG or IgG + complement antibodies. Conversely, those cases with only complement antibodies had minimal or no evidence of hemolysis. In nearly all cases there was an associated primary disease such as infection (especially viral), or inflammatory or neoplastic (especially myelo- and lymphoproliferative) diseases. The indirect Coombs' test was also uniformly negative in cases of complement antibodies.

2. Platelet Tests

If platelets are the target cells of immune-mediated destruction, one or more specific tests can be performed to determine the presence, type, and amount of antiplatelet activity in the blood.

The first test used routinely to detect antiplatelet activity was the platelet factor 3 (PF3) release test of Karpatkin and colleagues (Karpatkin, 1980). The assay was adapted for dogs (Wilkins *et al.*, 1973; Joshi and Jain, 1976; Jain and Kono, 1980) and other species (Dodds and Wilkins, 1977; Byars and Greene, 1982) by using species-specific platelet-rich plasma and control globulin fractions and substituting plasma for serum as the initial specimen. The latter change was made to reduce the possibility of obtaining false positive results from traces of thrombin in serum being transferred to the extracted globulin fraction. Being a potent promoter of the platelet release reaction, thrombin would cause nonspecific shortening of the clotting time end point in the test (Dodds and Wilkins, 1977). The collective experience of the author with over 200 cases of recurrent thrombocytopenia indicates that this test is the most practical and reliable overall for clinical use in animals (Dodds and Wilkins, 1977). Because 65–70% of recurrent cases of thrombocytopenia have an immunological basis (Karpatkin *et al.*, 1972; Wilkins *et al.*, 1973: Dodds and Wilkins, 1977: Karpatkin, 1980), a negative test result does not preclude this diagnosis. Serial monitoring may be required to detect the presence of antibody, and/or the circulating antiplatelet titer may be below the detection limits of the test. False positive test results may also be obtained in cases where a secondary tissue-inflammatory or stress-responsive disease is present (e.g., disseminated intravascular coagulation, acute sepsis) or when the test globulin fraction is contaminated with thrombin or endotoxin, which also induces platelet membrane injury and PF3 release (Karpatkin et al., 1972).

Several veterinary clinical pathology laboratories do use assays based on this test (Joshi and Jain, 1976; Jain and Kono, 1980; Wilkins and Hurvitz, 1981), although difficulties in standardizing the test have been encountered (Halliwell, 1978; Jain and Kono, 1980). The most commonly observed problem is an overly shortened clotting time endpoint for the control globulin fractions (i.e., less than 60 sec). This usually indicates that the normal platelet-rich plasma substrate has been activated during collection and/or preparation, thus causing premature release of PF3 and reduction in the amount of PF3 available for release from subsequent exposure to an immune globulin fraction. The ideal clotting time end point of the control specimen should be around 90 sec for dog samples and over 150 sec for equines. Another cause of foreshortening in the control specimens occurs if the globulin fraction used has been prepared by prior pooling of plasma from several healthy animals (Dodds and Wilkins, 1977). Apparently normal globulin extracts from different individuals can be sufficiently diverse to cause nonspecific interaction, inducing PF3 release. The problem is avoided by preparing a series of normal globulin fractions from several healthy dogs and testing each batch separately.

A variety of other tests have been developed in recent years for the identification of immune-mediated thrombocytopenia in humans (Cines and Schreiber, 1979; Hymes et al., 1979; Karpatkin, 1980; Sugiura et al., 1980; Morse et al., 1981, 1982; Myers et al., 1981) and animals (Shebani and Jain, 1983). Some of these, such as the platelet migration inhibition test (Duquesnoy, 1975), the antibody-dependent cellular toxicity test (Gengozian and Rice, 1982), and the lymphocyte transformation test (Wybran and Fudenberg, 1972), measure cellular involvement with antiplatelet activity; others are more specific and quantitate the amount and type of immune globulin bound to the platelet surface (Cines and Schreiber, 1979: Hymes et al., 1979; Sugiura et al., 1980; Morse et al., 1981, 1982; Myers et al., 1981). The latter tests are more sensitive than those based on measuring plasma or serum antibody levels. Some are simple and rapid (Sugiura et al.,

1980; Morse *et al.*, 1981, 1982), and results directly correlate with the degree of platelet destruction and severity of clinical disease, whereas plasma levels of antibody do not (Karpatkin, 1980). Unfortunately, such methods are not easily adapted for use in animals because highly purified radio or fluorescent-labeled, species-specific immunoglobulins or the active fragments of immunoglobulins are required. Development of these reagents would be most useful for research purposes but would be impractical for routine use because the assumption of an immune basis can safely be made for the majority of clinical cases of recurrent, severe thrombocytopenia.

Several simplified screening tests for circulating platelet antibodies are also available (Hirschman *et al.*, 1974) and have been used in dogs (Jain and Kono, 1980). Although promising, whether these are not only easier but also equally or more reliable than the established PF3-release test methods remains to be proven.

The antibodies present in immune thrombocytopenia are usually of the IgG type (75%); the remainder are usually IgM or IgA antibodies (Dodds and Wilkins, 1977; Karpatkin, 1980). The type of immunoglobulin involved can be identified by immunoprecipitation with specific immunoglobulins, in which case a positive PF3 test becomes negative upon removal of the specific immunoprecipitate (Karpatkin *et al.*, 1972; Wilkins *et al.*, 1973). This modification of the basic test can be used to confirm positive test results and avoid false positive diagnosis from nonspecific PF3 release.

In addition to specific tests for antiplatelet activity, other aids in establishing the diagnosis include serial monitoring of the platelet count, coagulation assays to rule out thrombocytopenias caused by the consumption coagulopathy phase of intravascular coagulation, bone marrow examination, and other immunological tests (e.g., Coombs' test, LE preparation, antinuclear antibody test) (Halliwell, 1978; Karpatkin, 1980). Generally, the lower the platelet count, the more severe the clinical entity (Karpatkin, 1980). Also, patients with platelet counts below 10,000 to 30,000 per mm^3 are usually destroying platelets preferentially in the liver rather than in the spleen (Dodds and Wilkins, 1977; Karpatkin, 1980; Pearson, 1980), although both organs frequently are involved. Bone marrow evaluations are usually nondiagnostic, because peripheral thrombocytopenia can result from reduced production and/or excessive destruction, utilization, or sequestration (Karpatkin *et al.*, 1972: Wilkins *et al.*, 1973). Thus, normal, reduced, or enhanced megakaryocytic activity may be present in marrow aspirates.

Because about two-thirds of cases of immune-mediated hemolytic disease also have thrombocytopenia at some point, it follows that patients with immune thrombocytopenia may also have positive direct Coombs' tests. Similarly, patients with SLE frequently show both antierythrocyte and antiplatelet antibodies (Karpatkin, 1980). Thus, tests for these other immunological disorders should also be performed on thrombocytopenic individuals.

3. Tests for SLE

In addition to the tests just described for antierythrocyte and antiplatelet antibodies, patients suspected of having SLE should be tested for the presence of LE cells and antinuclear antibodies (ANA). It may be necessary to monitor the patient on a serial basis to demonstrate the LE-cell phenomenon or ANA. The former test is based on the principle that *in vitro* incubation of antinuclear activity present in the patient's blood coats the nuclear material released from fragmenting cells, opsonizing it for phagocytosis by polymorphonuclear leukocytes. Thus the LE cell is a polymorph that has ingested coated nuclear material. Similar phagocytosis may occur *in vivo,* and about 75% of patients with SLE will have a positive LE test at some stage of their disease.

Improved specificity and sensitivity for the diagnosis of SLE is possible with quantitative ANA tests. Immunofluorescent and radioimmunoassay procedures are the most widely used and are quite specific. These detect the presence of circulating antibodies against native, double-stranded DNA. Antibodies against leukocytes and rheumatoid factor may also be present in SLE cases.

The criteria for establishing the diagnosis of SLE in dogs have been reviewed byHalliwell (1978) and Tizard (1978). These include one or more of the following: Coombs'-positive hemolytic anemia, thrombocytopenia (usually immune mediated), progressive renal failure with proteinuria, slowly progressive polyarthritis, skin lesions typical of SLE and usually on the muzzle, and the presence of LE cells, ANA, polyclonal gammopathy, or rheumatoid factor. Although Halliwell (1978) stresses that diagnosis of SLE is untenable without positive serological evidence of ANA titer greater than 1:100 or strongly positive LE preparation, there have been an increasing number of cases of so-called ANA-negative SLE, in which the clinical signs, other immunological tests, and response to treatment are typical of SLE (Dodds, 1982; R. J. Wilkins and A. I. Hurvitz, 1981, personal communication). Although the question of diagnosis remains to be resolved here, for all practical purposes these can be managed and treated similarly to proven cases of SLE.

C. Serial Monitoring

One mechanism for managing patients with immune-mediated diseases on a long-term basis is to monitor serially their clinical and clinicopathological status. Depending on the severity and nature of the illness, serial testing can be performed on a monthly or bimonthly basis, or it can be scheduled to coincide with each estrual and interestrual period for affected bitches. From the author's experience with several dog families apparently predisposed to immune-mediated anemia and/or thrombocytopenia, laboratory monitoring on a regular basis has been beneficial not only to identify animals newly converted from a negative to positive status, but also to initiate and adjust treatment regimens to optimize control of the disease process (Dodds, 1982).

IV. Findings

A. Family and Breed Histories

As mentioned earlier, we and other groups have experienced a large increase in the number of referrals of canine patients with immune-mediated diseases of the blood. The trend became noticeable in 1979, and the magnitude of the increase can best be appreciated if one considers that our laboratory studied over 200 animals referred for these diseases during an 18-month period between 1980 and 1982. In the past the average had been about one case per week; this increased to two to four cases per week, with the preponderance in the summer months. An apparent breed predilection has also been observed in our laboratory (Table II). The most frequently affected breed is the Old English sheepdog (57 cases), and the clinical course of the disease appears to be more severe and less responsive to treatment than expected.

In addition to certain breed predilections (discussed in detail in Section V,C), specific families of dogs also seem to have an increased tendency to develop these immune-mediated conditions. The following description summarizes our investigations of two purebred dog families with an abnormally high incidence of immune-mediated anemia and thrombocytopenia. Similar data (not shown) have been collected for families of American cocker spaniels and long-haired dachshunds, and are being assembled for the Old English sheepdog.

TABLE II

DOG BREEDS APPARENTLY PREDISPOSED
TO IMMUNE-MEDIATED BLOOD DISEASES

American cocker spaniels
German shepherds
Irish setters
Miniature and standard dachshunds
Miniature and toy poodles
Old English sheepdogs
Shetland sheepdogs
Scottish terriers
Vizslas

1. Vizsla Family

A four-generation pedigree of this family of Hungarian vizslas is shown in Fig. 1. The proband, a 5-year-old intact female, was presented to a local veterinarian approximately 2 weeks prepartum with anorexia of 3 days duration. One week later she had a packed-cell volume (PCV) of 18%, a platelet count of 156,000 per mm^3, and a "nonregenerative" anemia. A Coombs' test performed at this time was negative. She whelped 1 week later. Three weeks postpartum a diagnosis of pyometra was made, and the dog was spayed. One week later her PCV dropped to 11%, and a strong reticulocyte response was seen. The Coombs' test was strongly positive against both IgG and complement antibodies. The following week the patient remained Coombs' positive, and she died shortly thereafter. Postmortem histopathology revealed marked bone marrow hyperplasia, primarily of the granulocytic series, and hemosiderosis. The spleen was enlarged and found to be the site of active erythropoiesis and myelopoiesis. Megakaryocytes were present in the liver, as were macrophages filled with hemosiderin and red blood cells. Results of uterine histopathology included cystic endometrial hyperplasia and endometritis.

Six offspring and three siblings of the affected bitch as well as their progeny have been followed serially for evidence of hemolytic disease (Fig. 1). Of interest is the fact that the proband's 2 sisters and all 5 daughters had a history of reproductive abnormalities (irregular estrual intervals, pseudocyesis, infertility), and that 4 daughters and 1 sister were also Coombs' positive. Of 5 males tested in the family, two were Coombs' positive. Thus 9 of 12 tested females and 2 of 5 tested males had positive red cell antiglobulin tests on one or more occasions. Six family members (3 of each sex), including the proband, were also thrombocytopenic and had positive PF3-release tests for antiplatelet activity (in Fig. 1, dogs, II,2,6, and 9 and dogs III,4,11,14, and 16). One dog, a male, had mild thrombocytopenia but was PF3 negative (dog III,17).

When the proband's daughter (dog III,4) became Coombs' positive and remained so for a total of three serial tests (two in estrus and one between heats), and developed clinical signs during estrus like those of her dam, she was spayed. A pyosanguinous endometritis was found on histopathological examination of the extirpated tissues. Coombs' tests were then performed at regular intervals, and she became Coombs' negative 8 months after surgery and remained so as of 5 years later. The littermate of this bitch (dog III,3) and the proband's sister (dog II,9) were also considered at risk to develop clinical signs referable to immune-mediated hemolytic disease and/or thrombocytopenia, because they became consistently Coombs' positive. Following ovariohysterectomy, both dogs reverted to a negative antiglobulin status and remained so for 2 and 3 years, respectively, as of this writing. In both

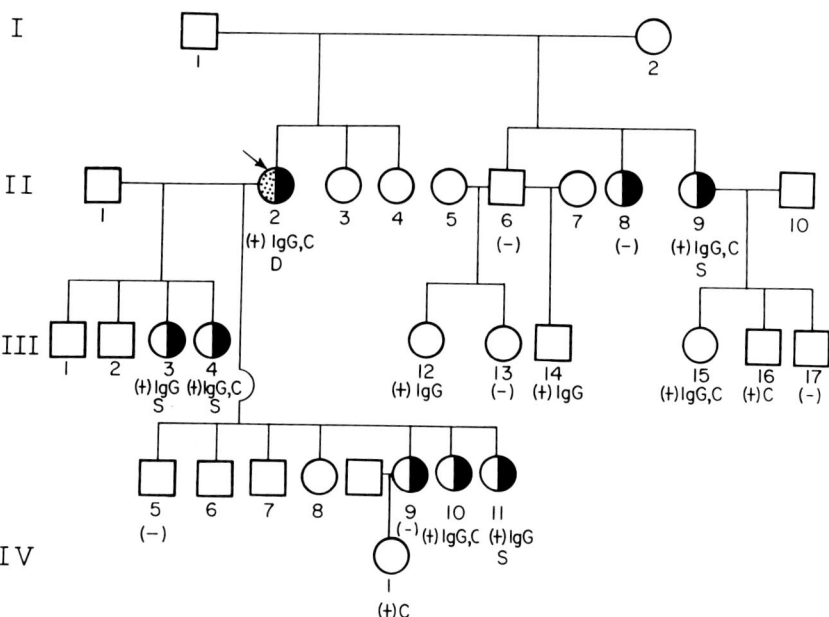

FIG. 1. Pedigree and relevant clinicopathological findings in vizsla family with immune-mediated anemia. The proband is indicated by the arrow. (+), Coombs' positive, IgG or C; (−), Coombs' negative: D, deceased; S, spayed; ◐, reproductive problems; ◉, immune-mediated anemia.

cases, the excised uterine tissues were engorged with uterine fluid. Other females in the family have experienced reproductive problems that include persistent vaginal discharge, irregular estrus cycles and behavior, and positive Coombs' tests. The breeder was advised not to breed females judged to be at risk for immune-mediated disease and to spay them. The immunological status of family members is currently monitored on a continuing basis. Whether spaying those bitches that became Coombs' positive aborted an impending disease problem remains to be proven, but at least none has developed clinical signs and all are Coombs' negative at this writing.

2. Scottish Terrier Family

The immunological status of this family of Scottish terriers was followed for several generations (Fig. 2).

The genetic background of this family was originally examined in relation to routine hematological screening procedures for the von Willebrand's disease gene (Dodds, 1980). During this period of testing the breeder was informed that an 8-month-old female puppy from a litter she had bred was acutely ill with a "blood-related" disease. The clinical history and postmortem histopathology suggested an episode of acute hemolytic anemia. A second closely related 11-month-old male

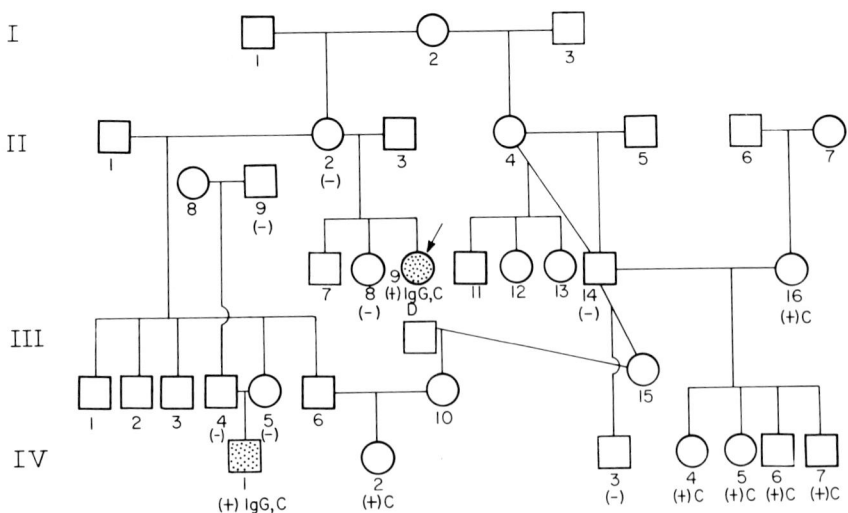

FIG. 2. Pedigree and relevant clinicopathological findings in Scottish terrier family with immune-mediated anemia. The proband is indicated by the arrow. ⊕ or ▨, Immune-mediated anemia; for other symbols, see Fig. 1.

puppy was presented to a veterinary hospital with a history of anorexia and lethargy. On initial examination the dog had a temperature of 104.4°F, pale mucous membranes, a bilirubinuria of 2+, and a PCV of 23%. Blood was submitted for analysis, and the dog was placed on antibiotics. A Coombs' test was not performed. Three days later the PCV had fallen to 8%. The dog received a transfusion of whole blood and underwent exploratory surgery the following day. Twenty-four hours later, with a PCV of 10% and evidence of jaundice, the dog died. Tissues submitted for histopathology revealed hepatitis with focal necrosis, splenitis, hemosiderosis, and extramedullary hematopoiesis.

Coombs' testing was initiated on dogs in the breeder's possession that were related to the two puppies that died. Several Coombs'-positive members were discovered (Fig. 2). Most of the antierythrocyte antibodies were directed against complement components. Eight of these animals were also thrombocytopenic, and five of them were positive for antiplatelet activity by the PF3-release test (dogs III,5,9, and 16 and dogs IV,1 and 2).

Examination of the pedigrees of this breeder's stock revealed a close relationship between the two clinically affected animals; the mother (dog II,2) of the proband (dog III,9) was also the grandmother of affected dog IV,1. Also, the brother (dog III,6) of this male's dam (dog III,5) sired a Coombs'-positive bitch puppy (dog IV,2). The sire of the litter in which all four puppies were Coombs' positive (dog III,14) had the same foundation grandmother (dog I,2) as the proband. Dog III,14 also had been bred back to his mother (dog II,4), but we have not located the three progeny for blood testing.

Since the first cases in Scottish terriers were brought to our attention, several other dogs of this breed with confirmed or presumed immune-mediated hematological disease have been discovered: an 8-year-old male that was euthanized after suffering a severe and unresponsive hemolytic crisis immediately following a second vaccination with modified live parvovirus vaccine of feline origin, a 4-year-old male with marked hepatomegaly that survived a hemolytic episode 2 weeks after receiving a modified live feline parvovirus vaccine, a 2-year-old female with PF3-positive immune thrombocytopenia, and two 6-week-old littermates that succumbed to acute hemolytic disease 9 days following vaccination with a combination of modified live distemper–hepatitis–leptospirosis–parainfluenza and feline parvovirus vaccines. Autopsies revealed distemper virus inclusions in the central nervous system. Blood samples from these puppies and their two surviving littermates were strongly Coombs' positive, with antibodies directed against IgG and complement. Parvovirus titers on the survivors were subsequently found to be in excess of 1:2000, indicating a recent viral exposure.

The pedigrees of these cases, except for that of the PF3-positive bitch, which was unavailable, were evaluated to search for common ancestry. The two littermate puppies that died after vaccination were not related to any of the others for at least 10 generations. The 4-year-old male with hepatomegaly and the older male were distantly related to the family shown in Fig. 2 through males I,3 and II,5.

B. Case Histories

Table III gives a breakdown of the 223 animals tested for immune-mediated hematological diseases by our laboratory in the 18 months between 1980 and mid-1982. Of these, 57 (26%) involved Old Inglish sheepdogs, 35 (16%) were long-haired dachshunds, 26 (12%) were Scottish terriers, 17 (8%) were vizslas, 15 (7%) were American cocker spaniels, and the remainder were other purebreds (8%) and mixed breeds (23%). Over 70% of these animals were females, which confirms the expected preponderance of females over males with respect to immune-mediated diseases (Dacie, 1967; Williams *et al.*, 1972; Schalm, 1975; Tizard, 1977; Halliwell, 1978). The ages of affected dogs varied from 6 weeks to 15 years, although most animals in this series were of middle age, as has been found previously (Halliwell, 1978).

Of the 214 dogs tested by the direct Coombs' test, 154 (72%) were positive. Of these, the majority (51%) had both IgG and complement attached to their red cells, whereas complement-mediated antibodies were the next most common (38%), with IgG antibodies being least frequent (11%). About one-half (109) of the total number of dogs tested were also thrombocytopenic, and of these, 68 (62%) were positive for antiplatelet activity by the PF3-release test (Wilkins *et al.*, 1973). A striking finding was observed in the Old English sheepdog breed; 39 of the 57 animals tested were thrombocytopenic, and 30 (77%) of these had circulating antiplatelet activity. Many of these affected animals were referred for severe thrombocytopenia without red cell involvement, although some cases also had strongly positive Coombs' tests and were seriously ill.

V. Predisposing Factors

Factors known to predispose to immune-mediated hematological diseases are listed in Table IV.

TABLE III
ANIMALS TESTED FOR IMMUNE-MEDIATED BLOOD DISEASES, 1980–1982

Breed	Number of animals	Sex (M/F)	Age range	Direct Coombs' test				PF3-Release test	
				(+IgG)	(+C)	(+IgG and C)	(−)	(+)	(−)
Old English sheepdog	57 (9 have same sire)	12/45	5 months to 12 years	5	7	24	18	30	9
Long-haired dachshund	35 (all related)	19/16	12 weeks to 5 years	0	18	5	14	3	7
Scottish terrier	26 (15 related)	7/19	6 weeks to 8 years	0	11	7	9	4	6
Vizsla	21 (all related)	5/16	8 months to 7 years	3	6	6	10	6	1
American cocker spaniel	15 (3 have same dam)	2/13	2–6 years	0	0	8	0	7	0
Other breeds	18	3/15	8 weeks to 14 years	2	4	12	0	3	0
Mixed breeds	51	12/39	5 months to 15 years	6	13	17	9	15	16
Totals	223	60/163	6 weeks to 15 years	16	59	79	60	68	41

TABLE IV

FACTORS THAT PREDISPOSE
TO IMMUNE-MEDIATED BLOOD DISEASES

Sex (females 2:1 over males)
Genetic or familial factors
Virus disease and possibly frequent use of modified live virus vaccines
Hormonal influences (pregnancy, abnormal estrous cycles, pyometra, and pseudocyesis)
Drug reactions
Stress (environmental, emotional, or physiological)
Underlying diseases (lymphoreticular malignancies and other autoimmune disorders)

A. Increased Frequency

The two- to threefold increase in our caseload between 1979 and mid-1982 was mentioned earlier and documented for the period after 1980 in Fig. 2. By comparison, Halliwell (1978) reported only 21 cases of immune-mediated hemolytic anemia and 15 cases of immune thrombocytopenia referred to the University of Pennsylvania School of Veterinary Medicine for the 6-year period from 1970 to 1976. Of these, there were 3 cockers and 5 poodles with red cell involvement, and 1 Old English sheepdog, 2 cockers, and 4 poodles with immune platelet destruction.

Nearly all the immune-mediated diseases studied have affected the blood at one time or another during the course of the disease. Other commonly associated problems were hepatosplenomegaly, hepatitis, splenomegaly, glomerulonephritis, and dermatitis. Occasionally (six cases) there was a painless and gradual sloughing of the toenails of all four feet. In each of these latter instances, the animal had received a modified live parvovirus vaccination of either feline or canine origin from 5 to 17 days beforehand.

An important question yet to be resolved is whether the observed increase in the number of referrals reflects a true increase in the frequency of these diseases and/or an increased awareness among dog owners, breeders, and veterinarians, who are recognizing and diagnosing such disorders more readily. Certainly, access to the laboratory tests required for diagnosis of immunological disorders in animals has improved in recent years, and this has facilitated accurate diagnosis and early treatment. It is our opinion, however, that the current influx of cases exceeds the number that can be explained on the basis of increased awareness alone.

B. Sex Predisposition

The predisposition of females to immune-mediated disease has been well established (Dacie, 1967; Williams *et al.*, 1972; Schalm, 1975; Dodds, 1977; Tizard, 1977; Halliwell, 1978; Karpatkin, 1980). This applies not only to SLE and immune-mediated anemias (Williams *et al.*, 1972) but also to thrombocytopenias of immunological causes (Karpatkin, 1980). The present canine data (Table III) are in agreement, because 163 of the animals tested were females whereas only 60 were males. Curiously, affected males—especially of the Old English sheepdog, dachshund, and Scottish terrier breeds—were very severely affected, and many were nonresponsive and succumbed despite vigorous treatment. In accordance with our previous studies (Wilkins *et al.*, 1973; Dodds, 1977), females were more often affected than males by a 2:1 or 3:1 ratio, whether intact or spayed.

C. Breed Predisposition

Breeds recognized by our laboratory and others to be predisposed to immune-mediated hematological diseases are listed in Table II (Wilkins *et al.*, 1973; Dodds, 1977; Halliwell, 1978; M. Estrin, 1982, personal communication). Data from specific dog families within the more commonly affected breeds have been collected for vizslas (Fig. 1), Scottish terriers (Fig. 2), American cocker spaniels, and long-haired dachshunds, and are presently being compiled for the Old English sheepdog. Whether certain bloodlines within these breeds will be found to have a significantly increased prevalence of immune disorders remains to be proven by statistical evaluation from pedigree analysis of the relationship between affected individuals. One way to accomplish this would be to compare the coefficients of inbreeding and commonality of ancestry of affected individuals to age- and geographically matched healthy animals of the same breed.

D. Genetic Influences

Familial tendencies are known to exist for several immune-mediated disorders of humans and animals including rheumatoid arthritis, Hashimoto's thyroiditis, SLE, AIHD, immune-mediated thrombocytopenia, and agamma-globulinemia (Bielschowsky *et al.*, 1959; Videbaek, 1962; Fialkow, 1964; Dobbs, 1965, Lewis *et al.*, 1965; Dacie, 1967; Robbins *et al.*, 1969: Schwartz, 1975; Dodds, 1977; Utroska, 1980). Hemolytic anemia can be associated with all types of immune-mediated disease and may be the first or only presenting clinical sign in SLE. In NZB/NZW hybrid mice, the AIHD can be directly transmitted from one generation to the next with clinical signs expressed by 6 months of age (Bielschowsky et al., 1959; Mellors, 1969). Affected females are highly susceptible to a nephritis similar to that found in patients with SLE.

In the human medical literature, several families are described with a history of AIHD (Videbaek, 1962; Fialkow, 1964; Dobbs, 1965: Dacie, 1967) or immune-mediated thrombocytopenia (Karpatkin, 1980). In one such family, the proband suffered from AIHD and had a strongly positive Coombs' test. The family history included members with increased levels of immunoglobulins, rheumatoid factor, ANA, positive Coombs' test, periarteritis nodosa, antibodies to thyroid and heart muscle, and clinical pancarditis and thyrotoxicosis. The blood from the proband's mother was strongly Coombs' and ANA positive. In another family, all the members with identifiable serological changes and evidence of AIHD had parents who both demonstrated serological abnormalities of AIHD. In this case, a recessive pattern of inheritance was proposed.

With respect to immune-mediated thrombocytopenia, there has been a strong association with the presence of an alloantigen of the HLA-D locus (called DRw2) and the genetic predisposition to this disease (Karpatkin, 1980). The DRw2 alloantigen was found in 75% of 20 consecutive patients in the New York City area with immune thrombocytopenia, whereas it was present in only 23% of an ethnically matched healthy control population. Of additional interest has been a parallel association of the DRw2 and DRw3 alloantigens of the major histocompatibility complex in patients with SLE (Karpatkin, 1980).

The most convincing evidence of genetic transmission of AIHD in dogs has involved the studies by Lewis and colleagues on a colony of animals with SLE (Lewis et al., 1965, 1973; Schwartz, 1975). Since then, the author has investigated several dog families with what appears to be a familial predisposition to immune-mediated hematological diseases. The cumulative data are shown in Figs. 1 and 2, and Table III. In addition, two 1-year-old littermate cats were reported to have a Coombs'-positive, feline leukemia virus-negative hemolytic anemia (Utroska, 1980).

E. Relationship to Viral Infections and Vaccinations

1. Viral Infections

Many diseases of immune-mediated origin are associated with or triggered by virus infections (Dacie, 1967; Williams et al., 1972; Lewis *et al.,* 1973; Tizard, 1977; Karpatkin, 1980). Viruses that infect lymphoid tissues are apparently capable of interfering with immunological control, thus leading to production of antibodies directed against self-antigens. This relationship has been the most clearly established for SLE.

The pathogenesis of SLE in humans and animals involves environmental influences, drugs such as procainamide, hydralazine, isoniazid, trimethadione, and primidone, and genetic predisposition (discussed in Section V,D), as well as viruses (Tizard, 1977; Halliwell, 1978). In the NZB/NZW mouse hybrid predisposed to develop SLE, breeding experiments suggested direct genetic transmission (Bielschowsky *et al.,* 1959), whereas infection with type C virus particles induced serological changes in other laboratory mice (Mellors, 1969). Type C virus-infected mice developed autoantibodies against nucleic acids and erythrocytes. In the dog, either type C or paromyxovirus (human measles or canine distemper viruses) infections have been associated with SLE (Lewis *et al.,* 1973; Schwartz, 1975). In experimental studies when SLE-affected dogs were bred, the number of serologically affected progeny was higher than could be accounted for by genetic influences alone (Lewis *et al.,* 1973). These findings suggested that vertical transmission was also involved. In other studies, when cell-free filtrates from healthy, LE-cell–positive dogs were administered to newborn mice and puppies, similar serological abnormalities were produced. However, despite the presence of a high incidence of ANA and positive LE preparations, neither the SLE-affected dogs nor those infected with virus developed clinical signs of SLE. Thus the question of the communicable nature of canine SLE is unresolved (Halliwell, 1978).

In humans a similar viral association has been proposed because individuals with SLE frequently have high titers to parainfluenza 1 and measles viruses (Tizard, 1977). Furthermore, myxovirus nucleoprotein strands have been observed in the endothelial cells of kidney biopsy specimens taken from SLE patients. With respect to AIHD in humans, several virus diseases, particularly infectious mononucleosis and mycoplasmal pneumonia, have been encountered (Dacie, 1967).

Acute-onset thrombocytopenic purpura in children is usually preceded by a seasonal (winter or spring) viral illness 1–3 weeks beforehand (Lusher and Iyer, 1977; Karpatkin, 1980). The most commonly associated viruses are varicella, rubella, rubeola, and pharyngitis. In a study of 305 children with idiopathic thrombocytopenic purpura, 80% had an antecedent viral infection (Luscher and Iyer, 1977). It has been postulated that the platelet membrane is altered by the virus or by soluble viral antigen–antibody complexes with an affinity for sites on the platelet surface. The platelets are thus susceptible to rapid destruction in the spleen or other parts of the reticuloendothelial system. Both sexes are equally affected in this situation, and the disease has an average duration of 1 to 2 months. From 7 to 28% of such children will subsequently develop a chronic thrombocytopenia syndrome. The chronic form of thrombocytopenia is more common in adults and usually occurs in females. Remissions in clinical signs occur, although the platelet count remains consistently at one-third to one-half of normal values (Karpatkin, 1980). Some patients have an intermittent form of thrombocytopenia with cyclical episodes occurring at 3- to 6-month intervals. The relationship of viral diseases to these latter two forms of thrombocytopenia is unclear.

2. Vaccinations

Recent vaccinations against viral diseases have been implicated as causes of acute-onset thrombocytopenia in children (Oski and Naiman, 1966; Bachand *et al.,* 1967; Lusher and Iyer, 1977; Karpatkin, 1980). The effect is seen during the period of viremia, 5–10 days after vaccination. Measles vaccine has been reported most frequently to cause such reactions (Oski and Naiman, 1966; Lusher and Iyer, 1977). Experimental studies in a variety of domestic and wild animals (bear, deer, fox, raccoon) have shown a consistent drop of about 100,000 per mm^3 in the circulating platelet count, beginning 3–5 days following use of modified live measles or canine distemper vaccines and lasting for as long as a week thereafter (Dodds, 1982). In clinical situations, a number of cases of bleeding tendency with petechiation and ecchymotic hemorrhages of the skin and mucous membranes have been reported following routine use of modified live measles and distemper virus vaccines in dogs (Dodds, 1980), and hog cholera vaccine in swine (Pilchard, 1966). In addition, animals with a preexisting congenital or hereditary hemostatic defect, such as hemophilia or von Willebrand's disease, frequently exhibit clinical signs of a bleeding tendency in the 5- to 10-day postvaccinal period. Elective surgery is thus contraindicated during this interval (Dodds, 1980).

Whether the vaccine-induced thrombocytopenia and thrombopathy are caused by an immunological mechanism is unknown, but many investigators and clinicians support this concept (Lusher and Iyer, 1977). Because the effect is not seen prior to the viremic phase postvaccination, one could postulate a hapten-mediated immune mechanism in which antibodies develop to the viral-coated or virus-infected cell. Immunofluorescent studies of the bone marrow of animals 7–10 days after viral infection or vaccination have located viral particles within megakaryocytes (Osborn and Shahidi, 1973), and megakaryocyte involvement and/or damage from viral infections have been implicated in the purpura associated with childhood varicella (Lusher and Iyer, 1977). Parallel studies of experimentally induced *Ehrlichia canis* infection in dogs have demonstrated increased platelet destruction by an immunological process primarily involving the spleen (Smith *et al.*, 1975).

The situations just described implicate vaccination with attenuated live viruses as one of the causative factors or "triggers" of immune-mediated disease in a susceptible host. That these adverse reactions can also occur in families provides evidence in support of genetic predisposition as an etiological factor. Although speculative at this point, the possibility exists that frequent exposure to monovalent or multivalent modified live vaccines sensitizes a susceptible host to viral antigen and increases the risk of developing immune-mediated reactions. There is a trend among virologists and immunologists to be cautious about the indiscriminate use of live virus vaccines, especially because of the risk of mutation or reversion of shed virus in vaccinated individuals to a virulent form. For example, could the current endemic of gastroenteric virus diseases of dogs (corona and parvoviruses) have resulted from mutated strains of vaccine viruses from this or other species? More specifically, could a mutant strain of cat enteritis (feline panleukopenia) virus have produced the highly infectious, virulent canine parvovirus (CPV)? In addition to the potential for viral reversion to a pathogenic form, mutated viruses could be recognized as new, foreign antigens to the host population, and the increased frequency of immune-mediated anemias and thrombocytopenias might thus be associated with the recent and concomitant widespread exposure to and vaccination against CPV.

Since the beginning of 1981, our laboratory and several other veterinary clinical pathology laboratories have been compiling careful histories of cases referred for immune-mediated blood diseases. In many cases there has been an association with recent exposure to CPV disease or vaccination 1 day to 3 weeks previously with modified live virus (MLV), feline panleukopenia virus (FPV), or CPV vaccine to protect against CPV disease (Young, 1981; Dodds, 1982; C. Pertz, 1981, personal communication; A. G. Ibsen, 1982, personal communication). In only a few instances did the recent history include vaccination with the killed form of FPV or CPV vaccine. A high percentage of these cases have been severe and resulted in permanent side effects, poor prognosis, or death. Some cases of immune-mediated anemia have progressed to a fatal dyplastic anemia-like syndrome whereby the marrow ceases to produce new red blood cells and/or platelets. In other recovered cases, the marrow remains dyplastic for about 3 weeks, after which there is a rapid, dramatic erythrogenic response, which behaves as though some "toxic" marrow suppression were suddenly lifted. Reticulocyte counts rebound from zero to over 20% of the blood smear in a matter of 3 to 4 days, once the marrow begins to respond (Dodds, 1982). This very serious syndrome has been particularly common in the Old English sheepdog, and several of these affected dogs have been younger than is usually encountered in immune-mediated disease (<2 years old) and were males. Nine affected sheepdogs had the same sire (Table III), and four were from the same litter of seven that had initial signs of disease from 5 to 10 months of age. Three of these dogs died as a result of nonresponsive erythroid dysplasia. In the Scottish terriers referred for immune-mediated anemia and thrombocytopenia (Section V,C), signs of disease in most cases followed recent vaccination with MLV, FPV, or CPV. Two 8-week-old golden retriever littermates were referred for profound anemia and jaundice. Both had strongly positive Coombs' tests directed against IgG + complement, and both responded dramatically to high doses of dexamethasone. Both pups had received MLV distemper–hepatitis–parainfluenza–CPV vaccinations 6 days previously. Another case involved a healthy 4-year-old poodle given a routine MLV–CPV vaccination. Within 24 hr the animal's skin and mucous membranes were covered with tiny purple bruises, and the platelet count was <10,000 per mm^3. The dog recovered uneventfully following aggressive treatment with dexamethasone.

Perhaps the most bizarre reactions observed to follow vaccination with MLV–FPV or –CPV vaccines have been pemphigus-like disorders. In six cases, the toenails on all four feet began to slough in a painless, nonswollen manner 7–10 days after vaccination (Dodds, 1982; C. Pertz, 1981, personal communication). All toenails eventually sloughed and had not regrown as of this writing. A widespread necrotizing dermatitis of the decubital areas of the limbs was reported in two litters of German shepherd puppies from the same sire (Ibsen, 1982). Both litters had been vaccinated 2 weeks previously with a multivalent product containing MLV–CPV. The third unusual finding has been an increase in the number of dogs referred with severe icterus, tender abdomens, swollen livers, and markedly elevated hepatic serum enzymes (Dodds, 1982; R. J. Wilkins and A. I. Hurvitz, 1981, personal communication; S. Crowe, 1982, personal communication). The history of such cases with a hepatitis-like syndrome has usually been a recent exposure to active cases of CPV disease or MLV–FPV or –CPV vaccination in the previous 1–4 weeks.

It cannot be concluded from these observations that MLV–FPV or –CPV vaccines are unsafe for dogs for several reasons. First, hundreds of thousands of dogs have been routinely and repeatedly vaccinated for

CPV with the feline and canine MLV and killed vaccines without obvious side effects. Thus the relatively few cases of documented or apparent reactions may have involved only those with a susceptible genetic or physiological makeup. Unfortunately, there is no way to predict or identify susceptible individuals. Avoiding the repeated use of MLV–FPV, or –CPV vaccines for close relatives of known immune reactors is one way to reduce the risk of immune-mediated problems. Such dogs should, of course, be given regular, spaced immunizations with the killed feline- or canine-origin vaccines to protect against overt CPV disease. Second, the fact that the observed reactions have frequently included a recent history of MLV, FPV, or CPV vaccination may be coincidental and not causally related for many of the cases. In a few situations, however, an immediate, severe febrile and immune-mediated destruction of red blood cells and/or platelets has followed vaccination within 24 to 48 hr. These reactions clearly were vaccine related, but it cannot be concluded that MLV, FPV, or CPV vaccine per se was the cause, because a similar reaction might have occurred if the dog had received another type of vaccine. Third, could the observed reactions result from the frequent revaccinations given to produce protective titers in relatively nonresponsive animals? Repeated exposure to viral antigen by frequent vaccinations could sensitize the host and eventually cause an immune-mediated reaction. In such dogs, what is a "safe" interval between vaccinations?

In summary, further research is necessary on the immune responses of dogs to vaccination procedures that would normally be considered to be routine. Whether immune-mediated reactions occur only in genetically predisposed or susceptible individuals needs to be clarified. Alternatively, certain types of viral antigens, such as CPV or FPV, may be more likely to trigger immune-mediated reactions. In this case, MLV vaccines may produce a severe immune reaction as the virus multiplies in the host and provides more antigenic stimulation. However, on this basis MLV vaccines produce higher antibody titers than killed vaccines, a factor that is beneficial to the host. The advantages and possible risks involved must be considered before a decision is made about the type and frequency of vaccines to be used. It is important that the veterinary profession record any usual drug or vaccine complications, especially those that produce immunological reactions.

F. Hormonal Influences

Traditionally, immune-mediated diseases are two to three times more common in females than in males, and this trend also applies to animals whether they are intact or neutered (Schalm, 1975; Dodds,

1977; Tizard, 1977; Halliwell, 1978). Our current data (Table III and Fig. 1) also support this sex predisposition. In acute idiopathic thrombocytopenic purpura of childhood, there is no sex difference (Lusher and Iyer, 1977; Karpatkin, 1980), but whether this applies to the similar syndrome in young animals is unknown. An interesting finding in the 305 cases of acute thrombocytopenia in childhood reviewed by Lusher and Iyer (1977) was an 87% preponderance in whites, with only 13% of black racial origin, although the pediatric hospital population at large was 55% black. These authors speculated that the less severe form of the disease with superficial petechiae and bruises might go unnoticed by the parents of a black child. However, only one child had a chronic, mild form of disease, thus a real difference in racial susceptibility was likely. A similar situation pertains in animals, especially of the poodle breed, in which acute-onset thrombocytopenic purpura is much more commonly seen in white, light-skinned animals than in grey or black dogs (Wilkins et al., 1973).

That the frequency of AIHD is similar in intact or spayed females is difficult to reconcile with the concept that hormonal influences are important in triggering or predisposing individuals to immune-mediated disease. Certainly our findings with the vizsla family (Fig. 1) strongly suggest an association between reproductive irregularities and the subsequent appearance of antierythrocyte and/or antiplatelet antibodies and overt hematological disease or the risk of such a disease.

Stress situations including pregnancy (Williams et al., 1972; Schalm, 1975; Dodds, 1977); hormonal imbalance such as abnormal or irregular estrous cycles, pyometra, and pseudocyesis (Fig. 1, Table IV; Dodds, 1977); and other underlying diseases precipitate episodes of disease in early or subclinical cases, and aggravate the preexisting disease of affected individuals. In our experience, spaying females in these instances has averted overt clinical disease.

G. Drug Reactions

Drug-induced immune hemolysis and/or thrombocytopenia occurs in humans and animals (Williams et al., 1972; Wilkins et al., 1973; Dodds, 1977; Schoen and Trentham, 1981). Three mechanisms have been proposed to account for the majority of these conditions: a haptene mechanism, immune-complex formation, and true autoantibody induction (Dodds, 1977). Schoen and Trentham (1981) have challenged the traditional theories and proposed that, for drug-induced SLE at least, the drug acts as an adjuvant or immunostimulant to trigger polyclonal Band T-lymphocyte activation and immune dysregulation; this would explain the widespread disruption of self-tolerance observed. They cite as evidence in support of the concept that experimental animal models of autoimmunity can readily be induced by injections of a variety of tissue components in complete Freund's adjuvant, thus producing allergic encephalomyelitis, thyroiditis, orchitis, uveitis, and polyarthritis (Schoen and Trentham, 1981).

The therapeutic agents implicated in provoking SLE in humans include hydralazine, procainamide, isoniazid, practolol, hydantoins, chlorpromazine, D-penicillamine, and nitrofurantoin (Schoen and Trentham, 1981). Other drugs that can produce AIHD and/or thrombocytopenia are quinine, quinidine, stibophen, sedormid, α-methyldopa, cephalothin, indomethacin, phenacetin, phenylbutazone, dilantin, streptomycin, and the most commonly recognized causative drugs, penicillin and heparin (Babcock et al., 1976; Dodds, 1977). Several of these drugs also produce a parallel disease entity in animals. It is generally believed that drug reactions of this type occur only in genetically susceptible subjects. An increased risk for the development of drug-induced SLE has been reported in persons with the alloantigen HLA-DRw4 (Schoen and Trentham, 1981).

Heparin-induced thrombocytopenia is a commonly reported disease in humans (Babcock et al., 1976). An immunological mechanism has been proposed for this effect in some patients, whereas in others and particularly in species such as the dog, hamster, rat, and guinea pig (Babcock et al., 1976; Dodds, 1980), heparin induces platelet aggregation *in vivo,* which causes thrombocytopenia.

H. STRESS AND UNDERLYING DISEASE

Immune-mediated diseases are associated with a variety of underlying diseases and are frequently precipitated by stress (environmental and hormonal influences) in genetically susceptible individuals (Dacie, 1967; Williams et al., 1972; Dodds, 1977). The most commonly associated diseases in humans and animals are lymphoreticular malignancies, especially lymphocytic leukemia, lymphosarcoma, and reticulum cell sarcoma, and other autoimmune disorders such as SLE, rheumatoid arthritis, and immune-mediated thrombocytopenias. Rarely, cases have occurred with carcinomas, viral diseases such as infectious mononucleosis, mycoplasmal pneumonia, severe bacterial infections, and inflammatory or granulomatous diseases (ulcerative colitis, rheumatic fever, acute and chronic liver disease, and sarcoidosis) (Dodds, 1977).

Extremes in temperature result in seasonal occurrences of AIHD and/or thrombocytopenia (Karpatkin, 1980). In our experience, chronic cases of canine AIHD or thrombocytopenia in remission or under control frequently relapse a few days to a week following a severe cold spell in winter or hot spell in summer (Dodds, 1982). Five dogs with chronic AIHD had a sudden relapse with *in vivo* hemagglutination and hemolysis 2–3 days following extremely hot weather. The blood of these animals had been monitored on a regular basis by laboratory testing for more than a year previously, and had been negative for serological evidence of antierythrocyte activity. All five dogs relapsed at the same time and were referred to our laboratory by three different veterinary clinics. This was a dramatic example of the effects of environmental stress in aggravating preexisting disease.

VI. Management and Treatment

Management of acute cases of immune-mediated anemia and/or thrombocytopenia consists mainly of reducing stress and restricting activity to reduce the chance of trauma, especially to the head. Although intracranial hemorrhage is a relatively rare complication, in severe thrombocytopenia bleeding into the central nervous system is a serious and often fatal occurrence.

Treatment should be directed at correcting the anemia and keeping the patient free of purpura, if thrombocytopenia is present. It is not necessary to restore the platelet count to normal for counts of 50,000 to 80,000 per mm^3 are usually sufficient in humans and animals (Lusher and Iyer, 1977; Dodds, 1980; Karpatkin, 1980) to prevent bleeding.

A. Red Cell Disorders

With respect to AIHD, transfusions should be avoided whenever possible because they accelerate hemolysis (Dacie, 1967; Williams *et al.*, 1972; Schalm, 1975; Dodds, 1977; Pearson, 1980). Individuals with chronic, compensated anemia can tolerate low hematocrits (12–20%) quite well and can be managed in a nonstressed environment without transfusions. If replacement is essential, it is crucial that transfusions be with typed, cross-matched red cells (Dodds, 1977). Truly serocompatible blood does not exist for these patients, and so the transfused cells will have a shortened *in vivo* survival.

The treatment of choice for immune-mediated anemias is corticosteroids (Williams *et al.*, 1972; Schalm, 1975; Schalm *et al.*, 1975; Dodds, 1977). The effect is quite rapid (24–48 hr); the mechanism whereby steroids ameliorate AIHD is unknown but may involve suppression of erythrophagocytosis as well as the immune response. Severely affected patients need high doses of parenteral steroids until the hematocrit has stabilized, followed by oral medication at reduced levels once the hematocrit starts to rise and the reticulocyte count falls. Maintenance doses of steroids are given every other day for the next 1–2 months. In some patients, low maintenance doses are required on a long-term basis to prevent relapses. Only minor side effects such as weight gain have been encountered with long-term treatment (2–3 years) in dogs (Dodds, 1982). In humans, about 75% of cases improve and/or stabilize even if they remain Coombs' positive, and only about 5–10% of cases are refractory to steroids. It is not advisable to treat Coombs'-positive cases that have no clinical signs with steroids.

In our collective experience with over 300 cases, the steroid of choice, especially in severe disease, is dexamethasone. In the rare but near-fatal cases of erythroid dysplasia syndrome mentioned earlier (Section V,E), aggressive therapy with dexamethasone was the only treatment to which the patients responded. Why this corticosteroid appears to be more efficacious that the commonly used prednisone or prednisolone is unknown, although we may now be encountering immune-mediated disorders of different etiology than were seen previously.

Our dosage of dexamethasone is calculated as follows: body weight divided by eight and given as milligrams of dexamethasone on a daily basis. This dosage is given in divided doses two to three times a day. For example, a 40-pound (18.4-kg) dog would receive a total of 5 mg dexamethasone daily as 2, 1, and 2 mg during the course of 24 hr. This amount is continued for 5 to 7 days and is roughly equivalent to 1 mg/pound/day of prednisone. The dosage is then reduced by one-third to one-half for another week and then again by one-third to one-half for the third week. After this time, treatment is maintained at 0.03 to 0.05 mg/pound/day every other day, as needed. Contrary to popular and pharmacological opinion, alternate-day dexamethasone treatment has worked well for our cases as well as for other clinicians. In some cases, veterinarians have switched their patients from dexamethasone to prednisone for long-term maintenance. In our experience, it probably is not important which steroid is used for most patients once the disease process is under control, but we do have a group of patients in which relapses occur within a week of discontinuing dexamethasone therapy and/or switching to prednisone or prednisolone. We therefore recommend maintaining dexamethasone as the steroid of choice as long as it is needed. Side effects of long-term therapy have not been a significant problem.

Splenectomy may be necessary or useful in steroid-refractory cases, in patients with frequent relapses, or when steroids are required continuously in high doses to maintain the patient. The use of splenectomy is still controversial, however, and recently has been called an obsolete concept for routine treatment (Pearson, 1980). Once splenectomy is performed, the patient is at risk for severe infection (especially pneumococcal) and rapid death from a disseminated intravascular coagulation syndrome. This postsplenectomy syndrome is uncommon in adults but is of concern in children, especially those with an underlying associated primary disease (Jiji *et al.*, 1973; Lusher and Iyer, 1977; Karpatkin, 1980; Pearson, 1980). Whether this syndrome occurs in animals is unknown, but it should be kept in mind that splenectomized animals are at risk to develop hemobartonellosis (Schalm *et al.*, 1975). In our experience, splenectomy has not been necessary in the management of chronic AIHD. The most important factor in successful management has been the immediate initiation of an appropriate steroid regimen.

Antimetabolite drugs or irradiation are also being used to treat AIHD in humans and animals. This treatment is reserved for cases that are steroid resistant, require very high doses of steroids, and/or did not respond to splenectomy. Use of such drugs requires careful monitoring of the patient because of the possibility of toxic side effects. The most commonly used drugs are the vinka alkaloids (Vincristine, vinblastine), cyclophosphamide, imuran, and 6-mercaptopurine (Dodds, 1977; Lusher and Iyer, 1977; Halliwell, 1978; Kelton *et al.*, 1981).

B. Platelet Disorders

The treatment of immune-mediated thrombocytopenia is basically the same as that discussed and recommended (Section VI,A) for red cell disorders. We have found dexamethasone to be consistently more successful in reversing thrombocytopenia than prednisone or prednisolone. If this treatment is to succeed, patients must be treated as soon as thrombocytopenia is discovered and not after several days or weeks of intermittent treatment with a variety of drugs or transfusions. Cases refractory to prednisone or prednisolone are usually responsive to aggressive dexamethasone therapy, but it takes higher doses for more extended periods than would have been needed if dexamethasone had been used at first. The more debilitated the patient and the more chronic the disease, the more difficult it will be to reverse the process with steroid therapy alone. Long-term maintenance with alternate-day dexamethasone has successfully controlled immune thrombocytopenia in dogs, cats, and horses, whereas prednisone has not been as effective in another series of cases (Dodds, 1982). As mentioned earlier, there is little value in bringing the platelet count to normal values with steroid therapy (Karpatkin, 1980). Bleeding is unlikely to occur with platelet counts above 50,000 to 80,000 per mm^3, provided that the available cells are functional. We aim with our animal patients to keep platelet counts around 100,000 per mm^3, because higher counts usually require doses of steroids, which place the patient at risk for hypercorticism.

Curiously, in acute childhood purpura, use of steroids is not routine other than for the first few days after onset, and, according to several experienced investigators (Lusher and Iyer, 1977; Karpatkin, 1980), there is no real evidence that they are of benefit in reducing the risk of serious complications such as intracranial hemorrhage. Perhaps the differing experience with thrombocytopenia in animals reflects the fact that most cases are not in neonates or young animals and represent models of the chronic thrombocytopenias of humans.

The case for splenectomy in acute and chronic immune thrombocytopenia in humans is more justified than in AIHD, although this is also controversial (Jiji et al., 1973; Lusher and Iyer, 1977; Karpatkin, 1980: Pearson, 1980). Certainly the majority of patients respond to corticosteroids, splenectomy, immunosuppressive therapy, or a combination thereof (Kelton et al., 1981). About 5 to 10% of childhood thrombocytopenias become chronic, and these respond best to splenectomy (Lusher and Iyer, 1977). A favorable response to moderate doses of steroids usually indicates that the spleen is the major site of platelet destruction, which suggests that the patient will benefit from splenectomy (Karpatkin, 1980). Splenectomy has been reported to be successful in 100% of such patients but has also been useful in 79% of patients who were refractory to steroids. The rationale for splenectomy is that it removes the potential site of platelet destruction as well as a major source of antiplatelet antibody production, and it restores to the body the active platelet pool (about 40%) normally sequestered in the spleen. Interestingly, the antiplatelet antibody frequently persists afterwards despite the apparent clinical remission (Karpatkin, 1980). In patients with severe thrombocytopenia the liver is also a major source of platelet destruction, and so patients who fail to respond to splenectomy may be exhibiting hepatic sequestration of platelets. The risk of infection and death postsplenectomy, especially in children, should be kept in mind (Jiji et al., 1973; Lusher and Iyer, 1977; Karpatkin, 1980; Pearson, 1980).

Despite the conclusions of many investigators concerning the benefits of splenectomy for immune thrombocytopenia in humans (Lusher and Iyer, 1977; Karpatkin, 1980) and animals (Halliwell, 1978), we have resorted to splenectomy in only 2 cases of the more than 200 studied (Dodds and Wilkins, 1977). Neither case responded to splenectomy. We also have not used antimetabolite drugs for these cases, although one problem case was nonresponsive to high doses of dexamethasone alone and responded to two, weekly spaced injections of vincristine along with the dexamethasone (Dodds, 1982). Use of antimetabolite drugs in humans and animals with thrombocytopenia has been increasing, and our recommendations are that clinicians rely on treatment regimen(s) that have been successful in their own experience.

Platelet transfusions with fresh platelet-rich plasma or fresh or frozen platelet concentrates have a very limited role in the management of acute thrombocytopenia of childhood (Lusher and Iyer, 1977). Usually such transfusions neither alleviate bleeding nor produce a detectable rise in platelet count, and the transfused platelets are rapidly destroyed. Therefore, platelet transfusions are reserved for cases of life-threatening bleeding or to cover the patients for surgical procedures. Occasionally platelet transfusions are needed in conjunction with high doses of steroids to protect the patient during splenectomy.

To summarize the information available for treatment of thrombocytopenia (Karpatkin, 1980), about 50% of patients respond to steroids alone. Long-term therapy is usually required because cessation results in eventual relapse in chronic cases. Splenectomy is successful in about 65 to 70% of human cases, but has not been needed in our experience with over 200 cases in dogs. Patients refractory to steroids and splenectomy present more serious problems. About a third of these are also refractory to immunosuppressive therapy and have frequent relapses.

VII. Prevention

Unfortunately, until affected patients are admitted with clinical signs of immune-mediated disease, there is no way to identify those at risk in the population at large. In families with an apparent genetic predisposition to such diseases, however, serial monitoring of the relatives, as discussed earlier (Section III,C), can be helpful in predicting eventual disease. It is important to remember that it is not uncommon for clinically healthy relatives of affected individuals to have positive serological evidence of AIHD and/or thrombocytopenia without disease. Thus, a safeguard for all breeding stock, especially females with reproductive irregularities, is to monitor them on a regular basis for serological changes compatible with impending immune-mediated disease. This approach has been used successfully in our laboratory for the past 5–6 years with several affected families of dogs (Figs. 1 and 2) (Dodds, 1982).

Acknowledgments

This work was supported in part by research grant HL09902 awarded by the National Heart, Lung, and Blood Institute, PHS/DHHS, and by grants from the Geraldine R. Dodge Foundation and the American Kennel Club. The author wishes to acknowledge the contributions of the numerous colleagues who shared case experiences, and the cooperation of the many owners and breeders whose animals were referred here for study. A special note of appreciation is extended to Cophelia Pertz, V.M.D., for her participation and contributions to this article.

References

Babcock, R. B., Dumper, C. W., and Scharfman, W. B. (1976). *N. Engl. J. Med.* **295**, 237–241.
Bachand, A. J., Rubenstein, J., and Morrison, A. N. (1967). *A. J. Dis. Child.* **113**, 283–285.
Bielschowsky, M., Helyer, B. J., and Howie, J. B. (1959). *Proc. Univ. Otago Med. Sch.* **37**, 9–14.
Branehog, I. (1975). *Br. J. Haematol.* **29**, 413–426.
Byars, T. D., and Greene, C. E. (1982). *J. Am. Vet. Med. Assoc.* **180**, 1422–1424.
Cines, D. B., and Schreiber, A. D. (1979). *N. Engl. J. Med.* **300**, 106–111.
Dacie, J. V. (1967). "The Haemolytic Anemias, Congenital and Acquired," 2nd ed. Grune & Stratton, New York.
Dacie, J. V., and Worlledge, S. M. (1968). *Prog. Hematol.* **6**, 82–120.
Dobbs, C. D. (1965). *Arch. Intern. Med.* **116**, 273–276.
Dodds, W. J. (1977). *J. Am. Anim. Hosp. Assoc.* **13**, 437–441.
Dodds, W. J. (1980). *In* "Clinical Biochemistry of Domestic Animals" (J. J. Kaneko, ed.), 3rd ed., pp. 701–712. Academic Press, New York.
Dodds, W. J. (1982). New York State Department of Health, Albany (unpublished data).
Dodds, W. J., and Wilkins, R. J. (1977). *Am. J. Pathol.* **86**, 489–491.
Duquesnoy, R. J., Lorentzen, D. F., and Aster, R. (1975). *Blood* **45**, 741–747.
Fialkow, P. J. (1964). *Am. J. Med.* **36**, 188–199.
Forget, B. G. (1980). *Hosp. Pract.* **15**, 67–78.
Gengozian, N., and Rice, D. T. (1982). *Clin. Exp. Immunol.* **47**, 431–434.
Halliwell, R. E. W. (1978). *Adv. Vet. Sci. Comp. Med.* **22**, 221–263.
Hirschman, R. J., Gralnick, H. R., and Schaff, F. (1974). *J. Lab. Clin. Med.* **84**, 292–297.
Hymes, K. H., Shulman, S., and Karpatkin, S. (1979). *J. Lab. Clin. Med.* **94**, 639–648.
Jain, N. C., and Kono, C. S. (1980). *Vet. Clin. Pathol.* **9**, 10–14.
Jiji, R. M., Firozvi, T., and Spurling, C. L. (1973). *Arch. Intern. Med.* **132**, 380–383.
Joshi, B. C., and Jain, N. C. (1976). *Am. J. Vet. Res.* **37**, 681–685.

Karpatkin, S. (1980). *Blood* **56**, 329–343.
Karpatkin, S., Strick, N., Karpatkin, M. B., and Siskind, G. W. (1972). *Am. J. Med.* **52**, 776–784.
Kelton, J. G., McDonald, J. W. D., Barr, R. M., Walker, I., Nicholson, W., Neame, P. B., Hamid, C., Wong, T. Y., and Hirsh, J. (1981). *Blood* **57**, 431–436.
Lewis, R. M., Schwartz, R., and Henry, W. B. (1965). *Blood* **23**, 143–160.
Lewis, R. M., Andre-Schwartz, J., Harris, G. S., Hirsch, M. S., Black, R. H., and Schwartz, R. S. (1973). *J. Clin. Invest.* **52**, 1893–1907.
Lusher, J. M., and Iyer, R. (1977). *Semin. Thromb. Hemostasis* **3**, 175–199.
Mellors, R. C. (1969). *J. Infect. Dis.* **120**, 480–487.
Morse, B. S., Giuliani, D., and Nussbaum, M. (1981). *Blood* **57**, 809–811.
Morse, B. S., Giuliani, D., and Nussbaum, M. (1982). *Am. J. Hematol.* **12**, 271–275.
Myers, T. J., Kim, B. K., Steiner, M., Bishop, J., and Baldini, M. G. (1981). *J. Lab. Clin. Med.* **97**, 854–863.
Newton, C. D., Lipowitz, A. J., Halliwell, R. E. W., Allen, H. L., Biery, D. N., and Schumacher, R. (1976). *J. Am. Vet. Med. Assoc.* **160**, 113–121.
Osborn, J. E., and Shahidi, N. T. (1973). *J. Lab. Clin. Med.* **81**, 53–63.
Osborne, C. A., Stevens, J. R., McClean, R., and Vernier, R. L. (1973). *J. Am. Anim. Hosp. Assoc.* **9**, 295–300.
Oski, F. A., and Naiman, J. K. (1966). *N. Engl. J. Med.* **275**, 352–356.
Pearson, H. A. (1980). *Hosp. Pract.* **15**, 85–94.
Pedersen, N. C., Pool, R. C., Castles, J. J., and Weisner, K. (1976). *J. Am. Vet. Med. Assoc.* **169**, 295–303.
Pilchard, E. I. (1966). *J. Am. Vet. Med. Assoc.* **148**, 48–51.
Robbins, J. B., Skinner, R. G., and Pearson, H. A. (1969). *N. Engl. J. Med.* **280**, 75–79.
Schalm, O. W. (1975). *Can. Pract.* **2**, 37–45.
Schalm, O. W., Jain, N. C., and Carroll, E. J. (1975). "Veterinary Hematology," 3rd ed., p. 644. Lea & Febiger, Philadelphia, Pennsylvania.
Schoen, R. T., and Trentham, D. E. (1981). *Am. J. Med.* **71**, 5–8.
Schultz, R. D. (1976). "Laboratory Diagnosis of Immunologic Disorders in the Dog and Cat." Miles Laboratories, Research Products, Elkhart, Indiana.
Schwartz, R. S. (1975). *N. Engl. J. Med.* **293**, 132–136.
Shebani, O. I., and Jain, N. C. (1983). *Vet. Clin. Pathol.* **11**, 23 (abstr.).
Slappendel, R. J. (1979). *Vet. Immunol. Immunopathol.* **1**, 49–59.
Slappendel, R. J., van Erp, C. L. G. M., Goudswaard, J., and Bethlehem, M. (1970). *Tijdschr. Diergeneeskd.* **100**, 445–460.
Smith, R. D., Ristic, M., Huxsoll, D. L., and Baylor, R. A. (1975). *Infect. Immun.* **11**, 1216–1221.
Sugiura, K., Steiner, M., and Baldini, M. G. (1980). *J. Lab. Clin. Med.* **96**, 640–653.
Tizard, I. R. (1977). *In* "Introduction to Veterinary Immunology," pp. 169–183. 279–288. 312–327. Saunders, Philadelphia, Pennsylvania.
Tizard, I. R. (1978). *Bi-Week. Small Anim. Vet. Med. Update Ser.* **16**, 1–8.
Utroska, B. (1980). *VM/SAC, Vet. Med. Small Anim. Clin.* **11**, 1699–1701.
Verheyden, C. N., Beart, R. W., Jr., Clifton, M. D., and Phyliky, R. L. (1978). *Mayo Clin. Proc.* **53**, 442–446.
Videbaek, A. (1962). *Acta Med. Scand.* **171**, 187–194, 449–462.
Wilkins, R. J., Hurvitz, A. I., and Dodds-Laffin, W. J. (1973). *J. Am. Vet. Med. Assoc.* **163**, 277–282.
Williams, W. J., Beutler, E., Erslev, A. J., and Rundles, R. W., eds. (1972). "Hematology," pp. 486–510. McGraw-Hill, New York.

Bovine Congenital Defects*

H. W. LEIPOLD, K. HUSTON, AND S. M. DENNIS

Department of Pathology, College of Veterinary Medicine, Kansas State University, Manhattan, Kansas

I.		Introduction	198
II.		Definitions	199
III.		Nature and Effect	199
IV.		Frequency	201
V.		Causes	203
	A.	Environmental Factors	203
	B.	Genetic Factors	212
VI.		Kansas Genetic Disease Program	215
	A.	Gathering and Recording	216
	B.	Analysis and Interpretation	216
	C.	Communicating and Using Results	217
VII.		Specific Defects	217
	A.	Skeletal Defects	218
	B.	Joint Defects	224
	C.	Muscular System Defects	225
	D.	Central Nervous System Defects	228
	E.	Ocular Defects	242
	F.	Skin Defects	243
	G.	Defects of Hair	247
	H.	Cardiovascular System Defects	249
	I.	Respiratory System Defects	250
	J.	Digestive System Defects	250
	K.	Hepatic Defects	251
	L.	Defects of Large Body Cavities	251
	M.	Reproductive System Defects	251
	N.	Metabolic Defects	255
	O.	Defective Twinning	256
VIII.		Conclusions	256
		References	258

*Supported by the Regional Dairy Cattle Breeding Project NC-2.

I. Introduction

A variety of structural and functional defects have been described in newborn calves. They range on a nominal scale of economic or biologic defectiveness from variant through blemish, imperfection, and deviant, to malformation and monstrosity. Until the 1980s, the study of such congenital defects has been an accepted, though little emphasized, opportunistic research activity of veterinarians and animal scientists. The limited emphasis undoubtedly reflected the general attitude of herd owners and others in the cattle industry. It also may have reflected the many and often insuperable difficulties encountered in such field research investigations.

Defective calves are rare, typically occurring in only 1 or 2 of every 500 births. Except in very large herds, most herd owners are unlikely to have a defective calf born in their herds more than once or possibly twice in a 5- to 10-year period. Only under unusual circumstances, as when the defect occurs repeatedly in the same herd, cattle family, or geographic area, is a defect likely to come to the attention of investigators concerned with such matters. Thus, most defective calves go unrecorded by the science community.

Until the 1960s, congenital defects of cattle were thought to be largely hereditary. Thus, they were of principal concern to geneticists. In the early 1960s, however, thalidomide-induced congenital defects in humans proved to the science community that defects need not be hereditary. This attracted the interest of a larger group of veterinary and animal science researchers to investigations of congenital defects. Still, only recently has there been a perceptible change in the attitude of the veterinary profession, geneticists, and cattle industry in general with regard to the importance of congenital and hereditary defects or diseases (Pearson, 1979; White *et al.*, 1981).

Much of the attitude change stemmed from experiences of large artificial insemination (AI) and breed registry organizations during the years since 1950. Sometime in that period, most such organizations have had one or more worrisome episodes involving congenital or hereditary defects. As those episodes unfolded, the organizations found that they required more scientific information than was available. Moreover, the threat of litigation became a reality; several organizations have faced million-dollar lawsuits. That altered the processes by which organizations reached and disseminated policy decisions relative to congenital and hereditary defects.

It is unfortunate that full accounts of those episodes will never be published in the scientific literature. Fragmentary accounts published here and there in trade publications often fail to impress even those few scientists who have occasion to read such materials with the seriousness of the issues and intensity of concern felt by the participants.

It is fortunate that organizations involved in those episodes shared their experiences with other organizations. As a consequence, most U.S. artificial insemination and cattle registry organizations have developed programs to monitor undesirable genetic traits and to control specific ones. Most programs include sharing with herd owners the names of animals known to transmit the defect.

This article is intended to be an update of our 1972 article (Leipold *et al.*, 1972a). Several newly discovered diseases have been the subject of intensive investigations, and those findings have been highlighted. Additional information on numerous other diseases and defects of cattle has been added to our earlier account; included also is information on other domestic, zoo, and feral animals (Leipold *et al.*, 1972a; Saperstein *et al.*, 1975, 1976; Huston *et al.*, 1977, 1978; Leipold, 1978a and b; Leipold, 1980; Leipold and Dennis, 1980). Yet, the current assessment reveals that the major problems of 1972 are still the major problems:

1. Inadequate information, that is, too few case reports
2. Inadequate anatomic and pathologic investigations or descriptions
3. Inadequate and inappropriate genetic analyses
4. Failure to integrate underlying processes of embryologic, pathologic, and genetic nature (Leipold *et al.*, 1972a)

II. Definitions

Congenital defects or diseases are abnormalities of structure or function present at birth. This definition excludes normal structural and functional variants, commonly identified as "defects" by cattle breeders. The distinction between abnormality and normal variants is not always obvious.

Regarding "congenital" as synonymous with "genetic" is no longer acceptable, because not all congenital defects are caused by genetic factors. Teratology is the division of embryology and pathology dealing with abnormal development and congenital defects. A teratogen is any agent causing abnormal development.

III. Nature and Effect

Congenitally defective calves pose a diagnostic challenge to the practicing veterinarian. They also may act as sentinels of our environment and are of comparative significance for other species. Many malformed calves are stillborn or die soon after birth. Some defects are linked with embryonic and fetal deaths, abortions, and resorptions, thus causing additional economic losses.

A defective neonate is an adapted survivor from a disruptive event of genetic or environmental nature or genetic–environmental interaction at one or more stages in the complexly integrated sequences of embryonic or fetal development. If the disruptive event is not immediately lethal, it is followed by the remaining normal developmental sequences, which must then accommodate the event and its sequelae. Often this is not possible, and the affected embryo or fetus dies before completing development and is resorbed or aborted, often undetected.

Susceptibility to injurious environmental or genetic agents varies with the stage of development and decreases with fetal age. Before Day 14 (period of preattachment), the zygote or embryo is resistant to teratogens but susceptible to genetic mutations and chromosomal aberrations. During the embryonic period (Days 14–42), the embryo is highly susceptible to teratogens, but this decreases with embryonic age as the critical periods for development of various organs or organ systems are passed. The fetus (Day 42 of pregnancy and onward) becomes increasingly resistant to the action of teratogenic agents with increasing fetal age, with the exception of later differentiating structures such as cerebellum, palate, and urogenital system. For instance, anagyrine contained in various lupines such as *Lupinus caudatus* or *Lupinus sericeus* may cause cleft palate in calves born to cows fed that plant between Days 40 and 60 of gestation.

Defects may affect only a single structure or function, or may involve several body systems, or may combine functional and structural defects (in which case it is called a syndrome). All body structures and functions may be affected. Some defects may be grossly obvious; others are not recognized without careful clinicopathologic and postmortem examination. The description of syndromes in veterinary medical genetics is important because it allows for more accurate diagnosis of some of these troublesome diseases.

The frequencies with which various parts of the body are affected vary according to breed, geographic location, season, sex, age of parent, and level of nutrition.

Developmental defects may be lethal, semilethal, or compatible with life; they may impair or have little effect on viability, or may have an esthetic effect and thus lower economic value. With the increasing use of artificial insemination and also embryo transfer, certain defects no longer are rare; all are important. Although economic losses due to congenital defects are less than losses due to clinical entities caused by nutritional deficiency, infectious agents, or neoplasia, defects may cause considerable economic losses to individual cattle breeders. Congenital defects cause economic losses not only by increasing perinatal calf mortality but also by decreasing the dam's productivity. In addition, loss of value of relatives of genetically defective calves can be serious. Productivity may be reduced by longer calving intervals. Additional economic losses occur when congenital defects are only one manifestation of a syndrome that also includes embryonic and fetal mortality. Therefore, new or more expensive management practices may be required. Herd improvement is hampered through loss of replacements and consequent reduction in culling potential. Congenital defects may be an added source of confusion in diagnosing other diseases or abortion. Finally, control measures may require extensive and expensive adjustments of breeding programs if the defect is genetically caused. These defects are particularly important because they are repeated generation after generation.

IV. Frequency

The frequency of congenital defects in animals is not a fixed proportion of all births but varies because congenital defects are caused by hereditary and environmental factors, or their interactions. The frequency of individual defects, defects of each body system, and total body defects will vary among breeds, geographic locations, and seasons. In addition, interest of the observer may bias data collection. Frequencies of all congenital defects as well as those of individual structures or functions are difficult to obtain, because many defects can be identified only by necropsy. Many defects go unnoticed; others are not reported for economic reasons; others occur so rarely as to defy accurate accounting. Frequent reporting of some defects may reflect high interest of the observer rather than high incidence of the defect.

The incidence of congenital defects among all calves seems to range from 1 in 500 to 3 in 100, with 40 to 50% born dead, and only a small fraction of the reported defects not being externally visible (Herschler et al., 1962; Helmig-Schumann, 1964; Priester et al., 1970; Bellows, 1971; Bonewitz, 1971; Leipold et al., 1972a; Rieck et al., 1972, 1973; Greene et al., 1973d; Rieck and Finger, 1973).

Losses of neonatal dairy calves due to stillbirths in Dairy Herd Improvement Association herds in the United States amounted to over 6% (Salisbury and Van Demark, 1961; Bonewitz, 1971). In 5258 births reported from Kansas herds in 1954 to 1955, 2.1 calves in every 1000 were affected with congenital defects, and another 5 calves in every 1000 had undesirable traits (Huston, 1957). Range herds of Angus and Hereford cattle involving 6409 calvings during 10 years listed 4.4% stillbirths; defective calves amounted to 28% of the stillbirths or 1% of the calves born (Bellows, 1971). In 4980 births in Ohio herds surveyed in 1957 to 1960, 36 calves in every 1000 had a congenital defect; stillbirth was treated as a congenital defect (Herschler et al., 1962). In two New Zealand surveys the incidence of defective calves reported was 3.5 in 1000 in 1957 and 2.4 in 1000 in 1960 (Anonymous, 1958, 1961). In English dairy herds, 6.8% of the perinatal mortality of 4.9% was defective (Sellers et al., 1968).

Bilateral dissection of 108 calves and unilateral dissection of 31 calves in Kansas identified 103 different defects: 58 angiologic, 23 neurologic, 8 splanchnic, 7 osteologic, 6 myologic, and 1 arthrologic. Only a few were recurrent. One or more defects were present in over two-thirds of the calves; most were unilateral. Evidence for genetic control of certain defects was present (Trotter et al., 1971).

A study of 1000 German calves included 532 stillbirths, of which 84% had signs of neonatal asphyxia, 6.9% were congenitally malformed, and the remaining 9.1% had evidence of infection. Of the remaining 468 malformed calves (all died within 3 months), 2.8% had congenital malformations that caused death within 3 days, and 5.1% had nonlethal malformations but died from some other cause (Helmig-Schumann, 1964).

In Hesse, Germany, a 9-year study counted a total of 2293 defective calves (German Black Pied, German Red Pied, Simmental, Yellow cattle, Red cattle, and crossbreds). Frequency of defects was estimated to be 0.25%. Relative frequencies of the various body systems affected were as follows: central nervous system (21.6%), musculature (13.7%), anomalous twins (10.0%), congenital systemic disturbances such as hydrops (9.5%), defects of large body cavities such as schistosomus reflexus (9.3%), facial skeleton (8.8%), leg bones including joints (6.9%), digestive (4.3%), urogenital (4.3%), bone and cartilage (2.8%), heart and vessels (2.7%), skin (2.0%), and others (1.7%) (Rieck and Finger, 1973; Rieck et al., 1972, 1973). Thus the majority of congenital defects noted in that study involved the central nervous system, and dysraphic changes made up a large part of these.

A total of 137,717 patients in veterinary college clinics in the United States and Canada included 6455 animals with congenital defects (Priester et al., 1970).

Four breeds were represented in a questionnaire on congenital defects in cattle. A total of 114 calves with congenital defects was reported over a 15-month period in the Bern area of Switzerland. Simmental cattle represented 83% of the calves born and 85% of the defects reported, followed by Brown Swiss (7.9% and 4.4%), Friesians (7.3% and 4.4%), and crossbred cattle (1.5% and 0.88%). Most calves revealed syndromes of various defects. Fifty percent of the calves had head defects combined with 19% of the brain defects. Heart defects were the next most common group with 10%. A number of rare defects were found. Overall incidence of defective calves in a cow population of 132,500 cows or 136,500 calvings was estimated at 0.08% (Konig et al., 1980).

V. Causes

Many congenital defects have no clearly established cause; others are caused by environmental factors, and others have genetic causes. In addition, interplay of environmental and genetic factors may account for a considerable proportion of the defects encountered.

A. Environmental Factors

Teratogenic factors reported in cattle include toxic plants, Akabane virus, bluetongue (BT) virus, bovine virus diarrhea (BVD) virus, drugs, trace elements, and irradiation.

Teratogenic agents are difficult to identify, but they often follow seasonal patterns and known stressful conditions, and they may be linked to maternal disease. They do not follow a familial pattern as do genetic causes. Maternal disease patterns vary, but calves from heifers are more frequently affected; fetal immunoglobulins are frequently detectable; abortion incidence is increased; and morbidity may be observed in the herd or in other animals on the farm.

1. Toxic Plants

Crooked calf disease in Utah and on Kodiak Island, Alaska, is characterized by contracture of joints of the legs. These contractures are usually discordant between right and left body halves. In addition, there may be torticollis, scoliosis, or kyphosis, as well as various degrees of cleft palate and combinations of these defects (Shupe et al., 1967a; Leipold et al., 1977; Keeler, 1978; Leipold, 1978a). The cause of this syndrome is ingestion of *Lupinus caudatus, L. sericeus,* or *L. nootkatensis* (Keeler, 1978). Arthrogryposis is the most common manifestation of lupine teratogenicity. Pregnant cows fed *L. sericeus* or *L. caudatus* produced these deformities when the plants were fed between Days 40 and 70 of pregnancy. In addition, the alkaloid anagyrine was identified as the teratogenic principle (Keeler, 1978). Fetal development is at greatest risk of being impaired when the pregnant cow grazes lupine early in growth of the plant or during formation of seed. Anagyrine content of lupines is low during early flower stages and when the postseed stage has been reached.

Not all cases of crooked calf disease can be explained by ingestion of lupines during the critical phases of development. Similar deformities, have been produced by feeding *Conium maculatum* to pregnant cows between Days 50 and 75 of pregnancy. Conium was identified as the possible teratogenic compound (Keeler, 1978). As knowledge expands, other plants may be identified as teratogenic in cattle. Plants suspected of causing deformities in calves are *Senecio, Indigofera spicata, Cycadales, Blighia,* loco plants, *Papaver, Colchicum, Vinca,* tobacco, and related plants (Keeler, 1978).

2. Rectal Palpation

Studies in Germany have revealed that atresia of the gut, particularly the colon, may be caused by pressure on the amnion. Rectal palpation between Days 35 and 40 of gestation may cause atresia coli (Müller *et al.*, 1982; Ness *et al.*, 1982). Calves affected with congenital intestinal atresia amounted to 1.39% of all calves necropsied in a region (Müller *et al.*, 1982). Bulls had from 0.237 to 6.4% affected progeny. The more calves a bull sired, the more defective calves he had. Jersey, Holstein, British Friesian, Black Pied, and various crossbred bulls were involved. Dams were also of various genotypes, and maternal influence was not demonstrable. Male calves were more frequently affected, because in one herd 134 defective calves (64.11%) were males as opposed to 75 females (35.89%). Genetic analyses yielded no results (Müller *et al.*, 1982). Exogenous factors were studied. On the basis of an earlier hypothesis (Bellows *et al.*, 1975), rectal palpation techniques and gestation times were studied (Müller *et al.*, 1982).

Palpation of the amniotic vesicle was considered a likely cause of congenital intestinal atresia, because affected calves were born to cows rectally palpated for pregnancy on Days 35, 36, and 37 after insemination. A subsequent study compared the effects of palpation prior to and after Day 42 after insemination. Of 125 calves born in the pre-Day 42 group, 6 had intestinal atresia, whereas not one of the 103 in the after-Day 43 group had atresia (Müller *et al.*, 1982).

Similar results were obtained in another study (Ness *et al.*, 1982).

Since 1975, increasing numbers of congenital intestinal atresias had been observed in a veterinary practice. From January 1, 1976 to March 31, 1977, 28 calves with atresia coli were observed from 524 cows and heifers. Clinical signs were anorexia and retention of meconium, and most affected calves died 3–8 days after birth. Some lived for 14 days, however, and these were euthanized. All were confirmed by necropsy. Early pregnancy diagnosis (Days 33–40 postinsemination) by palpation of the amniotic vesicle was suspected to be the cause. None of 995 cows and heifers examined after Day 40 produced calves with atresia coli. In additional work, 9 experimental cows underwent amniotic vesicle palpation 10 times daily, 45 experimental cows were palpated once for pregnancy before Day 41, and 14 controls were examined only by slipping the chorioallantois. Only the repeatedly palpated group produced atretic calves, 6 in all. The authors concluded that palpation and pressure applied to the amnion during organogenesis (Days 33–40) can cause atresia coli and occasionally, atresia jejuni. Palpation of the amniotic vesicle is apparently possible without hazard after Day 42 postinsemination (Ness et al., 1982).

3. Virus Infection

Prenatal viral infections may be teratogenic in cattle and may be of considerable economic importance.

a. *Akabane Virus.* Prenatal Akabane virus infection caused abortions, premature births, and congenital defects in cattle in Japan, Israel, Australia, and Kenya (Markusfeld and Mayer, 1971; Kurogi et al., 1975; Metselaar, 1976; Shepherd et al., 1978. Originally, the association of the triad of abortions, stillbirths, and congenital defects with Akabane virus was based on serologic studies (Miura et al., 1974). It was followed by isolating Akabane virus from two bovine fetuses, one collected at abortion and the other by cesarean section derived subsequent to serologic conversion of the dam to Akabane virus (Kurogi et al., 1976).

Hydranencephaly is defined as complete or almost complete absence of the cerebral hemispheres in a cranium of normal conformation, the spaces being filled with cerebrospinal fluid (CSF) and surrounded by a thin membrane of cerebral tissue (Kalter, 1968). In Australia, 30 cases of arthrogryposis and 5 of hydranencephaly were reported in several breeds of cattle during the years 1952–1955 (Blood, 1956), followed by another report of 29 cases in 1957 (Whittem, 1957). Arthrogryposis and hydranencephaly (A–H syndrome) of calves were considered to be different manifestations of a single disease (Blood, 1956; Whittem, 1957). Arthrogryposis was characterized by complete absence of ventral horn cells in the spinal cord, and the muscle fibers revealed neurogenic atrophy (Whittem, 1957). A report of other cases followed (Bonner et al., 1961). Another report of 62 cases of A–H syndrome between 1964 and 1973 contained 36 collected from epizootics in 1964; 4 came from small epizootics in 1966, and the others were sporadic. Arthrogryposis alone occurred first, followed by A–H syndrome, and finally by hydranencephaly alone. In the same area of Australia, congenital defects of sheep occurred, such as micrencephaly (Hartley and Haughey, 1974a). Attempted transmission of micrencephaly in newborn lambs using emulsion of cerebrum and spleen failed, however (Hartley and Haughey, 1974b). As these congenital defects seemed to be epizootic, viral infection was considered a possible cause. The relationship between these congenital deformities and ephemeral fever virus and hydranencephaly was found to be negative (Young, 1969).

In the spring of 1973, hydranencephaly was studied by subjecting samples of serum and central nervous system fluids (CSF) to serological assay for antibodies to bovine viral diarrhea (BVD), infectious bovine rhinotracheitis (IBR), parainfluenza (PI), and ephemeral fever viruses; negative results were obtained. Concentration of four immunoglobulins, IgG_1, IgG_2, IgM, and IgA, measured in serum and central nervous system fluids disclosed marked IgM levels in sera from affected calves and led to the conclusion that hydranencephaly may result from a specific infectious agent or toxin operative at a critical stage of gestation (Wanner and Husband, 1974).

The outbreak of A–H syndrome in 1969 to 1970 in Israel was estimated to affect 2–4% of all dairy calves born. Arthrogryposis had its peak occurrence in December and hydranencephaly in the following April (Markusfeld and Mayer, 1971).

Arthrogryposis was characterized by pathological changes in the limb muscles resulting in flexion or extension of various joints. Torticollis, scoliosis, and kyphosis were associated defects. Hydranencephaly varied in severity, without any concomitant changes in the bones of the skull. Depending on the part of the brain affected, a variety of clinical signs were exhibited: ataxia and lack of coordination, hemiplegia or paraplegia, blindness, dysphagia, regurgitation, stertorious breathing, and miscellaneous signs such as goose stepping, head pressing, continuous masticating movements, tongue paralysis, and tympany (Hartley et al., 1977).

Histologic examinations of 82 calves, 24 lambs, and 10 kids affected with A–H syndrome revealed either complete absence of ventral horn cells in the spinal cord, or fewer neurons and atrophy of the muscle fibers followed by replacement by fibrous and fat tissue. Two types of lesions were described: (1) muscular dysplasia due to atrophic innervation and (2) changes in the CNS from ependymal occlusion and consequent pressure atrophy (hydrocephalus and hydranencephaly) (Nobel et al., 1971).

In Japan, during a 1949–1950 outbreak, congenital defects in Japanese Black, Japanese Red, Shorthorn, and Holstein calves were hydromicrencephalia, hydrocephalus, or absence of cerebrum (Sugawa et al., 1951; Tajima et al., 1951; Sugiura and Fujio, 1961). During the period 1959–1960, outbreaks of congenital cerebral defects occurred again and included hydrocephalus, anencephaly, hydranencephaly, and porencephaly (Sugiura and Fujio, 1961; Inui and Maruyama, 1967). These epizootic congenital defects are now believed to have been partly due to various forms of Akabane disease (Konno, 1973, 1977). The outbreaks of abortions, premature births, stillbirths, and congenital A–H syndrome in Japan during the summer through winter of the years 1972–1973 and 1973–1974 affected over 40,000 fetuses and calves (Hamana et al., 1973, 1974a,b, 1975; Ohashi, 1973; Omori, 1973, 1977; Otsuka et al., 1973, 1975; Hamada, 1974; Miura et al., 1974; Omori et al., 1974; Konno et al., 1975; Moriguchi et al., 1976). Epizootic and seasonal occurrence, distribution only in the South and West of Japan, little or no recurrence in an area that experienced congenital defects in calves in the previous year, normal calves delivered by cows previously delivering abnormal calves, and periodic occurrence at intervals of several years all strongly suggested an environmental factor, especially viral infection (Otsuka et al., 1973; Inaba et al., 1975). Clinical findings were similar to those reported in Australia and Israel. The cow rarely had any clinical signs during pregnancy except for occasional cases of hydropic amnion. Recurrence of estrus and conception were generally normal in spite of delivery of defective calves. Dystocia and stillbirth were often encountered with arthrogrypotic calves; they were small and most were unable to stand. Some could stand and walk when helped. Arthrogryposis affected one, two, three, or four limbs and was often associated with single or multiple defects, such as torticollis, scoliosis, or hydranencephaly. Hydranencephaly occurred alone or together with arthrogryposis. Ocular anomalies included blindness, corneal opacity, inflammation, and lack of eye reflexes. Poorly calcified incisor teeth were often associated with gingivitis. Breathing difficulty was a clinical feature of hydranencephaly. Pathological changes were similar to those reported in Australia (Whittem, 1957; Hartley and Wanner, 1974) and Israel (Nobel et al., 1971). Although muscles of arthrogrypotic limbs were atrophic, generally the bones and joints had no marked changes. Hydranencephaly was characterized by a complete or partial absence of cerebral hemispheres; in partial hydranencephaly, the temporal lobe of the cerebrum primarily was affected (Tajima et al., 1951; Nosaka et al., 1973). The remainder of the brain of hydranencephalic calves revealed histologic degenerative changes and repair (Nosaka et al., 1973). Calves with mild A–H syndrome had little inflammatory reaction such as perivascular hemorrhage, infiltration of round cells, small hemorrhagic foci, and demyelinization of the ventral horn of the spinal cord. Another study reported hydranencephaly, porencephaly, gliosis, hypoplastic changes in the cerebellum, perivascular cuffing, various types of damage to the ventricular walls, and dilation of the perivascular spaces. Gliosis and associated findings were most characteristic; loss of neurons with gliosis were observed in the ventral horn of the spinal cord (Moriguchi et al., 1976).

Histopathological examination of calves either affected with A–H syndrome or delivered from a cow inoculated experimentally with Akabane virus revealed muscular changes. Initially, the term "runt muscle disease" was proposed. On the basis of marked progressive pathological changes, Akabane disease can be classified into three stages: early noninflammatory encephalomyelitis, "runt muscle disease" at the middle stage, and hydranencephaly in the late stage (Konno, 1973, 1977; Konno et al., 1975, 1982). Experimental reproduction of Akabane disease produced encephalomyelitis and polymyositis as primary lesions in cattle and goats (Konno and Nakagawa, 1982).

Epizootiological and pathological studies of A–H syndrome strongly indicated a viral cause. In the 1972–1973 outbreak in Japan, precolostral sera from calves with congenital A–H syndrome and from normal calves were examined for neutralizing antibodies against a group of arboviruses, such as Akabane, Aion, Geta, and Japanese encephalitis (JE) viruses. Only the antibody for Akabane virus was higher in calves with A–H syndrome, indicating a correlation between A–H syndrome and precolostral anti-Akabane antibody (Konno, 1973; Omori et al., 1974; Inaba, 1975; Inaba et al., 1975). The dams of these calves had high anti-Akabane antibodies, and few had antibodies to other viruses. Serological surveys indicated wide dissemination of Akabane virus in epizootic areas of Japan. All findings strongly suggested Akabane virus was the etiologic agent (Kurogi et al., 1975). Vertical transmission was demonstrated by experimentally inoculating pregnant cows, sheep, and goats with Akabane virus; A–H syndrome was thus experimentally produced in a calf and a kid (Omori, 1973; Omori et al., 1974; Inaba et al., 1975). It was concluded that outbreaks of A–H syndrome in Japan were caused by prenatal

Akabane virus infection and should be referred to as Akabane disease (Omori, 1977).

In Australia, neutralizing antibodies to Akabane virus were demonstrated in serum, collected prior to sucking, of calves with congenital A–H syndrome in 1964 and 1973 (Hartley and Wanner, 1974). Parsonson et al. (1981) were unable to transmit the virus via semen.

Akabane virus injected intravenously into 25 pregnant ewes produced lambs born with various degrees of A–H syndrome and also scoliosis, kyphosis, and brachygnathia. The inoculated ewes developed serum-neutralizing antibodies to Akabane virus; antibody also was detected in sera collected from the lambs (Parsonson et al., 1975). Distribution of Akabane virus in Australia, A–H syndrome, and the insect vector *Culicoides brevitarsis* overlapped (Della-Porta et al., 1976; St. George et al., 1978; Shephard et al., 1978).

A review of outbreaks involving more than 4000 newborn calves with A–H syndrome in Israel concluded that Akabane virus was the causative agent (Mayer, 1976). Persistence of antibodies for over 6 years and the total immunity they seem to confer were expected to lead to rapid development of an effective "lifelong" vaccine that would lead to elimination of rapidly spreading Akabane virus infection (Mayer, 1976).

The arthrogrypotic syndrome without hydranencephaly may include more than one etiologic or pathologic entity (Leipold et al., 1970c), for example, maternal ingestion of lupine (Shupe et al., 1967a) or manganese deficiency (Dyer et al., 1964). A hereditary example is arthrogryposis and cleft palate, inherited in the Charolais breed as an autosomal recessive (Nawrot et al., 1980).

b. Bovine Virus Diarrhea Virus. Bovine virus diarrhea (BVD) virus is fetopathogenic. Outcome of infection in pregnant and susceptible cows depends on the stage of pregnancy: (1) fetal death followed by abortion or mummification, (2) stillbirths, (3) neonates with various congenital defects such as cerebellar dysplasia, ocular defects, brachygnathia inferior, alopecia, dysmyelinogenesis, internal hydrocephalus, dysmaturity (intrauterine growth retardation), and impaired immunologic competence, and (4) immune viable neonates (Kahrs et al., 1970a,b; Casaro et al., 1971; Kendrick, 1971; Brown et al., 1973, 1974, 1975; Scott et al., 1973; Axthelm et al., 1980b, 1981a; Done et al., 1980; Kahrs, 1981). Different strains of BVD may have different effects on the developing bovine fetus (Done et al., 1980; Kahrs, 1981). Bovine virus diarrhea virus-induced congenital defects occur naturally and have been experimentally reproduced in calves and lambs (Ward, 1971; Scott et al., 1973; Done et al., 1980). Four of five susceptible pregnant heifers inoculated with the Studdert strain of BVD between Days 79 and 150 of gestation gave birth to calves affected with cerebellar degeneration. The calf from a dam inoculated at Day 79 of gestation revealed granuloprival hypoplasia, severe depletion of granule cells, clumping of granule cells, and ectopia of Purkinje cells. Calves whose dams had been inoculated after 100 days of gestation had more severe cerebellar changes, ranging from mild to severe depletion of the cortical layers, to complete destruction of cortex and folial white matter. Lesions in the folial white matter ranged from fiber-depleted streaks to irregular cavitation (Brown et al., 1973). During an epizootic of BVD, 29 pregnant cattle had 19 normal, 8 aborted, and 2 calves with cerebellar degeneration (Kahrs et al., 1970a). A study with a cytopathogenic strain of BVD used 14 pregnant susceptible heifers and 2 controls. The virus was inoculated at about 150 days of gestation, and subsequently fetuses were surgically recovered sequentially. There were no lesions between 4 and 14 days postinoculation (PI). Fetuses taken at 17 and 21 days PI had cerebellar lesions, such as leptomeningeal inflammation, cell necrosis in the external germinal layer, focal hemorrhages, and varying degrees of folial edema. By 42 days PI, the inflammatory response had subsided and the cerebellar lesion had completely evolved with folial degeneration and cavitation (Brown et al., 1974). Lesions induced by inoculation of 23 susceptible pregnant heifers at ~150 days of gestation revealed acute ocular lesions in fetuses taken 17–21 days PI. After 4 weeks, the acute lesions resolved, and focal or diffuse retinal atrophy was present in neonatal calves (Brown et al., 1975). In Great Britain, 10 antibody-free Jersey heifers were inoculated on gestation Day 100 with a mixture of 10 cytopathic strains of BVD virus. The heifers did not become infected, but all had seroconversion within 6 weeks. Six fetuses, including one set of twins, died *in utero;* 5 were aborted between Days 136 and 154, and 1 became mummified and was retained at Day 300. Of the remaining 10 fetuses born at term, 9 had evidence of dysmaturity. Three forms of dysmaturity were distinguished by Done et al. (1980):

1. Diffuse stunting in terms of crown–anus length and body weight. Such fetuses are identifiable by discrepancies between chronological and developmental age as estimated from long bone length
2. Selective stunting of vulnerable tissues, e.g., brain, lung, thymus
3. Sporadic checks to growth, e.g., growth arrest lines in long bones

Five of the six dead fetuses and one live calf had single or multiple growth arrest lines.

In addition, there were CNS defects in all 10 calves born at term; 4 had gross CNS lesions such as micrencephaly, internal hydrocephaly, cerebellar dysgenesis, and cerebellar hypoplasia. Furthermore, dysmyelination was seen in 2 of 10 calves by histochemical and by neurochemical studies in 9 calves at term. This was evidenced by low total lipids in 6 calves, low cholesterol in 4, and low lipid hexose in 7 (Done et al., 1980).

Experimental fetal infection with BVD virus caused characteristic changes in bovine fetuses: precocious development of secondary lymphoid tissue, cerebellar changes, and skin changes (Bielefeldt Ohmann, 1982).

Hydranencephaly with porencephalic cavitation was seen over a 2-year period in 5 calves from an 80-cow herd. The 5 calves were blind and had fine head tremors and limb rigidity. Bovine virus diarrhea was considered the likely cause of the defects because its antigens were present in tissues of 2 calves (Axthelm et al., 1981a).

Congenital internal hydrocephalus was diagnosed in two calves, 1 and 14 days old, respectively, associated with stenosis of the mesencephalic aqueduct and meningoencephalitis. Cerebellar hypoplasia was present in one calf. Bovine virus diarrhea virus was detected in the tissues of both calves and was thought to be the causative agent (Axthelm et al., 1980b). In contrast, recessive hereditary internal hydrocephalus in neonatal horned Hereford calves had other features, including small body size, cranial doming, and internal hydrocephalus characterized by maldevelopment of the mesencephalon. Microphthalmia and retinal dysplasia, cerebellar hypoplasia and dysplasia, and skeletal muscle myopathy were additional criteria that were useful for diagnosis. Herd histories of abortions, high neonatal mortality, and hydrocephalus in calves of common ancestry accompanied most of the 11 specimens submitted (Axthelm et al., 1980a).

c. Bluetongue Virus. Bluetongue (BT) virus has been found to be teratogenic in sheep, causing hydranencephaly and porencephaly (Osburn et al., 1971a,b). It also affects fetal calves (McKercher et al., 1970; Liendo and Castro, 1981; Luedke and Walton, 1981). Experimental transmission to pregnant heifers via insects resulted in abortions, stillbirths, and congenital defects such as arthrogryposis, campylognathia, and prognathia with domed cranium. In addition, excessive red to purple gingival tissue was observed (Luedke, 1977a,b; Luedke et al., 1977). Hydranencephaly and a "dummy-calf" syndrome (inactivity, dullness, behavioral disturbances) have also been associated with prenatal BT virus infection (McKercher et al., 1970; Richards et al., 1971). Fourteen heifers were bred to a bull shedding BT virus in his semen.

One heifer aborted at between 55 and 62 days gestation and remained in anestrus for 300 days; she was the only one to develop precipitating antibodies to BT virus 100 days after breeding. Of the 13 calves that went to term, 12 were born alive and were affected with congenital defects such as excessive gingival tissue, crooked legs, and deformed jaws. Five calves were weak and ataxic at birth. All calves were viremic at birth (Luedke and Walton, 1981). In Oklahoma, cattle herds infected with BT virus had abortions and congenital defects such as arthrogryposis, kyphosis, and scoliosis (Liendo and Castro, 1981).

d. Wesselsbron Virus. Wesselbron disease virus caused congenital porencephaly and cereballar hypoplasia in South Africa (Coetzer *et al.*, 1979).

B. Genetic Factors

Hereditary defects are pathologic or pathophysiologic results determined by mutant genes or chromosomal aberrations, the principal genetic factors. The term factor is used to identify the general class of genetic agents (genic and chromosomal), because the two usually cannot be distinguished in cattle. Chromosomal aberrations have been demonstrated, but as yet they have not attained the level of diagnostic prominence they have in humans. Genetic defects are commonly classified as lethal, semilethal, subvital (including compatibility with life), in accordance with survival of affected animals (0% survival, less than 50% survival, at least 50% survival) (Hadorn, 1961). The lists, particularly the list of lethals, are updated periodically (Stormont, 1958; Hutt, 1964; Fechheimer, 1968; Lauvergne, 1968). Early beliefs and continuing interest in genetic causes have resulted in the literature of congenital defects containing many genetic terms and points of emphasis not found in any other field of pathology.

The primary importance of diagnosis is prevention, particularly of defects impairing structure or function and hence the economic usefulness of the calf. Even undesirable inherited traits that do not impair usefulness should be listed on the pedigree or in any advertisement of breeding stock, in particular those for sires in artificial breeding or from which semen is sold.

Except for two brief discussions (Huston, 1966; Leipold and Huston, 1968b), there are no current guides to genetic diagnosis in cattle. There are, however, several for humans. *Human Genetics* (Li, 1961) is a book for the serious student; *Segregation and Linkage* (Morton, 1962) is highly advanced and thorough. Other useful works are by Cotterman (1954), Kempthorne (1957), and Edwards (1970). After 1970 there were a number of advances in both simple and complex segregation analysis in humans (Morton et al., 1971; Elston, 1981; Nicholas, 1982). A review by Elston (1981) demonstrates the complex analytical options already available for humans, options that one day may become useful in cattle. Whether the greater complexity and irregularity of cattle genealogies will limit these options remains to be discovered.

Diagnosis of genetically caused defects is based on the rule that genetic diseases run in families. Thus congenital defects occur in typical intergenerational and intragenerational patterns that require both enumeration of normal and abnormal offspring, and identification of their familial relationships. Various statistical methods are used to analyze such data. Breeding trials may be necessary to confirm inheritance patterns. For the study of skeletal defects, a combination of superovulation of homozygous affected cows, insemination with bulls of known or unknown genotype (to be tested), and preterminal gestation cesarian section have been used (Baker et al., 1980; Johnson et al., 1980, 1981; Castleberry et al., 1981; Leipold and Peeples, 1981).

Analysis is complicated when there are several diagnostic entities, as when a syndrome of defects is found. Several important analytical points should be noted. The family can be identified through one or more defective calves, the index cases (propositi or probands); this is important because under certain modes of inheritance some normal parents can produce both normal and abnormal young, whereas others can produce only normals. In genetic analysis only families from parents that produce a defective calf are included; families from parents that can but do not produce defects are excluded. This truncated selection increases the frequency of defectives over that expected theoretically from complete selection possible in experimental matings.

Although causes of many congenital diseases in cattle are not known, many follow simple Mendelian inheritance, mostly simple autosomal recessive patterns. Other monofactorial inheritance patterns are described as overdominant, dominant, or incompletely dominant, whereas only a few reports describe sex linkage. Congenital defects may also be inherited as polygenic traits.

The recessive inheritance pattern involves only two kinds of animals: normal and defective. Only a few normal carriers, or heterozygotes, can transmit the disease. Although two defective parents produce only defective calves, most defective animals do not reproduce; hence, most defectives are born to normal parents. Each normal parent (heterozygote) producing a defective calf transmits one of the two abnormal genes necessary to produce the defective offspring. However, most normal animals cannot transmit the disease. When the non-disease carriers are mated with other noncarriers, or even with normal carriers, they produce only normal offspring.

When normal cattle that produced a defective offspring are mated repeatedly, 25% of their progeny should be defective and 75% normal. Two of every three normal calves from such parents carry a hidden recessive gene that they may transmit to their progeny just as their parents transmitted the abnormal gene to them. Thus recessive defects are "carried" generation after generation by normal phenotypic cattle (carriers), resulting in insidious spread of the undesirable gene through the population. Carrier cattle (or heterozygotes) for a disease, transmitted as an autosomal recessive, are identified indirectly only after they have had defective offspring.

Eliminating defective progeny usually keeps recessive defects at low frequencies. However, breeds in which only a few animals produce most breeding animals, or in which many animals are closely related to some single outstanding animal, are vulnerable, and serious outbreaks of genetic defects may result. This happens when the foundation animal carries a recessive gene unknown to its owners. The defect is then exposed when descendants of such animals are mated. Inbreeding is therefore one way to expose the presence of abnormal recessive genes.

Other simple inheritance patterns include dominance, incomplete dominance, and overdominance. Dominance is the reverse of the recessive inheritance pattern. With dominant inheritance, normals breed true, but abnormals may produce both normals and abnormals. The defect does not skip generations as in recessive inheritance. Dominant defects are easily controlled by eliminating all defective animals.

Incomplete dominance creates three kinds of animals: normal, slightly abnormal, and severely abnormal. The normal and the severely abnormal animals breed true. The slightly abnormal animals, when mated together, produce 25% normal progeny, 50% slightly abnormal progeny, and 25% severely abnormal progeny. The disease is easily controlled by eliminating all abnormal progeny.

Overdominance is like incomplete dominance in that three kinds of animals are produced: normal, superior, and abnormal. Normal and abnormal animals breed true. The superior animals, when mated with other superiors, produce 25% normal, 50% superior, and 25% defective offspring. The superior animals are usually selected as replacements in preference to normal animals but at the cost of losing 25% of their offspring from like mates because they are defective. Overdominant traits are difficult to control, because all superior animals also carry the undesirable gene and owners are reluctant to choose inferior breeding animals.

Genetic analysis in a herd requires enumeration of normal and defective cattle as well as all of their family relationships. Analyses proceed along two important lines. Data on full-sib families containing one or more defective calves are subjected to segregation analysis; similar methods are being proposed for $\frac{3}{4}$- and $\frac{5}{8}$-sib families, which are larger and are common in cattle. These are the central and most critical analyses.

The remaining collateral evidence may be analyzed by a variety of comparisons. One demonstrates the compatibility of data with consequences of forces altering population gene frequencies. Another demonstrates that close relatives are more alike than more remote relatives, presumably because the close relative received copies of the same normal or mutant genes. Another analysis tests concordance with results of segregation analyses. Still others include searching for inbreeding in recessive inheritance or for homologous hereditary defects in experimentally more tractable species.

Analyses usually proceed from simplest modes of inheritance to the more complex ones. Modes based on two alleles at a single autosomal or sex-linked locus are tested first, then their modifications that are caused by the variable expressivity–incomplete penetrance phenomenon or by sporadic cases occurring as phenocopies, spontaneous mutations, or other sources of confusion. (Incomplete penetrance results when a genetically defective animal is itself normal.)

A few reports describe characteristics linked with sex; that is, the genes are carried on the sex chromosomes. Another class of genetic diseases is caused by chromosomal aberrations. However, structural and numerical aberrations of chromosomal material in cattle have not attained the diagnostic significance encountered in humans. One of the most common chromosomal defects in domestic animals encountered in high frequency in cattle is centric fusion of acrocentric chromosomes to form Robertsonian translocations. Chromosomal defects and aberrations in chromosomal number are becoming increasingly important for studying the etiology of congenital defects in cattle (Bruère, 1980; DiBerardino and Iannuzzi, 1982; Willer, 1982).

To summarize, genetically caused diseases run in families, in typical intergenerational patterns and intragenerational family frequencies. Various statistical methods are used to analyze such data. Test matings may be necessary to confirm the inheritance pattern.

VI. Kansas Genetic Disease Program

The Kansas State University (KSU) genetic disease program was initiated in the early 1930s and consists of gathering, recording, analyzing, and interpreting information, and communicating and using the results. Epizootiology of genetic defects has to be considered in three etiological contexts: unknown, suspected, and known causes. All three categories are handled in the KSU system.

A. Gathering and Recording

Initial case reports are received in many forms from veterinarians, breed organizations, artificial insemination organizations, extension personnel, and herd owners, and are recorded in chronologic order. Histories include breed, age of parents, parentage of affected and unaffected control calves, geographic region, season, type of pasture, soil type, exposure to or suspected exposure to teratogenic plants, feeding and management practices, breeding records, maternal medical and vaccination records, disease status of herd, periods of stress, drugs administered, congenital defects observed previously, and history of any similar congenital defects in neighboring herds.

All defective calves are subjected to standardized necropsy, and the defects are classified by the body system primarily involved. Serum samples are taken to check for bovine virus diarrhea and other viral antibodies. Samples of brain and other tissues are taken for possible virus isolation. Fluorescent antibody techniques are also employed. Histologic examination is done, and selected cases are submitted for electron microscopic studies.

Breeding records may be analyzed for evidence of inbreeding and for characteristic intergenerational transmission patterns and intragenerational frequencies. Etiologic diagnosis is made after the results of the tests have been carefully considered. Results are filed in a central congenital defects file.

B. Analysis and Interpretation

Preliminary analysis and interpretation are made during the gathering and recording phase, proceeding through the following steps:

1. Determine whether a similar defect has been reported among a bull's offspring.
2. Compare the case against similar cases recorded in central congenital defects file.
3. Search the literature file for reports of similar defects in cattle.
4. Search the literature on other species (human and animals).
5. Study all herd health data, necropsies, and other tests as outlined previously.

For decisions on breeding programs, the following steps should be taken. Most breed associations, such as the American Jersey Cattle Club, follow procedures similar to the following:

1. Blood typing should be utilized to establish verified parentage, especially where an AI sire is involved.
2. A certified statement by a veterinarian or a third-party witness should be obtained.
3. An extended pedigree chart should be made.
4. Laboratory examination by a pathologist should be performed where applicable.
5. A decision should be withheld until all reasonable doubt has been eliminated. This usually requires two or more thoroughly documented reports for bulls.

C. Communicating and Using Results

Communicating and using results include consideration of the following:

1. Many genetic defects have not been clearly identified to date and await description and clarification.
2. A single undesirable recessive trait can rapidly become a real problem in a breed of cattle.
3. Maintenance of a recording system by breed organizations, AI centers, and other institutions is the most efficient and least expensive way to monitor undesirable traits.

If evidence is presented that a bull carries an undesirable recessive gene, most organizations proceed to label the bull as a heterozygote and remove him from service. If he is not removed, advertisement material should carry information concerning the congenital defect. Sometimes it is desirable to test a bull for a recessive gene before using him. If the bull is of standard phenotype, he may be bred to unknown populations. Occurrence of defects would justify removal from AI service or at least labeling the bull. The suspected bull may be test-mated to known heterozygotes for a trait, to his own daughters, or to abnormal homozygous individuals that survive to reproduce.

VII. Specific Defects

It is difficult to arrive at a single system suitable for classifying congenital defects of cattle. Three principal systems have been used. Etiologic classification is useful for certain purposes but is not generally feasible. Classification has also been based on affected embryonic tissue (Herschler et al., 1962). Because primary classification on the basis of the principally defective body system is clinically most useful, that system is followed here.

This section defines defects of various body systems in cattle, placing emphasis on defects of current interest and concern, and contrasting them to defects of known environmental origin. The list is not complete but gives some insight into genetic diseases of beef and dairy cattle. Most breed organizations have listings of defects of special concern to their breeders and veterinarians. Most artificial breeding service units in the United States have monitoring systems for congenital defects.

A. Skeletal Defects

Each body system is susceptible to congenital defects, some more frequently than others. The skeletal system is involved in many congenital defects of cattle. Parts of the system may be affected with single, isolated, osseous defects, or the whole skeleton may be affected.

1. Single, Isolated Skeletal Defects

a. Face. Except for palatoschisis, congenital clefts of the face have been infrequently described (Shupe et al., 1968). Among 331 animals with cleft palate in a veterinary hospital population, cats, mixed-breed dogs, and German Shepherd dogs had low risk for cleft palate; high rates occur in English Bulldogs, some small purebred dogs, and in Charolais cattle, where cleft palate occurred as part of a syndrome of multiple malformations. The use of animal models for studying human cleft palate is recommended (Mulvihill et al., 1980). The association of palatoschisis with other congenital defects, particularly arthrogryposis, should be stressed (Leipold et al., 1970c; Nawrot et al., 1980). Recessive inheritance of cheilognathoschisis in Shorthorn calves has been reported (Wheat, 1960). Recessive inheritance could not be confirmed for cheilognathoschisis in two purebred Angus calves. Both calves (one male, one female) had unilateral cleft lip, and their karyotypes were normal (Swartz et al., 1982). References to other case reports are listed by Koch et al. (1957), Lauvergne (1968), Wiedeking (1968), and Wiesner and Willer (1974).

Several developmental defects of the jaws have been described. Campylognathia is lateral deviation of the face with normal development of the mandible. Abnormal length of the upper or lower jaw is termed superior or inferior prognathia, respectively; short upper and lower jaw are termed superior or inferior brachygnathia. Inferior brachygnathia (short lower jaw, parrot beak, parrot mouth) is a relatively common hereditary defect in cattle (Smith et al., 1961) and may vary considerably in degree. A lethal form involves impacted molar teeth (Grant, 1956). Brachygnathia inferior also may be due to a chromosomal aberration. Hohn and Herzog (1970) reported inferior brachygnathia combined with other defects in two calves that had autosomal trisomy. Inferior brachygnathia with molar teeth impaction is also one of the features of lethal hereditary osteopetrosis in Angus cattle (Leipold et al., 1970a).

Extreme hypoplasia to aplasia of the mandibles or agnathia is rare in cattle (Ely et al., 1939; Deniz, 1966). Agnathia, however, may be part of a mandibulofacial syndrome. Agnathia may involve the craniofacial skeleton and, in the extreme, merge into aprosopia or facelessness, which has been encountered rarely in cattle.

Craniofacial dysplasia was described in the Limousin breed in France by Blin and Lauvergne (1967) as "tête a mouton." The defect involved deficient ossification of the frontal sutures, convex profile of the nose, inferior brachygnathia, bilateral exophthalmus, scoliosis of the upperjaw, macroglossia, and associated defects of omasum and heart.

b. Vertebral Column. A severe but rare malformation resulting from a marked reduction in the axial skeleton is the short spine lethal, a recessive trait characterized by reduction and fusion of spines and ribs from 13 in normal calves to 6 or 7 (Mohr and Wriedt, 1930). Likewise, perosomus elumbis (agenesis of the caudal segments of the vertebral column) is rare (deBoom, 1965). Other spinal column defects include atlanto-occipital fusion (Leipold et al., 1972c), kyphosis (dorsal deviation), lordosis (ventral deviation), scoliosis (lateral deviation), and their combinations. Kyphoscoliotic deformities are commonly associated with arthrogryposis (Leipold et al., 1970c; Nawrot et al., 1980). Spina bifida is usually associated with abnormal development of the spinal cord. Lateral deviation of the neck is referred to as torticollis or wryneck (Whittem, 1957). Total agenesis (anury) and partial agenesis (brachyury) of the caudal part of the spinal column are found commonly in cattle and are often associated with defects in other organs such as eye and heart (Huston and Wearden, 1958; Rieck, 1965; Leipold and Huston, 1968a). Wrytail has been described in cattle (Atkeson et al., 1944a) as a recessive trait. Causes of anury and brachyury are unknown (Greene et al., 1973a).

c. Extremities. Duplication of a whole limb is polymelia. Heterotopic polymelia results when one or two additional legs are attached to various body regions and classified accordingly. The most common is notomelia, where the supernumerary leg is attached at the back. Other attachments include the occipital region of the head (cephalomelia), thorax (thoracomelia), and pelvic region (pygomelia).

In contrast to supernumerary extremities is a reduction in number. Agenesis of extremities is referred to as amelia; abrachia refers to front legs and apodia to hind legs. If only one leg is affected, the terms are monobrachia or monopodia, respectively. Calves with abrachia have dysplasia of the spinal cord segment corresponding to the leg defect (Goller, 1961, 1963).

In micromelia, all parts of the appendicular skeleton are present but hypoplastic. Peromelia is failure of the distal appendicular parts to develop, whereas phocomelia refers to absence of the proximal appendicular parts with distal parts developed (Fischer, 1951).

Localized defects of the appendicular skeleton are of various kinds, usually inherited, and some are of considerable economic importance. All appear to be significant as biomedical models (Leipold and Morris, 1979a,b; Morris and Leipold, 1979a,b). Reduced phalanges were described as lethal because of homozygosity of a recessive gene (Johannson, 1942). Tibial hemimelia in Scotland was described in a single calf as being caused by simple autosomal recessive inheritance (Young, 1951). Subsequently, tibial hemimelia became a commonly encountered defect in American Galloway herds (Ojo *et al.*, 1975a; Leipold *et al.*, 1978). Tibial hemimelia, a congenital syndrome affecting both sexes, may include the following defects: bilateral agenesis or reduction in length of the tibia, bilateral agenesis of the patella, nonclosure of the pelvic symphysis, cranioschisis, meningocele, internal hydrocephalus, ventral abdominal hernia, nonunion of the Müllerian ducts in females, and cryptorchidism in males. Most commonly, Galloway calves with tibial hemimelia are stillborn or die shortly after birth. Breeding trials with selected Galloway cattle indicated that tibial hemimelia is due to homozygosity of a simple autosomal recessive gene with variable expressivity in the tibial structure (usually bilateral agenesis) and pleiotropic effects on central nervous, reproductive, skeletal, and muscular systems (Leipold *et al.*, 1978). Tibial hemimelia has also been described in a Simmental calf (Doige *et al.*, 1978) and in a Bunaji calf (Salako and Abdullahi, 1982).

Rare congenital defects, like common ones, may be genetic or environmental in origin, or may reflect a combination of both. Although of modest economic importance, ectrodactyly, defined as partial or complete absence of phalanges, is such a defect (Leipold *et al.*, 1969b,d). Concern for this and other defects of similar nature is aroused because of external resemblance to hereditary bovine syndactyly.

Polydactyly, an increase in number of digits, is a genetic defect found in a number of species. Although all four feet may be affected, there is a tendency for only the front feet to be involved (Leipold et al., 1972b). Bovine polydactyly is considered to be genetic, but the mode of inheritance varies. It has been reported as a sex-linked recessive; males express the trait with one and two genes, but females need two (Morrill, 1945). In French Pied, polydactyly was inherited as an incomplete dominant (Lauvergne, 1962); a similar conclusion was reached for Swedish Red cattle (Dahlquist et al., 1962).

Five breeding trials were conducted to clarify the mode of inheritance of polydactyly in Simmental cattle. Two breeding trials involved superovulation of polydactylous females, embryo transfer, and early fetal recovery at 70 days of gestation. The other three breeding trials were father–daughter, mother–son, and polydactyly–polydactyly matings. The conclusion was that the mode of inheritance of bovine polydactylism may be polygenic. Expression of polydactyly seems to require a dominant gene at one locus and recessive genes at another locus (Johnson et al., 1981).

Syndactyly is defined as fusion or nondivision of functional digits. It is due to homozygosity of a simple autosomal recessive gene with incomplete penetrance and varying degrees of expressivity and pleiotrophic effect (Huston et al., 1961a; Leipold et al., 1969a,b,c, 1973a; Johnson et al., 1980; Leipold and Peeples, 1981). It is the most common inherited skeletal defect of Holstein cattle in the United States, but it is also encountered in Angus, Chianina, Simmental, and crossbred cattle (Leipold et al., 1973a; Ojo et al., 1975a). Simmental cattle in Europe also had syndactyly (Krölling, 1956).

Syndactyly in Holstein cattle usually follows a particular pattern of fusion or nondivision. If one leg is affected, it is the right front leg followed by the left front leg. If three legs are affected, the pattern is right and left front, followed by right hind leg. Rarely are all four feet affected. The degree of fusion or nondivision is always more advanced in the right front foot when more than one foot is affected (Leipold, 1968; Leipold et al., 1973a). Osteologic defects in syndactylous manus or pes have followed certain sequences: the second phalanges most frequently were horizontally synostotic, followed by the third, then the first. Osteologic defects paralleled the asymmetrical external pattern in that right–left and front–rear gradients were observed (Leipold et al., 1969c, 1973a). Muscles, blood vessels, and nerves accommodated the syndactylous deformities (Adrian et al., 1969a,b,c). The anatomical defects in hereditary bovine syndactyly are accompanied by a functional defect that requires special environmental conditions for expression (Leipold, 1968).

When syndactylous cattle and control cattle were subjected to controlled conditions in a climatic chamber, all five syndactylous Holstine–Friesian cattle developed signs of malignant hyperthermia (Leipold, 1968; Leipold et al., 1969a). This complemented experience with syndactylous cattle (kept at Kansas State University), which succumbed to environmental stresses such as higher ambient temperatures and calving (Huston and Leipold, 1968). Gruneberg and Huston (1965) studied the development of syndactylous carrier and normal Holstein–Friesian embryos, 31–45 days of age. The anlages of the metacarpal bones were close together in the 37-day syndactylous embryo, and the distal ends had started to fuse. The normal 39-day embryo had widely separated blastemata of the future phalanges, whereas the syndactylous embryo had a single mass of blastema.

A program to test syndactyly in Holstein and Angus cattle uses superovulation of homozygous, affected, syndactylous cows, insemination with semen of bulls to be tested, embryo transplant, and preterminal cesarian section (Baker et al., 1980; Johnson et al., 1980). Females may be tested by using semen from affected bulls, embryo transfers, and early fetal recovery (Leipold and Peeples, 1981). The defect seems to be allelic in Holstein, Angus, and Chianina breeds in the United States; however, beef breeds seem to be more severely affected (Ojo et al., 1975a).

2. Systemic Skeletal Defects

Many different types of systemic skeletal congenital diseases have been studied in humans (Rubin, 1969). Although similar regional skeletal defects occur in cattle, few (but including some economically important) have been described and still fewer adequately described. The latter are best illustrated by chondrodysplasia, which is a universal problem in all cattle breeds.

a. *Chondrodysplasia.* Various terms have been used in the past to describe genetic defective cartilage formation usually leading to reduction of body size. Dysplasia refers to embryonal or fetal dysmorphogenesis and thus is very applicable to these defects. Various classification schemes have been proposed for the chondrodysplasia– dwarfism complex. Julian's statement, "Dwarfism is complex and occurs in a variety of phenotypic forms," best describes the situation (Julian et al., 1959, p. 105). Various forms have been described on anatomic, histologic and genetic bases as Dexter-type, Telemark-type, and others as reviewed by Lauvergne (1968), Wiesner and Willer (1974), and Tucking (1976).

Chondrodysplasia is basically a defect of interstitial growth of epiphyseal, articular, and basocranial cartilages resulting in variable shortness of legs, cranial base, and vertebral column (Jubb and Kennedy, 1970a). Grossly, various types of dwarfism are distinguished such as short-headed, long-headed, and Telemark; all are considered to result from recessive genes. In addition, the Dexter, compressed, and compact mutants (generally considered to be dominants) are part of a complex of conditions from more than one locus and seem to be related to the recessive types (Gregory, 1955; Gregory et al., 1966, 1967).

Julian and co-workers (1959, 1964) distinguished the following types of dwarfs. The brachycephalic (short-headed) type is frequently referred to colloquially as the "snorter" dwarf because of its labored breathing. This type of dwarfism was formerly seen predominantly in Herefords and Angus, and was inherited as a simple autosomal recessive trait. Dolichocephalic (long-headed) dwarfs are characterized by a long and slender head and have been diagnosed in Hereford, Angus, and Shorthorn breeds. Intermediate dwarfism may be characterized by features of both short-headed and long-headed dwarfs, or by calves affected with compressed-type dwarfism. Compressed dwarfs reach 65–90% of normal body size. Overlapping with normal calves occurs, leading to three subgroups: heterozygous (carrier), homozygous normal, and genetically unclassifiable calves.

Jubb and Kennedy (1970a) distinguished Dexter-type, Telemark-type, and short-headed, the latter including the long-headed, compact, and compressed types. Stringam (1958) used the following two classifications for snorter dwarfs in Hereford, Angus, and Shorthorn cattle: (1) compressed (or compact) dwarfs of almost normal size and proportions but with shorter than normal legs; and (2) a miscellaneous group containing "long-headed," "pinheads," "ridgets," and crooked-leg dwarfs.

Several morphologic features can aid in the diagnosis of dwarfism:

1. Normal closure of the spheno-occipital synchondrosis occurs between 24 and 36 months in normal cattle, whereas in dwarfism it may occur from birth to 5 months of age (Julian et al., 1957).
2. Projection of the orbitosphenoid, ala minor, into the cranial cavity in a medial and dorsal direction is typical for dwarf cattle as compared to normal cattle (Tyler et al., 1959).
3. In calves younger than 10 days of age, compression of the ventral borderline of the lumbar and thoracic vertebrae can be of diagnostic help.
4. Three groups of calves may be distinguished: normal vertebral column, abnormal vertebral column, and intermediates with normal overlap (Emmerson and Hazel, 1956; High et al., 1959).

b. Osteopetrosis. Osteopetrosis, a recessive hereditary defect, has been encountered in Black and Red Angus calves. It is characterized grossly by small body size and weight, brachygnathia inferior with impacted molar teeth, misshapen coronoid and condyloid processes, open fontanelle, thickened cranial bones, agenesis or hypoplasia of major foramina of the skull, and lack of bone marrow cavities. The long bones lack strength and break under moderate lateral pressure. Radiographically, increased bone density is apparent. The basic microscopic feature is lack of remodeling of the primary spongiosa, persisting throughout the metaphyseal and diaphyseal areas (Thomson, 1966b; Leipold et al., 1970a, 1971b; Huston and Leipold, 1971). In one herd, calves affected with osteopetrosis were born prematurely at 251 to 272 days (mean 262) gestation. Observations in other herds have supported this finding and have emphasized that the disease is readily overlooked in the field and is sometimes mistaken for an abortion problem. Affected calves are stillborn, and the only external characteristics may be the body size and short lower jaw (Greene et al., 1974b). Osteopetrosis in Hereford calves had features similar to those described for Angus cattle (Ojo et al., 1975b). Recently, osteopetrosis has been described in a Dutch Holstein–Friesian and in a European Simmental calf (Goedegeburne et al., 1981).

c. *Crooked Calf Disease.* Crooked calf disease has been produced by feeding lupines (*L. sericeus* and *L. caudatus*) to pregnant cows between Days 40 and 70 of gestation (Shupe et al., 1967a). A similar skeletal defect syndrome of arthrogryposis, kyphosis, torticollis, scoliosis, and cleft palate may be due to homozygosity of recessive genes (Shupe et al., 1967b). The only distinction between the two conditions was the cleft palate, which was always manifested in the hereditary type but only occasionally in the lupine-induced disease. Calves born from cows fed a manganese-deficient diet had similar skeletal deformities (Dyer et al., 1964).

d. *Acroteriasis Congenita.* Acroteriasis congenita involves the entire skeleton and has been described several times, mainly in Europe. This recessive syndrome resulted in low birthweight, amputation of all four legs, defects of the facial skeleton, cleft palate, brachygnathia inferior, microtia, and hydrocephalus. Other findings included deficient ossification of the skeleton of the head, kyphosis or scoliosis of the vertebral column, and eye defects (Rieck and Bähr, 1967).

B. Joint Defects

Congenital disorders of joints may be generalized or restricted to a single joint. Ankylosis, abnormal union of the ends of bones forming the joint, may involve one or more joints. Arthrogryposis and congenital contracture of muscles have been reported many times as ankylosis.

From 15 cows irradiated with 200 roentgens between 27 and 34 days of gestation, 2 calves irradiated at Day 31 and 3 at Day 32 were born with osseous fusion of humeroradial joints (Erickson and Murphree, 1964). A hereditary type of ankylosis restricted to the mandibular joint has been encountered in calves and is listed under lethal factors (Koch et al., 1957).

Bilateral spontaneous osteoarthritis of the stifle joint in Holstein–Friesian and Jersey cattle has been described as an autosomal recessive trait (Sittmann and Kendrick, 1964). Occurrence of hip dysplasia in Hereford cattle is apparently hereditary (Carnahan et al., 1968).

Although joint diseases are of considerable importance, the shortness of this section indicates the scarcity of work on such diseases. The hereditary components and other etiologic factors remain unclassified.

C. Muscular System Defects

Congenital defects of muscle are common in cattle and are economically important.

1. Congenital Flexure of the Pasterns

This defect was studied in Jersey cattle and is reportedly a simple autosomal recessive trait; it occurs in all major breeds of cattle, however (Mead et al., 1943). Calves are usually affected bilaterally, and they knuckle over in the front pasterns; only occasionally are the hind legs also affected. The lesion is reversible, and calves usually recover in 2 to 8 weeks.

2. Arthrogryposis

One of the most frequent congenital defects in calves is arthrogryposis. Stern (1923) first used the term for infants and defined it as a permanent joint contracture present at birth. The arthrogrypotic syndrome includes more than one etiologic or pathologic entity. The problem is worldwide and has been described in all major breeds of cattle (Leipold et al., 1970a,b,c, 1973c; Greene et al., 1973c; Hartley et al., 1975, 1977). In humans, neuropathic arthrogryposis is characterized by normal to atrophic muscle fibers with replacement by fat cells and connective tissue. The myopathic form in humans has fibrous replacement (Adams et al., 1962). Spina bifida is a neurologic defect with bilateral arthrogryposis of the hind legs of calves of Scandinavian and

German breeds (Nes, 1959; Herzog and Adam, 1968); the cause is unknown.

Rieck (1965) listed segmental aplasia of the lumbar cord as the neurologic defect in a calf with arthrogryposis of the hind legs. Hydranencephaly and spinal cord lesions were described in Australia (Whittem, 1957). Spinal cord dysplasias were encountered in calves affected by arthrogryposis (Jubb and Kennedy, 1970b). Charolais calves with arthrogryposis revealed hydromyelia and syringomyelia of the cervical spinal cord (Leipold et al., 1970c).

Arthrogryposis and associated defects in newborn Charolais calves were studied (Leipold et al., 1970c). Usually all four legs were bilaterally and symmetrically arthrogrypotic. Cleft palate was associated with the defect. Scapulohumeral, humeroradial, and metacarpophalangeal joints were flexed and the carpal joints extended. Coxofemoral and tarsal joints were extended, and the femorotibial and metatarsophalangeal joints were flexed. Other calves had different symmetrical patterns of contracture. Metacarpophalangeal and metatarsophalangeal joint surfaces were incongruent. The distal trochlea of the femur and the patella were hypoplastic. Some calves also had kyphoscoliotic deformities of the vertebral column. The muscular system was characterized by moderate to marked wasting and widespread replacement of muscle fibers by fat cells. Congenital defects characterized by arthrogryposis or contracture of legs occur frequently in calves and may be inherited in Charolais as a simple autosomal recessive trait (Goonewardene and Berg, 1976; Nawrot et al., 1980). Nonhereditary examples of arthrogryposis have also been studied (Inaba, 1975; Hamana and Leipold, 1980).

Arthrogryposis syndrome of hereditary nature consists of tetramelic arthrogryposis and cleft palate; the leg contractures are symmetrical (Nawrot et al., 1980). Prenatal viral infection with Akabane virus can cause arthrogryposis, usually associated with hydranencephaly (Hartley et al., 1977).

A 3-year study summarized the importance of the arthrogryposis syndrome in cattle (Nawrot et al., 1980). Investigations for environmental factors were negative. However, analysis of pedigrees and matings that produced 76 arthrogrypotic calves confirmed that the arthrogryposis syndrome in Canadian Charolais calves was due to an autosomal recessive gene with complete penetrance. The findings were similar to those reported in the United States (Leipold et al., 1973c) and earlier in Canada (Goonewardene and Berg, 1976).

Differentiation of skeletal muscle tissue, neuromuscular junction, and peripheral nerves was studied in fetal and neonatal Charolais. It was concluded that muscular rigidity was caused by impaired neurogenic function involving mechanisms exerting influence on the motor activity of neurons in the spinal cord (Russell, 1980). However, another study in newborn Charolais calves affected with arthrogryposis syndrome described abnormal nerve–muscle interaction. Focal accumulation of 16 S acetylcholinesterase in end plate regions of the muscle was not observed as in the normal control calves. Silver nitrate impregnation of motor innervation revealed abnormal features such as preterminal branching and ultraterminal sprouting (Rieger et al., 1980). Several Charolais calves were born with tetramelic arthrogryposis and palatoschisis after introduction of a new Charolais bull. It was concluded that this syndrome is genetically transmitted and was possibly introduced into the herd by the new bull (Savey and Espinasse, 1980).

Records of 944 calves affected with arthrogryposis were compiled according to localization of the deformity, sex, Belgian province, month of birth, degree of retraction, therapy, and complications. In 50% of cases, the defects affected both carpi. The condition was more common (61%) in male calves, and in those born in December through April. Complications were tabulated, the most common being decubitus sores and omphalitis (De Kesel et al., 1981).

3. Muscular Hypertrophy

Another economically important congenital muscular disorder is muscular hypertrophy, also given other names including "Doppellender," double muscling, and muscular hyperplasia. The defect is encountered in all major beef breeds in the United States and is a problem in European breeds including Charolais (Lauvergne et al., 1963). One report summarized the historical aspects and genetic implications (Oliver and Cartwright, 1969).

The external appearance of muscular hypertrophy varies widely, and few calves have all the characteristics. However, a few characteristics in a herd indicates the presence of the trait, the most noticeable being the rounded outline of the hindquarters. The tail is attached more anteriorly than normal. The muscles of the shoulder, back, rump, and hindquarter are separated by deep creases; those between the semitendinosus and biceps femoris, and between the longissimus dorsi muscles of either side, are particularly noticeable. Necks of double-muscled cattle are shorter and thicker; their heads are smaller and lighter. Many double-muscled cattle stand in a stretched position. The diaphyses of the long bones tend to be shorter. Variable degree of macroglossia may be present. Additional pathological signs are infantile genital tracts, impaired reproduction, delayed sexual maturity, lengthened gestation, and high birthweight combined with dystocia (Oliver and Cartwright, 1969). Double-muscled calves are less viable and are particularly susceptible to rickets and joint problems (Lauvergne et al., 1963).

Oliver and Cartwright (1969) classified cattle populations into three groups: the majority with normal phenotypes, those with most or all characteristics of muscular hypertrophy, and those with some of the typical characteristics of double muscling. They noted that double muscling is mediated by a pair of incompletely recessive genes. Ashmore and Robinson (1969) used histochemical techniques to demonstrate by biopsy a significant decrease in succinic dehydrogenase activity in muscular hypertrophy. Fewer reacting fibers were observed, and the activity was less in fibers from double-muscled calves. They concluded that bovine hereditary muscular hypertrophy is associated with a disproportionate number of glycolytic-type fibers.

Myotonia congenita has been described only once in cattle, in a Holstein–Friesian calf (van Niekerk and Jaros, 1970).

D. Central Nervous System Defects

Congenital defects of the central nervous system (CNS) are common, and most can be recognized by a structural change that involves both the skeletal and central nervous systems, or only the latter. Functional defects have been encountered rarely in cattle (Saunders, 1965; Cho and Leipold, 1977b; Barlow, 1982).

Congenital CNS defects are the cause of a fairly significant percentage of neonatal loss and are important economically. Overall frequencies of congenital defects of the CNS are difficult to obtain, because many defects are identified only by necropsy.

Nature, cause, and frequency of congenital malformations of the CNS were studied in two separate studies. In the first, 117 congenital defects were recorded in 97 calves: 66 internal hydrocephalus, 14 spina bifida, 10 Arnold–Chiari malformation, 10 cerebellar defect, 5 meningoencephalocele, 4 anencephaly, 3 micranencephaly, 2 agenesis of corpus callosum, 2 hydranencephaly, and 1 arrhinencephaly. Common concurrent defects were internal hydrocephalus with multiple ocular defects and myopathy, internal hydrocephalus and arthrogryposis, Arnold–Chiari malformation with spina bifida and arthrogryposis, and anencephaly with meningoencephalocele. Other malformations had only a few associated defects (Cho and Leipold, 1977c; Cho et al., 1978). In the second group of 160 calves studied for causes of neonatal death,

35 calves were affected with CNS defects, internal hydrocephalus being the most common (Cho et al., 1978).

No satisfactory classification system has been established for CNS defects because multiple organ systems are also frequently involved, and causes may be unknown or diverse. Central nervous system defects are classified here into five groups by combining anatomical and functional approaches: (1) cerebral defects and malformations involving only or mainly the cerebrum, (2) defects of cerebellum and brain stem, involving only or mainly the cerebellum and brain stem, (3) spinal cord defects, (4) spastic and paralytic diseases, and (5) metabolic diseases (Cho and Leipold, 1978b; Jolly et al., 1981).

1. Cerebral Defects

a. Agenesis of Corpus Callosum. Isolated cases of this defect have been seen in various cattle breeds, usually in horned Hereford cattle (Cho and Leipold, 1978c). There are three types of abnormalities: (1) complete absence of the corpus callosum, (2) partial corpus callosum present anteriorly, and (3) partial corpus callosum present posteriorly. These variations may represent variable genic expressivity, possibly resulting from modifying genetic factors.

b. Anencephaly. Anencephaly is a malformation involving nonclosure of the anterior portion of the neutral tube and failure of the cranium to develop. Anencephaly is a misnomer for absence of the brain in neonatal calves, because a normal pons, medulla, and cerebellum or dysplastic vestiges are usually present (Kalter, 1968; Herzog, 1971; Cho and Leipold, 1978b).

c. Hydranencephaly. Hydranencephaly is complete or almost complete absence of cerebral hemispheres in a cranium of normal conformation, the space being filled with cerebrospinal fluid surrounded by a thin membranous cerebral tissue (Kalter, 1968). Congenital abnormality characterized by hydranencephaly or arthrogryposis, or both, occurs sporadically or epizootically in calves. The A–H syndrome was once considered to be different manifestations of a single disease (Blood, 1956; Whittem, 1957). Now it is known that hydranencephaly is caused by prenatal infection with Akabane virus (Hartley et al., 1977; Konno and Nakagawa, 1982; Konno et al.,1982).

d. Internal Hydrocephalus. Hydrocephalus, a common and well-documented CNS defect in cattle, results from excessive fluid accumulating in the cranial cavity within the ventricular system (internal hydrocephalus). Congenital internal hydrocephalus in cattle appears to be inherited in many breeds as a simple autosomal recessive trait.

The basic pathogenesis of hydrocephalus is considered to be a disturbance of the cerebrospinal fluid pathway, but in some cases the pathogenesis is obscure (Fankhauser and Luginbuhl, 1968; Greene et al., 1974a, 1978). Stenosis or obstruction of the aqueduct may be caused by an aberrant developmental defect, inflammation, neoplasia, parasitic cysts, or abnormal cranial bone development (Greene and Leipold, 1974). Hydrocephalus has been observed to be associated with dyschondroplasia and other forms of dwarfism, and also with the amputated syndrome.

Internal hydrocephalus may be congenital or acquired. Internal hydrocephalus, combined with defective development of skull and long bones, was described as a lethal recessive trait in Holstein–Friesian calves (Cole and Moore, 1942).

Six cases of internal hydrocephalus in Holstein–Friesian calves were reported by Gilman (1956) as a simple recessive genetic defect. Blackwell et al. (1959) reported a hydrocephalic lethal in Hereford calves in New Mexico and attributed it to a single autosomal recessive. Baker et al. (1961) in Nebraska also studied lethal internal hydrocephalus in Hereford calves in the field and in an experimental herd. Both Hereford studies supported a single autosomal recessive gene as the cause. Gross and dye injection studies indicated no obstruction in the fluid pathway of the CNS.

Variations and diagnostic problems encountered with internal hydrocephalus in 30 Hereford calves were summarized by Belling and Holland (1962). Urman and Grace (1964), in their morphological study of a hydrocephalic syndrome in newborn calves, reported multiple defects in the CNS and associated mesodermal defects. They found internal hydrocephalus combined with enlargement of the cranium, narrowing of the sylvian aqueduct as a result of malformation of the mesencephalon, hypoplasia or dysplasia of the cerebellum, myelin deficiency in the cerebellum, spinal cord, and cerebrum, and atrophy of the optic nerve. Eye defects such as microphthalmia, retinal detachment, cataract, and liquefaction of the vitrous body were consistently found. Urman and Grace (1964) also described generalized, progressive primary muscular dystrophy with the hydrocephalic syndrome.

Huston et al. (1961b) described hydrocephalic Ayrshire calves. Nuss (1966) reported a hydrocephalic syndrome in an Ayrshire herd that involved generalized edema, enlargement of thyroids and adrenals, and liver hemorrhage. The ratio of abnormal to normal calves was twice as high as would be expected if a single gene mutation was involved, and multiple gene action was postulated as the cause.

Congenital hydrocephalus in Hereford and Shorthorn calves was accompanied by a stenotic aqueduct, cerebellar hypoplasia, myopathy, and multiple ocular anomalies including retinal detachment and dysplasia, cataract, microphthalmia, and persistent pupillary membranes (Baker et al., 1961; Urman and Grace, 1964; Leipold et al., 1971a; Greene and Leipold, 1974; Greene et al., 1974a; Axthelm et al., 1980a). Calves affected with internal hydrocephalus are born dead or die within a few days. Results of breeding trials at Kansas State University with Hereford and Shorthorn cattle are compatible with a simple autosomal recessive gene. The homozygous affected calves were dead at birth and had internal hydrocephalus, myopathy, and bilateral microphthalmia.

Axthelm et al. (1980a) reported on a study of embryonic, fetal, and neonatal pathology of hydrocephalus in horned Herefords. Hydrocephalic horned Hereford calves had (1) reduced body size and weight, (2) narrow, refined facial features and cranial doming, (3) caudodorsal–rostroventral angulation of palpebral fissures, (4) microphthalmia, and (5) protruding edematous tongues. Micropolygyrus of the cerebral convexities appears to result from dorsal elevation of gyri located within the longitudinal fissure to the cerebral surface, and six shallow sulci form secondarily. Attenuation of the convolutions on the dorsal cerebral surface and cystic dilation of the optic chiasma were presumably the effects of pressure from severe internal hydrocephalus. Mesencephalic kinking at the anterior portion of the aqueduct, lateral splaying of the dorsal thalamus, and absence of the interthalamic adhesion were features. The sigmoid configuration of the brain and splaying configurations of the thalamus resembled the cephalic flexure and diencephalon of 40-day-old bovine embryos, respectively. Cerebellar hypoplasia and distribution of dysplastic lesions resembled findings of arrested development (Axthelm et al., 1980a).

Most major skeletal muscles were affected by degenerative lesions, and the quadriceps had the most consistent gross lesions. Although terminal nerve fibers and motor end plates were not examined, grouped distribution of atrophic fibers, preservation of neuromuscular spindles and cross striations, absence of lipid replacement, little or no inflammatory response, and lack of regeneration were compatible with neurogenic atrophy. Innervation of skeletal muscle occurs during early fetal life; however, it plays no part in muscle morphogenesis. Later in gestation, muscle becomes dependent on its nerve supply. Primary maldevelopment and hypoplasia of the mesencephalon is thought to cause the apparent neurogenic myopathy. Muscular development and movement in humans progresses from cephalic to caudal portions, providing a plausible explanation for the severe lesions in the quadriceps. In contrast to genetically caused internal hydrocephalus, BVD virus-induced hydrocephalus caused lesions such as porencephaly (Axthelm et al., 1980a,b, 1981a,b,c).

e. Meningoencephalocele. Meningoencephalocele is a protrusion of meninges and brain tissue through the cranial cleft, sometimes forming a large liquid-filled sac or hydrencephalocele (Schlegel, 1914). The malformation at times may form a complex, with spinal cord and meningeal protrusion through the vertebral defect (meningoencephalomyelocele) (Frauchiger and Fankhauser, 1957). Meningoencephalocele usually occurs in the frontal region (porencephaly), but sometimes is midfrontal, parietal, or occipital (Jubb and Kennedy, 1970b; Gopal and Leipold, 1979).

Tibial hemimelia is characterized by bilateral absence of tibias, but associated defects include meningoencephalocele and reproductive system anomalies.

f. Micrencephaly or Microcephaly. Micrencephaly or microcephaly refers to an abnormally small but not otherwise grossly deformed brain or head. It is a rare defect, but it has been described in seven Hereford calves (Fielden, 1959). The normal-sized cranial cavity was only partly filled by the brain, all parts of which were greatly reduced in size. The most striking abnormality was in the cerebrum, characterized by a decrease in number in gyri and absence of corpus callosum and fornix.

2. Defects of the Cerebellum and Brain Stem

a. Arnold–Chiari Malformation. The Arnold–Chiari malformation (ACM) consists of herniation of tonguelike processes of cerebellar tissue through the foramen magnum into the anterior cervical spinal canal with caudal displacement and elongation of the medulla oblongata, pons, and fourth ventricle (Chiari, 1891; Kalter, 1968). The malformation is often accompanied by spina bifida, hydrocephalus, and meningomyelocele (Ingraham and Scott, 1943; Frauchiger and Fankhauser, 1952; Cho and Leipold, 1977a,b,c).

b. Dandy–Walker Syndrome. The Dandy–Walker syndrome comprises a combination of defects consisting of hydrocephalus, aplasia or hypoplasia of the cerebellar vermis, cystic enlargement of the fourth ventricle covered by a greatly thinned medullary velum and associated tela chorioidea, and an inner ependymal layer representing the roof of the expanded fourth ventricle (Taggart and Walker, 1942). The pathogenesis of the syndrome is obscure.

c. Cerebellar Aplasia, or Hypoplasia and Degeneration. Since cerebellar hypoplasia was first described as a genetic defect in Hereford calves (Innes et al., 1940), many possibly hereditary cases have been documented in Hereford (Sippel, 1951; Belling and Holland, 1962), Ayrshire (Jennings and Sumner, 1951), Shorthorn (Finnie and Leaver, 1965; O'Sullivan and McPhee, 1975), Angus (Edmonds et al., 1973), and unknown breeds (Girgin, 1972). The mode of inheritance appears to be autosomal recessive (Innes et al., 1940; Johnson et al., 1958; Edmonds et al., 1973; O'Sullivan and McPhee, 1975). The clinical signs, usually present at birth, are characterized by recumbency with extended limbs, intermittent opisthotonus, and ataxia.

Macroscopically, the cerebellum is absent or small; its surface often appears smooth, and in cross-section the folia of the cortex are small and narrow. The cerebral hemispheres and brain stem appear normal. Microscopic changes are characterized by narrow and irregular folia, abnormally thin molecular and granular layers, and almost complete absence of Purkinje cells. In the most severely affected cases the cerebellum is not visible grossly (cerebellar aplasia), and rudimentary cerebellar tissue may be found only microscopically.

Congenital cerebellar defects in calves have been reported as single, isolated entities or associated with other brain defects such as hydrocephalus. Cerebellar agenesis has been observed rarely, and the cause is unknown (Fankhauser and Luginbuhl, 1968).

Innes et al. (1940) described clinical, gross, and histologic features of cerebellar hypoplasia in five Hereford calves. The cerebellum was abnormally small, tough, and leathery. Histological changes were confined to the cerebellar structures: narrow folia and gross disorganization of the cortex, thin molecular and granular layers, Purkinje cells almost completely absent, white matter reduced in amount but axis cylinders and myelin sheath preserved, and normal central nuclei. The entire process appeared to be arrested development and degeneration. Furthermore, the cases appeared to be familial. A genetic defect seemed likely because it occurred only in calves from a Hereford bull bred to Hereford cows, not in Shorthorn crossbreds with the same bull. Adjusting the breeding program by marketing the bull eliminated the defect.

Saunders et al. (1952) described hereditary congenital ataxia in Jersey calves. Gross lesions were minimal and consisted of wet, glossy-appearing cerebellar white matter that histologically had a lacy, loose, reticulated appearance. In addition, the medulla and midbrain were affected. The reticular formation had a few small misshapen neurons. The roof nuclei were also deficient. The lesions were interpreted as a failure of normal development. The defect was considered to be due to a single autosomal recessive.

Fankhauser (1957) and Hulland (1957) reported pathological findings in cases of congenital atrophy and aplasia of the cerebellum. Hereditary ataxia due to cerebellar hypoplasia combined with neuronal degeneration was considered genetic (Johnson et al., 1958). An inherited congenital nervous disorder in Hereford calves, referred to as "doddler cattle," caused calcifications of small vessels and neurons of the brain stem and cerebellum (High et al., 1958). Shorthorn–Angus crossbred calves with cerebellar ataxia had no gross lesions, but there was histologic evidence of depletion or absence of myelin in the cerebellum, pons, medulla, and other parts of the brain (Young, 1962). Finnie and Leaver (1965) found lesions in Shorthorn calves similar to those described (on a familial basis) in Hereford calves by Innes et al. (1940).

Two Ayrshire calves affected with gross cerebellar malformation had no familial relationships (Howell and Ritchie, 1966). Familial convulsions and ataxia appeared in Aberdeen Angus calves that had no gross CNS lesions, but histologic examination disclosed degeneration of Purkinje cells of the cerebellar cortex. The disease seemed to be transmitted as an incompletely dominant trait (Barlow et al., 1968; Barlow, 1981, 1982).

Barlow (1981) described a new familial cerebellar disorder characterized by recurrent episodic seizures in neonatal and young calves and by ataxia in survivors. Early lesions of the Purkinje cells were altered patterns of phosphatase reaction products. Purkinje cell axons in the outer half of the granular layer developed fusiform or spheroidal argyrophyllic swellings. Early lesions involved lingula and uvula, and more advanced cases involved other parts of the vermis. Ataxic calves had lesions in the cerebellar hemispheres. Axonal swellings revealed proliferation of tubulovesicular endoplasmic reticulum, neurofibrils, and mitochondria. Light microscopic examination revealed similar lesions in clinically normal adult transmitters (Barlow, 1981).

Whereas earlier investigators invariably incriminated hereditary causes in cerebellar disease, some evidence now points to intrauterine fetal infection with BVD virus causing cerebellar hypoplasia combined with ocular defects (Ward, 1969; Kahrs et al., 1970a,b). In light of their findings and the evolvement of more precise genetic analysis, the cause of cerebellar defects should be reevaluated.

The pathological changes in the allegedly genetic form of cerebellar aplasia or hypoplasia seem to differ from those of the BVD virus-induced cerebellar defect. The ocular lesions and large irregular cavities in the folial white matter and the inflammatory processes observed in cases of BVD viral origin have not been described in the genetic form, whereas cerebellar aplasia has not been seen in virus-induced cerebellar hypoplasia and degeneration (Cho and Leipold, 1977b; Swan and Taylor, 1982).

d. Cerebellar Ataxia. Cerebellar ataxia or hereditary hypomyelinogenesis congenita has been reported in Jerseys (Saunders, 1952; Saunders et al., 1952), Shorthorns (Hulland, 1957), Angus–Shorthorns (Young, 1962), Sofia Browns (Gerov et al., 1971), and an unknown breed (Cravero et al., 1976). The CNS appeared grossly normal. Common histopathologic changes were diffuse, spongy appearance in the white matter of the cerebellum, midbrain, and medulla due to paucity of nerve fibers and depletion or absence of myelin in many nerve sheaths. Purkinje cells and neurons appeared degenerative and fewer in number (Saunders et al., 1952; Hulland, 1957; Young, 1962; Gerov et al., 1971). Hypomyelinogenesis may be caused by prenatal BVD virus infection (Done et al., 1980).

e. Progressive Ataxia. Progressive ataxia has been described in Charolais cattle (Palmer et al., 1972; Ogden et al., 1974; Palmer, 1982). The clinical signs, primarily weakness of hind legs, were first noticed in animals 8–24 months of age, and in 1 to 2 years progressed from slight ataxia involving all four limbs to recumbency.

Nine Charolais cattle (three male, six female) were slaughtered because of a slowly developing paralysis or ataxia. Histologic examination revealed identical CNS lesions. There were multiple lesions throughout the white substance of the brain and spinal cord, all circular or ovoid areas of reduced density or stainability, often with one or more axons centrally or eccentrically placed (Mialot and Parodi, 1981).

f. Cerebellar Cortical Atrophy. Congenital cerebellar atrophy has been reported in Holstein calves with clinical and morphologic features comparable to the defect in lambs (daft lambs) and dogs (Jubb and Kennedy, 1970b). Nothing suggested heredity in Holsteins. The disease has also been described in a Charolais calf (Cho and Leipold, 1978a).

g. Hereditary Neuraxial Edema and Congenital Brain Edema. This disease, described in Polled Hereford calves by Cordy and associates (1969), was characterized clinically by extensor spasms and inability to stand. Histologically, it was characterized by edema of the terminal portions of myelinated bundles and by gray substances containing heavily myelinated fibers. Genetic analysis in two herds indicated autosomal recessive transmission (Cordy et al., 1969).

Polled Hereford calves affected with hereditary neuraxial edema were unable to raise their heads; they lay quietly without struggling and had incoordination and coarse muscular tonic contractions (Cordy *et al.*, 1969). A sudden touch or loud noise elicited vigorous extension of legs and neck. Withdrawal and patella reflexes were present. All were able to suckle their dams when aided. Macroscopically, most brains appeared normal, but the more severely affected appeared swollen. Microscopic spongy vacuolar appearance was widespread along the long axis of myelinated fibers in the white and gray matter. Myelination appeared slightly deficient, but glial or microglial reactions were not absent. The lesion was interpreted as being caused by edema.

Since the first report, the disease has been observed in other Polled Hereford (Blood and Gay, 1971; Weaver, 1975; Cho and Leipold, 1978d) and Polled Hereford–Friesian crossbred calves (Davis *et al.*, 1975). Some calves had no histologic lesions comparable to the clinical signs (Blood and Gay, 1971; Davis *et al.*, 1975).

Congenital brain edema has been described in an inbred-grade horned Hereford herd (Jolly, 1974). Calves had clinical signs almost identical to those of hereditary neuraxial edema but some differences in the pathologic changes. In hereditary neuraxial edema of Polled Hereford calves, the lesions were mainly in the white matter; this contrasted with vacuolations of both gray and white matter in the congenital brain edema of horned Herefords.

3. *Spinal Cord*

Various developmental spinal cord defects of calves have been described under the terms spina bifida and spinal dysraphism (status dysraphicus). Spina bifida (SB) implies a defect of vertebrae with or without spinal cord defects. Spinal dysraphism (SD) is a myelodysplasia or malformation of the spinal cord, especially of the central canal, with or without involvement of vertebrae.

Spina bifida, defective closure of the dorsal vertebral laminae, has been described infrequently in cattle. There are two types: SB occulta and SB aperta. Spina bifida cystica is a form of SB aperta in which there is a cyst filled with cerebrospinal fluid at the site of the defect.

Although SB occurs most frequently in the lumbar region, it may also occur at any point along the vertebral column. Although vertical skeletal defects are discussed under skeletal system, SB is emphasized here. Whittem (1957) described SB in the lumbar area; McFarland (1959) observed SB with meningomyelocele in an Aberdeen Angus calf; and Herzog and Adam (1968) found it combined with posterior arthrogryposis in various German breeds. Fankhauser (1959) reported a calf affected with sacral SB and Arnold–Chiari malformation of the cerebellum. It has been described in several cattle breeds: Angus (McFarland, 1959; Greene *et al.*, 1973b), Hereford (Greene *et al.*,

1973a; Doige, 1975; Cho and Leipold, 1977a), Zebu (Epstein, 1955), Ayrshire (Hughes, 1952), Norwegian Red and White (Nes, 1959), Holstein–Friesian (Goss and Hull, 1939), Charolais (Leipold et al., 1970c, 1973c; Singh and Little, 1972), Shorthorn (Greene et al., 1973b), Simmental (Herzog and Adam, 1968), and German Black and Red Pied (Herzog and Adam, 1968). Spina bifida in Zebu cattle consists of bifidity of the spinal process of vertebrae, but this is considered normal in Zebu cattle (Kalter, 1968).

Many anatomical variations of SB occur in cattle, including meningocele or meningomyelocele (Jackschath, 1899; Dobler, 1903; Magnusson, 1917; McFarland, 1959), syringomyelia and hydromyelia (Bullard, 1935; Martins and Ferri, 1951; Leipold et al., 1970c; Cho and Leipold, 1977a,b), diastematomyelia (Adelmann, 1920; Cho and Leipold, 1977a), and SB occulta (Keller and Niedoba, 1937; Goss and Hull, 1939; Nes, 1959).

Other defects associated with SB are hydrocephalus, ACM (Frauchiger and Fankhauser, 1952; Hughes, 1952; Gruys, 1973; Cho and Leipold, 1977a), arthrogryposis, neuromyodysplasia, kyphoscoliosis, lordosis, cleft palate, anury (Leipold et al., 1970c, 1973c; Singh and Little, 1972; Greene et al., 1973b,c; Hartley and Wanner, 1974; Doige, 1975), perosomus elumbis (Greene et al., 1973a), dicephalus (Krölling, 1922; Frauchiger and Hofmann, 1941; Tagand and Barone, 1942; Mammerickx and Leunen, 1964; Gruys, 1973), exencephaly (Taruffi, 1881–1894), and renal fusion (Doige, 1975).

One study presented 115 calves affected with spinal dysraphism. The cause was thought to be genetic, and polygenic inheritance seemed to be the best explanation. Cytogenetic studies on 20 of the calves revealed a significant increase of tetraploid cells in blood cell cultures (Vainas, 1980).

4. Spastic and Paralytic Diseases

This group of diseases includes those with clinical evidence implicating CNS involvement and genetic studies indicating a hereditary basis. The diseases in this group may be primarily functional disorders.

a. Spastic Paresis. Spastic paresis is characterized by spastic contracture of muscles and extension of the stifle and tarsal joints of the affected hind limb(s). It has been referred to as "contraction of the Achilles tendon," "straight hock," and "Elso-heel" (after the bull Elso) (Roberts, 1965; Baird et al., 1974). The contracted gastrocnemius muscle and superficial flexor tendons almost straighten the hock joint and draw the os calcaneus toward the tibia. Tension broadens the epiphyseal cartilage between the corpus and head of the calcis. The epiphysis may fail to unite and may even be separated from the head.

Although spasticity characteristically affects the gastrocnemius and superficial flexor muscles and tendons, in some cases the biceps femoris, semitendinosus, semimembranosus, quadriceps, and abductor muscles may be involved (Dirksen, 1970). Usually the clinical signs indicate a unilateral condition, with the right hind limb being frequently involved; bilateral involvement is rare (Leipold et al., 1967).

The progressive disease varies in severity and time of onset. In affected calves there may be only a straightened tarsus. In many, marked lameness develops, causing the limb to be stiff so that only the toe tips touch the ground and the affected limb appears shortened and swings freely. If both limbs are affected, the calf is usually unable to rise without assistance, and the limbs, even in recumbency, are extended. Accompanying signs are an arched back and a raised tail. The front limbs may bow at the carpal joints, and posterior parts of the hoofs may not touch the ground when the calf is standing (Leipold et al., 1967). It occurs at 3 to 6 months of age (Götze, 1932) or as late as at 2 years or older (Rosenberger, 1939). Sometimes the abnormality of gait is noticed in the first few days of life, but it usually is not seen until calves are 6 weeks to 8 months old, when it becomes obvious (Hickman, 1964; Dirksen, 1970). Severely affected calves may exhibit a pendulous, contracted limb that does not touch the ground.

Originally observed in German Friesian cattle (Götze, 1932), the disease has been subsequently reported in many breeds, including those in the United States (Rieck and Leipold, 1965; Roberts, 1965; Leipold et al., 1967). Although the primary lesion has not been identified, Chomiak and Milart (1971) indicated histological lesions in the CNS such as swelling of nerve fibers, degeneration and pigmentation of neurons, and glial infiltration. Other investigators considered innervation by an aberrant nerve to be the basic cause of spastic paresis (Greeley et al., 1968), whereas others regard it to be primarily myogenic (Schmahlstieg and Mätzke, 1962).

Although the disease is assumed to be genetic, the evidence is inconclusive. Initially it was thought to be inherited as a simple recessive. Breeding experiments and case studies indicate that spastic paresis is not inherited as a simple recessive (Stegenga, 1964; Engel, 1970; Dietz et al., 1971; Schönmuth et al., 1971; Stolzenburg and Schönmuth, 1971) and that genetic influence(s) as well as environmental factors play an important part in the incidence of the disease. A study of 100 cases of spastic paresis indicated some genetic influence but also possible environmental influences, because more paretics were conceived in winter than in other seasons (Engel, 1970).

The incidence is significantly higher in winter- or autumn-born calves than in calves born during other seasons, and the incidence is lowest in calves born to heifers (Stegenga, 1964; Engel, 1970). Some investigators advise that cattle with straight hocks (Schalk and Hoekstra, 1959; Baird *et al.*, 1974) and with greater hock joint angles (Rieck and Leipold, 1965; Dirksen, 1970) should not be bred, because both hock conditions predispose to spastic paresis. The role of trace elements such as lithium has also been discussed (Arnault, 1979, 1982).

b. Spastic Syndrome. Spastic syndrome, sometimes called "crampy" or posterior paralysis, is a chronic, progressive disease characterized by sudden spastic contraction of the muscles of both hind legs and often the muscles of the back, neck, and front legs (Becker *et al.*, 1961). The spastic syndrome is also referred to as remittent or periodic spastic syndrome, crampy neuromuscular spasticity, posterior paralysis, progressive posterior paralysis, or "stretches" (Becker *et al.*, 1961; Innes and Saunders, 1962).

Muscle function is normal between attacks but complete recovery never occurs (Roberts, 1965). Many cattle affected with spastic syndrome have straight rear limbs and weak hocks, the conformation observed in cattle affected with spastic paresis. Such confirmation appears to predispose to arthritis, foot diseases, and lameness (Smedegaard, 1964; Roberts, 1965). The spastic syndrome has been observed in some cattle with spondylosis (Roberts, 1965).

Clinical accounts of spastic syndrome are given by Smedegard (1964) and Roberts (1965). The condition occurs in mature cattle of both sexes, usually between 3 and 7 years of age. Spastic syndrome occurs in several European breeds and in the major beef and dairy breeds of the United States, but it is most common in Holstein–Friesian and Guernsey breeds (Frauchiger and Hofmann, 1941; Roberts, 1953; Becker *et al.*, 1961). Although the exact mode of inheritance has not been determined, it appears to be a single recessive with incomplete penetrance (Roberts, 1953; Becker *et al.*, 1961). Pathogenesis of the disease and its lesions has not been demonstrated (Innes and Saunders, 1962).

Histological examination of brain and spinal cord revealed no lesions of an etiological and pathogenetic nature (Innes and Saunders, 1962; Roberts, 1965). The disorder was believed to consist of a functional derangement of the postural reflex mechanism (Roberts, 1965).

c. Spastic Lethal. Spastic lethal (neonatal spasticity) has been recorded twice, in a grade Jersey (Gregory *et al.*, 1944) and in a Hereford (Gregory *et al.*, 1962), as a simple autosomal recessive trait. Spasms and incoordination involved all four legs at or shortly after birth, and the affected calves could not stand alone. The spasms also affected the head, neck, and back, and the calves trembled or shook from sudden touch or noise. They sometimes became extremely rigid with contracted muscles of the legs, back, and neck. They died about a week after onset of spasms. Although the CNS appeared to be implicated, histologic examination revealed no abnormality.

   d. *Neonatal Spasticity.* This defect has been recorded twice, once in Hereford and once in Jersey cattle (Gregory *et al.*, 1962). There were no lesions in the CNS; the condition is considered to be due to simple recessive inheritance.

   e. *Hereditary Epilepsy.* Epilepsy (idiopathic epilepsy) is defined as a convulsive state without discoverable etiologic factors or any definite underlying lesions (Innes and Saunders, 1962). Epileptic convulsions were recorded in Swedish Red cattle as an autosomal recessive trait (Isaksson, 1943), in Brown Swiss cattle as an autosomal dominant trait (Atkeson *et al.*, 1944b), and in purebred Brahman bulls as possibly hereditary (Palen, 1970).

   f. *Weaver.* The weaver condition is a familial neuromuscular disorder in Brown Swiss cattle. Clinical signs (a weaving gait) appear when calves are 6–8 months old and progress during the next 12–18 months to recumbency. Muscular lesions affect mainly the large muscle masses of the hind legs. The weaver condition is common in Brown Swiss cattle and is most likely inherited as an autosomal recessive trait (Leipold *et al.*, 1973b).

5. *Metabolic Diseases*

   a. *Storage Disease.* A lysosomal storage disease is associated with accumulation and storage of some substance within lysosomes because a specific enzyme deficiency is preventing specific catabolism. Criteria reviewed by Jolly (1982) for a disease to be classified as an inborn error of lysosomal catabolism are as follows:

1. It should be a storage disease.
2. It should be inherited.
3. The storage substance, not necessarily homogeneous, should be stored at least initially within lysosomes.
4. There should be partial or absolute deficiency of one lysosomal enzyme, normally responsible for hydrolyzing the storage material.

Among the recorded storage diseases involving the CNS of cattle are GM_1 gangliosidosis, glyconeogenesis, and mannosidosis.

   i. GM_1 *Gangliosidosis.* This condition occurs in Friesian calves of both sexes (Donnelly et al., 1972). The defect results from reduction (70–80%) in β-galactosidase activity (Donnelly et al., 1973a,b). It is probably analogous to type II GM_1 gangliosidosis (Derry's disease) in humans, because GM_1 ganglioside accumulates in the brain but not in liver and spleen of affected calves (Sheahan and Donnelly, 1974). Clinical signs, including slight swaying of the hindquarters, reluctance to move, and stiffness of gait, appear during the first few weeks of life. Circumstantial evidence indicates that the disease in Friesian calves may be hereditary, but the mode of inheritance has not been determined (Donnelly et al., 1972). The same defect in cats is inherited as a simple autosomal recessive trait (Baker et al., 1982). Microscopic lesions were a marked ballooning of neurons and slight glial reactions at all levels of the CNS, where the neuronal cytoplasm had foamy aggregates around displaced nuclei. The storage material stained intensely with Sudan black and Luxol fast blue (Donnelly et al., 1972, 1973b). Electron microscopy revealed membranous cytoplasmic bodies in neurons and glia. Electron-dense, membrane-bound inclusions were in perithelial cells (Sheahan and Donnelly, 1974).

ii. Glyconeogenesis. Generalized glyconeogenesis type II in cattle has been reported in Beef Shorthorn and Brahman (Howell et al., 1981; O'Sullivan et al., 1981).

iii. Mannosidosis. Mannosidosis, originally reported as pseudolipidosis (Whittem and Walker, 1957; Whittem, 1962; Jolly, 1982), is associated with a deficiency of α-mannosidase and occurs in Angus cattle as a simple recessive trait (Hocking et al., 1972; Phillips et al., 1974). A deficiency of mannosidase results in storage of an oligosaccharide containing glucosamine and mannose (Hocking et al., 1972).

Clinically, the disease is characterized by ataxia, incoordination, head tremor, aggression, and failure to thrive. Calves may be affected at birth, but clinical signs do not usually appear until they are several weeks or months old. Most affected cattle die within the first 12 months of life. However, α-mannosidosis is also a cause of neonatal mortality in Angus calves. The primary lesion is vacuolation of neurons, with vacuoles formed from saccular dilations of the Golgi apparatus. Secondary lesions include spheroidal swellings of axons due to local accumulations of electron-dense bodies, mitochondria, and local proliferation of neurofilaments. Globules that are PAS-positive and lipofuscin-like occur frequently within astrocytes, microglia, and pericytes of blood vessels. Vacuoles also occur in macrophages of the lymph nodes (Whittem and Walker, 1957; Whittem, 1962; Barlow et al., 1981; Jolly, 1982).

Because affected calves have an absolute deficiency of α-mannosidase and heterozygotes have a partial deficiency, mannosidosis can be controlled by identifying and eliminating heterozygotes (Thompson et al., 1976).

Mannosidosis in Angus and Murray Gray cattle, originally described in Australia and New Zealand, has recently been recognized in the United States. Mannosidase activity is used to test cattle for normal activity (homozygous) and reduced activity in heterozygous individuals (Leipold et al., 1979a; Jolly, 1982).

b. Other Metabolic Disease. Protoporphyria is a photosensitizing disease in Limousin cattle caused by homozygosity of a simple autosomal recessive gene. Heterozygote cattle may be detected by breeding trials, determination of ferrochelatase activity in a variety of tissues or fibroblast cultures, and quantitation of free protoporphyrin in circulating red blood cells (Ruth et al., 1980). Protoporphyric Limousin cattle kept at Kansas State University exhibited convulsions and ataxia.

c. Neuronal Lipodystrophy. Spontaneous neuronal lipodystrophy, characterized by neuronal inclusions resembling multilamellar cytosomes and curvilinear bodies in late infantile amaurotic idiocy, was described in an inbred bull (Read and Bridges, 1969).

E. Ocular Defects

Relatively few ocular defects have been described in cattle. Those described have been single or multiple defects restricted to the eye, or have been observed in conjunction with defects in other organs, or have been associated with pigment deficiencies. Bhatt and associates (1964) described ankyloblepharon combined with anophthalmia in Indian cattle. Palpebral agenesis combined with anophthalmia was noted in a calf by Kundu and Pandy (1967). Entropion is encountered rarely in cattle; Thier and Bay (1965) described six cases in the Simmental breed. Strabismus has been described in Jersey (Regan et al., 1944) and Shorthorn cattle (Holmes and Young, 1957). The condition seems to be conditioned by a simple autosomal recessive trait.

Hereditary opacity of the cornea has been reported on several occasions. Histologically, the lesions were restricted to the cornea and consisted of edema of the propria (Cohrs, 1955; Deas, 1960). Multiple ocular anomalies in Jersey cattle reported by Saunders and Fincher (1951) included irideremia, microphakia, ectopia lentis, and cataracts transmitted as a simple recessive trait. A similar condition had been described previously (Gregory et al., 1943).

Carter (1960) reported genetically induced cataract and glaucoma in Holstein–Friesian cattle in New Zealand. Ocular defects of incomplete albino Hereford cattle included iridic heterochromia, tapetum fibrosum hypoplasia, and typical coloboma of the nontapetal fundus (Gelatt et al., 1969; Ojo et al., 1982). Incomplete albinism in Hereford cattle was transmitted as an autosomal dominant trait (Leipold and Huston, 1969). The eyes of a complete albino Guernsey bull were normal except for pigment deficiency (Leipold and Huston, 1968b,c). Heterochromia irides has also been described in various breeds (Huston et al., 1968b).

Several descriptions of ocular defects in cattle included defects in other body organs, especially the CNS. Corneal opacity was observed in Norwegian Red Poll calves affected with posterior paralysis, an inherited defect (Tuff, 1948). Hereditary encephalomyopathy and internal hydrocephalus were combined with retinal dysplasia (Urman and Grace, 1964). Multiple ocular defects in grade Shorthorn calves, such as retinal detachment, cataract, microphthalmia, persistent pupillary membrane, and retinal dysplasia, were associated with internal hydrocephalus (Leipold et al., 1971a). The cause of the defect was unknown; however, it may have been genetic.

Although internal hydrocephaly in cattle has received considerable attention, relatively little information is available about the associated ocular lesions (Gibbons, 1966). Congenital defects of the caudal segments of the vertebral column and high ventricular septal defects occurred together with anophthalmia and microphthalmia (Leipold and Huston, 1968a). The frequency of ocular defects such as anophthalmia and microphthalmia was estimated in six U.S. breeds to be maximally 1 in 7,500 births and minimally 1 in 50,000 births. The cause of these bovine ocular defects is unknown (Leipold and Huston, 1968a). It has been demonstrated that BVD virus causes cerebellar hypoplasia combined with ocular defects such as retinal atrophy, acute and chronic neuritis, cataract, and microphthalmia with retinal dysplasia (Bistner et al., 1970).

F. Skin Defects

Developmental defects involving skin and adnexa are not uncommon in cattle and may be either generalized or localized. Deficiencies of skin pigmentation are included here. Most congenital skin diseases described in cattle have a genetic cause. Many more exist in various breeds of cattle and will be identified as knowledge expands. The nature, cause, and frequency of bovine skin defects have been studied (Leipold et al., 1979b). Coat color inheritance in cattle has also been reviewed (Olson and Willham, 1982).

1. Albinism

Albinism may be classified as partial, incomplete, and complete. In partial albinism, the iris is blue and white centrally and brown peripherally, and the coat color is usually either characteristic of the breed or dilute. Incomplete albinos have colobomas of the nontapetal fundus and tapetal fibrosum hypoplasia (Gelatt et al., 1969). Incomplete albinism is inherited as an autosomal dominant trait (Leipold and Huston, 1966, 1968b). A form of partial albinism is encountered in the Chediak–Higashi syndrome reported by Padgett et al. (1970). It is recessively inherited and includes, in addition to albinotic features, abnormally large membrane-bound organelles in various cell types and increased susceptibility to infection.

Complete albinos have pure white coats and white to pink irises, but a normal tapetum lucidum (Leipold et al., 1968). Complete albinism is a simple autosomal recessive trait. Albino calves were observed in two Charolais herds. The calves had pale skin and lacked pigment. The iris was pink; pupils were slitlike, and there was an albinotic reflex. The calves were blind in bright daylight because of photophobia. Histologic examination verified the complete absence of pigmentation in skin and eyes (Jayasekera and Leipold, 1981).

A new albinotic color deficiency has been identified in Angus cattle at KSU and appears to be inherited as a simple autosomal recessive trait. Heterochromia irides in Angus cattle is characterized by brown hair over the entire body surface instead of the typical black. The muzzle, hooves, and scrotum in males are also brown. The skin surface is brownish to gray, which is particularly obvious in the glabrous skin areas, such as around eyelids, ear openings, muzzle, anal, and reproductive openings. The most distinguishing factor involved iris color, the dark black iris of Angus cattle being replaced by a light, usually two-colored iris. This gives a double-ringed appearance to the iris when viewed closely: an outer, faintly brown ring surrounds an inner, light blue ring circling the pupil. The pupils appear constricted in daylight. From a distance the eyes appear white. The ocular fundus is albinotic.

2. Fragility of Skin

Two bulls, father and son, of the Middle and High Belgian breed, were identified as carriers of skin fragility similar to the Ehlers–Danlos syndrome in humans (Hanset and Ansay, 1967). Two similar cases in Hereford calves in Texas revealed hyperelasticity of skin and articular ligaments, cutaneous fragility, and delayed healing of skin wounds. Histologic and electron microscopic examination disclosed lack of mature collagen fibers. The calves resulted from a father–daughter and a half-sib mating (O'Hara et al., 1970).

Fragility of skin occurred in Simmental and Charolais calves from two different herds. It was characterized by extreme skin fragility and joint laxity. Collagenous tissues of the body exhibited fragmentation and disorganization of collagen fibers. Fibroblasts grown from diseased calves contained a relatively higher level of procollagen than fibroblasts from normal calves. Accumulation of procollagen may be due to an insufficiency of procollagen peptidase (Jayasekera et al., 1979b; Leipold et al., 1979b).

This hereditary defect in three German Black Pied cattle was characterized by excessive elasticity and fragility of skin on head, neck, and forelegs leading to traumatic skin wounds and formation of seromata. At necropsy the skin was easily detached. Histologic examination revealed edema in the stratum reticulare, with thinly distributed collagen fibers and aggregations of fibroblasts and fibrocytes. Biochemically, affected skin contained 12% less protein and 36% less glycine than normal skin (Stöber et al., 1982). Hegreberg (1982) has reviewed animal models of collagen diseases including skin fragility.

3. Epitheliogenesis Imperfecta

One of the more common skin defects is epitheliogenesis imperfecta, first described in Holstein–Friesian cattle in the United States (Hadley, 1927). Affected calves of either sex had large epithelial defects distal to the carpal and tarsal joints, and one or more defective claws. In addition, muzzle, nostril, tongue, hard palate, and cheeks had epithelial defects. The ears were deformed by rolled margins and adhesions on the contacted surfaces. Ayrshire calves had similar but less extensive lesions, and no horn or claw defects (Hutt and Frost, 1948). Jersey calves with extensive epithelial defects in the oral cavity, body, and legs were observed in Texas and California. Additionally, they had gross defects such as brachygnathia inferior and atresia ani (Regan et al., 1935; Wiprecht and Harlacher, 1935).

Calves affected with epitheliogenesis imperfecta either were born prematurely or died shortly after birth as a result of septicemia. Authors reported simple autosomal recessive inheritance of this lethal trait. Epitheliogenesis imperfecta also has been reported in various European breeds, and was reviewed by Straub (1969) and Jayasekera and Leipold (1979).

Shorthorn and Angus calves affected with epitheliogenesis imperfecta had extensive epithelial defects of skin, tongue, buccal mucosa, and hooves, and died from septicemia. Histologic examination disclosed abrupt transition from normal epidermis to lesions of epitheliogenesis imperfecta. The adjacent epidermis was hyperplastic with an increase in the germinal layer. Within the defect, the epidermis and adnexal structures were absent, and lymphocytes and polymorphonuclear leukocytes infiltrated the area. Genealogic data suggested simple autosomal recessive inheritance. Epitheliogenesis imperfecta is a rare defect in beef and dairy calves (Leipold et al., 1979b).

4. Imperfect Keratogenesis

Keratogenesis imperfecta hereditaria bovina (van't Hooft, 1959) is a lethal condition appearing a few months after birth and is characterized by erosions in the tongue, oral cavity, and esophagus, and around the claws.

McPherson et al. (1964) described a recessively inherited skin disease in British Friesian calves, involving lesions of exudative dermatitis of the legs and erosions of the mucosa of the oral cavity, esophagus, and forestomachs. A similar disease has been described in Danish Black Pied calves (Andresen et al., 1970). Affected calves appeared normal at birth and until 1 month of age, after which there were exanthema of the legs and symmetrical hair loss. Some calves developed diarrhea; others developed conjunctivitis, rhinitis, and bronchopneumonia; and still others developed CNS signs. Pedigree analysis of 24 affected calves indicated a simple autosomal lethal factor (Andresen et al., 1970).

Holstein–Friesian calves with a similar condition are referred to as baldy calves. They are born normal but develop scaly, thickened, and folded skin over neck and shoulders; there is also alopecia, and the horns fail to grow. This is followed by general body deterioration; therefore, affected calves are destroyed. The defect is inherited as an autosomal recessive trait.

Genetic etiology of parakeratosis, its pathogenesis due to deficient uptake of zinc in the intestinal tract and chromosomal defects, were reported in various European countries (van Adrichem et al., 1970; Brummerstedt et al., 1971; Bosma and Kroneman, 1979; Herzog et al., 1982).

5. Congenital Ichthyosis

Congenital ichthyosis has been described in cattle. Lueps (1963) reported 22 German Pinzgauer calves with ichthyosis and associated defects such as microtia, cataracts, and thyroid dysplasia. A less severe form of ichthyosis was described in Canadian Holstein–Friesians by Julian (1960).

The skin of two neonatal Chianina calves was hairless and covered with irregular large horny plates separated by deep fissures. The yellow-gray horn plates, ranging from 1 to 8 cm in diameter and 0.5 cm thick, had flat smooth surfaces. The fissures separating the horn plates were 2–8 mm deep. Histologically the bottoms of the fissures were covered with short stubby hairs, and excessive hyperkeratosis was evident. Father–daughter matings indicated that the defect was due to homozygosity of a simple autosomal recessive gene (Leipold et al., 1979b).

6. Protoporphyria

Protoporphyria, a photosensitizing disease in Limousin cattle, is caused by homozygosity of a simple autosomal recessive gene (Ruth et al., 1980). Limousin cattle affected with protoporphyria may have photodynamic dermatitis, ataxia, and seizures. Furthermore, liver cirrhosis may occur, indicating similarity to human protoporphyria, where a wide variation of clinical signs among patients has been noted (Wells et al., 1980).

Protoporphyria has been reported as an autosomal dominant disease in humans. Measurement of heme synthase activity in sonicates of cultured skin fibroblasts and whole-liver homogenates from protophorphyric, heterozygous, and normal cattle indicated the cause to be homozygosity of a simple autosomal recessive gene (Bloomer et al., 1982).

G. Defects of Hair

1. Hypertrichosis and Curliness

Congenital hypertrichosis has been described in European cattle and has been correlated with polypnea during hot weather (Helbig, 1958). Abnormal curliness of hair has been noted in Ayrshire calves and is transmitted as an autosomal dominant characteristic (Eldridge et al., 1949).

2. Hypotrichosis

According to Hutt (1963), six different kinds of hypotrichosis can be distinguished in cattle, all sensitive to environmental influences:

1. Hairless lethal is encountered in exotic breeds, with affected calves dying shortly after birth.

2. Semihairlessness has been reported only in Polled Herefords and is characterized by a thin hair coat at birth. Later, the hair coat is sparse and patchy, and the skin is wrinkled and scaly.
3. Hypotrichosis combined with anodontia has been described only in the Main–Anjou breed.
4. Viable hypotrichosis, encountered in Guernseys and exotic breeds, is characterized by partial to complete absence of hair at birth, but hair develops later. Histopathologically, an affected Jersey calf revealed poor development of hair follicles and associated sweat glands, as well as numerous abnormally complex arteriovenous anastomoses (Schleger et al., 1967).
5. A condition in which four to six incisor teeth are missing and patches of hair exist on the face and neck (later the hair coat is normal) has been reported only in Holstein–Friesian calves.
6. Streaked hairlessness in Holstein–Friesians is characterized by vertical hairless streaks over hip joints and sometimes over the body and legs.

The severity of hypotrichosis varies, some cases being lethal. All six types are inherited. Lethal hairless, semihairless, and viable hypotrichosis are simple autosomal recessive characters; hypotrichosis with anodontia is considered to be a sex-linked recessive trait; hypotrichosis with missing incisor teeth is possibly a dominant trait; streaked hairlessness is a dominant sex-linked gene (Hutt, 1963).

Hypotrichosis was studied in horned and in Polled Hereford cattle (Jayasekera et al., 1979a). The cases ranged from slightly to severely affected, and secondary skin changes were common. The skin was thin and pliable with only a few hairs observed per unit area on the lateral and ventral neck, face, ears, thorax, flank, rump, and forehead. The hair coat over the eyelids, around prepuce, umbilicus, and switch of tail was thin, wavy, and silky. Microscopic examination revealed an epidermis two to three cell layers thick and poorly differentiated dermal papillae. Frequently, the hair shafts were fragmented and did not conform to the internal contours of the hair follicles.

Hair follicles typically were shallow and evenly cylindrical. In sections stained with toluidine blue, Huxley's cells of the hair follicles contained spheroidal microdroplets of semitranslucent, pleomorphic material that was abundant in the region of differentiation and transformation of papillary cells into inner and outer hair sheaths. These microdroplets appeared to be electron-dense trichohyalin granules. The trichohyalin granules of hair follicle cells from hypotrichotic calves lacked the micro- and macrofilaments usually associated with normal animals. Hypotrichosis in Hereford calves is inherited as a simple autosomal recessive trait.

3. Interdigital Overgrowth

This condition has been reported mainly in Europe (Wegner, 1970), where it was considered that interdigital overgrowth was predisposed by genetic factors.

H. CARDIOVASCULAR SYSTEM DEFECTS

Like humans and other domestic animals, cattle are affected with several different cardiovascular defects. With few exceptions, most congenital cardiac defects were reported as single cases; there are few descriptions of series of cases. During routine meat inspection of 50,742 bovine hearts, van Nie (1966) found congenital anomalies in 88 (0.17%). The cause of cardiovascular defects has received little study.

1. Ectopia Cordis

Judging by the number of reports, ectopia cordis is a common defect; yet its cause is unknown. Herzog and Wiedeking (1970) reviewed the literature and added 12 new cases. The heart may be located in the cervical region, outside the thoracic cavity through a sternal fissure, or in the abdominal cavity. Various associated defects of the heart, its vessels, and the ribs and sternum have been observed.

2. Ventricular Septal Defects

Ventricular septal defects, common in cattle, may vary in size and location. They may be single and isolated, or they may be combined with abnormalities of the large vessels, which are referred to by using the nomenclature of their human counterparts. Fischer and Pirie (1964) reported 16 ventricular septal defects in common Scottish breeds: eight calves had no associated defects; four had pulmonary stenosis, dextraposition of aorta, and right ventricular hypertrophy (tetralogy of Fallot); and four had dextraposed aorta but no pulmonary stenosis. Only one case indicated familial incidence—a cow and her fetus affected with a ventricular septal defect.

Ventricular septal defects, associated with internal hydrocephalus in the French Limosin breed, were considered to be caused by an autosomal dominant gene (Lauvergne and Pavoux, 1969).

3. Vessels

Included here are persistence of the right aortic arch and double aortic arch. Transposition of vessels is usually encountered with other cardiac defects. One of the common defects in calves is patency of the ductus arteriosus; however, the cause is unknown. An interesting defect was described in Holland in which aneurysm-like lesions of the celiac artery and cranial mesenteric artery caused fatal hemorrhage (Schuiringa-Sybesma, 1961).

4. Lymphatics

Dysplasia of the lymphatics is an important autosomal recessive defect resulting in edema. It has been reported only in Ayrshire calves (Donald *et al.*, 1952; Herrick and Eldridge, 1955). The degree of edema varies, and it results in dystocia, stillbirths, or viable calves with edematous legs. A curious feature of the disease is accessory earlobes. Detailed pathological studies are lacking.

5. Blood

Familial bovine polycythemia has been reported in an inbred strain of Jersey cattle. There were no gross lesions at necropsy to account for the polycythemia. Clinically, the 14 affected calves had congested mucous membranes, dyspnea, and retarded growth; 9 calves died during calfhood. The defect was considered to be caused by homozygosity of a simple autosomal recessive gene (Tennant *et al.*, 1967).

I. Respiratory System Defects

Congenital defects of the respiratory system are rare and relatively unimportant in cattle. Congenital atresia of the nares has been described twice in European calves (Ilancic, 1940; Weber, 1946). Thomson (1966a) reviewed congenital lung defects in calves and added descriptions of two cases of accessory lungs and one of bronchial hypoplasia.

J. Digestive System Defects

Defects of the tongue are rare; one such defect is smooth tongue in Dutch Friesians. It is characterized by diminution of filiform papillae, fragility of the mucosa, velvety hair coat, soft horns, and microcytic hypochromic anemia (Gotink *et al.*, 1955). Dutch workers implicated a recessive mode of inheritance, but smooth tongue in American Brown Swiss was interpreted as being due to an incompletely penetrant, dominant gene (Huston *et al.*, 1968a).

Intestinal defects are usually localized and disrupt patency. Atresia of the ileum was described in Swedish cattle by Nihleen and Eriksson

(1958). Atresia of the colon in three Angus calves was listed by Maclellan and Martin (1956), and six calves with atresia coli were described by Osborne and Legates (1963). Atresia ani was reported in New Zealand (Rees and Boshier, 1966) and megacolon in Germany (Wiedeking, 1970; Wiesner and Willer, 1978).

Some work has indicated that atresia coli may be caused by rectal palpation. Results obtained thus far have incriminated palpation of the amniotic sac between Days 36 and 41 of gestation as a cause of atresia coli in calves (Müller *et al.*, 1982; Ness *et al.*, 1982).

K. Hepatic Defects

Little information is available on congenital defects of the liver in cattle. A commonly encountered incidental finding is subserosal cysts.

L. Defects of Large Body Cavities

Although hernias such as scrotal, inguinal, and in particular umbilical are considered common in cattle, little is known about their cause. Gilman and Stringam (1953) found progeny of four of seven Holstein–Friesian bulls with umbilical hernias (females 1.06%, males 0.51%). The closer familial relationship of the four bulls having affected offsprings was interpreted to be consistent with one or more pairs of recessive factors of low frequency. The introduction of American Holsteins into northern Germany has led to increasing reports of umbilical hernia (Suborg, 1976).

Clefts of the diaphragm may be encountered with or without herniation of abdominal organs. Troutt *et al.* (1967) discussed the surgical aspects of these defects.

Schistosomus reflexus, an extreme closure defect of the abdominal cavity, is a common lethal defect of cattle. Studies on its cause, however, are lacking.

M. Reproductive System Defects

1. Male

a. Penis and Prepuce. Various deviations of the penis and prepuce have been described; all are rare with unknown causes. Duplication of the penis has been described (Bosu and Barker, 1971). Persistent penile frenulum interfering with copulation was common in Shorthorn and Angus Aberdeen breeds. The condition is thought to be inherited (Carroll *et al.*, 1964).

b. Testicle. Since the study by Lagerloef and Settergren (1952) in Swedish Highland cattle, numerous other investigators have reported testicular hypoplasia (bilateral or unilateral, partial or complete). Galloway (1961) described bilateral testicular hypoplasia in a Jersey bull and a unilateral case in a Hereford bull. Markau (1963) and Christensen (1965) presented a series of 46 bilateral and 20 unilateral cases in European breeds. Chromosomal changes were demonstrated in testicular hypoplasia. König (1959) reported inversions and translocations, and Knudsen (1961a,b) described sticky chromosomes in squash preparations from hypoplastic testicles.

Cryptorchidism—incompletely descended testicle—may be unilateral or bilateral. Few studies indicate the cause in cattle, in contrast to the horse and pig. Wheat (1961) reported four cases of unilateral left cryptorchidism in purebred Hereford bulls; the available evidence indicated possible genetic transmission.

c. Wolffian Duct. The only important defect is segmental aplasia characterized by isolated lack of portions derived from the Wolffian duct, mostly located in the epididymal head. Christensen (1965) presented 83 cases of this defect, 79 unilateral (20 left, 59 right) and 4 bilateral.

Multiple defects of the male genital tract, including segmental aplasia of the Wolffian duct, gonadal hypoplasia, and intermittent cryptorchidism, were found to be due to a chromosomal constellation of XXY (Rieck et al., 1969; Rieck, 1970). Reproductive disturbances due to chromosomal defects were reviewed by Willer (1982).

2. Intersex

An intersex is an individual with congenital anatomical variations that confuse the diagnosis of sex; it may have some reproductive organs of both sexes, or be genetically one sex and phenotypically the other (Biggers and McFeely, 1966). Intersexuality has been reviewed by Biggers and McFeely (1966) and Hafez and Jainudeen (1966).

a. Hermaphrodite. Hermaphrodites have characteristics of both sexes. By definition a true hermaphrodite has gonads of both sexes, either as an ovary and testis, or combined into an ovotestis. A pseudohermaphrodite has the gonads of one sex and reproductive organs with some characteristics of the opposite sex (Biggers and McFeely, 1966); it is classified as a male or female by testis or ovaries. Pseudohermaphroditism is more common than hermaphroditism.

The tubular reproductive organs of a hermaphrodite vary. Chromosomal investigations in a true hermaphrodite (a cow with testes, uterus, and male ductal structures) revealed a chromosomal picture in the peripheral blood of predominantly XY and XX (McFeeley et al., 1967). Dunn et al. (1968) reported chromosomal findings in a hermaphrodite that was externally a male with an empty scrotum, a small vagina, one seminal vesicle, uterus, right oviduct and ovary, left spermatic cord, and ovotestis. Lung, muscle, and uterus revealed XX; blood, bone marrow, kidney, testis, and ovotestis had mainly XX but also XY cells.

b. Freemartinism. Freemartinism is a common defect of heifers born cotwin to a male; about 93% are affected with variable hypoplasia or agenesis of the organs developing from the Müllerian ducts and stimulated development of the Wolffian duct system. Freemartins have male characteristics and are usually sterile. Humoral factors passing from the male to the female through fused placenta circulation are considered to arrest development of the Müllerian duct system (Tandler and Keller, 1911; Lillie, 1919). Fechheimer et al. (1963) advanced the view that bovine freemartinism is not caused by humoral factors but may be a function of sex chromosome mosaicism. Benirschke (1970) did not consider blood cell chimerism (an individual with cell populations of more than one genotype arising through a mixture of different zygotic genotypes) to be the cause of the sterilizing effect in the female cotwin. He pointed out that we have no plausible explanation why freemartinism occurs in the cow but not in primates.

3. Female

a. Ovary. Ovarian aplasia has been reported with and without associated defects of the tubular reproductive structures. Haase (1967) reported ovarian aplasia combined with aplasia of uterus and cervix.

Ovarian hypoplasia has been extensively studied in the Swedish Highland breed; it may be total or partial, and unilateral or bilateral (Lagerloef and Settergren, 1953). Zemjanis et al. (1961) diagnosed an incidence of 1.9% ovarian hypoplasia in 20,913 clinical examinations in 14 Minnesota and Wisconsin herds.

b. Müllerian Ducts. Defects of oviducts, uterus, cervix, and vagina have been described in several breeds. In many, fusion of the Müllerian ducts is either lacking or exaggerated (Settergren and Galloway, 1965). They classified slaughterhouse specimens into three groups: partial or complete duplication of the uterine body and cervix, partial or complete duplication of cervix, and vaginal septa. Zemjanis and associates (1961) encountered, during 20,913 clinical examinations, three cases of uterus unicornis; Perkins et al. (1954) listed two cases among 1000 bovine reproductive tracts. Sittmann et al. (1961) reported a high incidence of duplication of the cervix in two closely related Hereford herds; they blamed a sex-limited, single, autosomal recessive gene with low penetrance and varying expressivity.

White heifer disease falls into two distinct classes of morphological aberrations, both with partial or total persistence of the hymen, and one with additional defects cranial to the hymen; common to both are functional ovaries and localized accumulation of secretion products (Hanset and Ansay, 1961). Although the defect is most common in White Shorthorn cattle, other breeds and colors have been reported (Ginther, 1965).

c. Rectovaginal Constriction in Jersey Cattle. Rectovaginal constriction affects the anus and vulvovestibular area of Jersey females as a result of a simple autosomal recessive inheritance. The defect is characterized by inelastic constrictions at the junction of the anus, rectum, vestibule, and vulva. Males are also involved, exhibiting anal stenosis. Affected cows are dystocic, and the calves are delivered following episiotomy or cesarian section. Rectal examinations are difficult to perform on affected cattle. In addition, Jersey cows affected with rectovaginal constriction are prone to develop udder edema at calving, followed frequently by severe mastitis (Leipold and Saperstein, 1975; Leipold et al., 1981).

The constricting tissues associated with rectovaginal constriction (RVC) in Jersey cattle were studied clinically, grossly, and microscopically in nine affected and two control cows. Common to RVC cows were nonelastic fibrous tissue bands located at the anorectal junction and within the vestibular muscularis. Light and scanning electron microscopic examination revealed variable amounts of fibrosis affecting the external anal sphincter muscle. Both tissue bands were composed of well-vascularized, irregular connective tissue containing randomly distributed myofibers and adipose tissue. No abnormalities in ultrastructure of the tissue bands were observed by transmission electron microscopy. The collagen had normal periodicity, and the striated muscle had normal cross banding (McGhee and Leipold, 1982).

Udder edema is a facultative factor associated with rectovaginal constriction in Jersey cattle. Sixteen Jersey cows, twelve affected with RVC and four normal controls, were used to study the pathological changes in the mammary gland associated with udder edema. Edema involved the entire udder but was more pronounced in the ventral aspects, and was due to increased vascular filtration of fluid and proteins. Microscopically, the edematous udder was characterized by excessive fluid infiltration between the muscle fibers of the subcutaneous tissues, into the interlobular and interalveolar interstitial spaces of udder parenchyma, and into the supramammary lymph nodes. Anatomical studies demonstrated abnormalities of the milk vein and milk wells in some RVC cows (Al-Ani et al., 1983).

d. *Prolonged Gestation.* Prolonged gestation has been recorded for most dairy breeds as hereditary. According to Kennedy (1971), it falls into two distinct classes on the basis of lesions. The first, reported in Holsteins and Ayrshires, is conditioned by a single autosomal recessive gene (Gregory et al., 1949–1951). The fetus continues to grow *in utero* and is carried as long as 100 days past term. Calves born or taken by cesarean section are weak and die in hypoglycemic crisis. Adrenals of such calves are hypoplastic (Holm, 1967). The second type of prolonged gestation is also caused by homozygosity of a recessive gene (Stormont et al., 1956). However, the fetus ceases to grow beyond 7 months, and gestation may last as long as 17 months. The fetus may be affected with craniofacial defects, disproportionate dwarfism, and other defects. In severely defective, as well as in nearly normal calves, the adenohypophysis was aplastic (Kennedy et al., 1957). This second type of prolonged gestation has been reported in Guernsey, Jersey, and Swedish Red and White breeds.

There are other incidental types of prolonged gestation, also due to adenohypophyseal aplasia, as described in a grade Holstein–Friesian by Huston and Gier (1958).

N. Metabolic Defects

1. Congenital Porphyria

The defect has been reported in a few breeds of cattle—most frequently in American Holstein–Friesians. It is transmitted as a simple recessive trait (Wass and Hoyt, 1965). In the homozygous state, affected cattle have pigmented teeth and increased porphyrins in blood and urine. Increased porphyrins accumulating in tissues may lead to erythrodontia, cutaneous photosensitization, and anemia. Porphyric calves from porphyric dams were weaker and had more severe metabolic acidosis at birth than control calves (Moore, 1970; Moore et al., 1970). The heterozygote is a clinically normal animal; however, studies have demonstrated that the ratios of urinary coproporphyrin isomers of normal Holstein–Friesian cattle, heterozygotes for congenital porphyria, and homozygotes differed significantly.

2. Congenital Goiter

Goiter is noninflammatory enlargement of the thyroid; it may be congenital or acquired. Van Zyl et al. (1965) reported a selectively bred herd of cattle with congenital goiter in a nongoiterous area. The condition was genetically determined; they concluded that the goiter could not be classified among the types reported elsewhere.

O. Defective Twinning

Defective twins are defined as partial or complete duplications of the axis of the body. Wiedeking (1968) proposed classifying twins as free symmetrical, free asymmetrical, attached symmetrical, and attached asymmetrical. Free and asymmetrical twins are, for instance, amorphus globosus and holocardius acephalus, both characterized by lack of a functional heart and always attached to the placental circulation of a normal twin. The body of such a calf is always extremely malformed. Karyotyping has shown such defective twins may be of opposite sexes (Dunn et al., 1967). Attached and symmetrical twins are usually mirror-like duplications, as encountered in a dicephalic calf. Attached and asymmetrical twins are characterized by attachment of a lesser developed parasite to the more or less normal twin or autosite. The body region of attachment is usually used to classify such defective calves. For example, attachment of a parasitic twin at the sacral area is referred to as parasitic pyopagus. Although defective twins are referred to as an unusual monster, there is little information available as to cause. Modrowich (1969), studying a series of 50 defective twins, found that more twins were conceived in winter than in other seasons, but was unable to find any genetic differences.

VIII. Conclusions

Animal breeders and veterinarians are involved in improving animal health and production. The goals are either to produce a quality pet or working animal, or to improve dairy and meat production. Accurate diagnosis of diseases and defects, partly or wholly caused by genetic factors, is necessary before control measures can be established. Such diagnosis involves understanding hereditary patterns of disease. Many different congenital defects of genetic, environmental, or unknown cause, or due to environmental–genetic interaction, have been identified in cattle. It is important to recognize that congenital defects are economically significant to the cattle breeding industry. Not only is diagnosis important; methods to control genetically induced defects in cattle should also be understood. Most cattle breeding associations and artificial insemination organizations have programs for controlling undesirable traits and genetic defects.

Many clinical reports of congenital defects contain little if any etiological information, particularly that which would be useful for genetic diagnosis. Most genetic diagnoses, naturally based on limited evidence because of the rarity of the defects, must be tentative. Many older genetic interpretations require reevaluation.

With the incrimination of viruses and plant toxins as causes of congenital defects, a concerted effort is needed to identify environmental agents that are teratogenic. The highly complex and poorly understood interactions between environmental and genetic factors require amplification.

Genetic diseases in cattle that are of concern include hypotrichosis, arthrogryposis with cleft palate, weaver condition, rectovaginal constriction, internal hydrocephalus, mannosidosis, osteopetrosis, tibial hemimelia, polydactyly, syndactyly, and umbilical hernia.

Greater use of cytogenetics may prove fruitful in studying congenital defects of cattle, particularly intersexuality defects. Detection of chromosomal aberrations in cattle should attain the same level of diagnostic significance that it has in humans.

Finally, there is an urgent need for more basic and planned research on congenital defects of cattle. Time and costs will unfortunately discourage experimental teratology in cattle. Meanwhile, expansion of our knowledge of congenital defects of cattle will result mainly from studying field cases—nature's experiments—by adequate description, detailed diagnostic examination, and genetic analyses.

Congenital defects are significant for the following reasons:

1. Congenital defects reduce the value of affected cattle and possibly that of their normal relatives.
2. Deaths of congenitally defective cattle and consequent loss of salvage value are of appreciable economic significance.
3. Economic losses occur when congenital defects are only a partial manifestation of a syndrome that also included embryonic and fetal mortality.
4. Productivity is reduced by longer calving intervals and by dystocia and infertility which are common maternal sequelae.
5. Herd improvement is hampered through loss of replacements and consequent reduction in culling potential.
6. Control measures may require alterations of breeding programs, including introducing less popular and less profitable breeding cattle.
7. New or more expensive management practices, such as artificial breeding under ranch conditions, may be required.
8. Congenital defects may be an added source of confusion in diag-

nosing other clinical entities, for example, osteopetrosis and abortion in Angus cattle.
9. All congenital defects of cattle have comparative biomedical significance.

Congenital defects, being essentially natural experiments, offer a correlative approach to the study of disease including genetic, biochemical, virologic, toxicologic, cytologic, and gross and histopathologic aspects.

REFERENCES

Adams, R. D., Denny-Brown, D., and Pearson, C. M. (1962). "Diseases of Muscle: A Study in Pathology," pp. 229–323. Harper (Hoeber), New York.
Adelmann, H. B. (1920). *Anat. Rec.* **19**, 29–34.
Adrian, R. W., Leipold, H. W., Huston, K., Trotter, D. M., and Dennis, S. M. (1969a). *J. Dairy Sci.* **52**, 1432–1435.
Adrian, R. W., Trotter, D. M., Leipold, H. W., and Huston, K. (1969b). *J. Dairy Sci.* **52**, 1436–1440.
Adrian, R. W., Trotter, D. M., Leipold, H. W., and Huston, K. (1969c). *J. Dairy Sci.* **52**, 1441–1444.
Al-Ani, F. K., Vestweber, J. G. E., and Leipold, H. W. (1983). *Bovine Pract.* (in press).
Andresen, E., Flagstadt, T., Basse, A., and Brummerstedt, E. (1970). *Nord. Veteringermed.* **22**, 473–485.
Anonymous (1958). *34th Annu. Rep., N.Z. Dairy Board* p. 83.
Anonymous (1961). *37th Annu. Rep., N.Z. Dairy Board* p. 81.
Arnault, G. A. (1979). "Etude de la parésie spastique des bovins," p. 97. Rivaton et Cie, France.
Arnault, G. A. (1982). *Proc. World Congr. Dis. Cattle, 12th, 1982* Vol. II, pp. 853–858.
Ashmore, C. R., and Robinson, D. W. (1969). *Proc. Soc. Exp. Biol. Med.* **132**, 548–554.
Atkeson, F. W., Eldridge, F., and Ibsen, H. L. (1944a). *J. Hered.* **35**, 11–14.
Atkeson, F. W., Ibsen, H. L., and Eldridge, F. (1944b). *J. Hered.* **35**, 45–48.
Axthelm, M. K., Leipold, H. W., Howard, D., and Kirkbride, C. A. (1980a). *Proc. Am. Assoc. Vet. Lab. Diagn.* **23**, 115–126.
Axthelm, M. K., Leipold, H. W., and Phillips, R. (1980b). *Bovine Pract.* **1**, 19–27.
Axthelm, M. K., Leipold, H. W., Jayasekera, U., and Phillips, R. M. (1981a). *Cornell Vet.* **71**, 164–174.
Axthelm, M. K., Leipold, H. W., and Phillips, R. M. (1981b). *Vet. Med. Small Anim. Clin.* **76**, 567–570.
Axthelm, M. K., Leipold, H. W., and Phillips, R. M. (1981c). *Kans. Vet.* **19**, 13–15.
Baird, J. D., Johnston, K. G., and Hartley, W. J. (1974). *Aust. Vet. J.* **50**, 239–245.
Baker, H. J., Walkley, S. N., Ratazzi, M. C., Singer, H. S., Watson, H. L., and Wood, P. A. (1982). *In* "Animal Models of Inherited Metabolic Diseases," (R. J. Desnich, D. F. Patterson, and D. S. Scarpelli, eds.) pp. 203–212. Alan R. Liss, Inc., New York.
Baker, M. L., Payne, L. C., and Baker, G. N. (1961). *J. Hered.* **52**, 135–138.
Baker, R. D., Snider, G. W., Leipold, H. W., and Johnson, J. L. (1980). *Theriogenology* **13**, 87.
Barlow, R. M. (1981). *Vet. Pathol.* **18**, 151–162.

Barlow, R. M. (1982). *Proc. World Congr. Dis. Cattle, 12th, 1982* Vol. II, pp. 859–863.
Barlow, R. M., Linklater, K. A., and Young, G. B. (1968). *Vet. Rec.* **83,** 60–65.
Barlow, R. M., Mackellar, A., Newlands, G., Wiseman, A., and Berrett, S. (1981). *Vet. Rec.* **109,** 441–445.
Becker, R. B., Wilcox, C. J., and Pritchard, W. R. (1961). *J. Dairy Sci.* **44,** 542–547.
Belling, T. H., and Holland, L. A. (1962). *Vet. Med. (Kansas City, Mo.)* **57,** 405–408.
Bellows, R. A. (1971). *Agric. Res.* **19,** 11.
Bellows, R. A., Rumsey, T. S., Kasson, C. W., Bond, J., Warwick, E. J., and Pahnish, D. F. (1975). *Am. J. Vet. Res.* **36,** 1133–1140.
Benirschke, K. (1970). *Curr. Top. Pathol.* **51,** 1–61.
Bhatt, P. L., Vyas, A. P., and Kohli, R. N. (1964). *Indian Vet. J.* **41,** 736–739.
Bielefeldt Ohmann, H. (1982). *Can. J. Comp. Med.* **46,** 363–369.
Biggers, J. D., and McFeely, R. A. (1966). *Adv. Reprod. Physiol.* **1,** 29–59.
Bistner, S. I., Rubin, L. F., and Saunders, L. Z. (1970). *Pathol. Vet.* **7,** 275–286.
Blackwell, R. L., Knox, J. H., and Cobb, H. E. (1959). *J. Hered.* **50,** 143–148.
Blin, P. C., and Lauvergne, J. J. (1967). *Ann. Zootech.* **16,** 65–68.
Blood, D. C. (1956). *Aust. Vet. J.* **32,** 125–131.
Blood, D. C., and Gay, C. C. (1971). *Aust. Vet. J.* **47,** 520.
Bloomer, J. R., Morton, K. O., Reuter, R. J., and Ruth, S. R. (1982). *Am. J. Hum. Genet.* **34,** 322–330.
Bonewitz, E. R. (1971). "Dairy Newsletter." Cooperative Extension Service, Kansas State University, Manhattan.
Bonner, R. B., Myrea, P. J., and Doyle, B. J. (1961). *Aust. Vet. J.* **37,** 160.
Bosma, A. A., and Kroneman, J. (1979). *Vet. Q.* **1,** 121–125.
Bosu, W. T. K., and Barker, C. V. A. (1971). *Can. Vet. J.* **11,** 21–23.
Brown, T. T., De Lahunta, A., Scott, F. W., Kahrs, R. F., McEntee, K., and Gillespie, J. (1973). *Cornell Vet.* **63,** 561–578.
Brown, T. T., De Lahunta, A., Bistner, S. I., Scott, F. W., and McEntee, K. (1974). *Vet. Pathol.* **11,** 486–505.
Brown, T. T., Bistner, S. I., De Lahunta, A., Scott, F. W., and McEntee, K. (1975). *Vet. Pathol.* **12,** 394–404.
Bruère, A. N. (1980). *Vet. Ann.* **20,** 29–40.
Brummerstedt, E., Flagstad, T., and Basse, A. (1971). *Acta Pathol. Microbiol. Scand.* **79,** 686–687.
Bullard, J. F. (1935). *J. Am. Vet. Med. Assoc.* **87,** 575–577.
Carnahan, D. L., Guffy, M. M., Hibbs, C. M., Leipold, H. W., and Huston, K. (1968). *J. Am. Vet. Med. Assoc.* **152,** 1550–1157.
Carroll, E. J., Aanes, W. A., and Ball, L. (1964). *J. Am. Vet. Med. Assoc.* **144,** 747–749.
Carter, A. H. (1960). *Proc. N. Z. Soc. Anim. Prod.* **20,** 108.
Casaro, A. P. E., Kendrick, J. W., and Kennedy, P. W. (1971). *Am. J. Vet. Res.* **32,** 1543–1561.
Castleberry, S., Johnson, J., Leipold, H. W., Peeples, G., and Schalles, R. (1981). *Theriogenology* **19,** 130.
Chiari, H. (1891). *Dtsch. Med. Wochenschr.* **17,** 1172–1175.
Cho, D. Y., and Leipold, H. W. (1977a). *Zentralbl. Veterinaermed., Reihe A* **24,** 680–695.
Cho, D. Y., and Leipold, H. W. (1977b). *Vet. Bull. (London)* **47,** 489–503.
Cho, D. Y., and Leipold, H. W. (1977c). *Acta Neuropathol.* **39,** 129–133.
Cho, D. Y., and Leipold, H. W. (1978a). *Vet. Pathol.* **15,** 264–266.
Cho, D. Y., and Leipold, H. W. (1978b). *Cornell Vet.* **68,** 60–69.
Cho, D. Y., and Leipold, H. W. (1978c). *Cornell Vet.* **68,** 99–107.

Cho, D. Y., and Leipold, H. W. (1978d). *Pathol., Res. Pract.* **163**, 158–162.
Cho, D. Y., Leipold, H. W., Gopal, T., Hibbs, C. M., and Anthony, H. (1978). *Proc. Am. Assoc. Vet. Lab. Diagn.* **21**, 103–116.
Chomiak, M., and Milart, Z. (1971). *Zentralbl. Veterinaermed., Reihe A* **18**, 48–54.
Christensen, N. O. (1965). *Zuchthyg., Fortpflanzungsstoer. Besamung Haust.* **2**, 145–166.
Coetzer, J. A. W., Theodaridis, A., Herr, S., and Kritzinger, L. (1979). *Onderstepoort J. Vet. Res.* **46**, 165–169.
Cohrs, P. (1955). *Dtsch. Tieraerztl. Wochenschr.* **62**, 82–83.
Cole, C. L., and Moore, L. A. (1942). *J. Agric. Res.* **65**, 483–491.
Cordy, D. R., Richards, W. P. C., and Stormont, C. (1969). *Pathol. Vet.* **6**, 487–501.
Cotterman, C. W. (1954). *In* "Statistics and Mathematics in Biology" (O. Kempthorne *et al.*, eds.), pp. 449–465. Iowa State Coll. Press, Ames.
Cravero, G. C., Cornaglia, E., and Fankhauser, R. (1976). *Schwiez. Arch. Tierheilkd.* **118**, 295–304.
Dahlquist, S., Henricson, B., and Hultnas, C. A. (1962). *Proc. Nord. Vet. Congr., 9th, 1962* Vol. 1, p. 118.
Davis, G. B., Thompson, E. J., and Kyle, R. J. (1975). *N.Z. Vet. J.* **23**, 181.
Deas, D. W. (1960). *Vet. Rec.* **30**, 619–620.
de Boom, H. P. A. (1965). *S. Afr. J. Sci.* **61**, 159–171.
De Kesel, A., Dewulf, M., and DeMoor, A. (1981). *Vlaams Diergeneeskd. Tijdschr.* **50**(1), 4–13.
Della-Porta, A. J., Murray, M. D., and Cybinski, D. H. (1976). *Aust. Vet. J.* **52**, 496–501.
Deniz, E. (1966). *Ankara Univ. Vet. Fak. Derg.* **13**, 281–291.
Di Berardino, D., and Iannuzzi, L. (1982). *J. Hered.* **73**, 434–438.
Dietz, O., Li, E., Berg, R., Schonmuth, G., and Stolzenburg, U. (1971). *Monatsh. Veterinaermed.* **26**, 24–30.
Dirksen, G. (1970). *In* "Krankheiten des Rindes" (G. Rosenberger, ed.) pp. 497–500. Parey, Berlin.
Dobler, R. (1903). *Mitt. Verbandes Badischer Tieraerzte* **3**, 65–66.
Doige, C. E. (1975). *Can. Vet. J.* **16**, 22–25.
Doige, C. E., Farrow, C. S., and Smart, M. E. (1978). *Can. Vet. J.* **19**, 230–233.
Donald, H. P., Deas, D. W., and Wilson, A. L. (1952). *Br. Vet. J.* **108**, 227–245.
Done, J. T., Terlecki, S., Richardson, C., Harkness, J. W., Sands, J. J., Patterson, D. S. P., Seweasey, D., Shaw, I. S., Winkler, C. E., and Duffel, S. J. (1980). *Vet. Rec.* **106**, 473–479.
Donnelly, W. J. C., Hannan, J., Sheahan, B. J., and O'Connor, P. J. (1972). *Vet. Rec.* **91**, 225–226.
Donnelly, W. J. C., Sheahan, B. J., and Kelly, M. (1973a). *Res. Vet. Sci.* **15**, 139–141.
Donnelly, W. J. C., Sheahan, B. J., and Rogers, T. A. (1973b). *J. Pathol. Bacteriol.* **111**, 173–179.
Dunn, H. O., Lein, D. H., and Kenney, R. M. (1967). *Cytogenetics* **6**, 413–419.
Dunn, H. O., Kenney, R. M., and Lein, D. H. (1968). *Cytogenetics* **7**, 390–402.
Dyer, I. A., Cossett, W. A., and Roa, R. R. (1964). *BioScience* **14**, 31–32.
Edmonds, L., Crenshaw, D., and Selby, L. A. (1973). *J. Hered.* **64**, 62–64.
Edwards, J. H. (1970). *Adv. Hum. Genet.* **1**, 1–34.
Eldridge, F. E., Atkeson, F. W., and Ibsen, H. L. (1949). *J. Hered.* **40**, 205–213.
Elston, R. C. (1981). *Adv. Hum. Genet.* **11**, 63–120.
Ely, F., Hull, F. W., and Morrison, H. B. (1939). *J. Hered.* **30**, 105–108.
Emmerson, M. A., and Hazel, L. N. (1956). *J. Am. Vet. Med. Assoc.* **128**, 381–390.

Engel, D. (1970). Ph.D. Dissertation, Justus Liebig-Universität, Giessen, Germany.
Epstein, H. (1955). *Indian J. Vet. Sci. Anim. Husb.* **25**, 313–316.
Erickson, B. H., and Murphree, R. L. (1964). *J. Anim. Sci.* **23**, 1066–1071.
Fankhauser, R. (1957). *Dtsch. Tieraerztl. Wochenschr.* **64**, 225–230.
Fankhauser, R. (1959). *Schweiz. Arch. Tierheilkd.* **101**, 407–416.
Fankhauser, R., and Luginbuhl, H. (1968). *In* "Handbuch der speziellen pathologischen Anatomie der Haustiere" (J. Dobberstein and H. Stünzi, eds.), Vol. 3 pp. 191–436. Parey, Berlin.
Fechheimer, N. S. (1968). *N.A.S.—N.R.C., Publ.* **1685**, 7–44.
Fechheimer, N. S, Herschler, M. S., and Gilmore, L. O. (1963). *In* "Genetics Today" (S. J. Geerts, ed.), Vol. 1, p. 265. Pergamon, Oxford.
Fielden, E. D. (1959). *N.Z. Vet. J.* **7**, 80–82.
Finnie, E. P., and Leaver, D. D. (1965). *Aust. Vet. J.* **41**, 287–288.
Fischer, E. W., and Pirie, H. M. (1964). *Br. Vet. J.* **120**, 253–272.
Fischer, H. (1951). *Berl. Muench. Tieraerztl. Wochenschr.* **10**, 202–204.
Frauchiger, E., and Fankhauser, R. (1952). *Schweiz. Arch. Tierheilkd.* **94**, 145–148.
Frauchiger, E., and Fankhauser, R. (1957). "Vergleichende Neuropathologie des Menschen und der Tiere." Springer-Verlag, Berlin and New York.
Frauchiger, E., and Hofmann, W. (1941). "Die Nervendrankheiten des Rindes." Huber, Bern.
Galloway, D. B. (1961). *Aust. Vet. J.* **37**, 335–341.
Gelatt, K. N., Huston, K., and Leipold, H. W. (1969). *Am. J. Vet. Res.* **30**, 1313–1316.
Gerov, K., Choushkov, P., and Dimitrov, A. (1971). *Vet. Med. (Prague)* **8**, 69–75.
Gibbons, W. J. (1966). *Mod. Vet. Pract.* **47**, 34–37.
Gilman, J. P. W. (1956). *Cornell Vet.* **45**, 487–499.
Gilman, J. P. W., and Stringam, E. W. (1953). *J. Hered.* **44**, 113–116.
Ginther, O. J. (1965). *J. Am. Vet. Med. Assoc.* **146**, 133–137.
Girgin, H. (1972). *Etlik. Vet. Bakteriol. Enstit. Dergisi.* **4**, 37–46.
Goedegeburne, S. A., Hani, H., and Poulos, P. W. (1981). *Zentralbl. Veterinaermed.* **28**, 345–356.
Goller, H. (1961). *Berl. Muench. Tieraerztl. Wochenschr.* **74**, 431–435.
Goller, H. (1963). *Anat. Anz.* **112**, 447–457.
Goonewardene, L. A., and Berg, R. T. (1976). *Ann. Genet. Sel. Anim.* **8**, 493–499.
Gopal, T., and Leipold, H. W. (1979). *Vet. Pathol.* **16**, 610–612.
Goss, L. J., and Hull, F. E. (1939). *Cornell Vet.* **29**, 239–240.
Gotink, W. M., Degroot, T., and Stegenga, T. (1955). *Landbouwk. Tijdschr.* **67**, 629–672.
Götze, R. (1932). *Dtsch. Tieraerztl. Wochenschr.* **40**, 197–200.
Grant, H. T. (1956). *J. Hered.* **47**, 165–170.
Greeley, R. G., Boyd, C. L., and Jolly, D. G. (1968). *Southwest. Vet.* **12**, 277–280.
Greene, H. J., and Leipold, H. W. (1974). *Cornell Vet.* **64**, 366–375.
Greene, H. J., Leipold, H. W., and Huston, K. (1973a). *Giessener Beitr. Erbpathol. Zuchthyg.* **5**, 158–169.
Greene, H. J., Leipold, H. W., and Dennis, S. M. (1973b). *VM/SAC, Vet. Med. Small Anim. Clin.* **68**, 167–168.
Greene, H. J., Leipold, H. W., Huston, K., and Guffy, M. M. (1973c). *Am. J. Vet. Res.* **34**, 887–891.
Greene, H. J., Leipold, H. W., Huston, K., Noordsdy, J. L., and Dennis, S. M. (1973d). *Ir. Vet. J.* **27**, 37–45.
Greene, H. J., Leipold, H. W., and Hibbs, C. M. (1974a). *Cornell Vet.* **64**, 596–616.

Greene, H. J., Leipold, H. W., Hibbs, C. M., and Kirkbride, C. N. (1974b). *J. Am. Vet. Med. Assoc.* **164,** 389–395.
Greene, H. J., Saperstein, G., Schalles, R., and Leipold, H. W. (1978). *Ir. Vet. J.* **32,** 65–69.
Gregory, K. E., Arthaud, V. H., Koch, R. M., and Swiger, L. A. (1962). *J. Hered.* **53,** 130–132.
Gregory, P. W. (1955). *J. Anim. Sci.* **14,** 1182–1183.
Gregory, P. W., Mead, S. W., and Regan, W. M. (1943). *J. Hered.* **34,** 125–128.
Gregory, P. W., Mead, S. W., and Regan, W. M. (1944). *J. Hered.* **35,** 195–200.
Gregory, P. W., Mead, S. W., and Regan, W. M. (1949–1951). *Port. Acta Biol., Ser. A: Goldschmidt Vol.* p. 861.
Gregory, P. W., Tyler, W. S., and Julian, L. M. (1966). *Growth* **30,** 343–369.
Gregory, P. W., Julian, L. M., and Tyler, W. S. (1967). *J. Hered.* **58,** 220–224.
Gruneberg, H., and Hutton, K. (1965). *J. Embryol. Exp. Morphol.* **19,** 251–259.
Gruys, E. (1973). *Zentralbl. Veterinaermed., Reihe A* **20,** 789–800.
Haase, H. (1967). *Monatsch. Veterinaermed.* **22,** 356.
Hadley, F. B. (1927). *J. Hered.* **18,** 487–495.
Hadorn, E. (1961). "Developmental Genetics and Lethal Factors." Methuen, London.
Hafez, E. S. E., and Jainudeen, M. R. (1966). *Anim. Breed. Abstr.* **34,** 1–15.
Hamada, T. (1974). *Vet. Rec.* **95,** 441.
Hamana, K., and Leipold, H. W. (1980). *Bovine Pract.* **1,** 18–32.
Hamana, K., Otsuka, H., Kaseda, Y., Nosaka, D., Usui, M., and Hataya, M. (1973). *Bull. Fac. Agric., Miyazaki Univ.* **20,** 293–310.
Hamana, K., Katayama, H., and Murata, K. (1974a). *Bull. Fac. Agric., Miyazaki Univ.* **21,** 135–143.
Hamana, K., Otsuka, H., Nosaka, D., Usui, M., and Hataya, M. (1974b). *Bull. Fac. Agric., Miyazaki Univ.* **21,** 145–160.
Hamana, K., Otsuka, H., and Nosaka, D. (1975). *Bull. Fac. Agric., Miyazaki Univ.* **22,** 115–129.
Hanset, R., and Ansay, M. (1961). *Ann. Med. Vet.* **105,** 443–449.
Hanset, R., and Ansay, M. (1967). *Ann. Med. Vet.* **7,** 451–470.
Hartley, W. J., and Haughey, K. G. (1974a). *Aust. Vet. J.* **50,** 55–58.
Hartley, W. J., and Haughey, K. G. (1974b). *Aust. Vet. J.* **50,** 323–324.
Hartley, W. J., and Wanner, R. A. (1974). *Aust. Vet. J.* **50,** 185–188.
Hartley, W. J., Wanner, R. A., Della-Porta, A. J., and Snowdon, W. A. (1975). *Aust. Vet. J.* **51,** 103–104.
Hartley, W. J., DeSaram, W. G., Della-Porta, A. J., Snowdon, W. A., and Shepherd, N. C. (1977). *Aust. Vet. J.* **53,** 319–325.
Hegreberg, G. A. (1982). *In* "Animal Models of Inherited Metabolic Diseases" (R. J. Desnick, D. F. Patterson, and D. G. Scarpelli, eds.), pp. 229–242. Alan R. Liss, Inc., New York.
Helbig, K. (1958). *Dtsch. Tieraerztl. Wochenschr.* **65,** 431–437.
Helmig-Schumann, H. (1964). *Zuchthyg.* **36,** 217–236.
Herrick, E. H., and Eldridge, F. E. (1955). *J. Dairy Sci.* **38,** 440–441.
Herschler, M. S., Fechheimer, N. S., and Gilmore, L. O. (1962). *J. Dairy Sci.* **45,** 1493–1499.
Herzog, A. (1971). *Giessener Beitr. Erbpathol. Buchthyg.,* Suppl. **2.**
Herzog, A., and Adam, R. (1968). *Dtsch. Tieraerztl. Wochenschr.* **75,** 237–243.
Herzog, A., and Wiedeking, J. F. (1970). *Giessener Beitr. Erbpathol. Zuchthyg.* **1/2,** 1–23.

Herzog, A., Hohn, H., and Kopp, U. (1982). *Berl. Muench. Tieraerztl. Wochenschr.* **95**, 284–287.
Hickman, J. (1964). "Veterinary Orthopaedics." Oliver & Boyd, Edinburgh.
High, J. W., Kincaid, C. M., and Smith, J. H. (1958). *J. Hered.* **49**, 250–252.
High, J. W., Smith, J. H., Kincaid, C. M., and Hobbs, C. S. (1959). *J. Anim. Sci.* **18**, 1438–1446.
Hocking, J. D., Jolly, R. D., and Batt, R. D. (1972). *Biochem. J.* **128**, 69–78.
Hohn, H., and Herzog, A. (1970). *Giessener Beitr. Erbpathol. Zuchthyg.* **3**, 1–7.
Holm, L. W. (1967). *Adv. Vet. Sci.* **11**, 159–205.
Holmes, J. R., and Young, G. B. (1957). *Vet. Rec.* **69**, 148–149.
Howell, J. McC., and Ritchie, H. E. (1966). *Pathol. Vet.* **3**, 159–168.
Howell, J., McC., Darling, P. R., Cook, R. D., Robinson, W. F., Bradley, S., and Gawthorne, J. M. (1981). *J. Pathol.* **134**, 266–277.
Hughes, H. V. (1952). *Vet. Rec.* **64**, 753–755.
Hulland, T. J. (1957). *Can. J. Comp. Med.* **21**, 72–76.
Huston, K. (1957). *Holstein-Friesian World* **54**, 26, 122–123.
Huston, K. (1966). *Kans. Vet.* **22**, 8, 10–15.
Huston, K., and Gier, H. T. (1958). *Cornell Vet.* **48**, 45–52.
Huston, K., and Leipold, H. W. (1968). *Holstein Friesian World* **64**, 2932–2934.
Huston, K., and Leipold, H. W. (1971). *Ann. Genet. Sel. Anim.* **3**, 419–423.
Huston, K., and Wearden, S. (1958). *J. Dairy Sci.* **41**, 1359–1370.
Huston, K., Eldridge, F. E., and Mudge, J. W. (1961a). *J. Dairy Sci.* **44**, 1197.
Huston, K., Eldridge, F. E., and Oberst, F. H. (1961b). *J. Anim. Sci.* **20**, 908.
Huston, K., Leipold, H. W., and MacFadden, D. L. (1968a). *J. Hered.* **59**, 65–67.
Huston, K., Leipold, H. W., and Freeman, A. E. (1968b). *J. Dairy Sci.* **51**, 1101–1102.
Huston, R., Saperstein, G., and Leipold, H. W. (1977). *Equine Vet. J.* **1**, 137–146.
Huston, R., Saperstein, G., Schoneweis, D., and Leipold, H. W. (1978). *Vet. Bull. (London)* **48**, 645–675.
Hutt, F. B. (1963). *J. Hered.* **54**, 186–187.
Hutt, F. B. (1964). "Animal Genetics." Ronald Press, New York.
Hutt, F. H., and Frost, J. M. (1948). *J. Hered.* **39**, 131–137.
Ilancic, D. (1940). *Zuchthyg.* **15**, 129–133.
Inaba, Y. (1975). *J. Jpn. Vet. Med. Assoc.* **28**, 457–461.
Inaba, Y., Kurogi, H., and Omori, T. (1975). *Aust. Vet. J.* **51**, 584–585.
Ingraham, F. D., and Scott, H. W., Jr. (1943). *N. Engl. J. Med.* **229**, 108–114.
Innes, J. R. M., and Saunders, L. Z. (1962). "Comparative Neuropathology." Academic Press, New York.
Innes, J. R. M., Russell, D. S., and Wilsdon, A. J. (1940). *J. Pathol. Bacteriol.* **50**, 455–461.
Inui, S., and Maruyama, Y. (1967). *Bull. Natl. Inst. Anim. Health* **55**, 63–73.
Isaksson, A. (1943). *Skand. Veterinaertidskr.* **33**, 1–27.
Jackschath, E. (1899). *Berl. Tieraerztl. Wochenschr.* **15**, 455–456.
Jayasekera, M. U., and Leipold, H. W. (1979). *Zentralbl. Veterinaermed.* **26**, 497–501.
Jayasekera, M. U., and Leipold, H. W. (1981). *Ann. Genet. Sel. Anim* **13**, 213–218.
Jayasekera, M. U., Leipold, H. W., and Cook, J. E. (1979a). *Zentralbl. Veterinaermed.* **26**, 744–753, 1979.
Jayasekera, M. U., Leipold, H. W., and Phillips, R. (1979b). *Z. Tierz. Zuechtungsbiol.* **96**, 100–107.
Jennings, A. R., and Sumner, G. R. (1951). *Vet. Rec.* **63**, 60–61.

Johannson, I. (1942). *Hereditas* **28**, 278–288.
Johnson, K. R., Fourt, D. L., Ross, R. H., and Bailey, J. W. (1958). *J. Dairy Sci.* **41**, 1371–1375.
Johnson, J. L., Leipold, H. W., Snider, G. W., and Baker, R. D. (1980). *J. Am. Vet. Med. Assoc.* **176**, 549–550.
Johnson, J. L., Leipold, H. W., Schalles, R. R., Guffy, M. M., Peeples, J. G., Castleberry, R. S., and Schneider, H. J. (1981). *J. Hered.* **72**, 205–208.
Jolly, R. D. (1974). *J. Pathol.* **114**, 199–204.
Jolly, R. D. (1982). *In* "Animal Models of Inherited Metabolic Diseases" (R. J. Desnick, D. F. Patterson, and D. G. Scarpelli, eds.), pp. 145–164. Alan R. Liss, Inc., New York.
Jolly, R. D., Dodds, W. J., Ruth, G. R., and Trauner, D. B. (1981). *Adv. Vet. Sci. Comp. Med.* **25**, 245–284.
Jubb, K. V. F., and Kennedy, P. C. (1970a). "Pathology of Domestic Animals," Vol. 1. Academic Press, New York.
Jubb, K. V. F., and Kennedy, P. C. (1970b). "Pathology of Domestic Animals," Vol. 2, Academic Press, New York.
Julian, L. M., Tyler, W. S., Hage, T. J., and Gregory, P. W. (1957). *Am. J. Anat.* **100**, 269–287.
Julian, L. M., Tyler, W. S., and Gregory, P. W. (1959). *J. Am. Vet. Med. Assoc.* **135**, 104–109.
Julian, L. M., Tyler, W. S., and Gregory, P. W. (1964). *Anat. Rec.* **148**, 296.
Julian, R. J. (1960). *Vet. Med. (Kansas City, Mo.)* **55**, 35–41.
Kahrs, R. F. (1981). "Viral Diseases of Cattle," pp. 89–106. Iowa State Univ. Press, Ames.
Kahrs, R. F., Scott, F. W., and De Lahunta, A. (1970a). *Teratology* **3**, 181–184.
Kahrs, R. F., Scott, F. W., and De Lahunta, A. (1970b). *J. Am. Vet. Med. Assoc.* **156**, 851–857.
Kalter, H. (1968). "Teratology of the Central Nervous System." Univ. of Chicago Press, Chicago, Illinois.
Keeler, R. F. (1978). *In* "Effects of Poisonous Plants on Livestock" pp. 397–408. Academic Press, New York.
Keller, K., and Niedoba, T. (1937). *Z. Zuecht., Reihe B* **37B**, 245–293.
Kempthorne, O. (1957). "An Introduction to Genetic Statistics." Wiley, New York.
Kendrick, J. W. (1971). *Am. J. Vet. Res.* **32**, 533–544.
Kennedy, P. C. (1971). *Fed. Proc., Fed. Am. Soc. Exp. Biol.* **30**, 110–113.
Kennedy, P. C., Kendrick, J. W., and Stormont, C. (1957). *Cornell Vet.* **47**, 160–178.
Knudsen, O. (1961a). *Acta Vet. Scand.* **2**, 1–14.
Knudsen, O. (1961b). *Acta Vet. Scand.* **2**, 199–209.
Koch, P., Fischer, H., and Schumann, H. (1957). "Erbpathologie der landwirtschaftlichen Haustiere." Parey, Berlin.
König, B., Tonitis, A., and Fatzer, R. (1980). *Schweiz. Arch. Tierheilkd.* **122**, 435–458.
König, H. (1959). *Dtsch. Tieraerztl. Wochenschr.* **66**, 65–70.
Konno, S. (1973). *J. Jpn. Vet. Med. Assoc.* **26**, 515–521.
Konno, S. (1977). *Jpn. J. Anim. Reprod.* **22**, 39–54.
Konno, S., and Nakagawa, M. (1982). *Vet. Pathol.* **19**, 267–279.
Konno, S., Moriwaki, M., Nakagawa, M., Uchimura, M., Kamimiyata, M., and Tojinbara, K. (1975). *Natl. Inst. Anim. Health Q.* **15**, 52–53. Tokoyo.
Konno, S., Moriwaki, M., and Nakagawa, M. (1982). *Vet. Pathol.* **19**, 246–266.
Krölling, O. (1922). *Wien. Tieraerztl. Monatsschr.* **9**, 140–143.

Krölling, O. (1956). *Wien. Tieraerztl. Monatsschr.* **3**, 129–139.
Kundu, P. B., and Pandy, S. K. (1967). *Vet. Rec.* **80**, 708–709.
Kurogi, H., Inaba, Y., Goto, Y., Miura, Y., Takahashi, H., Sato, K., Omori, T., and Matumoto, M. (1975). *Arch. Virol.* **47**, 71–83.
Kurogi, H., Inaba, Y., Takahashi, E., Sato, K., Omori, T., Miura, Y., Goto, Y., Fujiwara, Y., Hatano, Y., Kodama, K., Fukuyama, S., Sasaki, N., and Matumoto, M. (1976). *Arch. Virol.* **51**, 67–74.
Lagerloef, N., and Settergren, I. (1953). *Cornell Vet.* **43**, 52–64.
Lauvergne, J. J. (1962). *Ann. Zootech.* **11**, 151–156.
Lauvergne, J. J. (1968). *Bull. Tech. Dep. Genet. Anim.* p. 91.
Lauvergne, J. J., and Pavoux, C. (1969). *Ann. Genet. Sel. Anim.* **1**, 109–117.
Lauvergne, J. J., Vissac, B., and Perramon, A. (1963). *Ann. Zootech.* **12**, 133–156.
Leipold, H. W. (1968). Ph.D. Thesis, Kansas State University Library, Manhattan.
Leipold, H. W. (1978a). *Proc. Aust.—U.S. Conf. Poisonous Plants*, pp. 429–440.
Leipold, H. W. (1978b). *Vet. Clin. North Am.* **8**, 47–88.
Leipold, H. W. (1980). In "The Comparative Pathology of Zoo Animals." (R. J. Moutali and S. Migaki, eds.) Smithson. Inst. Press, Washington, D.C. pp. 497–470.
Leipold, H. W., and Dennis, S. M. (1980). *In* "Current Therapy in Theriogenology" (D. A. Morrow, ed.), pp. 410–441. Saunders, Philadelphia, Pennsylvania.
Leipold, H. W., and Huston, K. (1966). *J. Hered.* **57**, 179–181.
Leipold, H. W., and Huston, K. (1968a). *Pathol. Vet.* **5**, 407–418.
Leipold, H. W., and Huston, K. (1968b). *J. Hered.* **59**, 2–8.
Leipold, H. W., and Huston, K. (1968c). *J. Hered.* **59**, 223–224.
Leipold, H. W., and Huston, K. (1969). *J. Hered.* **59**, 222–224.
Leipold, H. W., and Morris, L. N. (1979a). *In* "Spontaneous Animal Models of Human Disease" (E. J. Andrews, B. C. Ward, and N. H. Altman, eds.), Vol. 2, pp. 213–214. Academic Press, New York.
Leipold, H. W., and Morris, L. N. (1979b). *In* "Spontaneous Animal Models of Human Disease" (E. J. Andrews, B. C. Ward, and N. H. Altman, eds.), Vol. 2, pp. 216–218. Academic Press, New York.
Leipold, H. W., and Peeples, J. S. (1981). *J. Am. Vet. Med. Assoc.* **179**, 69–70.
Leipold, H. W., and Saperstein, G. (1975). *J. Am. Vet. Med. Assoc.* **166**, 231–232.
Leipold, H. W., Huston, K., Guffy, M. M., and Noordsy, J. L. (1967). *J. Am. Vet. Med. Assoc.* **151**, 598–601.
Leipold, H. W., Huston, K., and Gelatt, K. N. (1968). *J. Hered.* **59**, 218–220.
Leipold, H. W., Huston, K., Dennis, S. M., and Farmer, E. L. (1969a). *J. Dairy Sci.* **52**, 923.
Leipold, H. W., Adrian, R. W., Huston, K., Trotter, D. M., Dennis, S. M., and Guffy, M. M. (1969b). *J. Dairy Sci.* **52**, 1422–1431.
Leipold, H. W., Huston, K., Guffy, M. M., and Dennis, S. M. (1969c). *Am. J. Vet. Res.* **30**, 1685–1687.
Leipold, H. W., Huston, K., Guffy, M. M., and Dennis, S. M. (1969d). *Am. J. Vet. Res.* **30**, 1689–1692.
Leipold, H. W., Doige, C. E., Kaye, M. M., and Cribb, P. H. (1970a). *Can. Vet. J.* **11**, 181–185.
Leipold, H. W., Cates, W. F., and Howell, W. E. (1970b). *Can. Vet. J.* **11**, 258–260.
Leipold, H. W., Cates, W. F., Radostits, O. M., and Howell, W. D. (1970c). *Am. J. Vet. Res.* **31**, 1367–1374.
Leipold, H. W., Gelatt, K. N., and Huston, K. (1971a). *Am. J. Vet. Res.* **32**, 1019–1026.

Leipold, H. W., Huston, K., Dennis, S. M., and Guffy, M. M. (1971b). *Ann. Sel. Genet. Anim.* **3,** 419–421.
Leipold, H. W., Dennis, S. M., and Huston, K. (1972a). *Adv. Vet. Sci. Comp. Med.* **16,** 103–150.
Leipold, H. W., Dennis, S. M., and Huston, K. (1972b). *Cornell Vet.* **62,** 338–345.
Leipold, H. W., Strafuss, A. C., Blauch, B., Olson, R., and Guffy, M. (1972c). *Cornell Vet.* **67,** 646–653.
Leipold, H. W., Dennis, S. M., and Huston, K. (1973a). *Vet. Bull. (London)* **43,** 339–403.
Leipold, H. W., Blauch, B., Huston, K., Edgerly, C. G. M., and Hibbs, C. M. (1973b). *Vet. Med. Small Anim. Clin.* **68,** 1040–1043.
Leipold, H. W., Greene, H. J., and Huston, K. (1973c). *Vet. Med. Small Anim. Clin.* **68,** 1140–1146.
Leipold, H. W., Husby, F., Brundage, A. L., and Shupe, J. L. (1977). *J. Am. Vet. Med. Assoc.* **170,** 1408–1410.
Leipold, H. W., Saperstein, G., Swanson, R. W., Schalles, R., and Guffy, M. (1978). *Z. Tierz. Zuechtungsbiol.* **34,** 291–295.
Leipold, H. W., Smith, J. E., Jolly, R. D., and Eldridge, F. (1979a). *J. Am. Vet. Med. Assoc.* **175,** 457–459.
Leipold, H. W., Jayasekera, U., and Cook, J. E. (1979b). *Proc. Am. Assoc. Vet. Lab. Diagn.* **22,** 69–76.
Leipold, H. W., Watt, B., Vestweber, J. G. E., and Dennis, S. M. (1981). *Bovine Pract.* **16,** 76–79.
Li, C. C. (1961). "Human Genetics." McGraw-Hill, New York.
Liendo, G., and Castro, A. E. (1981). *Bovine Pract.* **16,** 87–95.
Lillie, F. R. (1919). *Science* **43,** 611–613.
Luedke, A. J. (1977a). *Am. J. Vet. Res.* **38,** 1697–1700.
Luedke, A. J. (1977b). *Am. J. Vet. Res.* **38,** 1701–1704.
Luedke, A. J., and Walton, T. E. (1981). *Bovine Pract.* **16,** 96–100.
Luedke, A. J., Jochim, M. M., and Jones, R. H. (1977). *Am. J. Vet. Res.* **38,** 1687–1695.
Lueps, P. (1963). *Berl. Muench. Tieraerztl. Wochenschr.* **76,** 204–206.
McFarland, L. Z. (1959). *J. Am. Vet Med. Assoc.* **134,** 32–34.
McFeeley, R. A., Hare, W. C. D., and Biggers, J. D. (1967). *Cytogenetics* **6,** 242–253.
McGhee, C. C., and Leipold, H. W. (1982). *Cornell Vet.* **72,** 427–436.
McKercher, D. G., Saito, J. K., and Singh, K. V. (1970). *J. Am. Vet. Med. Assoc.* **156,** 1044–1047.
Maclellan, M., and Martin, J. A. (1956). *Vet. Rec.* **68,** 458–459.
McPherson, E. A., Beattie, I. S., and Young, G. B. (1964). *Nord. Veterinaermed.* **16,** 533–540.
Magnusson, H. (1917). *Berl. Tieraerztl. Wochenschr.* **33,** 533–534.
Mammerickx, M., and Leunen, J. (1964). *Rev. Agric. (Brussels)* **17,** 1007–1094.
Markau, W. (1963). *Monatsh. Veterinaermed.* **18,** Spec. No. 1, 23–25.
Markusfeld, O., and Mayer, E. (1971). *Refu. Vet.* **28,** 51–61.
Martins, E. O., and Ferri, A. G. (1951). *Rev. Fac. Med. Vet., Univ. Sao Paulo* **4,** 399–405.
Mayer, E. (1976). *Proc. World Conf. Buiatrics, 1976* pp. 229–234.
Mead, S. W., Gregory, P. W., and Regan, W. M. (1943). *J. Hered.* **34,** 367–372.
Metselaar, D. (1976). *Vet. Rec.* **99,** 86.
Mialot, M., and Parodi, A. L. (1981). *Recp. Med. Vet.* **157,** 339–345.
Miura, Y., Hayashi, S., Ishihara, T., Inaba, Y., Omori, T., and Matumoto, M. (1974). *Arch. Gesamte Virusforsch.* **46,** 377–380.
Modrowich, G. L. (1969). Dissertation, Giessen, Germany.

Mohr, O. L., and Wriedt, C. (1930). *J. Genet.* **22,** 279–297.
Moore, W. E. (1970). *Am. J. Vet. Res.* **31,** 1561–1567.
Moore, W. E., Stephenson, B. D., Anderson, A. S., and Swartz, S. (1970). *Proc. Soc. Exp. Biol. Med.* **134,** 926–929.
Moriguchi, R., Izawa, H., and Soekawa, M. (1976). *Zentralbl. Veterinaermed., Reihe B* **23,** 190–199.
Morrill, E. L. (1945). *J. Hered.* **36,** 81–82.
Morris, L. N., and Leipold, H. W. (1979a). *In* "Spontaneous Animal Models of Human Disease" (E. J. Andrews, B. C. Ward, and N. H. Altman, eds.), pp. 214–216. Academic Press, New York.
Morris, L. N., and Leipold, H. W. (1979b). *In* "Spontaneous Animal Models of Human-Disease" (E. J. Andrews, B. C. Ward, and N. H. Altman, eds.), Vol. 2, pp. 218–220. Academic Press, New York.
Morton, N. E. (1962). In "Methodology in Human Genetics" (W. J. Burdette, ed.), pp. 17–52, Holden Day, San Francisco, California.
Morton, N. E., Yee, S., and Lew, R. (1971). *J. Hum. Genet.* **23,** 602–611.
Müller, W., Kelker, L., Wünsche, K., Willer, S., Haase, H., and Barth, T. (1982). *Monatsh. Veterinaermed.* **37,** 84–89.
Mulvihill, J. J., Mulvihill, C. G., and Priester, W. (1980). *Teratology* **21**(1), 109–112.
Nawrot, P. S., Howell, W. E., and Leipold, H. W. (1980). *Aust. Vet. J.* **56,** 359–364.
Nes, N. (1959). *Nord. Veterinaermed.* **11,** 33–54.
Ness, H., Leopold, G., and Müller, W. (1982). *Monatsh. Veterinaermed.* **37,** 89–92.
Nicholas, F. W. (1982). *J. Hered.* **73,** 444–450.
Nihleen, B., and Eriksson, K. (1958). *Nord. Veterinaermed.* **10,** 113–127.
Nobel, T. A., Klopfer, U., and Neumann, F. (1971). *Ref. Vet.* **28,** 144–151.
Nosaka, D., Tateyama, S., Ashizawa, H., Hakamura, N., Yago, H., Shimizu, T., and Murakami, T. (1973). *Bull. Fac. Agric., Miyazaki Univ.* **20,** 311–344.
Nuss, J. I. L. (1966). *Diss. Abstr.* **26,** 6323–6324.
Ogden, A. L., Palmer, A. C., and Blakemore, W. F. (1974). *Vet. Rec.* **94,** 555.
O'Hara, P. J., Read, K. W., Romane, W. M., and Bridges, C. H. (1970). *Lab. Invest.* **23,** 307–314.
Ohashi, Y. (1973). *J. Jpn. Vet. Med. Assoc.* **26,** 487–490.
Ojo, S. A., Leipold, H. W., and Hibbs, C. M. (1975a). *J. Am. Vet. Med. Assoc.* **166,** 607–610.
Ojo, S. A., Leipold, H. W., Cho, D. Y., and Guffy, M. M. (1975b). *J. Am. Vet. Med. Assoc.* **166,** 781–783.
Ojo, S. A., Huston, K., Gelatt, K. N., and Leipold, H. W. (1982). *Bovine Pract.* **17,** 115–121.
Oliver, W. M., and Cartwright, T. C. (1969). *Tech. Rep.—Tex., Agric. Exp. Stn.* **12.**
Olson, T. A., and Willham, R. L. (1982). *Iowa State Univ., Agric. Home Econ. Exp. Stn., Res. Bull.* **595.**
Omori, T. (1973). *J. Jpn. Vet. Med. Assoc.* **26,** 510–515.
Omori, T. (1977). *Jpn. J. Anim. Reprod.* **22,** 25–38.
Omori, T., Inaba, Y., Kurogi, H., Miura, Y., Nobuto, K., Ohashi, Y., and Matsumoto, M. (1974). *Bull. Off. Int. Epizoot.* **81,** 447–458.
Osborne, J. C., and Legates, J. E. (1963). *J. Am. Vet. Med. Assoc.* **142,** 1104.
Osburn, B. I., Silverstein, A. M., Prendergast, R. A., Johnson, R. T., and Parshall, C. J. (1971a). *Lab. Invest.* **25,** 197–205.
Osburn, B. I., Johnson, R. T., Silverstein, A. M., Prendergast, R. A., Jochim, M. M., and Levy, S. E. (1971b). *Lab. Invest.* **25,** 206–210.

O'Sullivan, B. M., and McPhee, C. P. (1975). *Aust. Vet. J.* **51**, 469–471.
O'Sullivan, B. M., Healy, P. J., Fraser, I. R., Nieper, R. E., Whittle, R. J., and Sewell, C. A. (1981). *Aust. Vet. J.* **57**, 227–229.
Otsuka, H., Hamana, K., Hataya, M., Ohira, K., and Matsukata, Y. (1973). *Bull. Fac. Agric., Miyazaki Univ.* **20**, 273–291.
Otsuka, H., Hataya, M., Hamana, K., Ishiguro, Y., Taguma, S., and Kimoto, T. (1975). *Bull. Fac. Agric., Miyazaki Univ.* **22**, 107–114.
Padgett, G. A., Holland, J. M., Davis, W. C., and Henson, J. B. (1970). "Current Topics in Pathology." Springer-Verlag, Berlin and New York.
Palen, N. O. (1970). *Gac. Vet.* **32**, 158–159.
Palmer, A. C. (1982). *Proc. World Congr. Dis. Cattle, 12th, 1982* Vol. II, pp. 887–889.
Palmer, A. C., Blakemore, W. F., Barlow, R. M., Fraser, J. A., and Ogden, A. L. (1972). *Vet. Rec.* **91**, 592–594.
Parsonson, I. M., Della-Porta, A. J., and Snowdon, W. A. (1975). *Aust. Vet. J.* **51**, 585–586.
Parsonson, I. M., Della-Porta, A. J., Snowdon, W. A., and O'Halloran, M. L. (1981). *J. Comp. Pathol.* **91**, 611–619.
Pearson, H. (1979). *Vet. Rec.* **105**, 318–323.
Perkins, J. R., Olds, D., and Seath, D. M. (1954). *J. Dairy Sci.* **37**, 1158–1163.
Phillips, N. C., Robinson, D., Winchester, B. G., and Jolly, R. D. (1974). *Biochem. J.* **137**, 363–371.
Priester, W. A., Glass, G. G., and Waggoner, N. S. (1970). *Am. J. Vet. Res.* **31**, 1871–1879.
Read, W. K., and Bridges, C. H. (1969). *Pathol. Vet.* **6**, 235–243.
Rees, H. G., and Boshier, D. P. (1966). *N.Z. Vet. J.* **14**, 20–23.
Regan, W. W., Mead, S. W., and Gregory, P. W. (1935). *J. Hered.* **26**, 357–362.
Regan, W. M., Gregory, P. W., and Mead, S. W. (1944). *J. Hered.* **35**, 233–234.
Richards, W. P. C., Crenshaw, G. L., and Bushnell, R. B. (1971). *Cornell Vet.* **61**, 336–348.
Rieck, G. W. (1965). *Zuchthyg., Fortpflanzungsstör. Besamung Haust.* **1**, 326–342.
Rieck, G. W. (1970). *Sonderheft 1 Giessener Beitr. Erbpathol. Zuchthyg.* Spec. No. 1.
Rieck, G. W., and Bähr, H. (1967). *Dtsch. Tieraerztl. Wochenschr.* **74**, 356–364.
Rieck, G. W., and Finger, K. F. (1973). *Giessener Beitr. Erbpathol. Zuchthyg.* **5**, 71–138.
Rieck, G. W., and Leipold, H. W. (1965). *Zentralbl. Veterinaermed., Reihe A* **12**, 559–579.
Rieck, G. W., Hoehn, H., and Herzog, A. (1969). *Dtsch. Tieraerztl. Wochenschr.* **76**, 133–138.
Rieck, G. W., Finger, K. H., and Herzog, A. (1972). *Giessener Beitr. Erbpath. Zuchthyg.* **4**, 39–69.
Rieck, G. W., Herzog, A., and Rau, W. (1973). *Giessener Beitr. Erbpathol. Zuchthyg.* **5**, 1–70.
Rieger, F., Pincon-Raymond, M., Dreyfus, P., Guittard, M., and Fardeau, M. (1980). *Ann. Genet. Sel. Anim.* **11**(4), 371–380.
Roberts, S. J. (1953). *Cornell Vet.* **43**, 380–388.
Roberts, S. J. (1965). *Cornell Vet.* **55**, 639–644.
Rosenberger, G. (1939). *Dtsch. Tieraerztl. Wochenschr.* **47**, 18–23.
Rubin, P. (1969). "Dynamic Classification of Bone Dysplasias." Year Book Med. Publ., Chicago, Illinois.
Russell, R. G. (1980). *Diss. Abstr. Int. B* **41**, 487–488.
Ruth, J. R., Schwartz, S., and Stephenson, B. (1980). *Proc. Am. Assoc. Vet. Lab. Diagn.* **23**, 79–82.
St. George, T. D., Standfast, H. A., and Cybinski, D. H. (1978). *Aust. Vet. J.* **54**, 558–561.

Salako, M. A., and Abdullahi, U. S. (1982). *Vet. Rec.* **110**, 430.
Salisbury, G. W., and Van Demark, N. L. (1961). "Physiology of Reproduction and Artificial Insemination of Cattle." Freeman, San Francisco, California.
Saperstein, G., Leipold, H. W., and Dennis, S. M. (1975). *J. Am. Vet. Med. Assoc.* **167**, 314–322.
Saperstein, G., Harris, S., and Leipold, H. W. (1976). *Feline Pract.* **6**, 18–44.
Saunders, L. Z. (1952). *Cornell Vet.* **42**, 592–600.
Saunders, L. Z. (1965). *Pathol. Vet.* **2**, 97–100.
Saunders, L. Z., and Fincher, M. G. (1951). *Cornell Vet.* **41**, 351–366.
Saunders, L. Z., Sweet, J. D., Martin, S. M., Fox, F. H., and Fincher, M. G. (1952). *Cornell Vet.* **42**, 560–591.
Savey, M., and Espinasse, J. (1980). *Point Vet.* **10**(49), 27–30.
Schalk, C., and Hoekstra, P. (1959). *Tijdschr. Diergeneeskd.* **84**, 927–934.
Schlegel, M. (1914). *Z. Tiermed.* **18**, 364–405.
Schleger, A. V., Thompson, B. J., and Hewetson, R. W. (1967). *Biomed. Sci.* **20**, 661–668.
Schmahlstieg, R., and Maetzke, U. (1962). *Zentralbl. Veterinaermed.* **9**, 12–45.
Schönmuth, G., Stolzenburg, U., Dietz, O., Li, E., and Berg, R. (1971). *Monatsh Veterinaermed.* **26**, 17–24.
Schuiringa-Sybesma, A. M. (1961). *Tijdschr. Diergeneeskd.* **86**, 1192–1197.
Scott, F. W., Kahrs, R. F., De Lahunta, A., Brown, T. T., McEntee, K., and Gillespie, J. H. (1973). *Cornell Vet.* **63**, 536–560.
Sellers, K. C., Smith, G. F., and Wood, P. D. P. (1968). *Br. Vet. J.* **124**, 89–94.
Settergren, I., and Galloway, D. B. (1965). *Nord. Veterinaermed.* **17**, 9–16.
Sheahan, B. J., and Donnelly, W. J. C. (1974). *Acta Neuropathol.* **30**, 73–84. Berlin.
Shepherd, N. C., Gee, C. D., Jessep, T., Timmins, G., Carroll, S. N., and Bonner, R. B. (1978). *Aust. Vet. J.* **54**, 171–177.
Shupe, J. L., Binns, J. W., James, L. F., and Keller, R. F. (1967a). *J. Am. Vet. Med. Assoc.* **151**, 198–203.
Shupe, J. L., James, L. F., Balls, L. D., Binns, W., and Keller, R. F. (1967b). *J. Hered.* **58**, 311–313.
Shupe, J. L., James, L. F., Binns, W., and Keeler, R. F. (1968). *Cleft Palate J.* **1**, 346–355.
Singh, U. M., and Little, P. B. (1972). *Can. Vet. J.* **13**, 21–24.
Sippel, W. L. (1951). *G. Vet. J.* **3**, 4–5.
Sittmann, K., and Kendrick, J. W. (1964). *Genetica (The Hague)* **35**, 132–140.
Sittmann, K., Rollins, W. C., and Kendrick, J. W. (1961). *J. Hered.* **52**, 26–33.
Smedegaard, H. H. (1964). *Nord. Verinaermed.* **16**, 1029–1049.
Smith, S. T., Huston, K., Eldridge, F. E., and Mudge, J. W. (1961). *J. Anim. Sci.* **20**, 911.
Stegenga, T. (1964). *Tijdschr. Diergeneeskd.* **89**, 286–293.
Stern, W. G. (1923). *JAMA, J. Am. Med. Assoc.* **81**, 1507–1510.
Stöber, M., Trautwein, G., Scholz, H., and Munzenmayer, W. (1982). *Prakt. Tierarzt* **63**, 139–148.
Stolzenburg, U., and Schönmuth, G. (1971). *Wiss. Z. Humboldt-Univ. Berlin, Math.-Naturwiss. Reihe* **20**, 353–370.
Stormont, C. (1958). *Adv. Vet. Sci.* **4**, 137–162.
Stormont, C., Kendrick, J. W., and Kennedy, P. C. (1956). *Genetics* **41**, 663.
Straub, O. C. (1969). *Vet.-Med. Nachr.* **3**, 189–193.
Stringam, E. W. (1958). *Can. J. Comp. Med.* **22**, 400–403.
Suborg, H. (1976). Ph.D. Dissertation, University of Hanover.
Sugawa, Y., Mochizuki, H., and Tsubahara, H. (1951). *Bull. Natl. Inst. Anim. Health* **23**, 187–202.
Sugiura, K., and Fujio, S. (1961). *Bull. Natl. Inst. Anim. Health* **42**, 109–119.

Swan, R. A., and Taylor, E. G. (1982). *Aust. Vet. J.* **59**, 95–97.
Swartz, H. E., Vogt, D. W., and Kintner, L. D. (1982). *Am. J. Vet. Res.* **43**, 729–731.
Tagand, R., and Barone, R. (1942). *Bull. Soc. Sci. Vet. Med. Comp. Lyon* **43**, 118–123.
Taggart, J. K., Jr., and Walker, A. E. (1942). *Arch. Neurol. Psychiatry* **48**, 583–612.
Tajima, M., Yamagiwa, S., and Iwamori, H. (1951). *Jpn. J. Vet. Sci.* **13**, 43–54.
Tandler, J., and Keller, K. (1911). *Dtsch. Tieraerztl. Wochenschr.* **10**, 148–149.
Taruffi, C. (1881–1894). "Storia della teratologia," 8 vols. Regia Tipografia, Bologna.
Tennant, B., Asbury, A. C., Laben, R. C., Richards, W. P. C., Kaneko, J. J., and Cupps, P. T. (1967). *J. Am. Vet. Med. Assoc.* **150**, 1493–1508.
Thier, L., and Bay, F. (1965). *Berl. Muench. Tieraerztl. Wochenschr.* **78**, 328–329.
Thomson, R. G. (1966a). *Pathol. Vet.* **3**, 89–109.
Thomson, R. G. (1966b). *Pathol. Vet.* **3**, 234–246.
Thompson, K. G., Jolly, R. D., and Rammell, C. G. (1976). *N.Z. Vet. J.* **24**, 167–170.
Trotter, D. M., Huston, K., Leipold, H. W., Adrian, R. W., and Merriam, J. G. (1971). *Giessener Beitr. Erbpathol. Zuchthyg.* **3**, 31–54.
Troutt, H. F., Fessler, J. F., Page, E. H., and Amstutz, H. E. (1967). *J. Am. Vet. Med. Assoc.* **151**, 1421–1429.
Tucking, R. (1976). Ph.D. Dissertation, Justus Liebig-Universität Giessen, Germany.
Tuff, P. (1948). *Skand. Vet. Tidskr.* **38**, 379–395.
Tyler, W. S., Julian, L. M., McFarland, L. S., Evans, H. E., and Gregory, P. W. (1959). *Am. J. Vet. Res.* **20**, 702–707.
Urman, H. K., and Grace, O. D. (1964). *Cornell Vet.* **54**, 230–249.
Vainas, E. (1980). *Ph.D. Dissertation, Justus-Liebig University, Giessen, Germany.*
van Adrichem, P. W., van Leeuwen, J. M., and van Kluijue, J. J. (1970). *Tijdschr. Diergeneeskd.* **95**, 1170–1176.
van Nie, C. J. (1966). *Acta Morphol. Neth. Scand.* **6**, 387–393.
van Niekerk, I. J. M., and Jaros, G. G. (1970). *S. Afr. Med. J.* **44**, 898–899.
van't Hooft, A. J. G. (1959). *Tijdschr. Diergeneeskd.* **84**, 1556–1574.
van Zyl, A., Schulz, K., Wilson, B., and Pansegrouw, D. (1965). *Endocrinology* **76**, 353–361.
Wanner, R. A., and Husband, A. J. (1974). *Aust. Vet. J.* **50**, 560–562.
Ward, G. M. (1971). *Cornell Vet.* **61**, 179–191.
Ward, G. W. (1969). *Cornell Vet.* **59**, 570–576.
Wass, W. M., and Hoyt, H. (1965). *Am. J. Vet. Res.* **26**, 654–658.
Weaver, A. D. (1975). *Dtsch. Tieraerztl. Wochenschr.* **81**, 572–573.
Weber, W. (1946). *Schweiz. Arch. Tierheilkd.* **88**, 497–521.
Wegner, W. (1970). *Dtsch. Tieraerztl. Wochenschr.* **77**, 229–232.
Wells, M. M., Solitz, L. E., and Bender, B. B. (1980). *Arch. Dermatol.* **116**, 429–432.
Wheat, J. D. (1960). *J. Hered.* **51**, 99–101.
Wheat, J. D. (1961). *J. Hered.* **52**, 244–246.
White, J. M., Vinson, W. E., and Pearson, R. E. (1981). *J. Dairy Sci.* **64**, 1305–1317.
Whittem, J. H. (1957). *J. Pathol. Bacteriol.* **73**, 375–387.
Whittem, J. H. (1962). *Acta Neuropathol., Suppl.* **1**, 94–96.
Whittem, J. H., and Walker, D. (1957). *J. Pathol. Bacteriol.* **74**, 281–288.
Wiedeking, J. F. (1968). *Dissertation, Justus Liebig-University, Giessen, Germany.*
Wiedeking, J. F. (1970). *Giessener Beitr. Erbpathol. Zuchthyg.* **3**, 29–33.
Wiesner, E., and Willer, S. (1974). "Veterinärmedizinische Pathogenetik." Fischer, Jena.
Wiesner, E., and Willer, S. (1978). *Monatsh Veterinaermed.* **33**, 98–105.
Willer, S. (1982). *Monatsh. Veterinaermed.* **37**, 109–117.

Wiprecht, C., and Harlacher, W. R. (1935). *J. Hered.* **26,** 363–368.
Young, G. B. (1951). *Br. Vet. J.* **107,** 23–29.
Young, J. S. (1969). *Aust. Vet. J.* **45,** 574–576.
Young, S. (1962). *Cornell Vet.* **52,** 84–93.
Zemjanis, R., Larson, L. L., and Bhalla, R. P. S. (1961). *J. Am. Vet. Med. Assoc.* **139,** 1015–1018.

Acaricide Resistance in Ticks

KEITH R. SOLOMON

Department of Environmental Biology, University of Guelph, Guelph, Ontario, Canada

I.	Introduction	273
	A. Biology	273
	B. Importance to the Livestock Industry	274
	C. Resistance to Pesticides	275
	D. Acaricides for Tick Control	275
II.	Occurrence and Geographic Location of Tick Resistance	277
III.	Acaricide Resistance in Single-Host Ticks	277
	A. Inorganic Acaricides	277
	B. Chlorinated Acaricides	280
	C. Organophosphorus and Carbamate Acaricides	280
	D. Recently Introduced Acaricides	281
IV.	Acaricide Resistance in Multihost Ticks	282
	A. Inorganic Acaricides	282
	B. Chlorinated Acaricides	282
	C. Organophosphorus and Carbamate Acaricides	283
	D. Recently Introduced Acaricides	283
V.	Methods for Determining Resistance to Acaricides	284
	A. *In Vitro* Laboratory Methods	284
	B. Field Methods	286
	C. Interpretation of Resistance	286
VI.	Mechanisms of Resistance	288
	A. Inorganic Acaricides	288
	B. Organic Acaricides	288
VII.	Management of Resistance	290
	References	293

I. Introduction

A. Biology

Ticks are probably the most important problem affecting the livestock industry in subtropical and temperate regions of the world. They comprise approximately 800 known species, all of which are parasitic on terrestrial vertebrates. Some of the success of the ticks is probably due to their early emergence as parasites of reptiles in the Paleozoic and Mesozoic (Hoogstraal, 1976). This long history of parasitism, plus that they underwent extensive adaptive radiations during the development of the land mammals, have resulted in a seemingly ideally adapted ectoparasite. In addition, the activities of humans and the livestock industry have in many cases provided ideal conditions for the development of ticks and the problems associated with them.

Ticks are divided into two major taxonomic groups: the soft or argasid ticks and the hard or ixodid ticks. The former, comprising approximately 150 species, have a very different biology, physiology, and host–parasite relationship from the Ixodidae, of which approximately 650 species are known (Hoogstaal, 1976).

The tick life cycle is commonly 2–4 months in duration but may, under ideal conditions of humidity and temperature, be as short as 6 weeks in some species. Females, particularly in the family Ixodidae, produce large numbers of eggs that, under favorable environmental conditions, can result in a rapid increase in numbers. The ixodid ticks have three stages in the life cycle: larva, nymph, and adult. Each stage is parasitical, usually on a different host, and the females feed and produce eggs only once. Argasid ticks have a larval stage, several nymphal stages, and an adult stage, adult females being capable of feeding and laying eggs more than once, although in smaller numbers than the Ixodidae.

B. Importance to the Livestock Industry

The importance of ticks to the livestock industry was demonstrated to early pioneers who introduced host cattle into the grasslands of Africa, Australia, and North and South America. This introduction provided an additional food source for the ticks as well as aiding in transport from one area to another, as for example in the importation of *Boophilus microplus* into Australia (Harrison et al., 1973). Their impact on the livestock industry has been felt in a number of ways. Most ticks are parasitic on more than one host and can serve as both reservoirs and vectors of a number of diseases of animals and humans. Although disease transmission is probably their single most important characteristic, ticks also cause damage to the host through the removal of blood (in quantities several times the mass of the engorged female tick), by secondary infections resulting from the hosts' licking or scratching of the feeding site, and, in some cases, by the injection of toxins via the secretions of the tick's salivary glands.

It is not surprising that attempts were made to control ticks by chemical means. The chemicals used for tick control were (and in many cases still are) those used for the control of insects. As early as 1893 in South Africa and 1895 in Australia, arsenic in the form of sodium arsenate was introduced for the control of cattle ticks (Harrison et al., 1973). The inevitable outcome of this was the selection of individuals in the population that were resistant to the chemicals involved. Resistance to arsenic was reported in the 1930s in South Africa (DuToit et al., 1941), Australia, and Argentina (Wharton, 1976). Since that time, resistance has been reported to almost all chemicals used for the control of ticks and has been the subject of a number of reviews (Downing et al., 1952; Norris, 1956; Whitehead, 1958; Kerr, 1964; Wharton, 1967; Roulston, 1969; Wharton and Roulston, 1970; Shaw, 1970; Brown and Pal, 1971; Harrison et al., 1973; Gothe and Hartig, 1975; Wharton, 1976; Drummond, 1977; Baker et al., 1978a; Baker et al., 1979; Nolan and Roulston, 1979; World Health Organization, 1980).

C. Resistance to Pesticides

Resistance is the result of the selection of individuals in a population through the action of a pesticide that either kills or affects the reproduction of the more susceptible organisms. In order for the less susceptible individuals to survive and form the nucleus of a resistant strain of the organism, the mechanism by which resistance is conferred must be inheritable and must be passed on from one generation to another. Given time and random mutation, any organism can evolve resistance to a given pesticide. However, the rate of selection may be modified by properties of the population, such as the frequency of mutation, genetic variability, degree of dominance of the character, and genetically effective size of the population (Bishop, 1982). In addition to these internal factors, a number of external factors, such as persistence of the pesticide, number of times the pesticide is used, previous use of similar pesticides, and degree of genetic isolation in the population, may also influence the rate at which resistance develops.

D. Acaricides for Tick Control

Since the late 1800s, a number of pesticides have been used for the control of ticks. Most of these acaricides can be conveniently grouped into chemical classes; examples are shown in Table I. The physical acaricides were quite widely used before the introduction of arsenic, but, although these formulations were later improved by the addition of insecticides such as lindane, they have not been very successful. Use

TABLE I

Major Groups of Acaricides Currently Used for Tick Control

Group	Typical structure	Mode of action
Inorganic acaricides		
Metabolic poisons	As_2O_3	Metabolic poison
	Sodium arsenate	Inhibition of —SH-containing enzymes
Physical poisons	Grease, tar, creosote	Physical
Organic acaricides		
Organochlorine acaricides	DDT	Nerve axon, interference with nerve conduction
	LINDANE	
	TOXAPHENE	
Organophosphorus acaricides	CHLORFENVINPHOS	Acetylcholinesterase inhibitor
Carbamate acaricides	CARBARYL	Acetylcholinesterase inhibitor
Formamidine acaricides	CHLORDIMEFORM	Nervous system, possibly on octopamine receptors
Pyrethroid acaricides	PERMETHRIN	Nerve axon, similar to DDT
Cyclic amidines	CLENPYRIN	Metabolic inhibitor

of arsenic in tick control made possible the eradication of the single-host cattle tick *Boophilus* (*Margaropus*) *annulatus* in the southern United States (Graybill, 1912; Ellenberger and Chapin, 1919); however, it is now less widely used for reasons of resistance and toxicity except in parts of Africa and South America, where it is preferred because of its low cost and stability in the diptank. The organoclorine acaricides also are no longer used for reasons of resistance and environmental considerations. The most popular acaricides in current use are the organophosphates, carbamates, and formamidines. Recently introduced acaricides include the synthetic pyrethroids, the cyclic amidines, and, showing promise in laboratory trials, the avermectins (Drummond *et al.*, 1981).

II. Occurrence and Geographic Location of Tick Resistance

Generally speaking, acaricide resistance has occurred wherever acaricides have been used extensively. Wharton (1976) has listed those countries from which acaricide resistance has been reported, and these, plus more recent additions, are summarized in Table II.

III. Acaricide Resistance in Single-Host Ticks

The single-host ticks have led the field in developing resistance to acaricides. Although this is probably at least in part a result of the short life cycle of these ticks, there appear to be some marked differences in the rate of development of resistance in *B. microplus* in Australia and South Africa that are not explicable in these terms.

A. INORGANIC ACARICIDES

The observation of resistance to arsenic in *Boophilus decoloratus* in South Africa in the 1930s (DuToit *et al.*, 1941) was the first report of resistance to any acaricide, but similar observations were made in Australia shortly afterward (Legg, 1947) in *B. microplus*. Since that time resistance has been reported from almost all areas where arsenic is still used (Gothe and Hartig, 1975). Although *B. microplus* has been known in southern Africa for some 70 years (Baker *et al.*, 1981), the first reports of resistance to arsenic (and several other acaricides) in this species were only made in 1979 (Baker *et al.*, 1979). Although it is

TABLE II

Occurrence of Acaricide Resistance in Some Groups of Ticks[a]

	Pesticide (place and date of first reported occurrence of resistance)					
Group and species	Arsenic	DDT	Other organochlorines	Organophosphate–carbamate	Formamidines	Pyrethroids
Single-host ticks						
Boophilus microplus	Australia, 1936 Argentina, 1936 Brazil, 1948 Colombia, 1948 Jamaica, 1948 Uruguay, 1953 Venezuela, 1966 South Africa, 1979	Argentina, 1953 Australia, 1953 Brazil, 1953 Venezuela, 1966 South Africa, 1979	Argentina, 1953 Australia, 1953 Brazil, 1953 Guadeloupe, 1961 Martinique, 1961 Malagasy, 1963 India, 1964 Colombia, 1966 Ecuador, 1966 Venezuela, 1966 Malaysia, 1967 Trinidad, 1969 Uganda, 1970 South Africa, 1979	Australia, 1963 Brazil, 1963 Argentina, 1964 Colombia, 1967 Venezuela, 1967 South Africa, 1979 Brazil, 1980	Australia, 1981	Australia, 1965 (pyrethrum) Australia, 1978[b] (permethrin)
Boophilus decoloratus	South Africa, 1938 Kenya, 1953 Zimbabwe, 1963 Malawi, 1969	South Africa, 1954	South Africa, 1948 Kenya, 1964 Zimbabwe, 1969 Uganda, 1970	South Africa, 1966 Zimbabwe, 1976		South Africa, 1959 (pyrethrum)

Multihost ticks				
Amblyomma hebraeum	South Africa, 1975	South Africa, 1977	South Africa, 1975	South Africa, 1974
A. variegatum			Tanzania, 1973	
			Kenya, 1979	
			Spain, 1967	
Hyalomma marginatum	South Africa, 1975			
H. rufipes				
H. plumbeum			Soviet Union, 1974	Soviet Union, 1974
H. asiaticum			Soviet Union, 1974	Soviet Union, 1974
H. anatolicum			Soviet Union, 1974	Soviet Union, 1974
Rhipicephalus evertsi evertsi	South Africa, 1975		South Africa, 1959	South Africa, 1975
	Zimbabwe, 1972		Kenya, 1964	
			Zimbabwe, 1966	
			Tanzania, 1970	
			Uganda, 1970	
R. appendiculatus	South Africa, 1975		South Africa, 1964	South Africa, 1975
			Zimbabwe, 1966	
			Kenya, 1968	
			Uganda, 1968	
			Tanzania, 1971	

[a] Compiled from data obtained from Polyakov and Smirnova (1974); Gothe and Hartig (1975); Matthewson et al. (1976); Wharton (1976); Baker et al. (1979, 1978a, 1979); Crampton and Gichanga (1979); Patarroyo and Costa (1980).
[b] Demonstrated in laboratory selection only.

possible that resistance was present before this time and was obscured by resistance in the sympatric *B. decoloratus*, it is interesting to speculate on the apparently slower rate of development of resistance under essentially similar conditions to those in Australian *B. microplus*. Baker *et al.* (1981) suggest a rapid spread in the future of resistance in African *B. microplus*. Spickett and Malan (1978) have shown evidence of cytoplasmic and possibly genetic incompatibility between African and Australian (Yerongpilly) *B. microplus*, suggesting that the latency of resistance development in the former may be due partly to genetic differences.

B. Chlorinated Acaricides

Most of the single-host ticks developed resistance to the organochlorine acaricides within 5 to 6 years of their introduction in Africa, Australia, and South America (see reviews by Gothe and Hartig, 1975; Wharton and Roulston, 1970).

Resistance to these acaricides has also been reported from the Caribbean in *B. microplus* (Rawlins and Mansingh, 1977a,b; 1978a,b), with high resistance to lindane in some field strains. Baker *et al.* (1979, 1981) have shown resistance to DDT, toxaphene, lindane, and dieldrin in *B. microplus* from South Africa, even though the latter two compounds have not been registered for tick control. In surveys carried out in the years 1976–1977, Roulston *et al.* (1981) reported up to 49 and 9% of field samples of *B. microplus* showing resistance to dieldrin and DDT, respectively, in Australia.

C. Organophosphorus and Carbamate Acaricides

Some 5 years after the introduction of organophosphorus acaricides, resistance was reported in Australia (Shaw and Malcolm, 1964) and 2 years later in South Africa (Shaw *et al.*, 1967). Because the development and spread of resistance to the cholinesterase-inhibiting acaricides has been documented in reviews by Gothe and Hartig (1975), Wharton and Roulston (1970), Baker *et al.* (1978a, 1979), and Nolan and Roulston (1979), attention will be directed to more recent developments. Surveys of susceptibility to organophosphorus acaricides in *B. decoloratus* and *B. microplus* (Baker *et al.*, 1978b, 1979, 1981; Solomon *et al.*, 1979a,b) have indicated that the incidence of resistant field strains is increasing in South Africa.

Although the Berlin strain of *B. decoloratus* is also resistant to carbaryl (Shaw *et al.*, 1967), further bioassays using this compound have not been reported from South African ticks and no information on carbamate resistance patterns is available. Matthewson *et al.* (1976) reported organophosphorus and carbamate resistance in *B. decoloratus* in Zimbabwe and resistance to organophosphorus in Zambia (Matthewson and Blackman, 1980).

Rawlins and Mansingh (1977a,b, 1978a,b) reported the occurrence of resistance to organophosphorus compounds (dimethoate, chlorfenvinphos, crotoxyphos, and dicrotophos) in Caribbean *B. microplus* as well as less numerous instances of carbamate resistance. Further examples of resistance to organophosphorus acaricides have been reported from Argentina (Grillo Torrado and Arrieta Perez, 1977a; Perez Arrieta *et al.*, 1980), Brazil (Patarroyo and Costa, 1980), and New Caledonia (Daynes *et al.*, 1980).

The resistance spectra of the Australian *B. microplus* have been used to classify organophosphorus resistance into nine distinct types, the best biochemically and genetically characterized resistant strains of all ticks (Goethe and Hartig, 1975; Roulston *et al.*, 1981). Results of a tick resistance survey in the years 1976–1977 in Australia (Roulston *et al.*, 1981) showed that most types of organophosphorus resistance were present in all regions, but most common in North South Wales (100%), East Queensland (96%), and the North and Central Coastal regions (87 and 71%). Resistance appeared to have spread widely since an earlier survey done in 1970; however, no resistance to the carbamate, promacyl, was observed.

D. Recently Introduced Acaricides

Indications of resistance to the formamidine-type acaricides have only been received from Australia. Roulston *et al.* (1981) and Wharton and Norris (1980) reported indications of low levels of resistance or developing resistance to amidines in larval bioassays of *B. microplus*. These were not substantiated in *in vivo* trials; however, J. Nolan (personal communication, 1982) reports resistance to this class of acaricides.

Although cross-resistance between DDT and permethrin has been shown in laboratory selections of *B. microplus* (Nolan *et al.*, 1977), reports of field resistance have not been found in the literature.

Resistance to clenpyrin (as indicated by control failure) was reported in the Ingham strain of *B. microplus* (Roulston *et al.*, 1977).

IV. Acaricide Resistance in Multihost Ticks

It is apparent that resistance to acaricides in the multihost ticks has occurred more recently than in the single-host ticks discussed in Section III. The most likely reasons for this are these: the generation time is longer; only some stages of the life cycle may be exposed to the acaricide (Matthewson and Baker, 1975); and ticks are frequently found on wild animals and are thus more likely to show immigration of susceptible individuals. This may slow the rate of resistance development (Georghiou and Taylor, 1977a). Reports of resistance to acaricides in multihost ticks are sparse, and almost all of them refer to ixodid ticks. Only one reference to resistance in argasid ticks was mentioned by Gothe and Hartig (1975), and this has not been confirmed.

A. Inorganic Acaricides

Matthewson and Baker (1975) reported on the basis of larval bioassays that strains of *Amblyomma hebraeum, Rhipicephalus appendiculatus, R. evertsi evertsi, R. censis,* and *Hyalomma* spp. were resistant to arsenic. Certain ticks such as *Ixodes pilosus, Haemophysalis leachii,* and *H. silacea,* were classified as susceptible, although they and all other strains tested showed LC_{50} values in excess of the recommended field concentrations of 0.16% As_2O_3. However, a bioassay on a stage not normally exposed to the pesticide may be a poor indicator of resistance. Although adults of certain ticks such as *A. hebraeum* have not been well controlled by arsenic (Whitnall *et al.*, 1951), the author is not aware of reports or field observations of adult resistance to arsenic in these ticks. Polyakov and Smirnova (1979) reported strains of *Hyalomma detritum* resistant to arsenic in the Soviet Union.

B. Chlorinated Acaricides

Resistance to chlordane was reported first in the dog tick *Rhipicephalus sanguineus* (Hansens, 1956) in the United States, and to toxaphene in the cattle tick *R. evertsi evertsi* from South Africa (Whitehead and Baker, 1961). Reports by Baker and Shaw (1965) noted that strains of *R. appendiculatus* had developed resistance to lindane and toxaphene. Brown and Pal (1971) reported observations of resistance to DDT and lindane–dieldrin in *Dermacentor variabilis* and *R. sanguineus* in 1959 and 1954, respectively, and Baker *et al.* (1977) reported several strains of *A. hebraeum* resistant to toxaphene when larval, nymphal, and adult stages were bioassayed. One strain was subjected to screening with other acaricides and showed resistance to DDT and lindane. Lourens (1979a) and Lourens and Tachell (1979) reported the appearance of organochlorine-resistant strains of *R. evertsi evertsi* from Kenya and, in addition, Lourens and Tatchell (1979) showed that the genetic factors responsible for dieldrin, toxaphene, and lindane resistance were of intermediate dominance. Lourens (1979b) also showed the presence of lindane, toxaphene, and dieldrin resistance in *Amblyomma variegatum* but not in *A. lepidum* collected in Tanzania. The genetics of the resistant strain of *A. variegatum* showed that the gene was dominant and that the resistance factors were 10 for toxaphene, 385 for lindane, and unobtainably high for dieldrin. Similar studies on *R. appendiculatus* (Lourens, 1980a) also showed that resistance to toxaphene and lindane was dominant in three strains collected from East Africa. *Hyalomma detritum* has been reported to be resistant to DDT and lindane in the Soviet Union (Polyakov and Smirnova, 1979). Ziv (1979) reports no resistance to lindane in *Hyalomma excavatum, H. Marginatum rufipes,* or *H. detritum* from Israel.

C. Organophosphorus and Carbamate Acaricides

Baker *et al.* (1978b) bioassayed larvae from a number of field-collected strains of *A. hebraeum* and found that 5% showed resistance factors higher than 100 (at the LC_{99}) to dioxathion, chlorfenvinphos, quintiofos, and bromophosethyl. Dose–mortality plots of larval, nymphal, and adult bioassays of one strain did not show heterogeneity, suggesting dominance or the homozygosity of the strain.

Lourens (1979a, 1980b) reported the susceptibility of organochlorine-resistant strains of *R. evertsi evertsi* and *A. variegatum* to a number of organophosphates and carbaryl. Resistance was not found. Polyakov and Smirnova (1979) reported strains of *Rhipicephalus bursa* and *Hyalomma plumbeum* resistant to trichlorphon and carbaryl from the Soviet Union.

D. Recently Introduced Acaricides

Whereas resistance to the newly introduced formamidines has been reported in the single-host ticks, (J. Nolan, personal communication, 1982), this has not been noted in the multihost ticks; however, these compounds have only been in use for a short period, so that resistance would not be expected. Cross-resistance between organochlorines and the pyrethroids has not been shown in *R. appendiculatus* resistant to lindane and dieldrin (Jongejan and Lourens, 1980). The strain used was, however, not very resistant to DDT (with an LC_{50} ratio of 1.46) and was therefore a poor model to use in this investigation. Cross-resistance has been shown to be of significance in *B. microplus* (Nolan *et al.*, 1977) and is a possibility in other ticks exposed to DDT in the past. This should be taken into account before introducing the synthetic pyrethroids for the control of multihost ticks.

V. Methods for Determining Resistance to Acaricides

A. *In Vitro* Laboratory Methods

A number of methods have been developed for the estimation of susceptibility of ticks to acaricides. Laboratory techniques usually involve the use of either larval or adult ticks; however, most of the data involving resistance reports have unavoidably been obtained from larvae produced by a relatively small number of female ticks collected in the field. Practical difficulties often limit the use of larger numbers of field-collected individuals.

1. Larval Tests

These tests consist of two approaches: (1) immersion of the larvae in a commercial formulation of acaricide (Shaw, 1966; Fiedler, 1968) and (2) exposure of larvae to an acaricide-impregnated surface such as filter paper (Stone and Haydock, 1962), the similar techniques developed for the FAO resistance test kit (Harris, 1978; Food and Agriculture Organization, 1980), or glass such as in the pipet method used by Kigaye and Mattheysse (1973). Although the larval bioassay system does offer the advantage of larger numbers of test organisms, the methods do require incubation facilities as well as close attention to age of the larvae, conditions of incubation (Tatchell, 1974), and operator techniques. Another major drawback of a larval bioassay is that the data obtained may not apply to other stages in the life cycle. Although this is of lesser importance in the single-host ticks, where the larval bioassay has been successfully used for resistance tests and strain characterization in Australia, it is unlikely that a significant proportion of the larvae of multihost ticks will come into contact with acaricides. The validity of a larval bioassay is thus questionable.

Nari (1981) failed to show a correlation between mortality of larval *Boophilus microplus* assayed by the Shaw method (Shaw, 1966) and adult ticks of the same strains assayed by an immersion technique (Graham and Drummond, 1964). In a limited number of replicates, a poor correlation ($r = .896$), with little predictive value, was observed between the two tests. However, the correlation tested was that of percentage mortality at individual doses of acaricide. This difference in mortality is not unexpected in view of the different physiological states of the larva and adult ticks. The more practically important correlation that resistant larvae develop into resistant adults was not tested, but that is the basic assumption of larval tests and should be subjected to a statistical test for correlation in multihost ticks.

2. Adult Tests

As in the case of larvae, there are a number of bioassay methods for adult ticks. Immersion of adults in commercial formulations of acaricide has been proposed in a number of variations (Graham and Drummond, 1964; M. Van Orelli, personal communication). Contact with impregnated filter paper has been used to a limited extent for the screening of juvenile hormone mimics in engorged larvae of *Amblyomma hebraeum* (Solomon and Evans, 1978) and is possibly applicable to adults. Topical application of pesticides dissolved in an organic solvent has been recommended by the World Health Organization (1981). The bioassay of adult ticks is certainly of obvious advantage in screening for resistance in the case of multihost parasites; however, there are a number of drawbacks to the technique. It seldom is possible to obtain sufficient adult ticks from the field for a meaningful bioassay, and those that are obtained may be in different stages of engorgement and therefore of susceptibility. The criteria of evaluation of such assays are often complex. It is difficult to assess morbidity or death in a relatively immobile engorged female tick, thus a ratio of reproductive efficiency has been suggested as an assay criterion (Drummond *et al.*, 1973). Such ratios are not necessarily amenable to probit analysis (Finney, 1971), and the quantal response of ability to produce one or more viable eggs (Nari, 1981) is probably a better criterion.

3. In Vivo *Laboratory Methods*

Detection of resistance under field-simulated conditions is possible if ticks are bioassayed while they are feeding on a host. Roulston and Wilson (1964) initiated a method for treating and confining cattle ticks on the host in which a number of bioassays could be carried out with a single animal. The behavioral phenomenon of ticks tending to feed in areas of long hair has been exploited for efficacy trials by Downing *et al.* (1977), where patches of long hair are left on the skin of a closely clipped bovine. *Boophilus* spp. tend to attach and remain in these areas, which may then be used for replicate or dose–response assays without artificial confinement. Stendel (1980) reported that this technique is suitable for the identification of resistance. Matthewson (1977) has described a number of other *in vivo* techniques for use on single- and multihost ticks; however, these have not been used for resistance bioassay.

These *in vivo* assays offer the advantage of realistic testing procedures but require some time to carry out and invariably require the culture of the ticks for at least one generation. As such, they seem to have maximum utility in the study of resistance characteristics in established strains of ticks or in assays of those compounds, such as formamidines, which act as detaching agents and do not cause mortality directly.

B. Field Methods

No rapid and easy technique for evaluating pesticide susceptibility of ticks in the field has been reported. Many reports of putative resistance result from the field observation of inadequate tick control; however, such cases are often a result of poor pesticide use or farming practices. Howell (1977) has pointed out that many reports of "resistance" observed in the field are due to understrength dipping fluids or to unusually high loads of ticks, either because of infrequent winter dipping for control of juvenile multihost ticks or through favorable environmental conditions. Because of such errors in observations and interpretations, tick resistance is, as mentioned previously, usually confirmed by a laboratory bioassay of larvae or adults.

C. Interpretation of Resistance

The presence of resistance is usually determined by comparison of the susceptibility of the strain of ticks in question to that of a "reference" strain of the same species (for example the Yerongpilly strain of *B. microplus,* and the Kwanyanga and Lesotho strains of *B. decoloratus*). Where dose–mortality relationships have been statistically analyzed, the LC_{50} or LD_{50} is used for comparison purposes. Although use of the LC_{50} is based on the higher statistical certainty of the median response, it is of little significance in the field, where a much higher rate of mortality is desired (Matthewson, 1977). Added to this is the observation that dose–mortality lines from different strains of ticks are often of such different slopes (Solomon *et al.*, 1979a) that ratios of

LC_{50} values have little correlation with LC_{90} or higher mortalities. Perhaps in response to this obvious source of error, some reports of resistance have been based on LC_{99} data (Baker et al., 1977, 1978a,b, 1979, 1981).

Rather than comparing susceptibility of ticks to a known reference strain, Solomon et al. (1979a,b) have suggested using a frequency distribution technique to delineate the boundaries of the normal susceptibility of the species. This approach showed the expected normal distributions and also that the range of values for the LC_{50}, LC_{95}, and LC_{99} (from a larval bioassay according to Shaw, 1966) in the "susceptible" population extended over a concentration difference of 6- to 10-fold. This does suggest the possibility that, in choosing a susceptible reference strain of ticks, a strain from the lower end of the normal range would misleadingly suggest that all other strains were showing resistance. Similar approaches have not been reported in the literature, possibly because of the large amount of data required; however, frequency diagrams of data supplied by other bioassay units (J. A. F. Baker, personal communication) show similar patterns (Fig. 1). The use of this method to define the normal limits of the susceptible population may be applicable in cases where large collections of data are

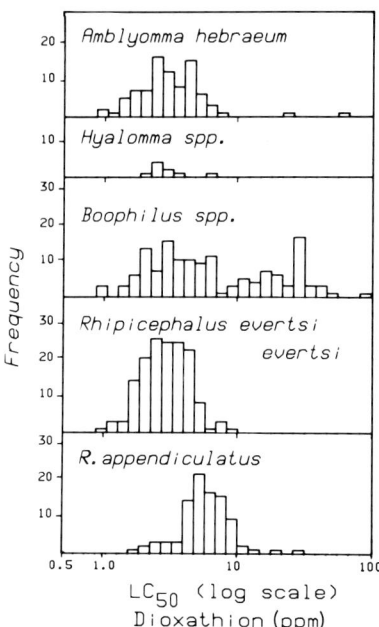

FIG. 1. LC_{50} values for Dioxathion in South African field strains of ticks (data from J. A. F. Baker, personal communication).

being assembled, as in the use of the proposed FAO resistance test kit (Harris, 1978). The establishment of a large data base on tick resistance does unfortunately require the use of a uniform method for bioassay; this has been the exception rather than the rule until the present time.

VI. Mechanisms of Resistance

The development and mechanism of resistance to insecticides in arthropods of veterinary and medical importance has been reviewed by Brown and Pal (1971), Gothe and Hartig (1975), Oppenoorth and Welling (1976), Drummond (1977), and Wilson (1978). On the basis of knowledge of resistance mechanisms in insects and ticks, three major mechanisms of resistance may be expected to occur: (1) a reduction in the rate of penetration of the pesticide into the animal, (2) changes in metabolism, storage, or excretion of the pesticide, and (3) changes in the site of action, which render the organism less sensitive to the effects of the pesticide. All of these have been studied in ticks, and both changes in site of action and increased detoxification have been reported. The following section is not intended to be a complete review of the work on mechanisms but rather a summary of the major findings.

A. Inorganic Acaricides

The only acaricide in this class is arsenic, and the mechanism has only been studied in *Boophilus decoloratus* and *B. microplus*. Work by Thompson and Johnston (1958), Harington (1959), and Whitehead (1961) has shown that resistant strains of ticks have higher levels of sulfhydryl (SH) group–containing compounds such as glutathion and cystein–cystine than do susceptible ticks. Because these free sulfhydryl groups had been observed to react with arsenic (Harington, 1959), it was suggested that this was a possible mechanism of resistance. Roulston and Schuntner (1960) were unable to demonstrate higher levels of sulfhydryl-containing compounds in arsenic-resistant *B. microplus* from Australia, suggesting the existence of another mechanism.

B. Organic Acaricides

The mechanism of resistance to DDT has been studied in ticks of the genus *Boophilus*. Studies by Roulston (1957) and Whitehead (1959a,

1965) failed to show increased metabolism of DDT by the enzyme DDT dehydrochlorinase in resistant strains of *Boophilus decoloratus* or *B. microplus*, suggesting that other mechanisms such as changes in the site of action were involved. This suggestion was supported by the observations of cross-resistance to pyrethrum (Whitehead, 1959b) and subsequently in studies by Schnitzerling *et al.* (1970), which showed that radiolabeled DDT penetrated as rapidly into resistant as into susceptible ticks. A later report of cross-resistance to the synthetic pyrethroids in DDT-resistant ticks (Nolan *et al.*, 1977) adds indirect evidence that the mechanism of DDT resistance is probably analogous to the well-known kdr-DDT resistance known from insects (Oppenoorth and Welling, 1976).

Resistance to lindane and other organochlorine acaricides has been less extensively studied, and the only experimental work reported (Wharton and Roulston, 1970) suggested that reduced penetration was not a mechanism.

Mechanisms of resistance to the acetylcholinesterase inhibitors have been most extensively studied in the genus *Boophilus*, and only in *B. microplus*. The major mechanisms involved in this resistance are varying combinations of increased ability to metabolize the inhibitor to less toxic products, as well as reduced sensitivity of acetylcholinesterase toward inhibition (Schnitzerling *et al.*, 1974; Nolan and Schnitzerling, 1975; Oppenoorth and Welling, 1976). Reduced reactivity of acetylcholinesterase was believed to result from changes in the active site of the enzyme that reduce reaction rates with both inhibitor and normal substrate (Nolan and Schnitzerling, 1976). In the Biarra strain of *B. microplus*, the sole mechanism of resistance appears to be a less sensitive acetylcholinesterase, but in the Mt. Alford strain the mechanism was a combination of increased detoxification and less sensitive enzyme (Schuntner and Thompson, 1978). The Tully and Ingham strains show slightly increased acetylcholinesterase activity (over the Yerongpilly susceptible strain) as well as increased rates of detoxification of organophosphates (Roulston *et al.*, 1977). Smallman and Riddles (1977) have shown that choline acetyltransferase activity in susceptible and resistant *B. microplus* is similar, indicating that the changes in acetylcholinesterase conferred by resistance have no genetic linkage to acetylcholine synthesis enzymes. Carbaryl resistance is conferred by changes in the sensitivity of acetylcholinesterase in the Ridgelands and Biarra strains, but a metabolic component appears to be important in the MacKay strain (Schuntner *et al.*, 1971).

Several of the resistant strains of *B. microplus* from Argentina also show decreased sensitivity of acetylcholinesterase (Grillo Torado and Perez Arrieta, 1977b; Reich *et al.*, 1978), suggesting similar mechanisms to the Australian Biarra strain. Both the Berlin strain of *B. decoloratus* from South Africa and the Alicedale West strain from Zimbabwe show reduced sensitivity of acetylcholinesterase to paraoxon inhibition, also suggesting a similar mechanism (Matthewson et al., 1976).

The mechanisms of resistance to clenpyrin in the Ingham strain of *B. microplus* (Roulston et al., 1977) are not known.

VII. Management of Resistance

Acaricides are an important and useful tool for the control of cattle ticks; however, the continuing appearance of resistance is gradually reducing the choice of pesticides available for control of these new resistant strains. At the same time, new pesticides seem to be appearing less frequently. Added to this dilemma is the possibility that cross-resistance and multiple-resistance phenomena will eliminate large groups of chemicals (having similar modes of action or detoxification) before these can be used in the field. It is obvious that the useful life of present acaricides must be extended for as long as possible. This can be done in a number of ways, many of which involve the integration of nonpesticidal, biological, or cultural methods into tick control programs. Such methods have been proposed and reviewed by Whitehead (1975), Baker (1976), Allen (1979), Obenchain (1979), Sutherst and Comins (1979), Sutherst et al. (1979), Wilkinson (1979), and Wharton and Norris (1980). The introduction of tick-resistant cattle such as the Zebu (*Bos indicus*) or Zebu–European cross cattle, and the use of pasture rotation in conjunction with proper acaricide use, have been found to be the most successful strategy for tick-resistance management in Australia (Sutherst and Comins, 1979; Wharton and Norris, 1980). However, the single-host tick *B. microplus* is the only major pest tick in Australia, and its simpler life cycle lends itself to such management.

In other areas where several species of multihost ticks may share hosts with single-host ticks, management strategies become more complex and less easy to apply. As a result, little extension of this Australian approach has occurred in other areas. This review will not cover these areas but will concentrate instead on those methods that involve the use of acaricides or acaricide management. It must be pointed out, however, that no single strategy for resistance management will succeed for any length of time and that a combination of strategies must be used, either together or in sequence.

Georghiou (1980) has reviewed the factors that influence the rate of development of resistance and has suggested a number of management strategies for resistance. Of those factors, some are dependent on the type of management system used and are thus under the control of the livestock producer. It has been suggested that the rate of resistance buildup will be slowest if:

1. The pesticide has a short environmental life.
2. The pesticide does not have a similar mechanism of action or is not degraded by similar pathways to earlier used pesticides.
3. Selection is directed mainly against the least numerous stage of the pest (i.e., adults).
4. The pesticide is not applied to large areas.
5. From time to time generations are left untreated to allow for selection by other environmental factors.

A combination of these strategies would be ideal but rarely attainable; however, it is possible to approximate some of these objectives. Use of low-persistence pesticides or formulations can be controlled through the choice of appropriate acaricides. However, the availability of a pesticide with a novel mechanism of action or degradation is not always predictable. A knowledge of the mechanism of action and degradation of the previously used pesticide would, however, allow for a more rational choice to be made. Selection of only adults is precluded in the case of the single-host ticks, and this may have been a contributing factor in the apparently more rapid rate of development of resistance in these ticks. Incomplete treatment of cattle either by not treating all animals or by allowing a treatment-free period is not always practicable when dealing with disease-carrying ticks. However, the release of susceptible, pathogen-free ticks as a means of maintaining heterogeneity in the population is one possible method of achieving a similar result (Georghiou and Taylor, 1977a).

A further operational influence on the rate of resistance development is the dose or concentration to which the organisms are exposed. Georghiou and Taylor (1977b) have simulated this, and their results suggest that a lower dose of pesticide will slow down the rate at which resistance develops. This will have little effect on the number of organisms, and ineffective control will be achieved. Use of higher doses will result in a rapid rate of selection of resistant individuals; however, numbers will increase so slowly that effective control will be achieved, even if for a limited time. During this period, resistant survivors may build up to economically significant levels; alternatively, it is possible that if the population is reduced to suboptimal numbers, the strain may become extinct.

This strategy of "management by saturation" is suggested by Sutherst and Comins (1979) as most suitable if eradication of the tick is possible. It does carry the added risk of "super resistance" being selected, but problems of host–animal toxicity and increased cost could make such an approach impractical.

The rate of resistance development is dependent on the frequency of selection, and a reduction in the latter would prolong the useful life of the acaricide. A reduced frequency of acaricide treatment of host animals is possible if an increased threshold of infestation is used or if other cultural methods of control are combined with acaricide use. This may not be possible in the case of disease vectors or multihost ticks.

Although some of these operational factors have yet to be field tested in the management of tick resistance, a number of chemical countermeasures are also possible, and some work has been done in this area.

The use of synergists to block detoxification pathways in resistant insects has been suggested by Georghiou (1980) and has been shown to function in ticks. Schuntner et al. (1974) reported that the commercially used synergist, piperonyl butoxide, increased the toxicity of carbaryl to the resistant Biarra strain of $B.$ $microplus.$ The use of S,S,S-tributylphosphorotrithioate (DEF) has reduced resistance factors in organophosphate-resistant insects (Ranasinghe and Georghiou, 1979), but has not been reported to be effective in ticks and may also introduce host toxicity problems (Nolan and Roulston, 1979). Metabolic interactions in currently used acaricides may be exploited in a similar manner as indicated by Nolan and Roulston (1979), who demonstrated synergism of pyrethroids by ethion and chlorfenvinphos in $B.$ $microplus.$

The use of mixtures or the alternation of pesticides of different mechanisms of action has been shown to decrease the rate at which resistance develops (Asquith, 1961; Pimentel and Bellotti, 1976; Georghiou, 1980; R. S. MacDonald, personal communication). Similar effects have been observed in $B.$ $microplus$ (Biarra strain) when chlordimeform was added to ethion in dipping vats in Australia (Roulston et al., 1971). The use of mixtures of pesticides with different modes of action is one means of approaching the "saturation management tactic" without undesirable host toxicity (Sutherst and Comins, 1979), but also may cause "super resistance." Alternation of chemicals has not been reported in tick control but in many cases would not be possible where dipping is used.

At the present time a number of methods for management of tick resistance are available, and a number of other approaches to tick control show promise but lack field application data. It is also apparent that resistance is a phenomenon that is virtually inseparable from acaricide use in the long term. In the face of increasing costs for pesticides, every method for postponing resistance must be employed, and every alternative method of tick control should be investigated. Once established in ticks, resistance appears to be stable even in the absence of selection. This is indicated by the high incidence of resistance to chlorinated hydrocarbons in *B. microplus* in Australia where these acaricides have not been used for 20 years (Roulston et al., 1981). Continued use of acaricides in a nonrational manner may eventually lead to the buildup of a completely stable resistance that may never disappear. Such phenomena are not unique (Bishop, 1982) and could occur in ticks.

ACKNOWLEDGMENTS

The author wishes to thank Linda Lepage for her typing skills and Jimmy Baker, Durr Bezuidenhout, Dr. R. O. Darwish, Ivan Horak, Mike Matthewson, Jim Nolan, and Jane Walker for their useful information, suggestions, and comments.

REFERENCES

Allen, J. R. (1979). *Recent Adv. Acarol.* **2,** 15–23.
Asquith, D. (1961). *J. Econ. Ent.* **54,** 439–441.
Baker, J. A. F. (1976). In "Tick-Borne Diseases and their Vectors" (J. K. H. Wilde, ed.), pp. 101–109. University Press, Edinburgh.
Baker, J. A. F., and Shaw, R. D. (1965). *J. S. Afr. Vet. Med. Assoc.* **36,** 321–330.
Baker, J. A. F., Thompson, G. E., and Miles, J. O. (1977). *J. S. Afr. Vet. Assoc.* **48,** 59–65.
Baker, J. A. F., Miles, J. O., Robertson, W. D., Stanford, G. D., and Taylor, R. J. (1978a). *J. S. Afr. Vet. Assoc.* **49,** 327–333.
Baker, J. A. F., Miles, J. O., and Robertson, W. D. (1978b). *J. S. Afr. Vet. Assoc.* **49,** 337–341.
Baker, J. A. F., Jordaan, J. O., and Robertson, W. D. (1979). *J. S. Afr. Vet. Assoc.* **50,** 296–301.
Baker, J. A. F., Jordaan, J. O., and Robertson, W. D. (1981). In "Tick Biology and Control" (G. B. Whitehead and J. D. Gibson, eds.), pp. 103–108. Tick Research Unit, Rhodes University, Grahamstown.
Bishop, J. (1982). *Pestic. Sci.* **13,** 97–103.
Brown, A. W. A., and Pal, R. (1971). *W.H.O. Monogr. Ser.* **38.**
Crampton, P. L., and Gichanga, M. M. (1979). *Bull. Entomol. Res.* **69,** 427–439.
Daynes, P., Brun, L., and Wilson, J. L. (1980). *Rev. Elev. Med. Vet. Pays Trop.* **33,** 339–399.
Downing, F. S., Stubbs, V. K., and Boyer, S. (1977). In "Crop Protection Agents" (N. R. McFarlane, ed.), pp. 609–622. Academic Press, New York.
Downing, W. H. E., Harbour, L. C., and Stones, L. C. (1952). *Vet. Rec.* **64,** 787–798.
Drummond, R. O. (1977). In "Pesticide Management and Insecticide Resistance" (D. L. Watson and A. W. A. Brown, eds.), pp. 303–319. Academic Press, New York.

Drummond, R. O., Ernst, S. E., Trevino, J. L., Gladney, W. J., and Graham, O. H. (1973). *J. Econ. Entomol.* **66**, 130–133.

Drummond, R. O., Whetstone, T. M., and Miller, J. (1981). *J. Econ. Entomol.* **74**, 432–436.

DuToit, R., Graf, H., and Bekker, P. M. (1941). *J. S. Afr. Vet. Med. Assoc.* **12**, 50–58.

Ellenberger, W. P., and Chapin, R. M. (1919). *Farmers' Bull.* **1057**, 3–32.

Fiedler, O. G. H. (1968). *J. S. Afr. Vet. Med. Assoc.* **39**, 84–87.

Finney, D. J. (1971). "Probit Analysis," 3rd ed. Cambridge Univ. Press, London and New York.

Food and Agriculture Organization (1980). "Recommended Methods for Measurement of Pest Resistance to Pesticides." FAO Plant Prod. Prot. Pap. No. 21. FAO, Rome.

Georghiou, G. P. (1980). *Residue Rev.* **79**, 131–145.

Georghiou, G. P., and Taylor, C. E. (1977a). *J. Econ. Entomol.* **70**, 319–323.

Georghiou, G. P., and Taylor, C. E. (1977b). *J. Econ. Entomol.* **70**, 653–658.

Graham, O. H., and Drummond, R. O. (1964). *J. Econ. Entomol.* **57**, 335–339.

Graybill, H. W. (1912). *Farmers' Bull.* **489**, 5–42.

Grillo Torrado, J. M., and Perez Arrieta, A. (1977a). *Rev. Med. Vet. (Buenos Aires)* **58**, 101–102, 105.

Grillo Torado, J. M., and Perez Arrieta, A. (1977b). *Rev. Med. Vet. (Buenos Aires)* **58**, 309–322.

Gothe, von R., and Hartig, M. (1975). *Dtsch. Tieraerztl. Wochenschr.* **82**, 385–420, 461–465.

Hansens, E. J. (1956). *J. Econ. Entomol.* **49**, 281–283.

Harington, J. S. (1959). *Nature (London)* **184**, 1739–1740.

Harris, E. G. (1978). "Center for Overseas Pest Research Annual Report," pp. 107–108.

Harrison, I. R., Palmer, B. H., and Wilmhurst, E. C. (1973). *Pestic. Sci.* **4**, 531–542.

Hoogstraal, H. (1976). *In* "Tick-Borne Diseases and their Vectors" (J. K. H. Wilde, ed.), pp. 3–14. University Press, Edinburgh.

Howell, C. J. (1977). *J. S. Afr. Vet. Assoc.* **48**, 11–12.

Jongejan, F., and Lourens, J. H. M. (1980). *Z. Angew. Entomol.* **89**, 321–323.

Kerr, R. W. (1964). *J. Aust. Agric. Sci.* **30**, 33–38.

Kigaye, M. K., and Matthysse, J. Y. (1973). *Bull. Epizoot. Dis. Afr.* **21**, 429–435.

Legg, J. (1947). *Aust. Vet. J.* **23**, 181–185.

Lourens, J. H. M. (1979a). *Pestic. Sci.* **10**, 495–401.

Lourens, J. H. M. (1979b). *J. Econ. Entomol.* **72**, 790–793.

Lourens, J. H. M. (1980a). *Bull. Entomol. Res.* **70**, 1–10.

Lourens, J. H. M. (1980b). *J. Med. Entomol.* **17**, 375–379.

Lourens, J. H. M., and Tatchell, R. J. (1979). *Bull. Entomol. Res.* **69**, 235–242.

Matthewson, M. D. (1977). *In* "Crop Protection Agents" (N. R. McFarlane, ed.), pp. 571–581. Academic Press, New York.

Matthewson, M. D., and Baker, J. A. F. (1975). *J. S. Afr. Vet. Assoc.* **46**, 341–344.

Matthewson, M. D., and Blackman, G. G. (1980). *Vet. Rec.* **107**, 491–491.

Matthewson, M. D., Wilson, R. G., and Hammant, C. A. (1976). *Bull. Entomol. Res.* **66**, 553–560.

Nari, A. J. (1981). "The evaluation of *in vitro* methods of testing acaricidal resistance in *Boophilus microplus*." Ph.D. Thesis, University of Pretoria, Pretoria, South Africa.

Nolan, J., and Roulston, W. J. (1979). *Recent Adv. Acarol.* **2**, 3–14.

Nolan, J., and Schnitzerling, H. J. (1975). *Pestic. Biochem. Physiol.* **5**, 178–188.

Nolan, J., and Schnitzerling, H. J. (1976). *Pestic. Biochem. Physiol.* **6**, 142–147.

Nolan, J., Roulston, W. J., and Wharton, R. H. (1977). *Pestic. Sci.* **8**, 484–486.

Norris, K. R. (1956). *Aust. Vet. J.* **32,** 177–182.
Obenchain, F. D. (1979). *Recent Adv. Acarol.* **2,** 35–43.
Oppenoorth, F. J., and Welling, W. (1976). *In* "Insecticide Biochemistry and Physiology" (C. F. Wilkinson, ed.), pp. 507–551. Academic Press, New York.
Patarroya, J. H., and Costa, J. O. (1980). *Trop. Anim. Health Prod.* **12,** 6–10.
Perez Arrieta, A., Marti Vidal, J. V., and Bulman, G. M. (1980). *Rev. Mil. Vet.* **26,** 275–283.
Pimentel, D. and Bellotti, A. C. (1976). *Am. Nat.* **110,** 877–888.
Polyakov, D. I., and Smirnova, O. J. (1979). *Proc. Int. Congr. Acarol., 4th, 1974* pp. 547–548.
Ranasinghe, R. E., and Georghiou, G. P. (1979). *Pestic. Sci.* **10,** 502–508.
Rawlins, S. C., and Mansingh, A. (1977a). *PANS* **23,** 137–141.
Rawlins, S. C., and Mansingh, A. (1977b). *J. Econ. Entomol.* **70,** 697–698.
Rawlins, S. C., and Mansingh, A. (1978a). *J. Econ. Entomol.* **71,** 142–144.
Rawlins, S. C., and Mansingh, A. (1978b). *J. Econ. Entomol.* **71,** 956–960.
Reich, C. I., Grillo Torrado, J. M., Perez Arrieta, A., and Zorzopulos, J. (1978). *Exp. Parasitol.* **44,** 50–55.
Roulston, W. J. (1957). "WHO Information Circular No. 5." W. H. O., Geneva (from Whitehead, 1965).
Roulston, W. J. (1969). *Proc. Int. Congr. Acarol., 2nd, 1967* pp. 515–521.
Roulston, W. J., and Schuntner, C. A. (1960). *Nature (London)* **186,** 1069–1070.
Roulston, W. J., and Wilson, J. T. (1964). *Bull. Entomol. Res.* **55,** 617–635.
Roulston, W. J., Wharton, R. H., Schnitzerling, H. J., Sutherst, R. W., and Sullivan, N. D. (1971). *Aust. Vet. J.* **47,** 521–528.
Roulston, W. J., Schuntner, C. A., Schnitzerling, H. J., Wilson, J. T., and Wharton, R. H. (1977). *Aust. J. Agric. Res.* **28,** 345–354.
Roulston, W. J., Wharton, R. H., Nolan, J., Kerr, J. D., Wilson, J. T., Thompson, P. G., and Schotz, M. (1981). *Aust. Vet. J.* **57,** 362–371.
Schnitzerling, H. J., Roulston, W. J., and Schuntner, C. A. (1970). *Aust. J. Biol. Sci.* **23,** 219–230.
Schnitzerling, H. J., Schuntner, C. A., Roulston, W. J., and Wilson, J. T. (1974). *Aust. J. Biol. Sci.* **27,** 397–408.
Schuntner, C. A., and Thompson, P. G. (1978). *Aust. J. Biol. Sci.* **31,** 317–325.
Schuntner, C. A., Schnitzerling, H. J., and Roulston, W. J. (1971). *Pestic. Biochem. Physiol.* **1,** 424–433.
Schuntner, C. A., Roulston, W. H., and Wharton, R. H. (1974). *Nature (London)* **249,** 386–387.
Shaw, R. D. (1966). *Bull. Entomol. Res.* **56,** 389–405.
Shaw, R. D. (1970). *Trop. Sci.* **12,** 29–36.
Shaw, R. D., and Malcolm, H. M. (1964). *Vet. Rec.* **76,** 210–211.
Shaw, R. D., Thompson, G. E., and Baker, J. A. F. (1967). *Vet. Rec.* **81,** 548–549.
Smallman, B. N., and Riddles, P. W. (1977). *Pestic. Biochem. Physiol.* **7,** 355–359.
Solomon, K. R., and Evans, A. A. (1978). *Onderstepoort J. Vet. Res.* **45,** 39–42.
Solomon, K. R., Baker, M. K., Heyne, H., and Van Kleef, J. (1979a). *Onderstepoort J. Vet. Res.* **46,** 171–177.
Solomon, K. R., Heyne, H., and Van Kleef, J. (1979b). *Recent Adv. Acarol.* **2,** 65–69.
Spickett, A. M., and Malan, J. R. (1978). *Onderstepoort J. Vet. Res.* **45,** 149–153.
Stendel, W. (1980). *J. S. Afr. Vet. Assoc.* **51,** 147–152.
Stone, B. F., and Haydock, H. P. (1962). *Bull. Entomol. Res.* **53,** 563–578.
Sutherst, R. W., and Comins, H. N. (1979). *Bull. Entomol. Res.* **69,** 519–537.

Sutherst, R. W., Norton, G. A., Barlow, N. D., Conway, G. R., Birley, M., and Comins, H. N. (1979). *J. Appl. Ecol.* **16**, 359–382.
Tatchell, R. J. (1974). *Proc. Int. Congr. Parasitol., 3rd, 1974* pp. 993–994.
Thompson, M. E., and Johnston, A. M. (1958). *Nature (London)* **181**, 647–648.
Wharton, R. H. (1967). *Aust. Vet. J.* **43**, 394–399.
Wharton, R. H. (1976). *World Anim. Rev.* **20**, 8–15.
Wharton, R. H., and Norris, K. R. (1980). *Vet. Parasitol.* **6**, 135–164.
Wharton, R. H., and Roulston, W. J. (1970). *Annu. Rev. Entomol.* **15**, 381–405.
Whitehead, G. B. (1958). *Bull. Entomol. Res.* **49**, 661–673.
Whitehead, G. B. (1959a). *J. S. Afr. Vet. Med. Assoc.* **30**, 221–234.
Whitehead, G. B. (1959b). *Nature (London)* **184**, 378–379.
Whitehead, G. B. (1961). *J. Insect Physiol.* **7**, 177–185.
Whitehead, G. B. (1965). *Adv. Acarol.* **2**, 53–70.
Whitehead, G. B. (1975). *Entomol. Mem. S. Afr., Dep. Agric. Tech. Serv.* **44**, 12–16.
Whitehead, G. B., and Baker, J. A. F. (1961). *Bull. Entomol. Res.* **51**, 755–764.
Whitnall, A. B. M., McHardy, W. M., Whitehead, G. B., and Meerholz, F. (1951). *Bull. Entomol. Res.* **41**, 577–591.
Wilkinson, P. R. (1979). *Recent Adv. Acarol.* **2**, 25–33.
Wilson, R. G. (1978). *J. S. Afr. Vet. Assoc.* **49**, 49–51.
World Health Organization (1980). "Resistance of Vectors of Disease to Pesticides," W. H. O. Tech. Rep. Ser. No. 655. W. H. O., Geneva.
World Health Organization (1981). World Health Organization unpublished document WHO/UBC/81.814.
Ziv, M. (1979). *Refu. Vet.* **36**, 114–116.

Control and Therapy of Fish Diseases

JOHN B. GRATZEK

Department of Medical Microbiology, College of Veterinary Medicine, University of Georgia, Athens, Georgia

I. Background 297
II. Veterinary Medicine and Fish Disease Control 298
    A. Diagnosis 299
    B. Principles of Disease Control 300
    C. Treatment of Fish Diseases................................... 304
    D. Common Therapeutic Agents Used in Parasite Control 307
    E. Antimicrobials Used in Control of Bacterial Diseases 311
    F. Vaccines Used in Disease Control 314
    G. Bacterins Used in Disease Control 315
    H. The Potential for Virus Vaccines............................... 318
    References 321

I. Background

The application of the principles of disease control and therapy to "aquaculture" requires definition of the field as to the basic requirements of availability of suitable water, fish, power, and land. Aquaculture encompasses a diversity of systems that can include the culture of both warm water and cold-water species such as catfish and trout, respectively. The culture of warm water species in the United States includes channel catfish, American eel, freshwater prawns (*Macrobrachium rosenbergii*), crayfish, and a variety of ornamental fish. Trout, goldfish, and bait fish represent some of the cold-water fish cultured. Brown (1980) has estimated the on-farm value of cultured freshwater species to be $50,000,000 for channel catfish, $35,000,000 for bait fish, $32,000,000 for trout and salmon, $21,000,000 for goldfish and Koi, $15,000,000 for ornamental varieties, and approximately $4,500,000 for other species such as bigmouth buffalo fish, tilapia, and American eel.

The culture of marine fish and invertebrates is referred to as mariculture. According to E. E. Brown (personal communication) the total on-farm value of propagated marine species amounts to approximately $60,000,000. Species cultured include oysters, penaeid shrimp mussels, abalone, and scallops. Other species that offer some potential for culture are blue crab and spiny lobsters. The continued development of mariculture will depend on wholesale prices as well as on socio-economic conditions such as the ability to lease bay areas for extended periods of time.

II. Veterinary Medicine and Fish Disease Control

In past years, the role of the veterinarian in fish disease control has been minimal. There have been notable exceptions where veterinarians, usually associated with state agencies, are delivering excellent services. The role of the veterinarian as a fish health specialist has been compared to that of the veterinarian in the poultry industry. In years past, veterinarians did not service the poultry industry. Today, with specialty postgraduate training programs available in poultry diseases, trained veterinarians are available and are in demand by the poultry and egg-producing industries. Whether this success story will be repeated with the aquaculture industry will be determined by a complex array of factors, including interest in diseases of aquatic species, availability of suitable training in veterinary colleges, availability of positions, and economic demand for services.

The interest in exotic species can be well documented from past experiences at the College of Veterinary Medicine at the University of Georgia. A 5-week elective study block that includes approximately 200 instructional hr of the diseases of fish, pet birds, and laboratory animals was selected by 80% of the last two graduating classes. At present, it appears that fish health management personnel are retained by federal or state agencies and, in some cases, by individual fish farms. Many of the fish health problems are handled by biologists affiliated with extension departments in land grant universities. The fish health biologist's availability depresses the demand for veterinarians with adequate training to handle problems in aquaculture.

A study by the National Research Council (1982) suggests that a modest surplus in the veterinary work force will occur by 1990. In this study, colleges of veterinary medicine are encouraged to anticipate this surplus by altering their program to meet societal needs in nontraditional fields. Relative to aquatic animal disease specialists, some veterinary colleges presently have active training programs at both the professional and graduate level. The future demand for the veterinarian trained in fish health management will depend on the economic viability of the aquaculture industry, available positions with adequate compensation, and the availability of trained veterinarians.

At this time, however, there appears to be a demand for services relative to fish health management problems of fish as pet animals. This need has been expressed by primary producers, fish wholesalers, retailers, and especially home aquarists.

In 1973, the size of the aquarium industry including sales of fish and all other fish-related products was estimated by Setzer (1974) to be $698 million. Axelrod (1971) estimates that there are 22 million aquarium owners in the United States. Over the 7 years from 1976 to 1982, referral calls from veterinarians across the country indicated that more and more veterinarians are engaging in fish health care in their practice areas. Interest has been increasing among veterinarians in continuing education courses in fish health. Finally, our graduates have reported that their fish health management training has assisted them in building and increasing the scope of their practices. The curricula of veterinary colleges provide an excellent basis for the study of fish health problems. Principles of physiology, pathology, epidemiology, infectious and noninfectious diseases, along with diagnostic methods, can be directly applied to fish health problems. Our experience with final-year veterinary students is that particular disease conditions unique to fish are easily grasped. However, it is obvious that few students are knowledgeable in the techniques of water-quality management in closed or open aquatic culture systems. Obviously, because of the fish's total dependence on water, a complete understanding of water management techniques is fundamental to fish health management. Fortunately, several excellent books are available (Letritz, 1969; Boyd, 1979; Spotte, 1979; Brown and Gratzek, 1980).

A. Diagnosis

Therapy and control of fish disease problems is dependent on establishing a specific diagnosis. In fish diseases where stressful conditions precipitate a disease outbreak, it is necessary to identify the primary stressor by taking a history or by doing laboratory tests. In general, the clinician involved in a fish disease problem will develop a mental diagnostic checklist. This checklist would include nutrition, environmental problems such as water quality, overcrowding, and toxicities, and infectious diseases such as those associated with parasites, bacteria, fungi, and viruses. A variety of books that provide information on fish diseases are available. Those covering general aspects of fish diseases include Reichenbach-Klinke and Elkan (1965), Amlacher (1970), and Sarig (1971). Specific information on bacterial diseases of fish can be found in Bullock et al. (1971) and Bullock (1971). Other specific subjects are covered in detail and include crustacean parasites by Kabata (1970), fish immunology by Anderson (1974), fungal diseases by Neish and Hughes (1980), and environmental stress by Wedemeyer et al. (1976). More current aspects of virus diseases of fish may be found in *Fish Diseases* edited by Ahne (1980). Two books that cover general fish diseases including some emphasis on histopathology are *The Pathology of Fishes* edited by Ribelin and Migaki (1975) and *Fish Pathology* edited by Roberts (1978). Books are available that specifically review diseases of trout and salmon (Roberts and Shepherd, 1974), channel catfish (Plumb, 1979), tropical fish (Schubert, 1974), and marine fish (Sinderman, 1966; Kingsford, 1975; Dulin, 1976; Reichenbach-Klinke, 1977). Articles on diseases of tropical fishes provide in-depth information on various problems (Gratzek, 1980; Scott, 1981; Sommerville, 1981).

B. Principles of Disease Control

Disease control in fish follows health management practices identical to those encountered with any other type of animal. Furthermore, it is important to establish that various types of fish are affected by closely related disease-producing parasites and microorganisms; therefore, disease avoidance procedures are essentially similar regardless of the species of fish cultured. The basic premise is that stressful conditions such as extremes of water pH, or the presence of ammonia or nitrites will exacerbate existing subclinical infestations to a point where fish become obviously sick. Consequently, disease control measures should be directed toward avoiding contact with a parasite or microorganism, avoiding stress, and augmenting the basic resistance of the fish through therapeutic agents or immunization. Specific therapy involves the use of medicants before stocking or during a disease outbreak. Therapeutic agents will be discussed in a later section.

1. Control by Avoidance

Control by avoidance of the offending parasite or microorganism is possible by a variety of methods, all dictated by the nature of the disease-producing agent. One of the safest methods for avoiding disease problems in fish stocked in ponds, raceways, or closed aquaria is to ensure that the stocked fish are free of specific parasites. In the case of trout, for instance, it is possible to purchase eggs from hatcheries that certify that the brood stock is free of the virus disease known as infectious pancreatic necrosis (IPN). If this virus is not introduced by addition of carrier fish or by contamination of stocked fish with virus from wild fish, the stocked fish should remain virus free.

In channel catfish production facilities, it is important that brood fish do not carry the virus of channel catfish virus disease (CCVD). Although it has not been definitely proven that the parental stock can serve as carriers, it is logical to assume so and to avoid possible shedding of virus by using brood fish with negative virus neutralization titers.

Parasites can be avoided by a variety of methods. In stocking a culture system with any species, the fish should, minimally, be held in quarantine and routinely treated for parasites before they are added to a culture system that has been drained and disinfected. In our experience, stocking ponds with catfish fry infested with *Scyphidia* results in a diminished harvest. If fry are treated before releasing them in ponds, production is increased considerably. Apparently the initial parasite load is directly or indirectly associated with mortality.

In fish culture, it is sound preventive medicine to practice the "all in, all out" method whenever possible. This means that a group of pretreated fish should be introduced into a previously cleaned culture system and allowed to grow without further additions of fish, including wild fish. When water supply is from a stream having a native fish population, there is considerable risk of the exposure of cultured fishes to various disease-causing agents. In trout raceway systems this method has been practiced for years. Raceways are relatively easy to clean, and water sources, at least in some areas of the northwestern United States, are devoid of fish as sources of parasites. In catfish culture, good managers drain ponds and remove accumulated organic debris before adding calcium oxide for disinfection purposes. Liming in conjunction with a drying period will ensure that parasites are not carried over when the pond is once again stocked. Presumably, once specific parasite-free fish are introduced into a system, they would remain parasite-free unless parasites were introduced by infested wild fish or by nets, pails, traps, and other implements found in fish farm areas. Wild birds can introduce eggs of digenetic trematodes. The "all in, all out" method does not preclude periodic grading of fish, with subsequent transfer of graded fish to other raceways or ponds.

Where pond drainage is not possible or practicable, introduced fish should be treated by the seller. Minimally, one should expect that common external protozoan and metazoan parasites are not introduced into the pond. Normally, a formalin bath treatment is effective in ridding fish of external parasites.

Disease control in the aquarium industry is complicated by the hundreds of different species of fish handled, as well as by the large number of holding units required and the labor required for handling and caring for fish. Generally, fish arrive at a wholesale supplier in closed plastic bags after being transported for 1 to 3 days. Transport water may be fouled by feces, ammonia, and high carbon dioxide levels. If such fish are medicated soon after arrival, the additional stress may prove fatal. Alert wholesalers of tropical fish realize that a slow acclimatization to a new water type is important in the avoidance of further stress. Normally, attention is given to temperature acclimatization and avoidance of radical pH changes. On arrival of shipments from fish farmers, most wholesalers clean aquaria, including a complete water change, before adding new fish. Fish may be routinely treated after being allowed to acclimate for a few days. Treatment schemes with medicants such as formalin, malachite green, methylene blue, or acriflavine are usually directed toward external parasites. Antibiotics are commonly used as a prophylactic measure against bacterial diseases. Introductions of parasites from contaminated nets or by addition of other fish should be avoided.

There are a few unique problems in the wholesale trade. Because of the demand for a vast variety of fish, the wholesaler must purchase from many different suppliers. Naturally, the quality of fish varies considerably, as do the nutritional and environmental requirements. Some producers are aware of disease problems and will treat prior to shipment. Others may not have the necessary personnel, knowledge, or desire to examine fish prior to distribution to wholesalers. Consequently, fish at the wholesale establishment often have a variety of inapparent problems. Such problems could include nematodes and metacercariae, as well as various sporozoans, *Hexamita*, and mycobacteria. In some cases these fish are not salable; in other cases, disease may be inapparent but slowly progressive, resulting in the distribution of potentially unhealthy fish to retailers and eventually to the public. These more complicated problems are inherent in the trade and cannot be completely avoided by management practices. It is at this point that accurate diagnosis and treatment recommendations are required.

2. Stress Control

Stress control is recognized by fish culturists as one of the principal ways to control disease outbreaks. Esch and Hazen (1978) define stress as the effect of any alteration or force that extends homeostatic or stabilizing processes beyond their normal limits at any level of biological organization. In fish culture, a stress can be any environmental change that affects the organism such that a physiological response is required. Changes could include transportation, low oxygen levels, high carbon dioxide levels, extremes of pH, high levels of ammonia, nitrites, nitrates, toxicants such as insecticides or heavy metals, and a variety of other changes including poor nutrition.

The stress response of fish is similar to that described for mammals (Selye, 1973). Adrenocorticotropic hormone from the pituitary gland controls the release of catecholamines (epinephrine and norepinephrine) and corticosteroids. In fish these hormones are released from chromaffin and interrenal tissues, which are analogous to the adrenal tissues in mammals. Among the physiological changes caused by the release of these hormones are dilation of the gill filamental arteries, an increase in the stroke volume of the heart, increased glycogen metabolism, and depression of the immune response.

Whether a disease outbreak will follow a period of stress may depend on the length of exposure to the particular stress. In the wild, the stress response is usually short-term and advantageous to the fish. When a fish needs additional energy for a short-term emergency, dilation of the filamental arteries and an increase in the heart's stroke volume will increase the uptake of oxygen. This, coupled with an increase in the breakdown of muscle glycogen, increases the available energy.

Under intensive fish culture conditions where fish are handled, transported, seined, graded, and often exposed to unfavorable water quality conditions, they are subjected to a series of stressors over prolonged periods. Fish can adapt to single stressors within physiological limits, but prolonged stress can lead to disease. For example, although increased blood flow through the gills increases the availability of oxygen, prolonged stress such as during extended handling eventually results in osmotic problems. Clinical experience suggests that bacterial disease follows stress periods. In mammals there is ample evidence to associate glucocorticoid activity with a depressed immune response (Levine and Claman, 1970; Gillis, 1979; Galili, 1980), but experimental evidence associating stress with immunological suppression is lacking in fish. An excellent review of the stress response in fish is found in *Stress and Fish* (Pickering, 1981).

C. Treatment of Fish Diseases

In a discussion of the principles of treating fish diseases, several factors must be taken into account. These are reviewed in the following paragraphs.

1. Legal Considerations

Drugs used for food fish are strictly regulated. For instance, malachite green, a drug that has been found to be particularly effective for the treatment of some external parasites, cannot be legally used for food fish.

2. Advisability of Treatment

In some cases where the majority of fish are moribund, it must be decided whether or not a treatment is economically feasible, in that the stress imposed by the treatment may add to the total mortality.

3. Drug Selection

When a diagnosis has been established, a specific therapeutic regimen can be initiated. Depending on the problem, the clinician has several choices as to which medicants to use. It is not enough to know that a particular drug is recommended for a particular disease. Various drugs may affect various species of fish differently. Malachite green, a common antiparasiticide, will kill fry and also is toxic when used to treat some scaleless fish. The conditions of the water may limit the selection of a drug. Copper sulfate has been used as an algicide in ponds; it is also effective in the treatment of external parasites of fish. In ponds with hard water (greater than 300 ppm as calcium carbonate), copper sulfate at 3 ppm is safe. However, if pond water is soft (50 ppm as calcium carbonate), more copper ions will be formed, resulting in toxicity to the fish.

Because of its oxidizing properties, potassium permanganate is frequently used as an algicide and a water clearant; it is also used as an external parasiticide. It is well known that in highly organic, murky water, relatively more drug must be used to elicit an antiparasitic effect. The reason for this is that the drug must oxidize the organic load in the culture water before affecting parasites on the surface of the fish. In practice, therefore, the dose must be adjusted depending on the natural conditions of the water. In water containing a high organic load, a given dose may not be effective in removing parasites; conversely, in water with a low organic load, that same dose may result in damage to the fish. In summary, the clinician must know the susceptibility of both the organism and the fish to a drug, and the drug's particular interactions with various types of water. Dosage guidelines for fish are available in several publications (Roberts and Shepherd, 1974; Plumb, 1979; Brown and Gratzek, 1980; Gratzek, 1980).

4. Environmental Response

The addition of a drug to a particular culture system may have a deleterious, indirect effect on the fish. During summer months, for example, the treatment of a pond with copper sulfate may kill enough algae to cause an eventual oxygen depletion problem. The dead algae sink to the bottom of the pond and, through the action of the oxygen-consuming decomposition process, oxygen depletion results. For this reason, treatment of ponds during summer months is dangerous unless ample surface agitation is provided.

Another example is provided by medication of aquaria. In home aquaria that have been in operation for a few months, gravel and other filter media develop a flora of nitrifying bacteria that functionally convert ammonia to nitrates. Collins *et al.* (1975) have shown that methylene blue, a commonly used parasiticide in home aquaria, will inhibit the nitrifying bacteria, leading to accumulation of ammonia and nitrites.

5. Type of Culture System

Fish culture systems can include individual aquaria, series of aquaria having a common central filtration unit, large vats, ponds, earthen or cement raceways, and fish cages or baskets floating in a freshwater pond or marine environment.

The selection of a particular drug may be limited by the culture system. For example, antibiotic powder may be added directly to small vats as a treatment for bacterial diseases; in contrast, pond-reared channel catfish or trout reared in raceways must be treated for bacterial problems by medicated feed.

6. Method of Administration

Depending on the specific diagnosis and culture system, fish can be treated in various ways. These are discussed next.

a. Localized Treatment. An example is the removal of a tumorous growth from an ornamental fish followed by topical disinfection. Localized ulcers can be topically disinfected using a suitable disinfectant on a swab.

b. Injection. Generally, drugs are injected in larger aquarium fish with signs suggestive of bacterial disease such as ulcerations or hemorrhages. Antibiotic injection may be indicated when fish are handled during spawning to prevent deaths from stress-induced generalized bacterial diseases.

c. Dips and Baths. A dip—immersion of fish for a short period of time (15–30 sec) in a relatively concentrated solution of drug—is frequently used to rid fish of external parasites. A bath usually suggests that fish be exposed to the medicant for a longer period of time (15–60 min). However, guidelines cannot be strict, because fish already weakened by disease may be able to withstand only a 10-min bath. Baths and dips are frequently used in conjunction with treatment of fish prior to shipment or after transfer. Generally, fish are allowed to acclimate during the postshipping period prior to a dip or bath treatment.

d. Flush Treatment. In cases where the fish culture system utilizes a continual flow of water such as in a trout hatchery, the addition of a concentrated solution of chemical at the water inlet without severely curtailing the normal flow constitutes a flush treatment.

e. Indefinite Treatment. The term "indefinite" regarding treatment time is an accurate description of the common therapeutic method of adding a chemical to a culture system where there is no significant inflow or outflow of water, such as in a pond or aquarium. In such treatments, especially those involving ponds, the dosage must be accurately determined and the environmental consequences must be carefully assessed, because rapid removal of the drug is impossible. Millions of fish have been inadvertently killed because of dosage miscalculations. Deleterious secondary effects on the environment have included oxygen depletion problems. For example, formalin can be used in a pond at 15 to 25 ppm for external parasites. However, if used during the summer months, it can lead to an oxygen depletion; formalin apparently interacts chemically with oxygen as well as accelerating the use of oxygen by killing planktonic growth resulting in the utilization of oxygen by decomposition. In aquarium systems, however, the clinician can exert some control over the termination of a long-term treatment. For example, if a 50-gallon aquarium is medicated with 25 ppm of formalin for the treatment of external parasites, the treatment can be terminated at will by changing water and/or filtering water with activated carbon, which removes organic compounds.

The term "indefinite" also suggests that the effective dosage over a period of time is decreased by combination or adsorption with organic detritus, bacteria, and other planktonic organisms.

f. Oral Treatment. Food fish are usually treated with antibiotics by the oral route; antibiotic-supplemented fish feeds are available commercially. Many medicants can be mixed with food to meet a particular need. These can include common anthelminthics such as di-*n*-butyl tin oxide or antiprotozoicides such as metronidazole. In some cases, brood fish can be administered drugs by balling gun.

D. Common Therapeutic Agents Used in Parasite Control

In this section, commonly used chemicals and drugs used in food fish culture and home aquaria will be covered, with emphasis on the best indicated uses for each drug. Descriptions of specific parasites can be found in other publications (Brown and Gratzek, 1980).

1. Acriflavine

Acriflavine has been used as a bacteriostatic and antiparasitic agent by both food and tropical fish farmers. It has been used specifically in transporting tropical fish or hauling fish, where it is used at 3 to 5 ppm in water. For aquarium usage, it may be one of the more effective drugs for the dinoflagellate *Oodinium;* however, acriflavine imparts a yellow color to water that is difficult to remove. Acriflavine is not used in commercial trout or catfish production because of its high cost.

2. Calcium Hydroxide

Calcium hydroxide (slaked or hydrated lime) is commonly used as a pond disinfectant after draining. It is used at the rate of 1000 to 2500 lb/acre.

3. Copper Sulfate

Copper sulfate is an effective algicide and has Food and Drug Administration (FDA) approval. It is not approved for use in food fish, but it is known to be an effective external parasiticide. In marine aquaria it has been shown to be effective for the prevention and treatment of two external protozoan parasites, *Cryptocaryon irritans* and *Oodinium*. One disadvantage to its use is its toxicity. Dosage must be regulated between 0.25 and 3 ppm of copper ions depending on the hardness of the water. Under soft water conditions, more copper ions are available. In marine aquaria Blasiola (1978) recommends a 10-day treatment period keeping the copper ion level between 0.115 and 0.15 ppm. According to Blasiola (personal communication), the copper ion concentration can be brought up to the upper limit of 0.18 ppm, but as the concentration nears 0.20 ppm, such marine fish as clownfish (Amphiprion), lionfish (Pterois), and certain butterflies (Chaetodon) will show signs of toxicity. Under practice conditions in which very valuable fish are being medicated, the use of a copper test kit on a daily basis to monitor dose is mandatory.

4. Di-n-Butyl Tin Oxide

This chemical has been in use for years for the treatment of helminth parasites found in the intestines of fish. It has been used successfully for tapeworms and could be effective against nematodes and acanthocephalans. Intestinal helminth infestations appear to be well tolerated by fish, and justification of treatment of food fish for optimal growth appears to be an open question. In aquarium systems, especially with marine fish, a cleansing therapeutic regimen for intestinal roundworms, tapeworms, and nematodes is advisable prior to stocking. Di-*n*-butyl tin oxide has not been shown definitely to be the best possible medicant for use in aquarium systems; however, it has been used at 0.3% in food for a period of 5 days. The chemical has not been approved for use in food fish by the FDA. Other drugs developed in recent years, such as levamisole, may also be useful for intestinal parasites. However, costs of developing FDA clearance for fish use may not be economically feasible.

5. Formalin

Formalin has been used for years to treat external parasites of fish, including ciliates (*Trichodina, Ichthyophthirius*), flagellates (*Ichthyobodo*), and monogenetic trematodes. Formalin is 37% formaldehyde by weight, and is supplied with 15% methanol to retard the development of paraformaldehyde, which is toxic to fish. Storage at temperatures below 40°F (5°C) will enhance the development of paraformaldehyde, which can be detected as a white precipitate at the bottom of a container. Dosages are based on the assumption that formalin is 100% active. Formalin is commonly used as a bath treatment and as an indefinite treatment. As a bath, the dosage is commonly between 125 and 250 ppm. Bath treatments should utilize a system where water can be flushed quickly; alternatively, fish can be removed from the bath. This treatment is very effective, but overtreatment is a problem if fish are not continually observed for signs of stress. Weaker fish may show signs of stress before stronger fish do during bath treatments, and the former should be removed immediately. At temperatures higher than 70°F (21°C), lower dosages (125–150 ppm) must be used because of the increased toxicity. Treatment should be terminated immediately at the first signs of stress, which can include surfacing, erratic swimming, loss of response to external stimuli, and attempts to jump out of the bath. Indefinite treatments for ponds or closed aquarium systems are commonly used at dosages between 15 and 25 ppm. Because formalin can remove oxygen from water, aeration is always recommended during and after treatment. Formalin has FDA approval for use on food fish.

6. Malachite Green

Malachite green has been used for control of fungus and external protozoan parasites. It is not approved for use in food fish by the FDA because it has been shown to be teratogenic. Malachite green is widely used in the aquarium industry for *Ichthyophthirius* infestations and for fungus. A very popular use is for controlling fungus development on fish eggs, where it is used as a 15–30-sec dip at 67 ppm. As an indefinite treatment, it is effective against external parasites at 0.1 ppm. Malachite green should be zinc-free for use in fish culture. Bass, bluegill, and some species of aquarium fish such as neon tetras, knife fish, and some scaleless fish are hypersensitive to normal therapeutic dosages.

7. Formalin–Malachite Green Mixtures

Mixtures of formalin and malachite green have been found to be an excellent treatment for external protozoan parasites of fish. Leteux and Meyer (1972) suggested that there was a synergistic effect when these two chemicals were used. Gilbert *et al.* (1979) demonstrated the synergistic effect in an *in vitro* system. Indefinite treatment dosages are 15–25 ppm formalin and 0.1 ppm malachite green. This formulation is particularly effective in the treatment of aquarium fish with external parasite problems. For *Ichthyophthirius,* three treatments on alternate days are recommended; other parasites such as *Ichthyobodo* or *Trichodina* can be controlled with one treatment.

8. Masoten

Masoten is an organophosphate that has been used to control external monogenetic trematodes, fish lice (*Argulus*), anchor worms, and leeches at a dosage of 0.25 ppm in freshwater. Organophosphates are inactivated by light, high water pH, and high temperature; consequently, variation in responses in various water systems may be encountered. In marine water systems where the pH of the water is maintained between 7.8 and 8.3, the drug is quickly inactivated, thus requiring saltwater aquaria dosages to be doubled to 0.5 ppm. Drug inactivation may also occur in freshwater ponds where, as a result of algae respiration, water pH in late afternoons may reach 9.0. Ponds should therefore be treated in the mornings. Curators of public aquaria have used Masoten with mixed results; apparently, some species of fish are adversely affected and develop central nervous system disturbances. Another problem is the development of resistant strains of parasites. Goven et al. (1980b) showed that monogenetic trematodes from a commercial goldfish farm were resistant to high levels of organophosphates. In pet supply stores, organophosphates are sold under a variety of trade names. Masoten is not approved for use on food fish.

There appears to be a need for a medicant that will circumvent the resistance problem. Goven and Amend (1982) used mebendazole–trichlorfon combinations for removal of monogenetic trematodes from the skin and gills of fish. They reported that this combination was toxic for channel catfish but was safe for other species tested in various areas within the United States.

9. Methylene Blue

Methylene blue has been used in the aquarium industry as an external parasiticide; however, formalin–malachite green mixtures are superior. One serious drawback to the use of methylene blue in home aquaria is that it has been shown to destroy nitrifying bacteria in filter systems, resulting in death of fish from nitrite toxicity. It has been used as an egg dip for fungus problems. Many importers consider methylene blue to be the chemical of choice for treatment of newly arrived fish, possibly because of its low toxicity to stressed fish. Other importers favor methylene blue because it imparts a very dark blue color to water, subduing light and assisting in acclimatization of fish. Some shippers of fish add both acriflavine and methylene blue to shipping water. A claim has been made but not verified that this chemical combination reduces postshipment losses caused by shipping stress.

10. Metronidazole

Hexamita is an intestinal flagellate found in food fish such as trout, and in ornamental fish including goldfish, angelfish, discus fish, gouramis, and a variety of cichlids. Metronidazole and metronidazole-related compounds under the trade names Flagyl, Ipropran, and Emtryl have been used to treat aquarium species where infections can be associated with debility and mortality. Our laboratory has consistently found that treatment of water with 5 ppm of active drug will rid fish of *Hexamita*. In our experience, there appears to be no effect on ciliate parasites infecting the skin or gills. Fish farmers report that Ipropran has less tendency to cloud water than other preparations.

11. Potassium Permanganate

Potassium permanganate is used extensively in pond culture. For aquaculture it is not classified as a pesticide but rather as an oxidizing agent used to reduce excessive accumulation of organic material and algae. The chemical is also used to treat external problems in pond fish. Its dosage in ponds varies according to the organic load in the pond. As mentioned previously, if the organic load is excessive, the oxidizing capacity of the chemical will be exhausted prior to parasiticidal activity. It has been suggested (Plumb, 1979) that in most situations a dosage of 2 ppm should be safe. Retreatment may be required if the organic load of the water is very high. If the normal red color that potassium permanganate imparts to water turns yellow within 12 hr, retreatment is indicated. With potentially toxic drugs such as potassium permanganate, biological tests must be done in pails filled with pond water to assess both toxicity and effectiveness.

12. Salt (Sodium Chloride)

Salt is probably the oldest general treatment for fish. It has been used in hauling tanks (Long *et al.*, 1977). A 3% salt dip has been used as a bath treatment for removal of external parasites. Treatment time should not exceed 30 min and should be terminated at the first signs of stress. The use of salt in cases where fish have been subjected to stress may be indicated as an osmoregulatory enhancer, because osmoregulation is severely affected during stress periods. For this purpose, a 0.3% salt concentration is recommended; however, some species of ornamental catfish, such as *Corydoras* spp., cannot tolerate this level of salt. Studies in our laboratory have suggested that channel catfish with open ulcers show a positive clinical response to 0.8% salt compared to control fish in freshwater. The results further indicate that this level of salt was not tolerated beyond a 14-day period. The use of salt is recommended more for its osmoregulatory-enhancing effect than for its antiparasitic effect. Whether the use of balanced salt solutions would be of additional benefit is a question worthy of further investigation.

E. Antimicrobials Used in Control of Bacterial Diseases

At present only a few antimicrobials are approved for food fish use; however, there appears to be no restriction for medicants including antimicrobials for pet fish.

1. Antibiotics

Sulfamerazine and oxytetracycline are currently approved for use in food fish. A nitrofuran, Furanace, is approved for nonfood fish use. In fish culture, antibiotics may be incorporated into feed, injected, or given as a bath treatment.

Antibiotic-supplemented feeds are recommended for bacterial disease problems or for use after handling and shipping to prevent stress-induced systemic bacterial disease. In commercial preparations, terramycin is incorporated at the rate of 84 to 117 gm of active antibiotic per 100 lb of feed. It is important to keep fish on medicated feed for 1 to 14 days to avoid emergence of antibiotic-resistant strains of bacteria.

On an experimental basis, our laboratory has incorporated a variety of antibiotics into aquarium fish food at the rate of 25 mg of antibiotic per 10 gm of food. Tetracyclines, chloramphenicol, sulfa drugs, and nitrofurans were studied. No adverse reactions among fish were observed when fed over a period of a week. Unfortunately, the inherent problem of feeding medicated food to fish during a disease episode is that sick fish seldom eat.

Bath treatments are particularly useful in various segments of aquaculture. Antibiotics are regularly used by the pet fish industry during transportation of fish. Fish kept in vats are easily medicated with a variety of antibiotics. In a study of antibiotic adsorption by channel catfish held in antibiotic baths, Nusbaum and Shotts (1981) exposed fish to therapeutic levels of chloramphenicol, erythromycin, Furanace, and oxytetracycline. They fould that after 5 hr of exposure, Furanace and oxytetracycline were adsorbed by the fish in proportion to the antimicrobial concentration in the water. Minimal inhibitory concentrations of Furanace and oxytetracycline were measured in blood 5 hr after exposure, but minimal inhibitory concentrations were not reached using either of the two antibiotics alone. Results further suggested that of the antimicrobials studied, both Furanace and tetracyclines gave good clinical responses. In an earlier study, Shotts *et al.* (1976) clearly demonstrated tetracycline resistance of isolates of *Aeromonas hydrophila* from both imported fish and fish from local pet stores given different antibiotics. They were further able to demonstrate the occurrence of plasmids imparting resistance to tetracycline in 25.5 and 1.2% of isolates of *A. hydrophila* from Southeast Asia and South America, respectively. This difference in resistance appears to be related to the fact that South American fish are caught in the wild and are shipped to foreign destinations in as short a time as possible, whereas fish from Hong Kong, Taiwan, and Singapore are intensively cultured and probably exposed to periodic doses of tetracycline. The continual use of tetracycline and antibiotics in general in any fish culture establishment has the potential of selecting antibiotic-resistant bacteria that could be pathogenic for fish.

Shotts et al. (1976) also demonstrated that when tetracyclines were used as "cure-alls" in pet shops over an extended period of time, there was a significant occurrence of tetracycline-resistant strains of *A. hydrophila.*

Antibiotic resistance can be circumvented in aquaculture systems by periodically changing to a different antimicrobial. This poses no problem in the pet fish market but would not be possible for food fish under FDA regulations, because only oxytetracycline and sulfamerazine are approved for food fish use. Various other antibiotics have been used as bath treatments with excellent results, including kanamycin (Gilmartin et al., 1976), oxolinic acid (Endo et al., 1973), and potentiated sulfonamides (McCarthy et al., 1974). Erythromycin may be useful in preventing the vertical spread of the gram-positive *Renibacterium salmoninarum,* the causative agent of kidney disease in salmon. Eggs dipped in solutions of erythromycin adsorb the antibiotic, but there is some question as to the efficacy of the treatment in preventing kidney disease (Meyer and Schnick, 1981). At present, a New Animal Drug Application has been filed with the FDA for a potentiated sulfa drug to treat enteric redmouth (ERM) disease of salmonid fish.

2. Quaternary Ammonium Compounds

Quaternary ammonium compounds have been used in aquaculture for disinfection and also for treating external bacterial infections. The compounds have proved to be useful in trout and salmon culture for the treatment of bacterial gill disease, which is associated with the gram-negative bacterium *Flexibacter columnaris.* Tropical fish farmers find quaternary ammonium compounds to be effective in the treatment of columnaris disease, which is also caused by *F. columnaris.* The dosage recommendation for bath treatments using quaternary ammonium compounds such as Roccal is 2 ppm as a 1-hr bath. Quaternary ammonium compounds are not registered for use for food fish. Apparently the difficulty in developing analytical methods for residue studies has impeded research required for registration (Meyer and Schnick, 1981).

Another chemical that appears to have antibacterial activity against *F. columnaris* is Diquat, a commonly used herbicide. Studies in our laboratory have shown that Diquat will inhibit the *in vitro* growth of *F.*

columnaris but not *A. hydrophila*. In practical use situations, Diquat as an indefinite treatment at 5 ppm has been effective in treating *F. columnaris* infections.

There is presently a need for the registration and clearance of drugs and chemicals for food fish use. In 1976, Meyer and Schnick emphasized the need for research for fish medicants that would be approved by the FDA. A principal stumbling block to obtaining drug approval is the unwillingness of industrial sponsors to provide support for the research required for registration.

F. Vaccines Used in Disease Control

The reader interested in an in-depth review of the current status of fish immunology, vaccines, and serological procedures is referred to *Developments in Biological Standardization* (International Association of Biological Standardization, 1981). It has been shown that fish possess both nonspecific and specific humoral and cell-mediated immune mechanisms that are similar to but not identical to immune systems of higher vertebrates. Sites of antibody production in fish are primarily the head kidney, thymus, spleen, and, in some fish, the intestines and gonads (Marchalonis, 1977). The diversity of leukocytes in fish is essentially similar to that of higher vertebrates (Ellis, 1977). From a functional basis, there appears to be T- and B-cell activity, but there is no clear differentiation of lymphocytes into T and B cells (Manning, 1980).

In fish culture, the development of vaccines depends on several important considerations. The need for the development of a vaccine is dependent on whether the disease is sufficiently widespread to be of real economic importance or could be controlled more effectively and less expensively by the use of chemotherapeutics. Fish vaccines, like those for higher vertebrates, must be developed and tested by the U.S. Department of Agriculture for efficacy prior to release.

That fish can be immunized has been known for some time. Hines and Spira (1974) showed that sublethal doses of the protozoan *Ichthyophthirius multifiliis* rendered fish immune to the disease ichthyophthiriasis on subsequent exposure to the parasite. Similarly, Bauer (1953), Beckert and Allison (1964), and Esch (1977) reported that fish treated for ichthyophthiriasis recovered and were temporarily refractory to reinfection. On the basis of the observations of Bauer (1953) and Beckert and Allison (1964), work toward the *in vitro* cultivation of *I. multifiliis* was initiated at our laboratory in 1970 utilizing fish cell culture systems. Failure to achieve *in vitro* replication of the parasite, which would have been suitable for vaccination trials, led to the hypothesis that fish could be immunized against *I. multifiliis* with closely related free-living and cultivatable nonpathogenic ciliates such as *Tetrahymena* spp. Using *Tetrahymena pyriformis*, Goven et al. (1980a) conclusively demonstrated that both ciliary and whole-cell preparations of *T. pyriformis* were able to confer immunity to channel catfish on subsequent challenge with *I. multifiliis*. The serological relationship between the two organisms was demonstrated by using various immunological tests *in vitro*. Rabbit anti-*Tetrahymena* serum was shown to immobilize both *I. multifiliis* tomites and *Tetrahymena* organisms. Serological relatedness was also shown by indirect fluorescent microscopy and by passive hemagglutination (Goven et al., 1981).

The work in progress on immunization of fish against ichthyophthiriasis by our research group has emphasized the need for standard challenge doses of tomites and the importance of the fish culture system in evaluation of the efficacy of the *Tetrahymena*-based vaccine (Dickerson et al., 1981). It appears that in small aquaria where fish are crowded, the parasite load can develop to a point where immunity can be shown only as a delay in death, whereas in open systems where tomites do not accumulate, death can be prevented. Most previous experiments with *I. multifiliis* have utilized quantitated amounts of antigen administered by injection. Experiments by Wolf (1981) using trout fry have suggested that immersion of fish in a culture of *Tetrahymena* organisms is adequate for immunization.

G. Bacterins Used in Disease Control

In aquaculture the need for a bacterin is dependent on whether a disease can be controlled by management practices alone or whether prophylactic treatments are as effective as vaccination. A very important feature of immunization of fish is the route of administration of the bacterin. In aquaculture, millions of fish are involved, and the stress induced by individual handling and injection would cancel any benefits of immunization. Additionally, the time and labor involved would be considerable. Incorporation of specific antigens against fish bacterial pathogens into fish food was attempted by Klontz (1966) using a cell wall extract of *Aeromonas salmonicida*. Under controlled conditions, 58% of the nonvaccinated fish died, as opposed to none of the vaccinated fish when subjected to natural challenge 90 days postvaccination. At present, no orally administered vaccines are available, possibly because of problems of antigen stability when mixed with food and the difficulty of regulating dosages.

Amend and Fender (1976) found that bovine serum albumin was

directly adsorbed into the bloodstream of trout if the fish were first immersed in a solution of either urea or salt. The primary route of bovine serum albumin entry into the fish was through the lateral line system. Presumably the mechanism of action was the initial dehydrating effect of the urea or salt solution followed by a rehydration with fluid containing bovine serum albumin. Croy and Amend (1977) used the hyperosmotic infiltration technique to immunize sockeye salmon (*Oncorhynchus nerka*) against vibriosis. They were able to demonstrate that this mass immunization technique was as effective as vaccination by injection.

Comparing the hyperosmotic infiltration technique with direct immersion of fish into a bacterin-containing solution, Antipa *et al.* (1980) demonstrated that the hyperosmotic infiltration method was not required for effective vaccination. Their results suggested that there were no differences in efficacy between the two methods, provided bacterins of sufficient potency were used; if diluted vaccines were used, the hyperosmotic immersion technique was slightly superior to the direct immersion method. The authors also observed that the hyperosmotic system resulted in greater stress to fish, providing additional support for use of the direct immersion method for mass immunization.

Gould *et al.* (1978) developed a method of vaccination utilizing a liquid spray apparatus that operates at pressures up to 7.0kg/cm^2. They demonstrated that a formalin-killed *Vibrio anguillarum* vaccine was both antigenic and immunogenic when sprayed directly on coho salmon and rainbow trout. Fish vaccinated by this technique, referred to as spray or shower vaccination, had higher levels of immunity against *V. anguillarum* than fish vaccinated by the oral method.

At this time, fish vaccines are being commercially produced primarily for bacterial problems associated with trout and salmon production. The vaccines are available as injectable, immersion, and spray preparations. Included in the following paragraphs are brief descriptions of diseases for which vaccines are available.

1. *Furunculosis*

Furunculosis is the common name for an acute to chronic disease caused by the bacterium, *A. salmonicida,* The name "furunculosis" refers to a boil-like condition that has been commonly associated with brook trout. In trout-raising areas of the United States, furunculosis is one of the principal disease entities on some fish farms. The disease is almost always associated with some stress situation such as overcrowding, low oxygen, or excessive water flow rates in rearing troughs. In the Hagerman Valley of Idaho, the condition can be seen in all ages of fish. According to R. Busch (personal communication), the lesion most characteristic of the disease in rainbow trout fry at 58°F is an external ulcer located ventral to the pectoral fin immediately adjacent to the sinus venosus of the heart. Studies conducted by Busch suggest that the bacteria colonize in the wall of the sinus venosus and extend directly to adjacent muscle. The vaccine is available only in injectable form. Use is therefore limited to injection of brood fish.

2. *Ulcer Disease of Goldfish*

In the years from 1977 to 1982, goldfish producers in Europe and the United States encountered a disease in all age groups of goldfish that is characterized by external hemorrhages and ulcers. The causative agent of this disease in goldfish was characterized by Shotts *et al.* (1980) as a strain of *Aeromonas salmonicida* that had distinct differences from strains isolated from salmonids. The disease is responsible for major losses of market-sized and brood fish in commercial goldfish hatcheries. The vaccine is available for injection only; consequently, its use for goldfish entering the retail trade is limited. The vaccine would be indicated for brood fish or fish selected as replacement brood stock. Our experience in treating infected fish in retail outlets suggests that one intraperitoneal injection of chloramphenicol (25 mg/kg) will ameliorate the disease and lead to full recovery.

3. *Enteric Redmouth Disease*

The disease of salmonids that is referred to as ERM is caused by a member of the Enterobactereaceae *Yersinia ruckevii*. In trout-producing areas of the northwestern United States, the disease ranges from acute to chronic, depending on the water temperature (R. Busch, personal communication). At 16 to 18°C, 2–5-gm trout may show no external lesions except ecchymotic hemorrhages at the bases of the fins. Internally, petechial hemorrhages may be seen on the liver and mesentery. A common lesion is flaccidity and hemmorhage of the lower intestine. A vaccine is available that can be administered by immersion or spray.

4. *Vibriosis*

Vibriosis is a potential problem whenever fish are cultured in marine or brackish water. *Vibrio anguillarum* causes the disease in cultured salmon especially when the fish are confined in large pens. Trout are especially susceptible to the disease when cultured in pens located in seawater or brackish water. Cultured eel are also susceptible (Chart and Munn, 1980), as are other important commercially raised fish such as milkfish (*Chanos chanos*) (Song *et al.*, 1980). Roberts and

Shepherd (1974) described the clinical picture in salmonids as being initiated by a brief period of inappetence. Dying fish are dark in color. On postmortem examination, internal organs appear hemorrhagic, and spleens are swollen. In chronic cases, ulcers develop deep in the musculature toward the bases of the fins. Immersion and spray vaccines are available.

5. *Present Status of Bacterins for Warm Water Fish*

Bacterial problems in cultured channel catfish invariably follow periods of stress such as handling, hauling, or suboptimal pond conditions. *Aeromonas hydrophila* is commonly isolated from diseased fish, causing a disease known as hemorrhagic septicemia. Clinical signs includes hemorrhages, exophthalmia, skin ulceration, and fin erosion. Because *A. hydrophila* is common in nature and its potential as a pathogen is dependent on avoidance of stress, it is doubtful whether a vaccine for *A. hydrophila* would be required. Undoubtedly there are some aquatic systems where stress conditions cannot be easily avoided, such as modified recirculating systems. In such unique situations, or in a situation where valuable brook stock or replacements need protection, vaccination may prove useful.

Flexibacter columnaris is the causative agent of "columnaris disease." Like *A. hydrophila,* it is found in nature, especially in water with high amounts of organic materials. The disease affects fish of all ages and is invariably associated with stress. Characteristics of the disease include whitish surface lesions of the fins, trunk, and mouth. The involved areas progress to frank ulcers that frequently harbor secondary bacterial pathogens and fungi. Columnaris disease is very common after transportation of fish. Generally, producers of fingerlings are aware of this and recommend food supplemented with antibiotics during the critical posthauling period. Columnaris disease can be a problem in high-production ponds, where the organic load and presumably bacterial proliferation are high. Vaccine trials under such conditions are being conducted by a commercial firm (G. Tebbit, personal communication).

H. THE POTENTIAL FOR VIRUS VACCINES

Readers interested in a comprehensive overview of fish viruses are referred to Pilcher and Fryer (1980), who have reviewed the known and suspected virus diseases of fish. In the United States there are three viruses that are of economic importance in aquaculture: channel catfish virus disease (CCVD), infectious pancreatic necrosis virus of salmonids (IPN), and infectious hematopoietic necrosis virus of salmonids (IHN). In Europe, viral hemorrhagic septicemia virus (VHS) causes a devastating disease of salmonids.

1. Channel Catfish Virus Disease

Fijan et al. (1970) first isolated CCVD virus from channel catfish fingerlings showing the following external signs of disease: hemorrhagic areas on the fins and body, ascites, pale gills with petechiations, and exophthalmia. Plumb et al. (1975) have shown that catfish fingerlings beyond the age of 3 months have a sharply reduced susceptibility to virus infection. Plumb (1973) had earlier demonstrated the restrictive effect that low water temperature had on mortalities and suggested that CCVD might be controlled by lowering ambient water temperature for rearing fry if sufficient well water was available. Observing that there were significant differences in mortality rates of fish from pond to pond during an active virus infection, he suggested that the differences in fish mortality rates might be explained by variation in the proliferation of the secondary bacterial invader, *F. columnaris*.

Channel catfish can be immunized against CCVD. Noga et al. (1978) showed that CCVD virus passed 59 times in a kidney cell line of the walking catfish (*Claria bactrachus*) was not pathogenic for channel catfish (*Ictarlus punctatus*), and the passed virus induced protection to immunized fish on challenge with wild-type virus.

At this point it appears that whereas CCVD may be an important disease where it strikes, the disease is not widespread enough to warrant control by vaccination. Because relatively simple and quick serological methods have been developed for the detection of channel catfish virus antibodies (Gratzek et al., 1973), a basic control measure would be to select brood stock without virus neutralization titers. The only known carriers of the disease are channel catfish. Plumb et al. (1981) demonstrated viral antigen in ovarian tissues from suspect carrier fish.

2. Infectious Pancreatic Necrosis Virus

Infectious pancreatic necrosis virus (IPN) was first described by McGonigle (1941) as an acute catarrhal enteritis. Today the virus is widespread throughout the trout-producing areas of the United States and Canada (Scherrer, 1973; Wolf, 1976).

The disease characteristically affects fry or fingerlings. Signs of the disease include corkscrew swimming, darkening in color, abdominal distension, hemorrhages at bases of fins, and occasional exophthalmia. On postmortem examination, petechiations are frequently found in the pyloric–cecal area. The digestive tract is devoid of food and frequently contains clear to opaque mucus. An outbread is confirmed by virus isolation and identification. The efficacy of vaccination of trout with either killed or modified live virus vaccines has been demonstrated (Hill et al., 1980), but there appear to be intrinsic problems that may weigh against the practicality of vaccination. The disease is known to affect juvenile fish until they are about 6 weeks of age, after which time susceptibility greatly decreases. To be successful a vaccination program would have to be initiated at a very early age, even though fish may not yet be immunocompetent (D. Amend, personal communication). Furthermore, it appears that there is considerable antigenic variation between strains of virus isolated from epizootics. Nicholson and Pochebit (1981) found that isolates of IPN fall into three serological groups by neutralization kinetic analysis. Obviously, a successful vaccine would have to include the principal serotypes.

Present management practices in a suspected epizootic generally include destruction of fry, disinfection, and restocking with eggs from virus-free brood stock. Amend (1976), who reviewed methods for the control of viral disease of salmonids, emphasized that procurement of specific pathogen-free eggs or fish is a necessity for avoidance of the disease. Methods for determining the absence of infectious pancreatic necrosis virus have been established (Amend and Wedemeyer, 1970). It appears that at least for the immediate future, methods other than vaccination will be more cost effective for the control of IPN.

3. Infectious Hematopoietic Necrosis Virus

The disease caused by infectious hematopoietic necrosis virus (IHN) is found in trout- and salmon-producing areas of the United States. The disease is characterized by a sudden increase in mortality accompanied by darkening in color, anemia, exophthalmia, and abdominal distension. Hemorrhages are frequently found at the bases of fins and in mesenteric tissue (Rucker et al., 1953; Ross et al., 1960). Histopathological changes occur in kidney, spleen, and pancreas. The disease is spread from adult carrier fish by virus contamination of eggs. Recommendations for control, with specific reference to Oregon but with potential universal application, are reviewed by Mulcahy et al. (1980). Central to their recommendations is the stocking of virus-free brood stock for production purposes.

The immunization of salmon and trout with modified live virus vaccines has been demonstrated by Fryer et al. (1976) and Amend and Smith (1974). The desirability of vaccination under some circumstances lies in the fact that IHN virus, unlike IPN virus, has the capacity to kill market-size fish, representing considerable financial losses (R. Busch, personal communication). An obvious problem in the development of a modified live virus vaccine is that it may have the potential to revert to the pathogenicity characteristic of wild-type virus. Another problem of a modified live virus vaccine for fish is that its potential pathogenicity must be determined for nontarget species in river systems receiving hatchery outflow water.

4. Viral Hemorrhagic Septicemia

Viral hemorrhagic septicemia (VHS) is the most important virus disease of trout in Europe. Losses in Europe have been estimated at between 20,000 and 30,000 tons of fish per year. De Kinkelin and Bearzotti (1981) have shown that immunization with a thermoresistant variant of the virus is feasible. The disease is particularly devastating because fish do not develop a natural resistance with age as they do with IPN virus and, to a degree, with IHN virus. Because VHS is considered to be an exotic disease, its entry into the United States is prevented by importation restrictions of living trout or fresh-killed products.

References

Ahne, W. (ed.) (1980). "Fish Diseases," pp. 3–29. Springer-Verlag, New York.
Amend, D. F. (1976). *J. Fish. Res. Board Can.* **33,** 1059–1066.
Amend, D. F., and Fender, D. C. (1976). *Science* **192,** 793–794.
Amend, D. F., and Smith, L. (1974). *J. Fish. Res. Board Can.* **31,** 1371–1378.
Amend, D. F., and Wedemeyer, G. (1970). *U.S. Bur. Sport Fish. Wildl.*, **FDL-27,** 1–4.
Amlacher, E. (1970). "Textbook of Fish Diseases" (transl. by D. A. Conroy and R. L. Herman). TFH Publications, Jersey City, New Jersey.
Anderson, D. P. (1974). "Fish Immunology, Book 4, Diseases of Fishes" (S. F. Snieszko and H. R. Axelrod, eds.). T.F.H. Publications, Jersey City.
Antipa, R., Gould, R., and Amend, D. F. (1980). *J. Fish Dis.* **3,** 161–165.
Axelrod, H. R. (1971). "The Aquarium Fish Industry—1971." TFH Publications, Jersey City, New Jersey.
Bauer, O. N. (1953). *Dokl. Akad. Nauk SSSR* **93,** 377–379.
Beckert, H., and Allison, R. (1964). *Proc. Southeast. Assoc. Game Fish Commissioners* **18,** 438–441.
Blasiola, G. C. (1978). *Mar. Aquarist* **8,** 50–59.
Boyd, C. E. (1979). "Water Quality in Warmwater Fish Ponds." Auburn University Agricultural Experiment Station, Auburn, Alabama.
Brown, E. E., and Gratzek, J. B. (1980). "Fish Farming Handbook." Avi Publ. Co., Westport, Connecticut.
Bullock, G. L. (1971). "Identification of Fish Pathogenic Bacteria. Book 2B. Diseases of Fishes" (S. F. Snieszko and H. R. Axelrod, eds.). T.F.H. Publications, Jersey City.
Bullock, G. L., Conroy, D. A., and Snieszko, S. F. (1971). "Bacterial Disease of Fishes. Book 2A. Diseases of Fishes" (S. F. Snieszko and H. R. Axelrod, eds.). T.F.H. Publications, Jersey City.
Chart, H., and Munn, C. B. (1980). *In* "Fish Diseases" (W. Ahne, ed.), pp. 39–44. Springer-Verlag, Berlin and New York.

Collins, M. T., Gratzek, J. B., Dawe, D. L., and Nemetz, T. G. (1975). *J. Fish. Res. Board Can.* **32**, 2033–2037.
Croy, T. R., and Amend, D. F. (1977). *Aquaculture* **12**, 317–325.
de Kinkelin, P., and Bearzotti, M. (1981). *Dev. Biol. Stand.* **39**, 431–439.
Dickerson, H. W., Dawe, D. L., Gratzek, J. B., Brown, J., and Pyle, S. W. (1981). *Dev. Biol. Stand.* **49**, 331–336.
Dulin, M. P. (1976). "Diseases of Marine Aquarium Fishes." T.F.H. Publications, Neptune, New Jersey.
Ellis, A. E. (1977). *J. Fish Biol.* **11**, 453–491.
Endo, T., Ogishima, K., Hayasaka, H., Kaneko, S., and Ohshima, S. (1973). *Bull. Jpn. Soc. Sci. Fish.* **39**, 165–171.
Esch, G. W. (1977). "Regulation of Parasite Populations." Academic Press, New York.
Esch, G. W., and Hazen, T. C. (1978). *DOE Symp. Ser.* **48**, 331–363.
Fijan, N. N., Wellborn, T. L., Jr., and Naftel, J. P. (1970). *Tech. Pap. Bur. Sport Fish. Wildl.* **43**, 1–11.
Fryer, J. L., Rohovec, J. S., Tebbit, G. L., McMichael, J.S., and Pilcher, K. S. (1976). *Fish Pathol.* **10**, 155–164.
Galili, N. (1980). *Cell. Immunol.* **50**, 440–444.
Gilbert, J. P., Gratzek, J. B., and Brown, J. (1979). *J. Fish Dis.* **2**, 191–196.
Gillis, S. (1979). *J. Immunol.* **123**, 1624–1631.
Gilmartin, W. G., Camp, B. J., and Lewis, D. H. (1976). *J. Wildl. Dis.* **12**, 555–559.
Gould, R. W., O'Leary, P. J., Garrison, R. L., Rohovec, J. S., and Fryer, J. L. (1978). *Fish Pathol.* **13**, 63–68.
Goven, B. A., and Amend, D. F. (1982). *J. Fish Biol.* **20**, 373–378.
Goven, B. A., Dawe, D. L., and Gratzek, J. B. (1980a). *J. Fish Biol.* **17**, 311–316.
Goven, B. A., Gilbert, J. P., and Gratzek, J. B. (1980b). *J. Wildl. Dis.* **16**, 343–346.
Goven, B. A., Dawe, D. L., and Gratzek, J. B. (1981). *Dev. Comp. Immunol.* **5**, 283–289.
Gratzek, J. B. (1981). *In* "Proceedings of the Fourth Kal Kan Symposium for the Treatment of Small Animal Diseases," Kal Kan Foods Inc., Vernon, California (L. D. Howell, ed.), pp. 25–39. Columbus, Ohio.
Gratzek, J. B. (1981). *J. Small Anim. Pract.* **22**, 345–366.
Gratzek, J. B., McGlamery, M. H., Dawe, D. L., and Scott, T. (1973). *J. Fish. Res. Board Can.* **30**, 1641–1645.
Hill, B. J., Dorson, M., and Dixon, P. F. (1980). *In* "Fish Diseases, Third COPRAQ-Session" (W. Ahne, ed.), pp. 29–36. Springer-Verlag, Berlin and New York.
Hines, R. S., and Spira, D. T. (1974). *J. Fish Biol.* **6**, 373–378.
International Association of Biological Standardization (1981). "Developments in Biological Standardization. Fish Biologics: Serodiagnostics and Vaccines," Vol. 39. Karger, Basel.
Kabata, Z. (1970). "Crustacea as Enemies of Fishes, Book 1, Diseases of Fishes" (S. F. Snieszko and H. R. Axelrod, eds.). T.F.H. Publications, Jersey City.
Kingsford, E. (1975). "Treatment of Exotic Marine Fish Diseases." Palmetto Publishing Company, St. Petersburg.
Klontz, G. W. (1966). *Resour. Publ.—Bur. Sport Fish. Wild.* **17**, 11–12.
Leteux, F., and Meyer, F. P. (1972). *Prog. Fish-Cult.* **34**, 21–26.
Letritz, E. (1969). Fish Bull. No. 107. Dept. of Fish and Game, State of California.
Levine, M., and Claman, H. (1970). *Science* **16**, 1515–1516.
Long, C. W., McComas, J. R., and Monk, B. H. (1977). *Mar. Fish. Rev.* Pap. 1255, pp. 6–9.
McCarthy, D. H., Stevenson, J. P., and Salsbury, A. W. (1974). *Aquaculture* **4**, 407–410.
McGonigle, R. H. (1941). *Trans. Am. Fish. Soc.* **70**, 297–300.

Manning, M. J. (1980). "Phylogeny of Immunological Memory." Elsevier/ North-Holland Biomedical Press, Amsterdam.
Marchalonis, J. J. (1977). "Immunity in Evolution." Arnold, London.
Meyer, F. P., and Schnick, R. A. (1976). *Proc. Southeast. Assoc. Game Fish Commissioners* **30**, 5–14.
Meyer, F. P., and Schnick, R. A. (1981). *5th Annu. Meet. Fish Health Sect. (AFS), Miss. State Univ.* p. 1–13.
Mulcahy, D. M., Tebbit, G. L., Grobert, W. J., Jr., McMichael, J. S., Winton, J. R., Hedric, R. P., Philippon-Fried, M., Pilcher, K. S., and Fryer, J. L. (1980). *Tech. Pap.*—**5504**, *Oreg. Agric. Exp. Stn.* 1–71.
National Research Council (1982). "Specialized Veterinary Manpower Needs Through 1990." A Report Prepared by the Committee On Veterinary Medical Sciences, Commission on Life Sciences. National Academy Press, Washington.
Neish, G. A. and G. C. Hughes (1980). "Fungal Diseases of Fishes, Book 6, Diseases of Fishes" (S. F. Snieszko and H. R. Axelrod, eds.). T.F.H. Publications, Jersey City.
Nicholson, B. L., and Pochebit, S. (1981). *Dev. Biol. Stand.* **39**, 35–41.
Noga, E. T., Walczak, E. M., and Hartmann, J. X. (1978). *Proc. Jt. 3rd Bienn. Fish Health Sect. 9th Annu. Midwest Fish Dis. Workshops, 1978* p. 48.
Nusbaum, K. E., and Shotts, E. B., Jr. (1981). *Can. J. Fish Aquat. Sci.* **38**, 993–996.
Pickering, A. D., ed. (1981). "Stress and Fish." Academic Press, New York.
Pilcher, K. S., and Fryer, J. L. (1980). *CRC Crit. Rev. Microbiol.* **7**, 287–364.
Plumb, J. A. (1973). *J. Fish. Res. Board Can.* **30**, 568–570.
Plumb, J. A., ed. (1979). *South. Coop. Ser. Bull.* **225**, 1–92.
Plumb, J. A., Green, O. L., Smitherman, R. O., and Pardue, G. B. (1975). *Trans. Am. Fish. Soc.* **104**, 140–143.
Plumb, J. A., Thune, R. L., and Klesius, P. H. (1981). *Dev. Biol. Stand.* **39**, 29–34.
Reichenbach-Klinke, H. H. (1977). "All About Marine Aquarium Fish Diseases" (M. P. Dulin, ed.). T.F.H. Publications, Jersey City.
Reichenbach-Klinke, H., and Elkan, E. (1965). "The Principal Diseases of Lower Vertebrates," Part I. Academic Press, New York.
Ribelin, W. E. and Migaki, G. (eds.) (1975). "The Pathology of Fishes." University of Wisconsin Press, Madison.
Roberts, R. J. (ed.) (1978). "Fish Pathology." Bailliere Tindall, London.
Roberts, R. J., and Shepherd, C. J. (1974). "Handbook of Trout and Salmon Diseases." Fishing News (Books) Ltd., Surrey, England.
Ross, A. J., Pelnar, J., and Rucker, R. R. (1960). *Trans. Am. Fish. Soc.* **89**, 160–163.
Rucker, R. R., Whipple, W. J., Parvin, J. R., and Evans, C. A. (1953). *Fish. Bull.* **54** (76), 35.
Sarig, S. (1971) "The Prevention and Treatment of Diseases of Warmwater Fishes Under Subtropical Conditions, with Special Emphasis on Intensive Fish Farming. Book 3. Diseases of Fishes" (S. F. Snieszko and H. R. Axelrod, eds.). T.F.H. Publications, Jersey City.
Scherrer, R. (1973). *EIFAC Tech. Pap.* **17**, 51.
Schubert, G. (1974). "Cure and Recognize Aquarium Fish Diseases" (transl. by C. Ahrens). TFH Publications, Jersey City, New Jersey.
Scott, P. W. (1981). *J. Small Anim. Pract.* **22**, 331–343.
Selye, H. (1973). *Am. Sci.* **61**, 692–699.
Setzer, P. A. (1974). "Pets/Supplies/Marketing," 2nd Annual State of the Pet Industry Report, pp. 42–50, Harcourt Brace Jovanovich.
Shotts, E. B., Vanderwork, V. L., and Long, W. J. (1976). *In* "Wildlife Diseases" (L. A. Page, ed.), pp. 493–501. Plenum, New York.

Shotts, E. B., Jr., Talkington, F. D., Elliott, D. G., and McCarthy, D. H. (1980). *J. Fish Dis.* **3,** 181–186.

Sindermann, C. J. (1966). " Diseases of Marine Fishes." T.F.H. Publications, Jersey City.

Sommerville, C. (1981). *J. Small Anim. Pract.* **22,** 367–376.

Song, Y., Chen, S., Kou, G., Lin, C., and Ting, Y. (1980). *In* "Reports on Fish Disease Research (III), "CAPD Fish. Ser. No.3, pp. 101–108.

Spotte, S. (1979). "Fish and Invertebrate Culture," 2nd ed. Wiley, New York.

Wedemeyer, G. A., Meyer, F. P., and Smith L. (1976). "Environmental Stress and Fish Diseases, Book 5, Diseases of Fishes" (S. F. Snieszko and H. R. Axelrod, eds.). T.F.H. Publications, Jersey City.

Wolf, K. (1976). *Fish Pathol.* **10,** 135–154.

Wolf, K. (1981). *U.S. Fish Wildl. Serv., Res. Inf. Bull.* **81-28.**

Avian Lymphoproliferative Diseases and Their Virus Associations

K. PERK

The Hebrew University of Jerusalem, Rehovot Campus, Rehovot, Israel

I. Introduction 325
II. Classification 326
III. Avian Retroviruses 327
IV. Clinical and Pathological Features 330
  A. Pathogenesis of Lymphoproliferative Disease of Turkeys 330
  B. Pathogenesis of Reticuloendotheliosis 332
  C. Pathogenesis of Avian Lymphoid Leukosis 334
  D. Pathogenesis of Marek's Disease 335
V. Epidemiology, Virology, and Oncogenesis 336
  A. Lymphoproliferative Disease Virus of Turkeys 336
  B. Reticuloendotheliosis Viruses 338
  C. Avian Lymphoid Leukosis Viruses 340
  D. Marek's Disease Herpesvirus 341
VI. Relationship of LPD to RE 342
VII. Concluding Comments 343
  References 343

I. Introduction

Avian lymphoproliferative diseases (leukosis-sarcoma, Marek's disease, reticuloendotheliosis, and lymphoproliferative disease of turkeys) are the most frequently occurring neoplasms in poultry. These diseases have important economic implications for the poultry industry and, additionally, provide model systems of great usefulness for studies in comparative and basic medicine.

Avian lymphoproliferative diseases are naturally occurring viral-induced neoplasms. The mode of infection may be horizontal, congenital, or genetic. With the developments in viral oncology and the recognition of two new disease complex entities, reticuloendotheliosis (RE) and lymphoproliferative disease of turkeys (LPD), new light has been thrown on the complicated relationships, pathogenesis, and etiology of lymphoproliferative disorders in poultry.

Because the study of RE and LPD is a relatively new field, this article will present a more comprehensive comparison and discussion of these two diseases, with emphasis on their retrovirus association. Lymphoid leukosis and Marek's disease will only be briefly reviewed. The reader seeking more extensive information on the latter two disease complexes may refer to the following reviews (Hanafusa, 1977; Vogt, 1977; Bishop, 1978; Calnek and Witter, 1978; Graf and Beug, 1978; Purchase and Burmester, 1978; Wang, 1978; Taylor, 1979).

II. Classification

Avian neoplasms can be categorized into four disease complexes, based on the terminology adopted by the World Veterinary Poultry Association and including modifications in current usage (Calnek, 1978). The first is the leukosis-sarcoma group, referred to also as leukemia sarcoma, which are induced by a number of RNA tumor viruses (retroviruses, REV). This avian leukemia virus group can be subdivided further:

1. The nondefective leukemia viruses predominantly induce lymphoid leukosis (LL) after a long latency period and primarily involve the bursa of Fabricius and visceral organs.
2. The defective leukemia viruses predominantly cause acute erythroid and myeloid leukemias, which have short latency periods.

The latter are beyond the scope of this article (Graf and Beug, 1978; Purchase and Burmester, 1978).

The second group of avian lymphoproliferative diseases is Marek's disease, which is caused by a DNA herpesvirus and is characterized by lymphoproliferative involvements of the peripheral nervous system and visceral organs (Marek, 1907; Calnek and Witter, 1978).

The third disease group is the avian reticuloendotheliosis complex, induced by RNA tumor viruses totally unrelated to the avian leukosis sarcoma retroviruses. The reticuloendotheliosis (RE) group of avian viruses include five different pathogenetic types: duck spleen necrosis virus (SNV), duck infectious anemia virus (DIAV), chicken syncytial virus (CSV), and the reticuloendotheliosis virus strain T (REV-T), which was originally isolated from turkeys with leukotic disease by Twiehaus in 1958 (Sevoian et al., 1964; Theilen et al., 1966; Purchase et al., 1973; Robinson and Twiehaus, 1974; Witter, 1978). The latter (REV-T) is the only member of the RE group with the ability to cause lymphoproliferative neoplasm *in vivo* and to transform hematopoietic cells or fibroblasts *in vitro* (Franklin et al., 1974; Hoelzer et al., 1979, 1980). Also included in this group is a reticuloendotheliosis virus complex characterized by its ability to induce an undifferentiated acute lymphoblastic leukemia in the Muscovy duck (Perk et al., 1982).

The fourth group is a recently recognized lymphoproliferative disease complex in turkeys, designated lymphoproliferative disease of turkeys (LPD) (Biggs et al., 1978; McDougall et al., 1978). This disease is caused also by an RNA tumor virus unrelated to the retroviruses of the avian leukosis-sarcoma group or to the RE viruses. Considerable heterogeneity of the lymphoid cell types characterizes LPD, and the pancreas and thymus are primarily involved.

III. Avian Retroviruses

Before reviewing the four lymphoproliferative disease entities, some characteristics of retroviruses (RNA tumor viruses, oncorna viruses) should be discussed. Members of this virus family are proven agents of oncogenesis in several species (Gross, 1970). Except for Marek's disease, the avian lymphoproliferative diseases are caused by C-type retroviruses (Beard, 1973; Dalton et al., 1974; Perk, 1980). The retrovirus prototype, Rous chicken sarcoma virus (RSV), was discovered by Peyton Rous in 1911 at the Rockefeller Institute (Rous, 1911). An RNA tumor virus had actually been discovered earlier in 1908 at the Royal Veterinary School in Copenhagen by Ellerman and Bang. They were successful in transmitting leukemia to healthy birds, using cell-free filtrates from diseased fowls (Ellerman and Bang, 1908). Their virus, however, was little studied because it was harder to work with than the Rous sarcoma virus, which became the prototype retrovirus for subsequent studies.

Retroviruses are approximately 100 nm in diameter and are surrounded by an envelope consisting of a lipid bilayer and external glycoproteins (derived by budding from the host cell membrane) (Fig. 1). The core contains a ribonucleoprotein particle, 60–70 S RNA, basic

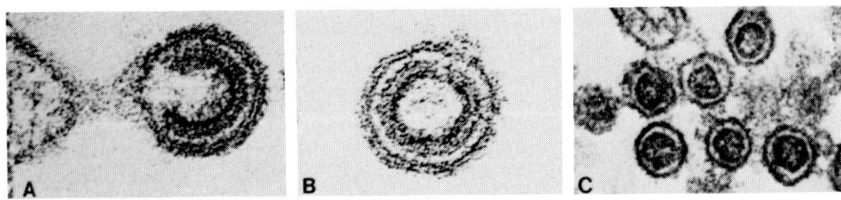

FIG. 1. Retrovirus C–type morphogenesis. (A) Typical budding virion; (B) extracellular "immature" form; (C) extracellular "mature" form.

proteins, and the unique RNA-directed DNA polymerase (reverse transcriptase) (Baltimore, 1970; Temin and Mizutani, 1970). Several characteristics distinguish retroviruses from other known animal viruses. Most RNA viruses replicate RNA directly into new copies of RNA and translate information from RNA to protein with no direct involvement of DNA. In contrast, a central event in the genesis of retroviruses is the RNA-directed DNA polymerase ("reverse flow"), which initiates infection by copying the RNA viral genome into DNA. The viral DNA intermediate (provirus) resides inside the infected cell genome, rarely kills the cell, and joins the genetic entity of the cell. Once integrated, many alternative pathways are possible. Proliferation of the infected cell results in the transmission of the provirus to the daughter cells without the appearance of the intact virus. If retroviruses find their way into the germ cells, they are transmitted from one generation to another, resulting in endogenous viruses (vertical transmission). Thus the ability of retroviruses to become established in cells as integrated proviral DNA can be either by infection or by inheritance.

If the viral genome is introduced into somatic cells of an animal, the infection is terminated by the death of the host; if established in the germ cells, it can be passed from generation to generation indefinitely. Under certain circumstances the DNA provirus can be expressed, and the cell begins producing new viral particles that may infect neighboring cells or other animals (horizontal transmission) (Bishop, 1980).

Three viral genes participate in the replication of the retroviruses: *gag*, the genetic regions encoding the precursor to all of the major internal structural viral proteins, *pol*, which encodes the reverse transcriptase, and *env*, the gene responsible for specifying the amino acid sequence of the major glycoprotein found on the surface of the envelope of the virion. In addition, the retroviruses possess a genetic region termed "C" (constant) that does not appear to encode a protein (Wang,

1978; Czernilovsky *et al.*, 1980). Certain retroviruses possess genes that may directly mediate neoplastic trnasformation of the host cell. This unique class of genes was termed *onc* genes (Baltimore, 1975). The *onc* genes of RSV have been termed *src* (Bishop, 1978; Graf and Beug, 1978) (Fig. 2).

The retroviruses can be classified into strong, weak, and nononcogenic viruses (Hanafusa, 1977; Graf and Beug, 1978; Shih and Scolnik, 1980). The strongly oncogenic retroviruses cause tumors rapidly and elicit transformation in cell cultures. All but Rous sarcoma virus are defective. The weakly oncogenic viruses cause tumors only after a long latent period; they do not cause transformation *in vitro* and are not defective. This group of viruses exists in natural situations and is transmitted either vertically or horizontally. There appears to be an evolutionary relationship between the two classes. Strongly oncogenic viruses may evolve from weakly oncogenic retroviruses and cellular DNA (Temin, 1980).

Based on the types of neoplasms they induce, the avian retroviruses can be assigned to subgroups;

1. Sarcoma viruses (RSV) are strongly oncogenic viruses and cause sarcoma.
2. Acute leukemia viruses, also strongly oncogenic, are also referred to as defective leukemia viruses (DLV). These cause acute erythroid or myeloid leukemias and reticuloendotheliosis after short periods of latency.
3. The lymphatic leukemia (lymphoid leukosis) viruses are weakly oncogenic viruses, referred to also as nondefective leukemia viruses, and predominantly induce lymphatic leukemias usually only after long latent periods (Bister and Duesberg, 1980).

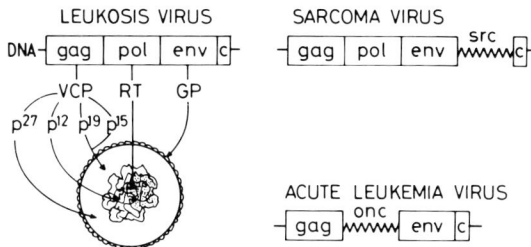

FIG. 2. Schematic diagram of the topography of avian retrovirus genome. p^{27}, etc represent the specific viral core proteins; GP, glycoproteins; RT, reverse transcriptase; VCP, viral core proteins.

IV. Clinical and Pathological Features

A. Pathogenesis of Lymphoproliferative Disease of Turkeys

1. Introduction and History

Lymphoproliferative disease of turkeys (LPD) has been described by Biggs *et al.* (1978) and McDougall *et al.* (1978) as a naturally occurring entity. However, during the years since 1940, sporadic cases or small outbreaks of lymphoproliferative diseases in turkeys have been reported under various names, such as neurolymphomatosis, visceral lymphomatosis, and Marek's-like disease (Biggs *et al.*, 1978; Ianconescu *et al.*, 1980). No attempt was made to distinguish between the etiological agents of these diseases in turkeys and in chickens, and it was assumed that they were identical.

Isolation and characterization of the etiological agents of the leukotic conditions in turkeys revealed that RE and LPD are the main leukotic diseases in turkeys. However, experimental inoculation of pathogenic Marek's disease virus in turkeys also resulted in tumor formation (Elmubarak *et al.*, 1981).

Sporadic cases of LPD were observed by Biggs *et al.* (1978) during the 1960s, but the first naturally occurring outbreaks of LPD in several commercial flocks were reported in England in 1973. Subsequently, sporadic outbreaks have been observed in additional flocks under different conditions, and soon after the disease was reported in England, it appeared in other countries in Europe and in Israel (Biggs *et al.*, 1978; Ianconescu *et al.*, 1979).

2. Clinical Aspects

Cases of LPD are usually observed as small outbreaks starting in turkeys at the age of 8 to 10 weeks, with a mortality rate of 2% per week. Thereafter, mortality continues at this level until slaughter at 16 to 18 weeks of age. The cumulative mortality losses in a flock can reach 15–25% (Biggs *et al.*, 1978; Ianconescu *et al.*, 1979). The clinical course of the disease is usually acute, with practically no premonitory signs of the disease prior to death.

3. Gross Lesions

Macroscopically, LPD in turkeys is characterized by spleen and liver enlargement. The spleen may reach the weight of 40 to 60 gm. Its color is whitish or pale pink, and on cutting the pulp has a uniform or marbled discoloration. The liver is also enlarged, but not so greatly as the spleen, with milliary, grayish white foci appearing throughout the liver parenchyma. The pancreas and thymus are usually enlarged; the lungs, kidneys, gonads, intestinal wall, and heart may also be involved, showing milliary or diffuse grayish white lesions, but these lesions are less common.

4. Microscopic Lesions

Histologically, the affected organs show infiltration of pleomorphic cells of the lymphoid series: different-sized lymphoblasts, lymphocytes, reticulum, plasma, and fusiform giant cells (Fig. 3). The proliferating cells appear either as cords or nests, or they may have a tendency toward nodular architecture; areas with randomly distributed proliferative cells are also found. Because of infiltration, normal organ structure is changed to varying degrees; for example, in the spleen the architecture of the white and red pulp is obliterated. The cortex of the thymus may disappear or be reduced to a thin layer of cells (Biggs *et al.*, 1978; McDougall *et al.*, 1978; Perk *et al.*, 1979).

Variations in the LPD lesions correspond to the different stages of the disease (Ianconescu *et al.*, 1979). At early stages, 2 weeks after

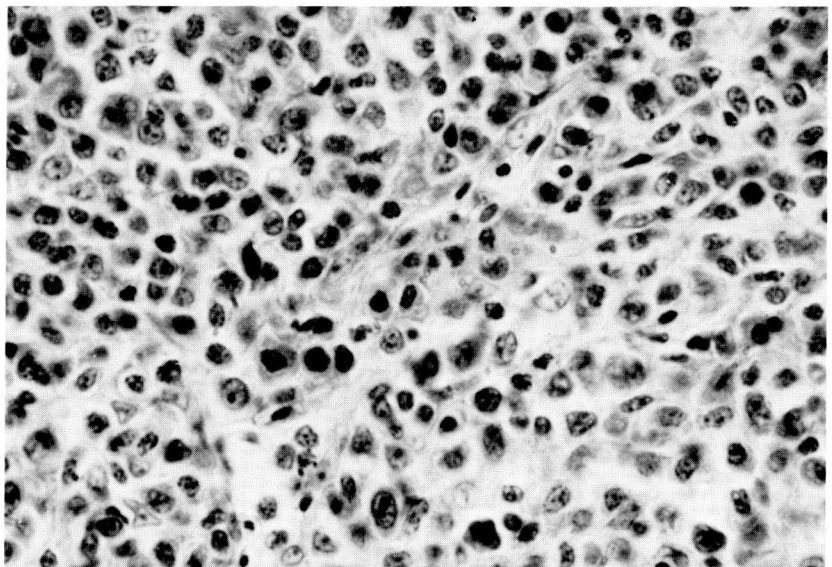

FIG. 3. Photomicrograph showing the histopathology of the lesion of LPD. Note the pleomorphic cytology of the tumor.

experimental LPD virus inoculation, the lesions consist mainly of lymphocytic infiltrations with few lymphoblasts or plasma cells. Gross lesions found in dead turkeys consist of the typical pleomorphic infiltrate, that is, a high proportion of lymphoblasts and plasma cells, with numerous mitoses indicating the proliferative character of the tumoral process.

In experimental cases, regressive lesions are also found. They consist of discrete infiltrations with mature lymphocytes and well-demarcated areas of fibroblastic infiltration. Birds having such lesions were not found dead. These findings suggest that some of the birds, even in nature, can overcome the proliferative process and experience its regression (Ianconescu et al., 1979).

5. Ultrastructure

The histological pleomorphism of the proliferating cells also became evident when the cells were examined by transmission electron microscopy (Perk et al., 1978, 1979). Although the cells vary greatly in their nuclear size and shape, and differences are found in organelle development and distribution, the proliferating cells display basically similar morphological features.

The proliferating lymphoid cells are larger than the normal turkey lymphocytes and exhibit a much higher cytoplasmic:nuclear ratio. Most are irregularly shaped, with pseudopodal extensions. Nuclei show irregularities such as nuclear pockets or indentations. Albeit displaying marked variations in shape, the chromatin is arranged in small aggregates at the nuclear membrane, which is characteristic for the lymphoid series. The nucleoli are distinct in most of the tumor cells. Frequently, nuclear bodies are present. Polyribosomes are prominent in the cytoplasm. Long, thin channels of rough endoplasmic reticulum, frequent vacuoles, and lipid droplets are also present in the cytoplasm. The fusciform tumor cells have ultrastructural features similar to other proliferating cells (Perk et al., 1979).

B. Pathogenesis of Reticuloendotheliosis

1. Introduction and History

Reticuloendotheliosis (RE) was recognized initially as a sporadic neoplastic disease of turkeys resembling lymphoid leukosis (Sevoian et al., 1964; Theilen et al., 1966; Robinson and Twiehaus, 1974). The etiological agent, a retrovirus (REV), was originally isolated from an adult turkey with leukosis-like lesions (Theilen et al., 1966; Robinson and Twiehaus, 1974). This isolate, designated REV-T strain, when inoculated into turkeys, quail, chickens, ducklings, pheasant, and guinea keets, produced a proliferative and/or invasive reticuloendotheliosis (Sevoian et al., 1964; Larose and Sevoian, 1965; Theilen et al., 1966; Purchase and Witter, 1975).

The disease, although expressing symptoms of a generalized undifferentiated lymphoid leukemia, displayed some morphological indications of reticuloendothelial cell origin and was thus referred to as reticuloendotheliosis, a designation that found worldwide acceptance. Using sets of antigenic and functional differentiation markers characteristic of mature and immature myeloid, erythroid, and lymphoid cells, it was found that this neoplastic disease is derived from very immature lymphoid precursor cells, corresponding to a pre-B-, pre-T-like cell type (Beug et al., 1981). The REV-T strain became the prototype of a new group of avian retroviruses, the REV group, which induce in their hosts a variety of diseases referred to as spleen necrosis disease, duck infectious anemia, lymphoblastic leukemia, visceral and neural reticuloendotheliosis, and duck lymphoblastic leukemia (Purchase et al., 1973; Purchase and Witter, 1975; Witter, 1978; see Section II).

The type of reticuloendotheliosis that is induced by the REV-T strain will be the form mainly discussed in this article.

2. Clinical Aspects

Although reticuloendotheliosis is considered by many to be primarily of research interest, outbreaks and infections commonly occur, inflicting major economic losses. The severity of the disease in turkeys, chickens, and ducks varies. Experimentally inoculated chickens, turkeys, or ducks, like naturally occurring cases on poultry farms, show similar clinicopathological changes (Paul et al., 1976). Illness is either acute or chronic. The acute form of RE may result in death even before specific clinical signs develop, within an average period of less than 10 days. In chronic cases, birds show poor feather development, growth retraction, emaciation, and anemia.

3. Gross and Microscopic Lesions

Gross and microscopic lesions vary with the acuteness of the disease, but consist of both splenomegaly and hepatomegaly. Small, irregular, grayish foci may also be seen in spleen, liver, or in other visceral organs. In diseased birds the bursa of Fabricius and the thymus are frequently atrophied, but cases with tumor involvement of these organs have also been frequently observed. Although paralysis and

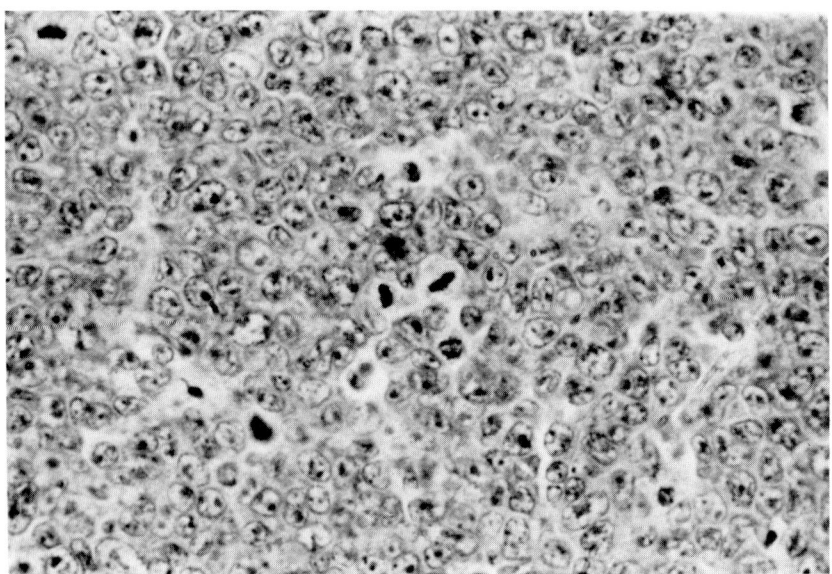

FIG. 4. Photomicrograph showing the histopathology of the lesion of RE. Note the highly undifferentiated lymphoid cells.

incoordination are rarely seen, microscopic neural lesions are often found (Witter et al., 1970). This nerve involvement is microscopically indistinguishable from that seen in Marek's disease (Witter et al., 1970). Thus it is virtually impossible to distinguish RE from Marek's disease on the basis of pathology alone. Infection with REV should be confirmed by virus isolation or antibody identification.

The proliferative lesions consist of morphologically undifferentiated lymphoblastoid cells (Fig. 4). In this regard, the study of Beug et al. (1981) is of great interest. They report that the REV-transformed hematopoietic cells express antigenic markers common to B and T lymphoid cells, and provide evidence that the transformed cells represent every immature B- and/or T-lymphocyte precursor (Keller et al., 1979; Beug et al., 1981).

C. Pathogenesis of Avian Lymphoid Leukosis

Avian lymphoid leukosis (ALL) is a naturally occurring neoplastic disease of the sexually mature chicken; it is caused by replication-competent members of the exogenous leukosis retrovirus group (Graf and Beug, 1978; Purchase and Burmester, 1978). The earliest changes found in lymphoid leukosis are observed in the bursa of Fabricius (Peterson et al., 1966; Cooper et al., 1968; Purchase and Gilmour, 1975; Romero et al., 1978). They consist of larger than normal lymphoblasts grouped together in nests, in an otherwise normal bursal follicle. Transformed bursa cells usually metastasize to the liver, spleen, gonads, and other visceral organs, leading to death of the host at the onset of sexual maturity. The proliferative lymphoblasts possess large vesicular nuclei, one or several prominent nucleoli, an abundance of cytoplasmic ribosomes, and scattered strands of rough endoplasmic reticulum. Regardless of their location, the lymphoblasts have detectable surface immunoglobulin, indicative of a B-cell origin. Occasionally virus particles, C-type retroviruses, may be seen budding from the cell membrane of tumor cells, but virions are more abundant in the nontumorous cell types. In considering the outcome of the virus–host interaction, the dose size and source of the virus, and the age, breed, sex, route of infection, and immune status of the host are all determining factors in oncogenicity. The most common route of infection on poultry farms occurs through infected eggs, that is, from dam to offspring (Burmester, 1962), but the disease rarely develops before the chickens are 14 weeks old (Crittenden and Witter, 1978). The causes of this prolonged tumor latency are still not completely understood. It was suggested that it is host-controlled, because metastasis occurs at the time that the bursa of Fabricius is undergoing its most rapid regression at the onset of sexual maturity (Purchase, 1976). However, Fadly et al. (1981) have shown in cell transfer studies that the long latency period in ALL is determined by intrinsic properties of the bursa target B cells and not by other features of host physiology. It has been shown that inherited postinfection resistance to ALL is also an intrinsic property of bursa target cells (Purchase et al., 1977). Further, it was demonstrated that tumors are clonal. Unique proviral integration sites were detected by restriction analysis in the DNA of bursal tumors (Neel et al., 1981). Moreover, metastases have the same restrictive pattern as bursal tumors from the same animal, again suggesting that primary and metastatic tumors are clonal and thus presumably derived from a single infected transformed cell. Therefore, the initiation event in tumorigenesis is probably a rare one (Neiman et al., 1980; Neel et al., 1981).

D. Pathogenesis of Marek's Disease

Marek's disease (MD), in contrast to LPD, RE, and ALL, is caused by a DNA herpesvirus. It primarily infects young chickens and includes both inflammatory and neoplastic elements. The inflammatory lesions consist mainly of small lymphocytes and plasma cells, and are often accompanied by interneuritic edema. The herpesvirus infection persists, leading to neoplastic transformation, mainly of T lymphocytes (Akiyama and Kato, 1974; Powell et al., 1974; Nazerian et al., 1977; Calnek et al., 1978). All lymphoblastoid cell lines established from MD tumors in chickens are transformed T lymphocytes and are positive for MD tumor-associated surface antigen (Powell et al., 1974; Witter et al., 1975). The proliferative T lymphoblasts infiltrate mainly the peripheral nerves, resulting in the typical paralysis syndrome of Marek's disease.

In addition, multifocal lymphoid proliferation may be found in the gonads, liver, spleen, kidneys, heart proventiculus, and even in skeletal muscles. Marek's disease viral infections usually occur in the poultry house via the airborne route (i.e., by inhalation of infectious material derived from feathers, dander, and dust). The latent period is relatively short (Payne and Biggs, 1967; Calnek et al., 1970).

Although there are no confirmed reports of MD outbreaks in commercial turkey flocks, experimental inoculation of MD virus in turkeys induces the disease, characterized by extensive lymphoproliferation, gross tumor formation, and death (Elmubarak et al., 1981; Nazerian et al., 1982). It is of interest to note that the lymphoblastoid cells of the turkey tumor lines are positive for Marek's disease tumor-associated surface antigen, bearing B-cell surface markers (Nazerian et al., 1982). Thus MD virus, apparently in contrast to chickens, transforms B cells in turkeys.

V. Epidemiology, Virology, and Oncogenesis

A. Lymphoproliferative Disease Virus of Turkeys

1. Virus Morphology and Morphogenesis

Virus particles morphologically characteristic of Retroviridae, resembling murine C-type particles, have been demonstrated in thin sections of tissues with proliferating lesions (Fig. 5) (Biggs et al., 1978; McDougall et al., 1978; Perk et al., 1978, 1979). These isolates were found to be the infective agents of LPD in turkeys. Similar to type C retroviruses, the virus buds from the plasma membrane, with crescent-shaped cores (~70–80 nm in diameter) formed during the process of budding. The inner layers form concomitantly with the bud. The elec-

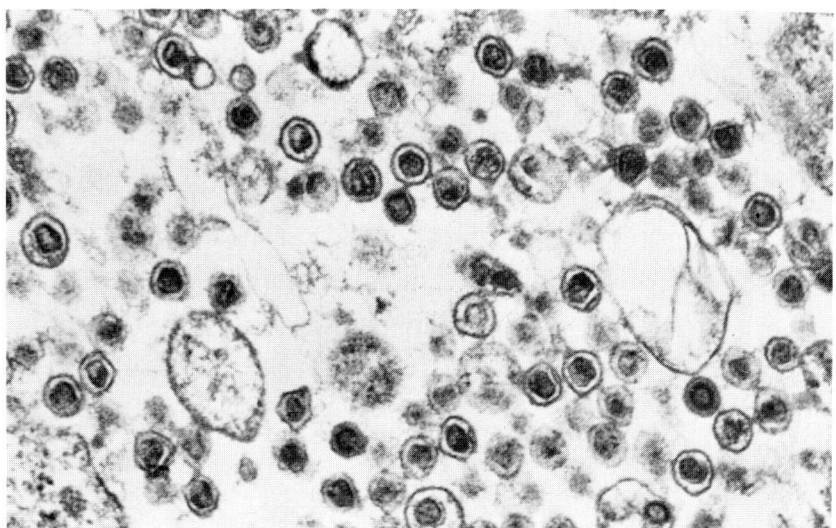

FIG. 5. Electron micrograph showing extracellular typical type C mature and immature virus particles of LPD.

tron density of the inner components of the virus is in most instances greater than that of the intermediate layers. With further maturation, the buds protrude into the extracellular space. Extracellular mature virions (100–120 nm in diameter), typical of type C retroviruses in appearance, show a distinct intermediate layer and a centrally located core. However, significant differences in diameter and density of the cores set the LPD virus apart from the avian leukosis-sarcoma viruses (Perk et al., 1979). On the other hand, the ultrastructure and development of the LPD viruses resemble those of the RE virus group.

2. Biochemical and Biophysical Characterization of LPD Virus

Velocity and equilibrium sucrose density gradient centrifugation showed that the infective LPD virus particles sediment at a density similar to that of the retroviruses (i.e., 1.16–1.18 gm/ml) (Yaniv et al., 1979). Like the retroviruses, LPD virions contain an RNA-dependent DNA polymerase. The enzyme in its exogenous reaction demonstrates a preference for ribohomopolymers over deoxyribohomopolymers as templates (Schwarzbard et al., 1980). Furthermore, the LPD virus polymerase is preferentially activated by magnesium ions. Cross-virus nucleic acid hybridization assays revealed no sequence homology between the viral genome of LPD and avian myeloblastosis virus or reticuloendotheliosis virus, thus indicating that the LPD virus belongs to a distinct, unrelated group (Gazit et al., 1979; Yaniv et al., 1979).

3. Molecular Evidence for LPD Virus in the Lymphoproliferative Disease

Using complementary DNA of LPD viral RNA, it was found that the LPD viral genome is specifically and efficiently transcribed (2500 copies per cell) in LPD tumor cells (Gazit et al., 1979). These cells contain newly inserted LPD viral information. The absence of LPD virus-specific sequences in the normal cell genome of turkeys indicates that LPD virus is not an endogenous virus residing in latent form within the normal DNA and also that it does not originate in this species (Gazit et al., 1979). Thus, like other important type C retroviruses of farm animals, bovine leukemia virus (Kettman et al., 1976), visna-maedi (Weiss et al., 1975; Perk, 1983), and reticuloendotheliosis (Barbacid et al., 1979), LPD virus originated in another presently unknown animal species.

Quantitation of viral RNA expression in various organs established the bone marrow and the lymphoid organs as targets for LPD virus replication. The bone marrow was the first organ to be infected prior to histopathological changes, and subsequently virus replication extended to the thymus, spleen, and bursa of Fabricius. Further, it was found that LPD virus organotropism is regulated at the level of integration; that is, LPD proviruses can integrate only into the DNA of lymphoid cells, whereas cells of nonlymphatic origin seem to restrict LPD virus productive infection at any of the stages prior to integration (Gazit et al., 1982).

4. Structural Polypeptide Composition of LPD Virus

The polypeptide composition of LPD virions as analyzed by 6 M guanidine hydrochloride–agarose gel chromatography and sodium dodecyl sulfate–polyacrylamide gel electrophoresis consists of polypeptides with molecular weights of 77,000, 43,000, 31,000, 28,000, 20,000, and 14,000. Prolonged electrophoresis through 15% polyacrylamide gels reveals that, in addition to the 14,000-dalton protein, there are two other distinct polypeptides with low molecular weights of 13,000 and 4500 (Gazit et al., 1983).

B. Reticuloendotheliosis Viruses

Reticuloendotheliosis viruses (REVs) are a group of avian retroviruses (Sections II and IV,B,1) morphologically and antigenically different from avian leukosis virus (Ziegel et al., 1966; Purchase et al., 1973). Reticuloendotheliosis viruses also do not share genetic homology with ALL or LPD virus. Several investigations indicate that the REV group is more closely related to mammalian C retroviruses than to the ALL virus (Maldonado and Bose, 1973; Mizutani and Temin, 1973; Moelling et al., 1975; Witter, 1978; Barbacid et al., 1979). The RE and LPD viruses possess ultrastructural features that resemble those of mammalian type C viruses (Kang et al., 1975). Furthermore, the REVs have an RNA-dependent DNA polymerase complex; its molecular weight and cation preference are similar to those of murine leukemia viruses. The major structural proteins possess antigenic determinants common to known mammalian type C viruses (Barbacid et al., 1979). It is of interest that a close antigenic relationship has been established between the major structural retrovirus type C proteins of an owl monkey, an endogenous virus of deer, and REV (Barbacid et al., 1980). In addition, the major core protein (P28) of MMC-1, an endogenous type C virus of the rhesus monkey, and REV-A P30 share a specific subset of antigenic determinants not present in any other avian or mammalian type C virus (Oroszlan et al., 1981). These studies implicate mammalian retrovirus in the evolutionary linkage leading to the generation of the avian RE virus.

In tissue culture, REV-T strain is the only member of the RE group that transforms fibroblasts, spleen cells, and bone marrow cells (Franklin et al., 1974; Hoelzer et al., 1979, 1980). It has been shown that the infective virus preparation consists of two viral components. The first is a replication-defective but transforming virus, referred to as REV_T, which contains a 28 S RNA and causes the acute neoplasia but requires the presence of a helper virus (REV-A) for replication. The second is the nondefective associated helper virus, referred to as nd REV or REV-A, which contains a 35 S RNA and cannot transform cells in vitro (Breitman et al., 1980). In vivo it may cause an immunodepressive runting disease (Bülow, 1977; Carpenter et al., 1977; Hoeltzer et al., 1979; Witter et al., 1979, 1981). It has been reported that after a long latent period (17–93 weeks), the nondefective REV may induce lymphomas in chickens, involving the bursa of Fabricius and other visceral organs (Witter et al., 1981). Nucleic acid hybridization experiments revealed that approximately 70% of the REV_T genome is related to REV-A (Breitman et al., 1980). The remaining sequences are unique to REV_T (ret) and presumably encode the transformation-specific functions of the virus. These transforming oncogenic-specific sequences have not been found in other RE viruses (i.e., spleen necrosis virus, duck infectious anemia virus, and chick syncytial virus), or in all other known viral oncogenic sequences (Cohen *et al.,* 1981; Wong and Lai, 1981). It was further shown that the REV_T-specific sequences are localized as a contiguous stretch, possibly interrupted by a short stretch of REV-A–related sequences. Analogous to all the known leukemia- and sarcoma-specific sequences, *erb, myb, mac,* and *src,* the REV_T-related transforming sequences, *ret,* also have cellular counterparts in normal avian cells (Cohen *et al.,* 1981; Wong and Lai, 1981). This suggests that REV-T was probably derived from recombination between an RE virus and cellular *ret* sequences.

C. Avian Lymphoid Leukosis Viruses

Because this topic has been extensively reviewed (Hanafusa, 1977; Vogt, 1977; Bishop, 1978; Graf and Beug, 1978; Wang, 1978), only some fundamental facts and reports of recent studies will be presented here. On the basis of their biological and oncogenic properties, avian leukosis-sarcoma retroviruses can be assigned to either of two major classes. The first includes the acute viruses, which include replication-competent RSV and replication-defective viruses, the acute leukemia viruses such as avian erythroblastosis virus (AEV), avian myeloblastosis virus (AMV), and avian myelocytomatosis virus. It now is known that all of these strains consist of mixtures of a defective leukemia virus and one or more nondefective leukemia viruses acting as "helpers." The acute leukemia viruses induce neoplastic diseases in host animals rapidly (2–4 weeks) and with high efficiency, and transform appropriate target cells in tissue culture. It has been established that the transforming ability of the acute viruses is due to the presence of a specific "transforming gene," an oncogene, within the viral genome (Hanafusa, 1977; Vogt, 1977; Beug *et al.,* 1981; Bishop, 1978).

Studies during the 1970s presented evidence that the retrovirus oncogenes are merely cellular genes, "passengers," acquired from the animals in which the viruses replicate (Section III). These cellular "relatives" of retroviral oncogenes have the structural organization of cellular genes rather than that of viral genes, have survived long periods of evolution, and are active in normal cells (Stehelin *et al.,* 1980).

The viruses of the second category, nondefective leukemia viruses (the chronic viruses), can be further subdivided into seven subgroups, A–G, as typified by their viral envelope antigen. Subgroups A–E consist of viruses isolated from the chicken; subgroups F and G come from pheasant (Vogt, 1977). They are competent for replication; they may induce neoplasia only after prolonged latent periods (4–12 months) and with lower efficiency in tumor induction (Fadly *et al.,* 1981). They fail to transform any target cell thus far tested in cell cultures. No transforming gene(s) has been identified in the chronic avian retroviruses, suggesting that the mechanism of neoplasia by chronic viruses is different from that of the acute viruses. The genome of the ALL virus possesses genes *gag, pol,* and *env,* which encode only the replication and structural functions of the virus. In addition, there is the sequence termed "C" (for constant), which maps at the 3' end of the viral RNA genome (Wang, 1978) but does not appear to encode protein (Czernilovsky *et al.,* 1980) (Fig. 2). Neel *et al.* (1981), in their important study, revealed that ALL viral gene products are not required for maintenance of neoplastic transformation. Furthermore, in the lymphoid tumors, the ALL provirus is integrated adjacent to a specific cellular gene, more recently recognized as similar to the oncogene known as c-*myc.* The previous ALL insertion adjacent to this gene may suggest its enhanced expression leading to neoplasia. These findings have important general implications for a common pathway for the mechanism of viral and nonviral carcinogenesis (Bishop, 1982).

D. Marek's Disease Herpesvirus

The causal agent of Marek's disease (MD) is a DNA virus of the herpesvirus group, first isolated from chickens independently by Churchill and Biggs (1967), Nazerian *et al.* (1968), and Solomon *et al.* (1968). Each group observed cytopathic effects and herpesvirus particles in cell cultures inoculated with material from diseased chickens. The morphology and chemical composition have been extensively studied and reviewed (Ahmed and Schidlovsky, 1968; Calnek *et al.,* 1970; Nazerian and Witter, 1970; Roizman and Spear, 1973; Calnek and Witter, 1978). In negatively stained preparations, the nucleocapsid was observed to have cubic icosahedral symmetry and to possess 162 hollow-centered capsomes. Viral DNA appears to be wound around a central structure connecting the two inner poles of the capsid (Nazerian, 1974).

The incidence of MD has been greatly decreased by the development of effective vaccines that are antigenically related to Marek's disease virus (MDV) and derived from turkey herpesvirus or a live, attenuated MD virus (Churchill and Biggs, 1967; Churchill *et al.,* 1969). It should be noted that in contrast to MD virus, turkey herpesvirus is not highly contagious among chickens, even though it spreads rapidly among turkeys. Turkey herpesvirus does not induce gross lymphomas in chickens or turkeys, but minor microscopic lymphoproliferative nerve lesions have been reported.

Lymphoblastoid cell lines, established from Marek's disease tumors, contain multiple copies of MD viral genome. However, only a small population of certain cell lines spontaneously produces virus particles in contrast to most lines, which are viral nonproducers. The latent viral DNA in these cells is present in the plasmid state—not covalently integrated into the host DNA. Marek's disease viral DNA replicates during the early S phase of the cell cycle, which occurs prior to the onset of active cellular DNA synthesis (Lau and Nonoyama, 1980). Thus there is a restricted control in the transcription of viral genomes in these generally nonproducer cells. Induction of latent virus by different methods, such as the use of iododeoxyuridine, has been successfully achieved.

VI. Relationship of LPD to RE

Although it is morphologically similar to REV, the LPD type C virus does not share any antigenic properties with REV or with ALL virus complexes (McDougall *et al.*, 1978; Ianconescu *et al.*, 1979) (Section V,A and B). Furthermore, whereas REV replicates productively *in vitro* in a wide range of avian cells, attempts to propagate the LPD virus in a variety of cell cultures have so far been unsuccessful. The LPD and RE viruses differ also in their viral polymerase: whereas REV polymerase requires only manganese, the LPD virus enzyme is preferentially activated by magnesium ions (Schwarzbard *et al.*, 1980). Cross-virus nucleic acid hybridization experiments reveal the absence of sequence homology between the viral genome of LPD and ALL viruses (Gazit *et al.*, 1979; Yaniv *et al.*, 1979). These biological, morphological, and molecular data suggest that LPD virus belongs to a group genetically distinct from the ALL or the RE group of viruses. The conclusion that RE and LPD represent two different diseases caused by two different viruses finds its support in numerous dissimilarities between the two disease complexes. Under natural or experimental conditions, RE virus causes neoplastic diseases in a wide range of birds, whereas so far LPD virus has been found to be pathogenic under natural conditions only to turkeys. Even if the gross lesions are found in the same organs in both diseases, the main target organ in RE is the liver, followed by the spleen and, to a lesser degree, the pancreas, heart, gonads, and lungs. In LPD, the spleen and pancreas are the principal organs affected, followed by liver, thymus, and gonads. Tumors of the intestine and prominent nodular tumors in the liver are indicators for a diagnosis of RE; in contrast, a pale spleen, mottled pancreas, and congested thymus point to LPD. Histopathology provides useful criteria for differential diagnosis between the two diseases. In RE the neoplastic cells, the infiltrative lesions, consist of a homogeneous population of highly undifferentiated lymphoblasts; in LPD the lesions consist of a mixed population of mature lymphocytes with relatively few undifferentiated lymphoblasts, plasma cells, and reticular cells (cf. Figs. 3 and 4) (Biggs et al., 1978; Perk et al., 1979).

VII. Concluding Comments

Research on avian lymphoproliferative diseases provides the basis for methods of disease control for the benefit of the poultry industry, including a Marek's disease vaccine and the development of serological and pathological diagnostic procedures. In addition, study of these diseases and their virus association has introduced revolutionary new vistas in biology and serves as a basis for valuable insights into molecular genetics and genetic engineering. Moreover, avian leukemia viruses are excellent models for analysis of the interaction of viruses with various types of differentiating cells, for elucidation of problems of target cell specificity, and for understanding the process of hematopoietic cell differentiation.

Although retroviruses do not seem to be a major cause of human cancer, they illuminate central mechanisms whereby the disease arises, and much has been learned from avian tumor virology about the mechanisms by which animal and human tumors may develop.

REFERENCES

Ahmed, M., and Schidlovsky, T. (1968). *J. Virol.* **2**, 1443–1457.
Akiyama, Y., and Kato, S. (1974). *Biken J.* **17**, 105–116.
Baltimore, D. (1970). *Nature (London)* **226**, 1209–1211.
Baltimore, D. (1975). *Cold Spring Harbor Symp. Quant. Biol.* **39**, 1187–1200.
Barbacid, M., Hunter, E., and Aaronson, S. A. (1979). *J. Virol.* **30**, 508–514.
Barbacid, M., Daniel, M. D., and Aaronson, S. A. (1980). *J. Virol.* **33**, 561–566.
Beard, J. M. (1973). *In* "Ultrastructure of Animal Viruses and Bacteriophages" (A. J. Dalton and E. Haguenau, eds.), pp. 26–281. Academic Press, New York.
Beug, H., Müller, H., Grieser, S., Doederlein, G., and Graf, T. (1981). *Virology* **115**, 295–309.
Biggs, F. M., McDougall, J. S., Frazier, J. A., and Milne, B. S. (1978). *Avian Pathol.* **7**, 131–139.
Bishop, J. B. (1978). *Annu. Rev. Biochem.* **47**, 35–88.
Bishop, J. M. (1980). *N. Engl. J. Med.* **303**, 675–682.
Bishop, J. M. (1982). *Sci. Am.* **246**, 69–78.

Bister, K., and Duesberg, P. H. (1980). *Cold Spring Harbor Symp. Quant. Biol.* **44**, 801–821.
Breitman, M. L., Lai, M. M., and Vogt, P. K. (1980). *Virology* **100**, 450–461.
Bülow, V. (1977). *Avian Pathol.* **6**, 383–393.
Burmester, B. R. (1962). *Cold Spring Harbor Symp. Quant. Biol.* **27**, 471–478.
Calnek, B. W. (1978). *In* "Diseases of Poultry" (M. S. Hofstand, B. W. Calnek, C. F. Helmbolt, W. M. Reid, and H. W. Yoder, eds.), pp. 383–385. Iowa State Univ. Press, Ames.
Calnek, B. W., and Witter, R. L. (1978). *In* "Diseases of Poultry" (M. S. Hofstand, B. W. Calnek, C. F. Helmbolt, W. M. Reid, and H. W. Yoder, eds.), pp. 385–418. Iowa State Univ. Press, Ames.
Calnek, B. W., Adldinger, H. K., and Kahn, D. E. (1970). *Avian Dis.* **14**, 219–233.
Calnek, B. W., Murthy, K. K., and Schat, K. A. (1978). *Int. J. Cancer* **21**, 100–107.
Carpenter, C. R., Rose, H. R., and Rubin, A. S. (1977). *Cell. Immunol.* **33**, 392–401.
Churchill, A. E., and Biggs, P. M. (1967). *Nature (London)* **215**, 528–531.
Churchill, A. E., Payne, C. N., and Chubb, R. C. (1969). *Nature (London)* **221**, 744–747.
Cohen, R. S., Wang, T. C., and Lai, M. M. C. (1981). *Virology* **113**, 672–685.
Cooper, M. D., Payne, N. L., Dent, P. B., Burmester, B. R., and Good, R. A. (1968). *JNCI, J. Natl. Cancer Inst.* **41**, 373–389.
Crittenden, L. B., and Witter, L. B. (1978). *Avian Dis.* **22**, 16–23.
Czernilovsky, A. P., DeLorbe, W., Swanstrom, R., Varmus, H. E., Bishop, J. M., Tischer, E., and Goodman, H. M. (1980). *Nucleic Acids Res.* **13**, 2967–2984.
Dalton, A. J., Melnik, J. L., and Bauer, H. (1974). *Intervirology* **4**, 201–206.
Ellerman, J., and Bang, D. (1908). *Zentralbl. Bakteriol., Parasitenkd., Infektionskr. Hyg., Abt. 1:Orig.* **46**, 595–609.
Elmubarak, A. K., Sharma, J. M., Witter, R. L., Nazerian, K., and Sanger, V. L. (1981). *Avian Dis.* **25**, 911–926.
Fadly, A. M., Purchase, H. G., and Gilmour, (1981). *JNCI, J. Natl. Cancer Inst.* **66**, 549–552.
Fanklin, R. B., Maldonado, R. L., and Bose, H. R. (1974). *Intervirology* **3**, 342–352.
Gazit, A., Yaniv, A., Ianconescu, M., Perk, K., Aizenberg, B., and Zimber, A. (1979). *J. Virol.* **31**, 639–644.
Gazit, A., Schwarzbard, Z., Yaniv, A., Ianconescu, M., Perk, K., and Zimber, A. (1982). *Int. J. Cancer* **29**, 599–604.
Gazit, A., Basri, R., Yaniv, A., Ianconescu, M., Perk, K., and Zimber, A. (1982). In preparation.
Graf, T., and Beug, H. (1978). *Biochim. Biophys. Acta* **516**, 269–299.
Gross, L. (1970). "Oncogenic Viruses," 2nd ed. Pergamon, Oxford.
Hanafusa, H. (1977). *Compr. Virol.* **10**, 401–483.
Hoelzer, G. D., Franklin, R. B., and Bose, H. R. (1979). *Virology* **93**, 20–30.
Hoelzer, G. D., Lewis, R. B., Wasmuth, C. R., and Bose, H. R. (1980). *Virology* **100**, 462–472.
Ianconescu, M., Perk, K., Zimber, A., and Yaniv, A. (1979). *Refu. Vet.* **36**, 1–12.
Kang, C. Y., Wong, T. C., and Holmes, K. V. (1975). *J. Virol.* **16**, 1027–1038.
Keller, L. H., Rufner, R., and Sevoian, M. (1979). *Infect. Immun.* **25**, 694–701.
Kettman, R., Portetelle, D., Mammericlex, M., Cleuter, Y., DeKegel, D., Galoux, M., Ghysdael, J., and Burny, A. (1976). *Proc. Natl. Acad. Sci. U.S.A.* **73**, 1014–1018.
Larose, R. N., and Sevoian, M. (1965). *Avian Dis.* **9**, 604–610.
Lau, R. Y., and Nonoyama, H. (1980). *J. Virol.* **33**, 912–914.
McDougall, J. S., Biggs, P. M., Shilleto, R. W., and Milne, B. S. (1978). *Avian Pathol.* **7**, 141–155.

Maldonado, R. L., and Bose, H. R. (1973). *J. Virol.* **11**, 741–747.
Marek, J. (1907). *Dtsch. Tieraerztl. Wochenschr.* **15**, 417–421.
Mizutani, S., and Temin, H. M. (1973). *J. Virol.* **12**, 440–448.
Moelling, K., Gelderblom, H., Pauli, G., Friis, R., and Bauer, H. (1975). *Virology* **65**, 546–557.
Nazerian, K. (1974). *J. Virol.* **13**, 1148–1150.
Nazerian, K., and Witter, R. L. (1970). *J. Virol.* **5**, 388–397.
Nazerian, K., Solomon, J. J., Witter, R. L., and Burmester, B. R. (1968). *Proc. Soc. Exp. Biol. Med.* **127**, 177–182.
Nazerian, K., Stephens, E. A., Sharma, J. M., Lee, L. F., Gailitis, M., and Witter, R. L. (1977). *Avian Dis.* **21**, 69–76.
Nazerian, K., Elmubarak, A., and Sharma, J. M. (1982). *Int. J. Cancer* **29**, 63–68.
Neel, B. G., Hayward, W. S., Robinson, H. L., Fang, J., and Astrin, S. M. (1981). *Cell* **23**, 323–334.
Neiman, P., Payne, L. N., and Weiss, R. A. (1980). *J. Virol.* **34**, 178–186.
Oroszlan, S., Barbacid, M., Copeland, T. D., Aaronson, S. A., and Gilden, R. V. (1981). *J. Virol.* **39**, 845–854.
Paul, P. S., Pomeroy, K. A., Sarma, P. S., Johnson, K. H., Barnes, D. M., Kumar, M. C., and Pomeroy, B. S. (1976). *JNCI, J. Natl. Cancer Inst.* **56**, 419–421.
Payne, L. N., and Biggs, P. M. (1967). *JNCI, J. Natl. Cancer Inst.* **39**, 281–302.
Perk, K. (1980). *Comped. Contin. Educ.* **2**, 729–737.
Perk, K. (1983). *Adv. Vet. Sci. Comp. Med.* **26**, 267–287.
Perk, K., Ianconescu, M., Yaniv, A., and Zimber, A. (1978). *Refu. Vet.* **35**, 29–30.
Perk, K., Ianconescu, M., Yaniv, A., and Zimber, A. (1979). *JNCI, J. Natl. Cancer Inst.* **62**, 1483–1487.
Perk, K., Malkinosn, M., Gazit, A., Yaniv, A., and Zimber, A. (1982). *Adv. Comp. Leuk. Res., 1981* pp. 369–371.
Peterson, R. D., Purchase, H. G., Burmester, B. R., Cooper, M. D., and Good, R. A. (1966). *JNCI, J. Natl. Cancer Inst.* **36**, 585–598.
Powell, P. C., Payne, L. N., Frazier, J., and Rennie, M. (1974). *Nature (London)* **251**, 79–80.
Purchase, H. G. (1976). *In* "Differential Diagnosis of Avian Lymphoid Leukosis and Marek's Disease," EUR Publ. 549e, pp. 55–65. Luxemburg.
Purchase, H. G., and Burmester, B. R. (1978). *In* "Diseases of Poultry" (M. S. Hofstand, B. W. Calnek, C. F. Helmbolt, W. M. Reid, and H. W. Yoder, eds.), pp. 418–468. Iowa State Univ. Press, Ames.
Purchase, H. G., and Gilmour, D. G. (1975). *JNCI, J. Natl. Cancer Inst.* **55**, 851–855.
Purchase, H. G., and Witter, R. L. (1975). *Curr. Top. Microbiol. Immunol.* **71**, 103–125.
Purchase, H. G., Ludford, C., Nazerian, K., and Cox, H. W. (1973). *JNCI, J. Natl. Cancer Inst.* **51**, 489–499.
Purchase, H. G., Gilmour, D. G., Romero, C. H., and Okazaki, W. (1977). *Nature (London)* **270**, 61–62.
Robinson, F. R., and Twiehaus, M. J. (1974). *Avian Dis.* **18**, 278–288.
Roizman, B., and Spear, P. G. (1973). *In* "Ultrastructure of Animal Viruses and Bacteriophages" (J. A. Dalton and F. Haguenau, eds.), pp. 83–90. Academic Press, New York.
Romero, C. H., Purchase, H. G., Frank, F., Crittenden, L. B., and Chang, T. S. (1978). *Avian Pathol.* **7**, 87–103.
Rous, P. (1911). *J. Exp. Med.* **13**, 397–411.
Schwarzbard, T., Yaniv, A., Ianconescu, M., Perk, K., and Zimber, A. (1980). *Avian Pathol.* **9**, 481–487.

Sevoian, M., Larose, R. N., and Chamberlain, D. M. (1964). *Avian Dis.* **8,** 336–347.
Shih, T. Y., and Scolnik, E. M. (1980). *In* "Viral Oncology" (G. Klein, ed.), pp. 135–160. Raven Press, New York.
Solomon, J. J., Witter, R. L., Nazerian, K., and Burmester, B. R. (1968). *Proc. Soc. Exp. Biol. Med.* **127,** 173–177.
Stehelin, D., Rousell, S. S. M., Sergeant, A., Lagrou, C., Rommes, C., and Raes, M. B. (1980). *Cold Spring Harbor Symp. Quant. Biol.* **44,** 1215–1223.
Taylor, J. M. (1979). *Curr. Top. Microbiol. Immunol.* **87,** 23–41.
Temin, H. M. (1980). *Cold Spring Harbor Symp. Quant. Biol.* **44,** 1–7.
Temin, H. M., and Mizutani, S. (1970). *Nature (London)* **226,** 1211–1213.
Theilen, G. H., Zeigel, R. F., and Twiehaus, M. J. (1966). *JNCI, J. Natl. Cancer Inst.* **37,** 731–743.
Vogt, P. K. (1977). *Compre. Virol.* **9,** 341–430.
Wang, L. H. (1978). *Annu. Rev. Microbiol.* **32,** 561–592.
Weiss, M. J., Gulatic, S. C., Harter, D. H., Sweat, R. W., Spiegelman, S., and Lopez, C. (1975). *J. Gen. Virol.* **29,** 335–339.
Witter, R. L. (1978). *In* "Diseases in Poultry" (M. S. Hofstand, B. W. Calneck, C. F. Helmboldt, W. H. Reid, and H. W. Yoder, eds.), pp. 480–486. Iowa State Univ. Press, Ames.
Witter, R. L., Purchase, L. G., and Burgoyne, G. H. (1970). *JNCI, J. Natl. Cancer Inst.* **45,** 567–577.
Witter, R. L., Stephens, E. A., Sharma, J. M., and Nazerian, K. (1975). *J. Immunol.* **115,** 177–183.
Witter, R. L., Lee, L. F., Bacon, L. D., and Smith, E. J. (1979). *Infect. Immun.* **26,** 90–98.
Witter, R. L., Smith, E. J., and Crittenden, L. B. (1981). *Avian Dis.* **25,** 374–394.
Wong, T. C., and Lai, M. M. C. (1981). *Virology* **111,** 289–293.
Yaniv, A., Gazit, A., Ianconescu, M., Perk, K., Aizenberg, B., and Zimber, A. (1979). *J. Virol.* **30,** 351–357.
Ziegel, R. F., Theilen, G. H., and Twiehaus, M. J. (1966). *JNCI, J. Natl. Cancer Inst.* **37,** 709–729.

Rift Valley Fever

ARNON SHIMSHONY* and ROY BARZILAI†

Veterinary Services and Animal Health, Beit Dagan, Israel and †Israel Institute for Biological Research, Ness Ziona, Israel

I.	Introduction and History	347
II.	The Etiological Agent	349
	A. Classification	349
	B. The Virion	350
	C. Biosynthesis and Morphogenesis of RVFV	352
	D. Isolation, Propagation, and Assay of RVFV	354
	E. Immunological Identification of RVFV	357
	F. Strains	362
III.	The Host	366
	A. Host Range and Susceptibility	366
	B. Clinical Disease	367
	C. Pathological Changes	378
	D. Differential Diagnosis	387
IV.	Epidemiological Features	390
	A. Epizootiology and Epidemiology	390
	B. Vectorial Transmission	397
	C. Nonvectorial Transmission	402
	D. Virus Maintenance in Mammals	405
V.	Prevention and Control Measures	408
	A. Live Vaccines	408
	B. Inactivated Vaccines for Humans	411
	C. Inactivated Veterinary Vaccines	411
	D. Unorthodox Vaccines	413
	E. Treatment and Laboratory Safety Precautions	414
	F. Prevention and Control	415
	References	416
	Note Added in Proof	425

I. Introduction and History

During the first week of October 1977, physicians reported to the Egyptian Ministry of Health that an unusual "dengue-like illness" was rife among residents of villages near Inshas, in the southeastern sector of the Nile Delta. The morbidity reached extreme proportions and by the third week of October, the area of the epidemic had spread northward and southward. "Village streets usually bustling with activity at every hour of the day were all but deserted when much of the population suddenly became ill or stayed indoors to tend sick relatives (Darwish and Hoogstraal, 1981, p. 49)." The human disease continued to spread until the onset of cooler weather in early December. On October 10, agents from sera of 11 patients were isolated in white mice (Imam and Darwish, 1977). On October 30, one isolate was brought to the Yale Arbovirus Research Unit (YARU) in New Haven, Connecticut, which is the Arbovirus Reference Center of the World Health Organization. The specific diagnosis of Rift Valley fever (RVF) was made about 30 hr after reception of the specimen in the laboratory (Casals, 1978; Meegan, 1979).

It soon became apparent that widespread abortions and mortality in sheep, cattle, and buffalo had been devastating the livestock in various areas in Egypt for some time before RVF was diagnosed in humans. The epizootic represented also the first identified extension of RVF virus beyond the sub-Saharan range. It manifested a major human involvement, including many fatalities and complications that had not previously been observed during the African epizootics. Rift Valley fever has come into prominence as a potential international zoonotic virus disease problem, and has become an important topic of surveillance, research, and contingency activities of both vererinary and public health agencies.

This dramatic change represents a new chapter in the history of a virus first isolated by Daubney *et al.* (1931) near Lake Naivasha in the Rift Valley area of Kenya. They demonstrated in their classic work its characteristic destructive action on hepatic cells of susceptible animals, mainly newborn ovines and bovines, its abortifacient activity, possible mosquito transmission, and the resemblance of the human disease to "true dengue" and to yellow fever. They proposed the name "Rift Valley fever" as a "popular alternative to our first suggestion *enzootic hepatitis,* which was originally applied to the disease in sheep . . . since we have as yet no evidence that the liver is involved in man [p. 578]." They also remarked that the disease had undoubtedly existed in the Rift Valley for some time, causing extensive losses in sheep and cattle as well as dengue-like fever in humans in certain wet years, one of which was 1926. Indeed, later cited reports indicate that Montgomery (1912) and Stordy (1913) had observed epizootics in sheep on the government farm at Naivasha and on other farms in the Rift

Valley. Lambs inoculated by Montgomery with infective serum collapsed and died, revealing necrotic livers at necropsy; he suggested that the disease was distinct from Nairobi sheep disease. After 1931, laboratory studies and field observations revealed the wide host range of RVF—including domestic, wild, and laboratory animals—as well as the transmission of RVF virus by numerous mosquito species and the wide distribution of the virus within sub-Saharan African countries. Prior to 1977, RVF was recognized in at least 18 countries, and epizootics, encountered after periods of excessive rainfall and often separated by periods of as long as 10 or 15 years without any case of RVF, were reported from at least 8 countries and mainly from Kenya, South Africa, and Zimbabwe. Humans became infected whenever they came into close contact with diseased or dead animals, as well as in laboratories involved in RVF diagnosis or research. An inactivated lyophilized vaccine was produced and used for the protection of laboratory personnel at risk; attenuated neurotropic and inactivated vaccines for animal protection were developed and proved to be a successful control measure.

The virus has now spread in a 7000-km (4200-mile) north–south range throughout Africa, circulating in a number of differing climatic and geographical settings; its penetration into Egypt means successful amplification in a totally new ecosystem. Combined with the unprecedented severity of the epidemic in humans, it demonstrates the significance of this disease as a potential human and animal pathogen outside Africa.

Current knowledge of the properties of RVF virus and its epidemiology and pathogenesis are to be summarized in this article. The reader is referred to previous published review of RVF (Henning, 1956; Weiss, 1957; Easterday, 1965; Peters and Meegan, 1981) and to the proceedings of a workshop on Rift Valley fever, held in 1980 in Israel (Swartz *et al.*, 1981).

II. The Etiological Agent

A. Classification

For about three decades after its isolation by Daubney *et al.* (1931), Rift Valley fever virus (RVFV) was a unique species. By the standard arbovirus serological techniques (hemagglutination inhibition, neutralization, and complement fixation; Casals, 1967), no antigenic relationship was found between RVFV and any other arbovirus (Casals, 1963, 1971). Murphy *et al.* (1973) have shown by electron microscopic studies that RVFV is very similar in morphology and morphogenesis to other viruses of the Bunyamwera supergroup. Because of this similarity, Berge (1975) and Karabatsos (1978) listed RVFV as a "bunya-like virus." Antigenically, however, RVFV remained unrelated to any other agent as yet classified (Berge, 1975). Shope *et al.* (1980) reported serological cross-reactivity between RVFV and some members of the phlebotomus fever group.

Further serological confirmation was obtained by Shope *et al.* (1981) and Tesh *et al.* (1982). Biochemical proof that RVFV should be included in the phlebotomus fever group of viruses (composed of over 30 members) has been provided by Rice *et al.* (1980) and by Cash *et al.* (1981). Current classification of the Bunyaviridae family recognizes four genera: *Bunyavirus, Phlebovirus, Nairovirus,* and *Uukuvirus,* with RVFV as a member of the *Phlebovirus* genus (Bishop *et al.*, 1980).

B. The Virion

1. Size

The earliest estimation of the RVF virion's diameter was given by Broom and Findlay (1933). Based on filtration through collodion membrane, their estimation was 23–35 nm. Polson (1953) reported a diameter of 48.9 nm, as a result of ultracentrifugation studies. Naudè *et al* (1954), using the same methodology, observed some heterogenicity in the virions' size. The diameter of the pantropic virion was 49.7 nm. A similar value, 50 nm, was recorded for virions of the Smithburn neurotropic strain, at the 102nd mouse brain passage. In contrast, a derivative of the Smithburn strain, which had undergone 106 mouse brain plus 50 embryonated egg plus 9 mouse brain passages, revealed two populations of virions with diameters of 51.8 and 30.9 nm. Using electron microscopy (EM), Levitt *et al.* (1963) estimated a diameter of 60 to 75 nm for virions from serum of infected mice. McGavran and Easterday (1963), using the same technique, extended the size to about 90 nm for virions from infected mouse liver cells or from lamb serum. Levitt (1964) reported homogeneous diameter of about 100 nm for unpurified virions in mouse serum. Lecatsas and Weiss (1968), investigating RVFV-infected BHK cells by EM, reported that the diameter of the extracellular virion was 94 nm, with a core component of about 77 nm and capsid structure of about 9 nm. Murphy *et al.* (1973), also using EM, reported the size to be 90–110 nm. The same values were obtained by Ellis *et al.* (1979) for virions of the Egyptian isolate.

2. Molecular Analysis

The study by Rice et al. (1980) is essentially the chief comprehensive analysis of RVFV at the molecular level. The data obtained can be summarized as follows: the density of the virion in CsCl is 1.21 gm/ml. The density of the nucleocapsid (or "core component") is 1.29 gm/ml. As is typical for all members of the Bunyaviridae, the genome of RVFV is single-stranded RNA, in three segments. Polyacrylamide gel electrophoresis (PAGE) of the viral genome yields three classes of molecular weights: the large (L) segment of 2.7×10^6, the medium (M) segment of 1.7×10^6, and the small (S) segment of 0.6×10^6. This size distribution is similar to the distribution found in other phleboviruses (Cash et al., 1981). The virion contains three major structural proteins. The molecular weights of the virion proteins by PAGE are 65,000, 56,000, and 25,000. The 65,000 and the 56,000 MW proteins are glycosylated and are the structural components of the envelope. The 25,000-MW protein is nonglycosylated and is the major component of the nucleocapsid. There is an additional glycoprotein with a molecular weight of 100,000, which appears erratically in varying amounts in different preparations. The structural proteins of several different RVFV isolates migrate at an identical velocity in PAGE. The data provided by Rice et al. (1980) have been confirmed and extended by Cash et al. (1981).

No genome–product relationship is known for RVFV. By analogy, however, to other members of the Bunyaviridae that have been studied extensively, the following relationship can be surmised. The S-RNA segment codes for the nucleocapsid protein (Gentsch and Bishop, 1978). The M-RNA segment codes for the two envelope glycoproteins (Gentsch and Bishop, 1979), and these gene products are responsible for the induction of neutralizing antibodies in recipient animals (Gentsch et al., 1980). Moreover, as shown by Beaty et al. (1981), M-RNA codes for the structural components that determine transmissibility by the natural vector. The nucleocapsid (core) protein is probably the viral antigen that elicits complement-fixing antibodies (Lindsey et al., 1977).

In accordance with all other members of the Bunyaviridae, the RNA of RVFV should be of negative sense (Bishop and Shope, 1979). Viruses with genomes of negative-sense RNA depend on a structural RNA-dependent RNA polymerase for generating early viral m-RNA. Such an enzymatic activity has been demonstrated in Uukuniemi virus (Ranki and Pettersson, 1975) and in Lumbo virus (Bouloy and Hannoun, 1976). Neither the negativity of the RNA genome nor the polymerase activity has been demonstrated in RVFV.

3. Physicochemical properties

Rift Valley fever virus lyophilizes well and is very stable in liquid serum (Berge, 1975). Findlay (1932) found that blood preserved in oxalate–carbol–glycerin retained virulence after 8 months at 4°C. Easterday (1961) reported on sheep plasma that retained infectivity after 8 years of storage and shipment under a variety of refrigeration conditions. The virus is very resistant to temperatures lower than 60°C and will readily be recovered from serum after several months of storage at 4°C or after 3 hr at 56°C (Smithburn et al., 1949b; Mims and Mason, 1956; Craig et al., 1967; Klein et al., 1969).

The virus is inactivated by fixation in acetone at −30°C overnight (Easterday and Jaeger, 1963), by 0.25% solution of 10% commercial formalin at 4°C for 3 days, and by methylene blue in the presence of light (MacKenzie, 1935). Lipid solvents such as ether (Andrewes and Horstmann, 1949; Findlay and Howard, 1951) and sodium deoxycholate (Theiler, 1957) inactivate the virus, indicating the presence of lipid envelope. Thomas et al. (1978) reported that RVF antigen was susceptible to tryptic digestion at trypsin levels of 8 to 16 µg/ml. In cell monolayers, the virus is not completely inactivated by the addition of acetone at −60°C for 48 hr (Hahon and Zimmerman, 1969). The virus is inactivated rapidly at pH below 6.8 (Mims, 1956b). Rift Valley fever virus is highly stable in aerosol form at temperatures of 23°C and at relative humidity of 50 or 85% (Miller et al., 1963).

C. Biosynthesis and Morphogenesis of RVFV

Very little is known about the biosynthesis of RVFV-directed macromolecules and the biochemical stages in virus replication. Most of the available information has been derived from ultrastructural studies by EM. McGavran and Easterday (1963), who were first to investigate by EM thin sections of liver cells from RVFV-infected mice. The main findings were that RVFV replicates in the cytoplasm, that virions are assembled in a membrane-limited system, and that the site of assembly is closely associated with the Golgi apparatus. Lecatsas and Weiss (1968) conducted a similar investigation in BHK cells infected with a pantropic or a neurotropic strain of RVFV. Both virus strains produced the same ultrastructural effects in the infected cells. The finding in general agreed with McGavran and Easterday's observations (1963). Lecatsas and Weiss (1968) stressed the finding that "no envelope derived from the cell membrane is present on virus particles inside or outside the cell." Murphy et al. (1973) reported similar findings and have shown that the morphogenesis of RVFV proceeds along the general replication pattern of all bunyaviruses. It is generally assumed today that RVFV is a typical Bunyaviridae member (Bishop and Shope, 1979), and it is inferred that intracellular events during RVFV replication would be similar to those known for other better studied members of this family. The reader is referred to Bishop and Shope (1979) for a detailed life history of the bunyaviruses.

A singular feature of RVFV replication is the appearance of nuclear inclusion bodies (NIB) in virus-infected cells. Again, the first to observe and describe NIB were Daubney et al. (1931). These structures were noted in liver cells from RVFV-infected sheep. They were heavily eosinophilic on staining and were globular in shape. Findlay (1933) extended this finding to liver cells of other species, noting that NIB appeared in hepatocytes but not in Kupffer cells. Horning and Findlay (1934) tried to analyze these structures but were unable to stain them for lipids, "thymonucleic acid" (DNA), or iron. MacKenzie and Findlay (1936) described NIB in brain tissue from mice infected with neurotropic RVFV; similar findings were reported by Smithburn (1949). Mims (1957) noted that under condition of infection with "saturation dose," NIB appeared as early as 1 hr post inoculation. Plowright and Ferris (1957) were the first to observe NIB in RVFV-infected monolayer cultures of sheep kidney cells. In addition to the known globular form of NIB, they have encountered an elongated, fibrous form of NIB. Coackley (1963) found both types of NIB in cultures of lamb testis cells infected with pantropic or neurotropic RVFV strains.

The fibrous form was more prominent in cells that were infected with the pantropic strains. In the wake of the South African RVF outbreak in 1975, Coetzer (1977) reported that NIB were visualized in 49% of all positive cases in newborn lambs. Van Velden et al. (1977) have encountered NIB in histological sections of livers from fatal human cases. Eisa and Obeid (1977) reported NIB in livers from sheep infected during the 1973 RVF epizootic in Sudan, as well as in livers of mice inoculated with Sudanese isolates of RVFV. Tomori and Kasali (1979) demonstrated that NIB appeared in liver or brain cells of mice that were infected with Lunyo virus, thereby substantiating the notion that the Lunyo virus may be a natural derivative of RVFV. Nuclear inclusion bodies were encountered with such regularity in RVFV-infected cells that their presence in histological sections of animal tissues became indicative of RVF. The nature of NIB, however, remained enigmatic for a long time. Failing to stain NIB with fluorescent anti-RVFV antibodies or to react them positively in the Feulgen reaction for DNA, Easterday and Jaeger (1963) and McGavran and

Easterday (1963) concluded that NIB were the manifestation of some degenerative process in the cell. Lecatsas and Weiss (1968) did not rule out the possibility that NIB were some sort of ribonucleoproteins of cellular or of viral origin.

In 1977, Swanepoel and Blackburn reported that fibrous NIB appeared in BHK, Vero, or lamb testis cell cultures after infection with several Zimbabwean isolates of RVFV. They also reported, in contrast to previous findings of other investigators, the indirect staining of the infected nuclei by anti-RVFV sheep serum and fluorescent anti-sheep antibodies. Ellis *et al.* (1979) also found the fibrous NIB in Vero or in mouse hepatocytes after infection with an Egyptian isolate of RVFV. They agreed with Swanepoel and Blackburn (1977) that the fibrous NIB may be virus related and "probably precursor material for virus cores to be assembled later in the cytoplasm (Ellis *et al.*, 1979, p. 336)."

Struthers and Swanepoel (1982) were again able to demonstrate virus-specific fluorescence in the nuclei of Vero cells infected with several Zimbabwean isolates of RVFV. Moreover, they were able to demonstrate by immunoprecipitation the intranuclear existence of a virus-specific protein with a molecular weight of 25,000. They considered this molecule as virus-specific, thus implicating the nucleus at some stage in the biosynthesis of an otherwise cytoplasmic virus.

D. Isolation, Propagation, and Assay of RVFV

1. Isolation

The first isolation of RVFV (Daubney *et al.*, 1931) was accomplished by inoculating lambs with serum from a moribund sheep. After Findlay and Daubney (1931) had shown that mice were susceptible to RVFV by any inoculation route, mouse inoculation became the primary tool for virus isolation. Because viremia in moribund cases of RVF reaches very high levels and closely follows the clinical signs, whole blood, plasma, or serum samples have generally been used as virus source. The virus was isolated in this way during the RVF epizootics in 1973 (Sudan; Eisa and Obeid, 1977), 1975 (South Africa; Van Velden *et al.*, 1977), and 1977 (Egypt; Imam and Darwish, 1977; Abdel Wahab *et al.*, 1978).

Rift Valley fever virus has usually been isolated from whole blood, plasma, or serum sampled during the febrile period of the disease. The virus can be isolated from various body organs, preferably liver, spleen, kidneys, and fetal tissues (Peters and Meegan, 1981). Aqueous suspensions of insect tissues are (since the original isolation by Smithburn *et al.*, 1948) the standard source of virus in vector studies.

Intracerebral (ic) inoculation of suckling mice is standard procedure for virus isolation for many arboviruses. Because RVFV is pantropic, intraperitoneal (ip) inoculation in weaned mice is also effective. Swanepoel (1981) stressed that virus isolation by ip inoculation has the added advantage of presumptive RVF diagnosis. During the 1973 RVF epizootic in the Sudan, however, Eisa and Obeid (1977) were unable to isolate the virus by the ip inoculation of weaned mice. Virus was isolated only by ic inoculations (any age) or ip in suckling mice.

There are few modifications of this basic isolation scheme. Kaschula (1953) used embryonated eggs. Johnson *et al.* (1978) used Vero cell cultures in addition to mouse inoculation. Imam *et al.* (1981a) recommended that clinical specimens first be inoculated into cultures of CER cells and that the medium from these cultures should be used in mouse inoculations. El-Mekki and van der Groen (1981) isolated and identified RVFV in serum samples within 24 hr, by immunofluorescence staining of infected BHK, Vero, or CV-1 cell cultures.

2. Propagation and Assay

RVFV can be propagated in various *in vivo* or *in vitro* systems. Virus yields are assayed by usual virus titrations, with titers expressed (per unit volume) in MIC LD_{50} (mouse ic dose 50%), MIP LD_{50} (same, ip), TC ID_{50} (tissue culture-infecting dose 50%; productive infection being determined by cytopathic effects in the cell monolayer), or PFU (plaque-forming units). The arithmetic method of finding the 50% is based mainly on Reed and Muench (1938). With all its inaccuracies, it is sufficient for "end point" (50% effect level) along a 7- or 8-log scale. Mice are still utilized extensively as the main *in vivo* system for propagating most strains of RVFV, with up to 10^{10} MIP LD_{50}/ml yields (Mims, 1956a–d).

Embryonated eggs, minced chick embryos, or cultures of chick embryo fibroblasts have been repeatedly used for RVF propagation (MacKenzie, 1933; Saddington, 1934; Endo, 1951; Kaschula, 1953; Matumoto *et al.*, 1959; Easterday, 1961; Randall *et al.*, 1962; Binn *et al.*, 1963a). Virus yields from these substrates were usually lower than in other systems. Vaccines obtained from RVFV grown in embryonated eggs or chick cells were of poor antigenicity. Eisa and Obeid (1977) reported that they were able to demonstrate RVFV activity by lethality to chick embryos *in ovo,* but not in chick embryo fibroblasts. It is of interest to note that Saddington (1934) was unable to find any nuclear inclusion bodies in chick cells exposed to RVFV.

Various malignant cells, of mammalian origin, proved to be good propagators of RVFV, *in vivo* or *in vitro* (rat sarcoma, mouse sarcoma, and Ehrlich ascites, Takemori et al., 1954; rat hepatoma, Takemori et al., 1955a; plaque formation, Takemori et al., 1955b).

Several primary cultures of mammalian cells were extensively used for propagation and study of RVFV. These include sheep kidney cells (Weiss, 1956, cited by Weiss, 1957; Plowright and Ferris, 1957), lamb testis cells (Hess et al., 1963; Coackley, 1963; Swanepoel and Blackburn, 1977), goat kidney cells (Imam and El-Karamany, 1978), and kidney cells from *Macaca mulata* or *Cercopithecus aethiops* (rhesus and African green monkey, respectively, Randall et al., 1962, 1963). In contrast to these cells, which proved excellent propagators for RVFV, calf kidney cells are apparently poor substrate (Eisa and Obeid, 1977).

The use of established cell lines was started by Iwasa (1959), who had utilized an established cell line of human origin (Chang liver) for virus propagation, for plaque formation, and for immunofluorescence studies. Titration in mice was more sensitive than the plaque assay by a factor of $10^{2.3}$. When the virus had undergone successive passages, the sensitivity gap decreased to a factor of $10^{1.1}$ to $10^{0.4}$, with mouse titration being more sensitive. Several cell lines were examined by Easterday and Murphy (1963a) for their ability to propagate the pantropic van Wyk strain (Chang liver and HeLa, of human origin; L cells from mice; guinea pig lung cell line; hamster kidney line). In most cases, better yields were obtained when low-input multiplicities were used. Maximal titer was obtained in the hamster kidney line, about $10^{8.2}$ MIP LD_{50}/ml, which represented a 380-fold increase over the inoculum. Boyle (1965) titrated the van Wyk strain of RVFV in hamster kidney cell line by TC ID_{50} and PFU, as well as in mice by the cerebral and peritoneal routes. For the same virus suspension, he obtained titers (per milliliter) of $10^{8.1}$ TC ID_{50}, $10^{8.2}$ PFU, 10^7 MIC LD_{50}, and $10^{6.5}$ MIP LD_{50}. Boyle (1967) reported that after three serial passages of the van Wyk virus in mouse fibroblast line, he was able to observe and isolate plaques of distinctly different sizes. The small-plaque (SP) variant was more stable at 56°C than the large plaque (LP). Maximal yield after propagation were higher by a factor of 16 for SP than for LP. The SP variant was 100-fold more virulent to mice by the ip route than the LP variant. Again, titrations in tissue cultures generally gave higher titers than mouse titrations. By comparison to the parental strain, however, the SP was found to be 100-fold less virulent by the mouse ip inoculation. In contrast, Moussa et al. (1982) reported that their SP variant appeared to be less pathogenic to mice than the parental, LP ZH501 strain. Orlando et al. (1967) and Johnson and Orlando (1968) reported the propagation of the van Wyk strain in suspended culture of L cells, reaching yields of over 10^9 MIC LD_{50}/ml. This system was further investigated and optimized by Walker et al.

(1969). They used suspended L cells and the small-plaque variant of the van Wyk strain. Klein et al. (1970) found, in contrast to Boyle's results, that the titration of van Wyk SP yields from suspended cultures of L cells was 30-fold more sensitive by MIC LD_{50} than by PFU. Klein et al. (1971) propagated the original van Wyk strain in 20 and 40 liters of suspended L-cell cultures, with yields in the range of 10^8 to 10^9 MIC LD_{50}/ml. Again, titers by PFU were about 10-fold lower than by MIC LD_{50}.

The MBDK cell line was used by Prozeski (1972) to plaque-purify a wild-type strain of RVFV and to propagate the cloned strain. Temperature-sensitive mutants were searched for after mutagenesis by nitrosoguanidine. One plaque, called ts-1, proved to be a true ts mutant. This is the only work of its kind with RVFV. The Vero cell line was used by Koyama and Higashihara (1974) to propagate the pantropic Daubney strain and to clone variants by plaque-to-plaque purification. Four derivatives were obtained, three of which were nonpathogenic to mice by subcutaneous (sc) or intravenous (iv) routes.

Cultures of BHK cell line were used by Barnard and Botha (1977) to propagate the Smithburn strain and a pantropic field isolate for vaccine production. Monolayer cultures of BHK cells were used (Yedloutschnig et al., 1980) to produce an inactivated vaccine from the Entebbe strain. Barzilai and Ben-Nathan (1982a) used BHK cells for plaque assay and plaque purification of the Smithburn strain.

The FRhL-2 cell line (from fetal rhesus monkey lung; also called DBS-103) has been used by Eddy et al. (1981) to grow the Entebbe strain for the production of an inactivated vaccine. The ZH-501 strain was also propagated in FRhL-2 cells, and yields used for animal challenge (Harrington et al., 1980; Yedloutschnig et al., 1980, 1981a–d). Several clones of ZH-501 were plaque-purified in FRhL-2 cells (Peters and Anderson, 1981). The CER cell line has been extensively studied in Egypt by El-Karamany et al. (1979, 1981) and was utilized for vaccine production from Egyptian RVFV isolates.

E. Immunological Identification of RVFV

1. Neutralization

Findlay (1932) performed the first serum neutralization test (SNT) for RVFV. He had used the constant virus–serum dilution procedure and ip inoculation of adult mice for the neutralization index (NI). With minor modifications (e.g., Kitchen, 1950), this procedure has been extensively used by most laboratories. The NI is still a prime characteristic of a successful vaccine (Randall et al., 1962; Weiss, 1962; Coackley *et al.*, 1967a,b; Barnard and Botha, 1977; El-Karamani *et al.*, 1981). The SNT was utilized for the detection of antibodies in humans and animals by Findlay (1936), Sabin and Blumberg (1947), and Smithburn *et al.* (1949b). Gear *et al.* (1951) used SNT for the diagnosis of suspected RVF cases. Eisa and Obeid (1977) identified RVFV as the etiological agent responsible for the epizootic outbreak in Sudan in 1973, by SNT. This procedure, however, is applicable only when pantropic strains are utilized. With the advent of neurotropic strains, the NI could have been estimated only by ic inoculation of the virus–serum mixture. Kaschula (1953, cited by Weiss, 1957), however, preferred ip inoculation of suckling mice. Randall *et al.* (1962) also concluded that the NT using suckling mice inoculated ip was consistently more sensitive than the test employing the ic route in adult mice. Kasahara and Koyama (1973) noted that "the intracerebral injection is more sensitive for virus detection and is particularly suitable for recovering active virus from materials containing active virus and neutralizing antibodies [p. 106]." Currently, the constant virus–serum dilution is being utilized, in the plaque-reduction neutralization test (PRNT) format (Harrington *et al.*, 1980; Eddy *et al.*, 1981). Abdel-Wahab *et al.* (1978) and Johnson *et al.* (1978) used a qualitative SNT in Vero cells for the identification of RVF cases in Egypt during the years 1977–1978.

2. Complement Fixation

The first RVF complement fixation test (CFT) was carried out by Broom and Findlay (1932), using 2% saline extract of infected liver as antigen. This test detected RVFV antibodies in convalescent sera from human cases and various animals. Matumoto *et al.* (1950) demonstrated that their pantropic and neurotropic strains were antigenically identical by CFT. Gear *et al.* (1951) used this test for the diagnosis of RVF cases. They also reported that there was an exact correlation between results obtained by CFT and SNT. Due to the rather high laboratory hazard of the pantropic strains, they preferred CFT over SNT as the diagnostic procedure of choice. Haig and Kaschula (1952, cited by Weiss, 1957), however, found that immunization by neurotropic RVF did not always elicit detectable levels of CF antibodies. Henning (1956) pointed out that the antigen utilized in these cases was not prepared from the homologous strain but from a virulent field isolate. Weiss (1956) found that a CF antigen (CF-Ag) prepared from lamb kidney tissue culture infected with a neurotropic strain was effective in detecting CF antibodies (at a low titer) in sera of sheep immunized with a neurotropic RVFV. Iwasa (1959) found CF antigen in RVFV-infected Chang human liver cells and determined that his fluorescent antibodies were actually directed against this antigen. Randall et al (1962) used CF-Ag from a neurotropic RVFV strain. They reported that sera from mice immunized with inactivated pantropic RVFV failed to yield CF reaction with this antigen compared to sera from mice immunized with inactivated neurotropic RVFV.

Levitt and Polson (1964) compared soluble CF antigens extracted from mice infected with four different RVFV strains and concluded that they were immunologically identical. The pantropic CF-Ag was consistently obtained in greater amounts than neurotropic CF-Ag.

In 1975 CFT was used to identify RVFV as the pathogen responsible for the 1975 South African epizootic (Van Velden et al., 1977). Casals (1978) reported that CFT was the first step in the identification of the Egyptian epizootic in 1977 as RVF. Abdel-Wahab et al. (1978) and Johnson et al. (1978) similarly used CFT as an initial step in RVFV identification. Shope (1978) reported that by CFT, RVFV was still in splendid antigenic isolation, different from all other Bunyamwera or bunya-like viruses.

3. Hemagglutination and Hemagglutination Inhibition

The first demonstration that RVFV was able to agglutinate erythrocytes was accomplished by Mims and Mason (1956). They also characterized the inhibition of that reaction by specific antisera. Because antisera specific to group A or group B arboviruses failed to inhibit the hemagglutination (H) reaction, they concluded rather prophetically that "serologically, therefore, RVF, like Bunyamwera and sandfly fever virus, must be placed in a group of miscellaneous viruses [p. 430]." Because the hemagglutination inhibition (HI) test or reaction proved later to be important for RVFV classification (Shope et al., 1980), this subject will be discussed in somewhat greater detail. The initial H antigen (H-Ag) was obtained by acetone–ether extraction of serum from RVFV-infected mice (Mims and Mason, 1956). This extract agglutinated only erythrocytes obtained from 24-hr-old chickens. In contrast, untreated serum from infected mice agglutinated erythrocytes from cock, <24-hr-old mice (also from adult mice, but at eightfold lesser efficiency), guinea pig, and human group A. The pH of the reaction was found to be rather critical, with maximal agglutination taking place at pH 6.5. In the wake of Porterfield's report (1957) that erythrocytes from an adult goose were an excellent indicator for H activity of arboviruses, and in fact even better than the 1-day-old chick erythrocytes, Clarke and Casals (1958) included these cells in their standard procedure. They recommended the sucrose–acetone extraction procedure for obtaining high-titered preparations of H-Ag. This work, however, dealt with RVFV only by reference to Mims and Mason's report (1956). In 1978, Thomas et al. compared H-Ag obtained from livers of RVFV-infected suckling mice according to Clarke and Casals (1958), with mouse serum antigen obtained according to Mims and Mason (1956).

The sucrose–acetone extracted liver antigen had a 10-fold greater H activity than the acetone–ether antigen. In both cases, however, maximum activity was obtained at pH 6.0. Sucrose–acetone extract prepared by Imam and Darwish (1977) from brains of infected mice was active only as a CF antigen, with no H activity at all. Imam et al. (1981b) obtained large amounts of H-Ag at very high titers and in short time from the amniotic fluids of pregnant sheep that were infected in utero with RVFV. The HI technique (HIT) has been employed for monitoring seroconversion after vaccination by various investigators (Randall et al., 1962; Binn et al., 1963b). It has been extensively used in Egypt for serosurveys during and after the 1977–1978 epizootic (see Darwish and Hoogstraal, 1981, for comprehensive summary), and in Israel as part of the contingency activities (Shimshony et al., 1981b).

In 1980, Shope et al. reported that for the first time, some antigenic relationship had been established between RVFV and other viruses. Using HIT, they were able to demonstrate cross-reactivity between RVFV and several members of the phlebotomus fever group. This finding was corroborated later by fluorescent antibodies (Shope et al., 1981; Tesh et al., 1982) and other techniques (Rice et al., 1980; Cash et al., 1981).

4. Fluorescent Antibody Technique

As early as 1959 Iwasa was able to apply fluorescent antibodies (FA) to RVFV-infected Chang human liver cells and to identify virus-specific components. According to Iwasa, the component responsible for uptake of anti-RVFV FA was identical to the virus CF antigen. Easterday and Jaeger (1963) used the same "direct" FA test (FAT) to monitor time sequences in RVFV replication. They were able to detect the production of RVFV-specific antigens in infected cells as early as 6 hr postinoculation. Hahon (1969) corroborated these findings. Ohder et al. (1970) utilized FA to follow the growth of various viruses, including RVFV, in tissue cultures. Pini et al. (1970) used the "indirect" FA technique (IFAT) for the detection of RVFV-specific antigens in frozen sections of tissues from experimentally infected animals. The IFAT was equally effective in visualizing antigens induced by two neurotropic strains (Smithburn, IB 8) and the pantropic strains (Kabete, van Wyk). (The differences encountered were only in the tissue distributions of the antigens.) Neurotropic antigens were generally limited to the brain, whereas the pantropic antigens were encountered in visceral organs. Davies *et al.* (1972) utilized FAT and IFAT to demonstrate viremia and circulating antibodies, respectively, in baboons. These investigators considered IFAT to be at least as sensitive as the neutralization test to detect antibodies produced by the pantropic virus. This statement was substantiated later by Pini *et al.* (1973). Antibodies to Smithburn neurotropic strains were found only in cattle, at low level and for short duration.

El-Mekki and van der Groen (1981) tried to isolate and identify RVFV (among other viruses) directly from infected mouse brain material. They inoculated tissue cultures with the infective material at a very low initial multiplicity. With IFAT, they were able to detect and identify RVFV as early as 22 hr postinfection. Shope *et al.* (1981) and Tesh *et al.* (1982) further demonstrated the antigenic relationship between RVFV and the phleboviruses, utilizing IFAT.

5. Gel Diffusion Precipitation (GDP)

Mansy (1955, cited by Weiss, 1957) has shown that a number of viruses could be recognized by using precipitin reaction in agar. Weiss (1956) demonstrated this reaction using RVFV. Levitt and Polson (1964) were able to isolate a soluble antigen with CF activity from brains or livers infected with neurotropic or pantropic RVFV strains. They were able to produce precipitation lines with specific antisera. They concluded that all of their strains were antigenically identical, irrespective of the source organs or the tropism of the strain. Irregularities in line numbers were explained on various quantitative grounds. Because both CF activity and precipitability in GDP tests (GDPT) comigrated in an electrophoretic column, Levitt and Polson (1964) concluded that the CF antigen is the precipitate material in GDP. Swanepoel (1976) has used GDPT for RVFV identification. A plain 10–20% suspension of an organ obtained by necropsy proved to be a relatively good antigen for this test. A total of 102 samples considered RVFV-positive by histology were analyzed by both CFT and GDPT; 93 samples were positive by CFT, and 52 were positive by GDPT. None of an additional 53 necropsies judged as RVFV-negative by histology gave identity lines. Ayoub and Allam (1981) found that infected livers or brains were good sources of antigen for GDPT, whereas infected tissue cultures were not. Also, they reported that GDPT detected RVF antibodies only in sera from convalescent sheep, but not from actively immunized animals. Tomori (1979b) used GDPT to study the antigenic relationship of the Nigerian RVFV, the Smithburn strain, and the Lunyo virus. All the strains were indistinguishable from each other by CFT. Also, at least one line of identity was common to all strains, from any source. Peters and Anderson (1981) reported that three lines of identity were formed when Lunyo and Zagazig RVFV strains were compared in GDPT.

6. The Antigenic Activities of RVFV

The response of RVFV strains in various immunological test systems present a slight confusion. It is generally agreed that for the bunyaviruses, neutralizing and HI activities are displayed by antibodies directed against the envelope glycoproteins. Complement fixation activity is displayed by antibodies directed against the nucleocapsid (see Bishop and Shope, 1979). Also, as a rule, SNT and HIT coincide in specificity. The CFT, however, sometimes coincides with the specificity of SNT and HIT (Bishop and Shope, 1979). For RVFV, SNT apparently coincides with CFT in specificity, whereas HIT reveals cross-reactivity with other viruses.

According to Iwassa (1959), FAT is based on the intracellular CF antigen. If so, then FAT should have the same specificity as CFT, but in fact it is as cross-reactive as the HIT. Apparently, the antigenic structure of RVFV is not as yet completely clear.

F. Strains

1. Field Isolates of RVFV

Pantropic RVFV has been isolated repeatedly from domestic ruminants, arthropod vectors, and humans. Some of these isolates have been employed more extensively than others in various laboratories or have special significance in RVFV research. A partial list is presented in Table I. Additional strains were listed by Peters and Anderson (1981). El-Karamany *et al.* (1981) list a collection of 103 Egyptian isolates. The Lunyo isolate, although different in some respects from other RVFV strains, was considered sufficiently similar to prototype strains to be included in this table. Peters and Meegan (1981) reported that serial mouse liver passages result in the emergence of classical

TABLE I

WILD-TYPE ISOLATES OF RVFV FREQUENTLY ENCOUNTERED IN PUBLISHED REPORTS

Virus name	Country	Year	Source	Reference
Daubney	Kenya	1930	Sheep	Daubney et al. (1931)
Kabete	Kenya	?	?	Coackley (1965)
Chu	Kenya	?	Cattle	Coackley et al. (1967a,b)
Entebbe[a]	Uganda	1944	*Eretmapodites*	Smithburn et al. (1948)
Lunyo[b]	Uganda	1954	*Aedes africanus*	Weinbren et al. (1956, 1957)
Ib-Ar 5171	Nigeria	1967–1970	*Culex antennatus*	Lee (1970)
Ib-Ar 5172	Nigeria	1967–1970	*Culicoides* spp.	Lee (1970)
Van Wyk	South Africa	1951	Sheep	Kaschula (1953)
Field strain	South Africa	1974	Cattle	Barnard and Botha (1977)
SA-75	South Africa	1975	Human	Rice et al. (1980)
ZW-(Several)	Zimbabwe	several	Cattle	Swanepoel (1976, 1981)
Zagazig series				
ZH-41	Egypt	1977	Human	Imam and Darwish (1977); Casals (1978)
ZH-501	Egypt	1977	Human	Meegan et al. (1979)

[a] Findlay and Howard (1951) used this name for two neurotropic strains, produced and dried in 1945 by the Yellow Fever Research Laboratory, Entebbe, Uganda.
[b] See text.

RVF virus. Several pantropic strains, well separated by time, space, and source of isolation, have been compared by various criteria. Nigerian, Smithburn, and Lunyo strains were shown to be identical by CF test (Tomori, 1979a,b). Antibodies against Lunyo virus neutralized both the Nigerian and the Smithburn strain, but antisera that were raised against these strains failed to neutralize Lunyo (Tomori, 1979a,b). Also, the Lunyo virus was shown to lack hemagglutinating activity for chick or goose erythrocytes (Tomori, 1979a,b). Van Wyk, Entebbe, Zagazig 501, and SA-75 (a South African isolate from humans; Peters and Anderson, 1981) were indistinguishable by cross-neutralization, by PAGE analysis of structural proteins (Rice et al., 1980; Peters and Meegan, 1981), or by infective dose by aerosol inoculation (Brown et al., 1981).

Cash et al. (1981) compared the viral RNA fingerprints of two Egyptian (Zagazig) isolates, Entebbe, van Wyk, and two Zimbabwean isolates from 1970 and 1974. With one exception, all displayed unique oligonucleotide patterns, significantly different from each other. The exception was the two Zagazig series isolates, which appeared identical by this analysis.

Most wild-type isolates are basically pantropic. Lunyo is an exception, being more neurotropic (Weinbren et al., 1957). Some differences were noted in the host range of various isolates: the Egyptian isolates were shown to be lethal to Wistar-Furth rats whereas other African isolates were innocuous. All pantropic strains are characterized by being highly pathogenic after inoculation by any route, exhibiting high-titered viremia and causing death by major liver necrosis. Various conditions may alter the pathogenesis by an otherwise pantropic strain. In most cases, the altered pathogenesis is expressed by lethal encephalitis, with average survival time significantly longer than that observed in liver necrosis. Bennett et al. (1965) reported that when immune serum was administered at 16 hr postinfection or later to van Wyk-infected mice, a significant number of the treated mice developed lethal encephalitis. When examined for virus, the brain content was 10^7–10^8 MIP LD_{50}, with $\sim 10^3$ MIP LD_{50} in the liver.

Eddy et al. (1981) were able to protect mice with antiserum or interferon inducers against sc inoculation with $10^{5.4}$ PFU of ZH-501. The protection was not complete and 10–20% mortality was recorded, with encephalitis as the cause of death. Peters and Anderson (1981) have shown that ZH-501 exhibited a typically neurotropic behavior on infection of a nonpermissive host. "Incomplete viruses" (Mims, 1956d), accumulated during low-dilution passages of the Entebbe strain, caused on occasion a typically neurotropic behavior of the pantropic strain. (For a review on the subject of interference, see Easterday, 1965.)

2. Neurotropic Derivatives of Pantropic RVFV

Table II lists several attempts to obtain neurotropic strains. The common denominator to all these attempts was the repeated propagation of the virus in a highly permissive system (mouse brain or tissue culture). Kaschula's strains $NRVF_1$ and $NRVF_2$ were actually the 86th and the 102nd passages of the Smithburn strain, and therefore already neurotropic before egg passages had commenced (Weiss, 1957). Kaschula's strains $RRVF_1$, $PRVF_2$, and PRVFM were the only ones in which the starting strain was pantropic. Except the citation by Weiss (1957), the published data about these strains are insufficient to describe their tropism. The mechanisms by which a pantropic strain acquires neurotropic properties are not known. Apparently the various

TABLE II

NEUROTROPIC DERIVATIVES OF PANTROPIC RVFV STRAINS

Method	Derived strain	Reference
Serial passages of the Daubney strain in mouse brains; the first inoculations carried out in passively immunized mice		MacKenzie and Findlay (1936); MacKenzie et al., (1936)
Serial passages of the Entebbe strain in mouse brains, without initial step of passive immunity	Smithburn	Smithburn (1949)
Serial passages in mice as above		Kitchen (1950)
Serial passages of Daubney strain in tissue-cultured chick brain	Endo	Endo (1951)
Serial passages of a pantropic strain isolated from cattle, in tissue-cultured lamb testis cells	IB 8	Coackley (1965)
Serial plaque-to-plaque transfer of Daubney strain in vero cell line	E Plaques	Koyama and Higashihara (1974)
Cloning by plaque to plaque and terminal dilution of ZH-501 in FRhL cell line	205514 and other clones	Peters and Anderson (1981)

systems listed in Table II selected preexisting variants that could no longer replicate to the same extent as the wild-type strains. The brain, however, affords an ideal replication site, even to otherwise enfeebled viruses. When such viruses replicate freely under "virotropic" conditions, new variants with improved growth characteristics may be generated. Within one passage in rat hepatoma cells, progeny viruses of the Endo strain exhibited pathogenicity by the sc route (Takemori *et al.*, 1955a). These investigators did not attempt the isolation of variants capable of causing a visceral disease. Tomori and Kasali (1979) reported that by two cycles of collecting sera from suckling mice inoculated ic with the Lunyo or the Smithburn strains, pantropic variants were obtained. Barzilai and Ben Nathan (1982b) observed ascending infection by Smithburn strain after its ic inoculation into suckling mice. The passaged virus showed enhanced virulence for adult mice by ip inoculation.

III. The Host

A. Host Range and Susceptibility

The host range of RVF, on the basis of direct and indirect evidence of natural infection as well as experimental infection trials, was reviewed and summarized according to degrees of susceptibility by Weiss (1957), Easterday (1965), and Provost (1981). The modified data are represented in Table III. There is serological evidence that RVFV might also infect hippopotamus (Weinbren and Hewitt, 1958), donkeys (Meegan, 1981), and weaverbirds (Davies and Addy, 1979).

The susceptibility of various species has been reviewed by Peters and Anderson (1981) in light of their experiments with various inbred strains of rats and their crosses. Susceptible rat strains, such as Brown-Norway or Wistar-Furth, developed fulminant liver necrosis within 3 to 5 days when inoculated with less than 5 PFU virus dose of

TABLE III

Host Range of Rift Valley Fever Virus

100% Fatal	High mortality	Severe, mostly nonfatal	Subclinical	Refractory to experimental infection
Lamb (1)[a]	Sheep (1)	Human (1)	Monkey (African) (1)	Mongoose (1)
Kid (1)	Calf (1)	Monkey (Indian and South American) (1)	Wild rodents (6)	Hedgehog (1)
White mouse (1)	Rat[b] (1)	Cattle (1)	Rabbit (1)	Spider monkey (1)
Hamster (1)	Gerbil (3)	Goat (1)	Pig (1)	Tortoise (1)
Field mouse (1)	Laucha (3)	Sheep[b] (4)	Dog (2)	Frog (1)
Dormouse (1)	Puppy (2)	Buffalo (African) (1)	Cat (2)	Hedgehog (1)
Field vole (1)	Kitten (2)	Buffalo (Asian) (5)	Horse (7)	Geckos (8)
Rat[b] (3)		Gray squirrel (1)	Rat[b] (3)	Hen (1)(9)
		Wild rodents (6)	Guinea pig (3)	Canary (1)
		Camel (5)		Pigeon (1)
				Parakeet (1)

[a]References: (1) Easterday (1965); (2) Walker et al. (1970a, b); (3) Peters and Anderson (1981); (4) Fagbami et al. (1975); (5) Meegan (1981); (6) McIntosh (1961), Swanepoel et al. (1978); (7) Erasmus and Coetzer (1981), Yedloutschnig et al. (1981b); (8) Williams et al. (1960); (9) Davies and Addy (1979).

[b]Certain species or breeds.

the ZH-501 RVFV strain. Resistant strains, such as Lewis, Buffalo, and F344, developed viremia and later antibody, but no overt disease, when inoculated with more than 500,000 PFU virus dose. "Encephalitic strains," such as ACI and Maxx, developed encephalitis within 7 to 14 days when inoculated with 5000 to 500,000 PFU virus dose. They found that resistance to fatal hepatic lesions was inherited as a simple Mendelian dominant gene. Susceptibility was age and sex related: resistant strains showed marked susceptibility in younger age, males at all ages were less resistant, and castrated males showed resistance similar to females. Syrian hamsters, Sprague-Dawley rats, and ICF Swiss mice were shown to be highly susceptible, with ascending rate of dose resistance; cotton rats (*Sigmodon hispidus*), lauchas (*Calomys callosus*), and gerbils (*Meriones unguiculatus*) were "encephalitic"; guinea pigs were found to be resistant even to the highest infective dose (10^7 PFU), with antibody production. Age-dependent resistance had been demonstrated in rats by Findlay and Howard (1952) and is seen in various species (see Table III). Differential susceptibility of various breeds of domestic animals has been mentioned (Fagbami *et al.*, 1975; Kamel, 1981; World Health Organization, 1982b). Peters and Anderson (1981) suggested that perhaps two-thirds of sheep are genetically resistant to fulminant hepatic disease. They also suspected that the pathogenesis of the rat and human infections may share critical features. Rosebrock and Peters (1982) demonstrated that RVFV replicated in cultured macrophages from genetically susceptible rat strains. Macrophages from genetically resistant rat strains, however, were restrictive for virus growth. During the outbreak in Egypt, the disease was prevalent in all age groups with a predominance in adults, and in both sexes with a predominance in males (El-Akkad, 1978).

B. CLINICAL DISEASE

1. Domestic Animals

a. Sheep. Sheep and their progeny were the first animal species in which RVF was described in detail, and are regarded as the most susceptible domestic animal with heavy losses during recorded epizootics. Since the first description, by Daubney *et al.* (1931), of the natural disease that "was causing a heavy mortality in newly born lambs on a farm in the Rift Valley [p. 545]," various authors have described the disease in the field. Dickson (1951) classified the symptomatology of the disease as observed during the outbreak in South Africa, describing the peracute, acute, subacute, and inapparent courses of RVF.

The peracute form was most commonly found in lambs, where after an incubation period of about 12 hr, collapse and death followed within 36 hr, with a mortality rate of 95 to 100%. The acute form was encountered in young lambs and to a lesser extent in adult sheep. Rapid febrile reaction was seen in both; death, mostly in lambs, occurred within 24 to 48 hr. The symptoms, in adult sheep less regular, included vomiting, rapid pulse, mucopurulent nasal discharge, unsteady gait, often a hemorrhagic diarrhea, and abortion in pregnant ewes. The mortality rate was high in lambs; in adult sheep it did not exceed 20–30%. Henning (1952) added that affected animals were disinclined to move and often exhibited some form of abdominal pain. They went down very soon, and when in recumbent state they were unable to rise. In adult sheep, vomiting was sometimes the only clinical symptom observed, yet the sheep might be found dead a few hours later. The subacute form of RVF was common in adult sheep. A febrile reaction of 40 to 41°C that lasted 24–96 hr was accompanied by anorexia and general weakness. Abortions in pregnant ewes were a prominent symptom and occurred either during the acute or convalescent phases of the disease. In the mild or inapparent form of RVF, which involved adult sheep, there was only slight febrile reaction, and the disease was usually detected only by serological examination.

Barnard and Botha (1977) reported that during the course of disease in a flock of 110 adult merino ewes, mortality and abortion rates were 50 and 37%, respectively. Lewis *et al.* (1978) reported that all pregnant ewes in an infected flock aborted over a 4-day period. Approximately 25 of 150 sheep died, and later more than 60% of the sheep were shown to have HI antibodies to RVF. In this respect it might be mentioned that Yedloutschnig *et al.* (1981a) demonstrated high levels of RVF virus in aborted fetuses and fetal membranes. Eisa (1981) reported mortality rates of 96 and 70%, in young lambs and in adult sheep, respectively. The disease course in Sudan was very short, extending from 2 to 7 days; prominent clinical manifestations were severe icterus and abortions. Meegan (1981) reported that on four sheep farms studied in Egypt, 80–100% of ewes aborted, 8–60% of the adult animals died, and mortality in the few lambs present approached 100%. Kamel (1981) reported that in some areas sheep were the only species affected.

Indigenous sheep in Kenya have been found to be relatively resistant to RVF in comparison to the exotic breeds that had been introduced for genetic ungrading (Davies, 1981a). It was in these breeds and their crosses that the most dramatic effects were seen in epizootics, both in Kenya and in South Africa.

Experimental disease in sheep of various breeds and ages has been reported by various authors (Daubney et al., 1931; Findlay, 1932; Easterday et al., 1962c; Fagbami et al., 1975; Coetzer and Barnard, 1977; Harrington et al., 1980; Scott, 1981; Yedloutschnig et al., 1981a,d). The disease could be experimentally produced by subcutaneous, intratesticular, intracerebral, intramuscular, and intravenous inoculations, as well as intranasal instillation and application of the virus to scarified skin and conjunctiva. Vector transmission was experimentally carried out by Smithburn et al. (1949a), Easterday et al. (1962c), and McIntosh et al. (1980a). Aerosol transmission was reported by Easterday et al. (1962c). Contact transmission was suspected by Weiss (1957) and experimentally demonstrated by Yedloutschnig et al. (1981a).

The incubation period in lambs was found to be as short as 12 hr, with very high mortality within 24 to 72 hr after infection. Easterday et al. (1962c) infected crossbred, medium-type wool sheep of various ages, with the van Wyk RVFV strain, subcutaneously. Viremia in lambs less than 7 days old commenced 16–72 hr after infection, depending on the dose inoculated; a similar dose–course relationship could be seen in lambs 6–12 weeks old, but not in adult sheep. Viremia extended to Day 5 and Day 7 postinfection in young and adult animals, respectively. Peak titers in lambs were $10^{3.3}$–$10^{10.1}$, and in adult sheep $10^{5.5}$–$10^{7.6}$ MIP LD_{50}/ml.

Febrile response of 41 to 42°C was first noted 24–36 hr after inoculation. The onset of viremia and febrile response was earlier in young lambs than in adults. The mortality rate in lambs less than 1 week old was 90%, whereas in animals older than 1 week it was 20%. Lambs were fatally infected when exposed to aerosol of the virus; viremia, febrile response, and mortality were somewhat delayed in the aerosol-infected lambs. The development of leukopenia was shown to be very common in lambs (Daubney et al., 1931; Findlay, 1932; Easterday, 1965).

Several investigators recorded the relatively low pathogenicity of various RVFV strains to adult nonpregnant sheep. Fagbami et al. (1975) challenged sc West African dwarf sheep, 6–10 months old, with 6.0×10^4 M LD_{50} of Ib-AR 55172 RVFV strain, isolated in Nigeria from Culicoides. Viremia, slight febrile reaction, and neutralizing antibodies were demonstrated. Harrington et al. (1980) challenged susceptible adult crossbred sheep of both sexes sc with 10^6 PFU Zagazig 501 RVFV strain, which had been isolated from a fatal human case of hemorrhagic fever. Clinical symptoms were pyrexia and listlessness for 1 to 8 days; no mortality occurred. The viremia lasted for 1 to 8 days, peak titers being $10^{1.9}$–$10^{7.5}$ PFU/ml. Yedloutschnig (1981c) challenged susceptible adult crossbred sheep sc with 10^5 PFU of the

Zagazig 501 RVFV strain. By Day 6 postinfection 2 out of 63 sheep died. The others showed febrile reaction of 40 to 41°C on Days 1 and 2, accompanied by hyperemia of the buccal cavity and conjunctivitis. Viremia was shown on Days 1–4 postinfection. Scott (1981) compared the pathogenicity of the OM/7 strain of RVFV to that of Nairobi sheep disease virus in susceptible adult nonpregnant sheep. Rift Valley fever virus caused only transient pyrexia. Tomori (1979a) compared the responses of 11 adult West African dwarf sheep of both sexes to challenge with three strains of RVFV. One ewe, which aborted at Day 17 postinfection, died. The others showed transient febrile response and viremia. The severity of clinical response seemed milder in animals inoculated with Smithburn's neuroadapted strain than in those inoculated with either the Ib-AR 55172 (Nigerian) strain or Lunyo strain.

Attenuated RVFV inoculated in ewes 42–74 days pregnant could cause abortion, prolonged gestation, hydrops amnii, and arthrogryposis with micrencephalic brain, as well as hydranencephaly and arthrogryposis of the fetus without hydrops amnii (Coetzer and Barnard, 1977). The differential breed susceptibility to RVF that has been mentioned in field observations concerning sheep is still to be experimentally examined; it has been demonstrated in rats by Peters and Anderson (1981).

b. Cattle. The symptomatology of RVF in cattle following natural infection was described in various countries. Daubney *et al.* (1931) described morbidity and mortality in a dairy herd in Kenya during the 1930 epizootic. No definite symptoms were observed. The initial pronounced sign of illness was more or less complete dysgalactia, followed by pyrexia, anorexia, profuse salivation, abortions, staring coat, and fetid diarrhea. Contrary to their observations in sheep, no lameness or motor disturbances were recorded. The mortality, including deaths from complications following abortions, was about 10%.

Dickson (1951) described subacute symptoms in cattle, as observed during the outbreak in South Africa in the years 1950–1951. A febrile reaction that lasted 24–96 hr was accompanied by anorexia and general weakness. Abortions were numerous and occurred during the acute or convalescent phases of the disease. Kaschula (1953) reported mortality rate of less than 10%, abortion being in many cases the only clinical manifestation of the disease. Abortions or infertility were also the main obvious RVF symptoms in cattle in Zimbabwe (Shone, 1958; Swanepoel *et al.*, 1975) and in Malawi (Klastrup and Halliwell, 1977). During the major outbreak in Zimbabwe in 1978, 15% of all the cows in the affected areas aborted, the average mortality being less than 5%. In one, closely inspected herd, 28 of 1000 cows died and 85% of the remainder aborted (Swanepoel, 1981). Few abortions were reported in Namibia (Schneider, 1977).

The outbreak in the Kosti district in Sudan in 1973 was characterized by symptoms resembling those just described, but in addition severe icterus was described (Eisa et al., 1977). In adult cattle the disease duration was 10–20 days, and spontaneous recovery was common. In calves, the clinical signs invariably included febrile reaction, inappetence, general weakness, salivation, slight lachrymation, bloodstained fetid diarrhea, and dryness of the skin; in advanced stages of the disease, the calves were laterally recumbent, with stiff and extended legs and necks. Mortality in calves was about 20%.

The epizootic in Egypt in the years 1977–1978 was characterized by extensive losses in foreign and crossbreeds of cattle, due to abortions and mortality. The abortions in dams were preceded by a short pyrexia, nasal mucous or mucopurulent discharge, and fetid bloody diarrhea. Mortality in infected aborting cattle was about 30% (Kamel, 1981).

Experimental infection was described in detail by Easterday et al. (1962b), who infected 14 Holstein–Friesian calves less than 1 week old. Viremia was observed from 1 to 7 days postinoculation. Peak viremia occurred on Days 2–5, and was $10^{7.5}$ MIP LD_{50}/ml. The temperature responses, viremia, and leukopenia were distinct. During the height of the disease, most of the calves became laterally recumbent with extended legs and neck. Elevated icterus indices were recorded. Seventy percent of the calves died 2–8 days postinoculation; the course of the disease was not influenced by the doses of virus inoculated, which were $10^{4.3}$–$10^{7.3}$ MIP LD_{50} of the van Wyk strain isolated from sheep in South Africa; onset of the febrile response and viremia tends to be earlier in animals receiving higher doses of the virus. In the animals that survived, recovery was rapid and appeared to be complete by the ninth day after inoculation.

Coackley et al. (1967a) inoculated 59 susceptible grade cattle with two pantropic virus strains, 1119 and Chu, which had been isolated from naturally infected cattle in Kenya. Results of infections with both strains were similar. During the course of these experiments, none of the cattle inoculated showed any overt signs of disease. Pyrexia of 40.0 to 41.5°C was first seen on Days 2–6 postinoculation, in most animals on Day 3 or 4. The duration of the pyrexia was 24–96 hr, in most animals only 24 hr. Viremia was noted 1 day prior to pyrexia and remained for 1 to 4 days, in most animals 2–3 days. The intensity of the response did not appear to depend on the amount of virus inoculated.

Yedloutschnig et al. (1980) challenged five susceptible pregnant Hereford cows sc with 10^5 PFU of Zagazig 501 strain. Viremia was observed on Days 1–5 postinoculation. Peak viremia, of 10^6 to $10^{8.6}$ MIP LD_{50}/ml, was observed on Days 2–5 postinoculation, corresponding with elevated temperatures of 39.8 to 41.3°C. They developed a mild rhinitis and conjunctivitis. One cow died on Day 6 postinoculation, and one aborted. All of the remaining three cows revealed dead fetuses when killed and examined 11 days after inoculation, the fetuses were found viremic; each gram of the tissue had at least $10^{4.5}$ MIP LD_{50} of RVFV. In vaccinated, pregnant Hereford cows, which were also challenged, 50% of the live, apparently normal fetuses were *found* viremic when examined 10 days postinoculation (Yedloutschnig et al., 1981d).

c. *Goats.* Daubney et al. (1931) reported that during the epizootic in Kenya in 1930, no outbreaks in goats were reported although abortions in pregnant goats were suspected. The only goat inoculated by them with the virus reacted similarly to inoculated sheep and recovered. Findlay (1932) indicated that the leukopenia in goats was more pronounced than in sheep. Extensive experimental infection trials with goats were reported by Easterday et al. (1962b), who inoculated 15 goats ip with various doses of virus. It was observed that the course of RVF in young goats was not as predictable as the course in lambs. In goats less than 1 week of age, the onset of viremia, its concentration, and its duration were variable; virus levels in blood were significantly lower than levels recorded in lambs of comparable age when exposed to similar doses. Young goats could be infected by very low doses of virus. Definite febrile responses or leukopenia were not consistently observed; mortality rate was very high. The lesions observed in the goats were essentially the same as those observed in lambs. In an older, lactating goat, febrile reaction (41–42°C) and viremia appeared 60–72 hr postinoculation. Virus could not be demonstrated in the milk during viremia; this goat, as well as two kids about 4 weeks old, did not show any signs of illness besides the febrile reaction.

Eisa (1981) described an epizootic in Sudan in 1973, where goats of all ages were involved; morbidity was estimated at 100%, mortality in goats reported as 50%, compared to 90% in young lambs, around 70% in adult sheep, and 20% in calves. The symptoms in adult goats were icterus and abortion, thermal reaction, anorexia, bilateral mucopurulent nasal discharge, dyspnea, hematuria, unsteady gait, diarrhea, and agalactia.

Kamel (1981) reported that goats appeared to be resistant to RVF during the outbreak in Egypt in 1978. The number of goats found to be serologically positive in field surveys was lower in goats than in cattle and sheep, both in Egypt and Sudan (Eisa, 1981; Kamel, 1981). Schneider (1977) reported abortions in goats and mortality in their offspring in Namibia. Van Tonder (1975) reported the susceptibility of Angora goats. During limited studies on experimentally infected 2- to 3-month-old goats in Egypt (Imam et al., 1978), variable febrile reactions were observed; incubation time was 24 hr, the duration of viremia 3 days.

d. *Buffalo.* Daubney and Hudson (1933) found the cape buffalo, *Syncerus caffer,* to be susceptible to RVFV. Experimental infection of this species was carried out by Davies and Karstad (1981). Five adult female buffalo, two of them pregnant, were inoculated intradermally, $10^{7.7}$ TC ID$_{50}$ of the Kabete strain of RVFV being given at multiple sites. Four of the five developed a viremia on the second day after inoculation, persisting for 48 hr with an antibody response comparable to that found in cattle after RVF infection. One of the two pregnant animals aborted. No other clinical symptoms were recorded.

The Asian buffalo, *Bubalus bubalus,* is bred in large numbers in Egypt and was found to be involved in the outbreak there during the years 1977–1978. Of the tested buffalo sera 21.9% were found positive to RVF. Moderate or low mortality, mainly in calves, and numerous abortions were reported (Kamel, 1981; Meegan, 1981) and resembled the data collected in cattle. Consequently, the Egyptian authorities decided to include buffalo in the vaccination scheme, together with cattle and sheep.

e. *Camels.* Scott et al. (1963) demonstrated RVF-neutralizing antibodies in sera of 27 camels (*Camelus dromedarius*) in various age groups, originating from the northern frontier of Kenya. The observation followed a report on many abortions in camels that were 6–8 months pregnant, occurring simultaneously with an outbreak of RVF in cattle during the same rainy season (1961–1962). There were no other signs of illness. Other possible causes of abortion (trypanosomiasis, leptospirosis, brucellosis) were excluded, but no conclusive diagnosis could be achieved.

Eisa (1981) reported that during an outbreak of RVF in cattle and sheep in Sudan, no clinical disease was reported in camels, though 22.2% of the tested camels were found CF-positive, compared to 30.6% of sheep and 1.6% of cattle, sampled there (Bucci et al., 1980). During the large epizootic of RVF in Egypt (1977–1978), serological evidence for the involvement of camels was gathered in various regions; over 30% of the camels sampled at the southern border of Egypt were serologically positive for antibodies to RVFV (Hoogstraal et al., 1979). Virus was isolated from a camel's serum. There are no reports on clinical disease in camels during the said outbreak. An inactivated RVF vaccine was administered to 16,000 camels during a prevention scheme in Sinai, 1978–1979 (Shimshony et al., 1981a). No HI antibodies could be detected at 6 and 14 months postvaccination, contrary to cattle, sheep, and goats (Klopfer-Orgad et al., 1981).

The possible role of camels as transmitters of RVF virus has been discussed; it has been reported that the incubation time in camels is 2 days and that virus has been found to a titer of 10^3/ml, the viremia lasting 2 days (Sellers et al., 1982, citing U.S. Navy Medical Research Unit No. 3, 1981, unpublished results. Units of viral titers, not specified).

f. Pigs. Pigs have been found to be refractory to RVF virus by Daubney et al. (1931), who failed to elicit a clinical response in two pigs they injected. Weiss (1957) directed attention to the circumstantial field evidence that sows had aborted on farms in South Africa where sheep had died. Easterday et al. (1962b) injected three young pigs intraperitoneally with doses of $10^{2.2}$ and $10^{3.2}$ mouse LD_{50} of RVF virus; no clinical response, viremia, or antibody development followed. Scott (1963) showed that if pigs were inoculated with higher doses of virus, namely 10^5–10^6 hamster LD_{50} units, virus could be recovered on the second and fourth days after inoculation and antibodies detected. The pigs remained clinically healthy in spite of the large quantities of virus inoculated.

g. Horses. Although horses have been regarded as refractory to RVF (Weiss, 1957), it was reported that equines seroconverted (Hoogstraal et al., 1979) and RVFV was isolated from horse serum (Imam et al., 1979) during the 1977–1978 outbreak in Egypt. Despite relatively high positive CF rates in donkeys, no clinical disease in these animals was reported during an outbreak of RVF in Sudan (Eisa, 1981).

Experimental infection trials supported the field observations: Erasmus and Coetzer (1981) reported that infection with a high dose of virus (10^8 M LD_{50}) does lead to the formation of antibodies in the horse. Yedloutchnig et al. (1981b) infected eight ponies with 10^5 to 10^7 PFU/ml. No clinical signs were observed, but five of the animals had low levels of viremia, less than $10^{2.5}$ M LD_{50}/ml, which lasted for 3 to 8 days after an incubation period of 1 to 4 days. All eight ponies seroconverted, producing relatively low and refractory serological titers.

h. Dogs. No natural infection of dogs has been reported. Walker et al. (1970a) described experimental infection of dogs. Inoculation of pups, 1–21 days of age, with various doses of RVF virus ($10^{2.2}$–$10^{8.2}$

MIC LD_{50}), did not regularly produce pyrexia. Incubation time was 2–4 days. One-day-old pups died following inoculation with $10^{0.2}$ MIC LD_{50}. Viremia lasted 4–6 days; in older pups and in adult dogs it had levels of $\sim 10^3$ MIC LD_{50}/ml blood without significant clinical response. Until 18 to 24 hr before death, when most young puppies became comatose, no clinical signs of illness were expressed. Some pups showed ataxia, paddling, and opisthotonus. The mortality rate in young puppies was very high, and pups were invariably hypothermic at death. Older animals showed no signs of infection, although 50% of them developed antibodies. Transmission of RVFV from pup to mother and from pup to pup was demonstrated. There was evidence of passive immunity through colostrum. Keefer *et al.* (1972) reported experimental infection of 8- to 10-week-old puppies by inhalation. Hoogstraal *et al.* (1979) reported on serological evidence for RVF infection in a dog during the 1977–78 epizootic in Egypt.

i. Cats. Findlay (1932) showed that RVFV could be reisolated from the blood of kittens for 48 to 72 hr after experimental inoculation. A febrile reaction associated with changes in the total leukocyte count was noticed. Walker *et al.* (1970b) proved that challenge with various doses of RVFV ($10^{2.2}$–$10^{8.2}$ MIC LD_{50}) resulted in an 81% mortality in kittens under 3 weeks of age, which are thus as susceptible as lambs. Some kittens developed pyrexia; clinical signs of central nervous involvement, such as ataxia and paddling, preceded death. Adult cats and 12-week-old kittens showed no clinical signs of infection but did develop antibodies. Keefer *et al.* (1972) reported the susceptibility of 8- to 10-week-old kittens to experimental infection by inhalation with the van Wyk strain of RVFV. Infection did not occur following ingestion of infected skim milk.

2. In Humans

The course of the disease in humans was first described by Daubney *et al.* (1931) during the outbreak in Kenya; consequently, cases were described in detail by Findlay (1932), Schwentker and Rivers (1933), Kitchen (1934), and Francis and Magill (1935). Incubation period was 3–6 days. Viremia in a human volunteer (Daubney *et al.*, 1931) commenced 4 days after inoculation and lasted for 6 days. The symptoms were quite similar to dengue and sandfly fever. The uncomplicated disease had a sudden onset with pyrexia that sometimes was biphasic, followed by headache, muscular and articular pains, photophobia, and weakness of a relatively short course. Complete recovery sometimes required some weeks. In less benign cases, the pyrexia persisted for several days after the initial attack, the symptoms including epistaxis, retroorbital pain, vomiting, abdominal pain, and vertigo. In some cases headache continued for some weeks, accompanied by defective vision and a prolonged convalescence period.

During the epizootics in South Africa in 1951 and 1953, serious ocular complications were observed (Freed, 1951; Schrire, 1951; Gear et al., 1955). In many cases, visual problems were the first RVF symptom reported to clinicians, with serological confirmation. A central serous retinopathy followed the acute RVF; the ocular involvement corresponded with the initial febrile period or began during the 3 following weeks. Visual defects persisted for very long periods. The ophthalmic complications were unilateral or bilateral, and consisted of white patches of retinitis near the macula, retinal hemorrhage, iritis, and papillitis.

The course of disease in 12 male and 5 female hospitalized patients was described in detail by Van Velden et al. (1977). After an incubation period of 4 to 6 days, the onset of illness was sudden, with chills, headache, painful eyes, backache, tender muscles, diarrhea, vomiting, and fever that often showed a biphasic pattern. Several patients, during the recrudescence of fever, developed signs of involvement of the central nervous system, including meningeal irritation, confusion, stupor and coma, hypersalivation with teeth-grinding, visual hallucinations, lock-in syndrome, and choreiform movements. Lumbar puncture revealed pleocytosis. Four patients developed a hemorrhagic state with epistaxis, hematemeses, melena, and hematuria, from which they died. Postmortem examination revealed profuse gastrointestinal hemorrhage associated with extensive typical liver degeneration, showing eosinophilic intranuclear inclusions in the parenchymal cells. It was further stated (McIntosh et al., 1980b) that during the said outbreak, retinitis clinically associated with defective vision occurred in about 20% of the patients. In one fatal case, the brain showed perivascular cuffing and round-cell infiltration. Maar et al. (1979) described a human case of encephalitis.

The course of disease and clinicopathological findings in numerous human patients infected during the outbreak in Egypt (1977–1978) was described by various authors (Abdel-Wahab et al., 1978; Boctor, 1978; Shousha, 1978; Laughlin et al., 1979; Siam and Meegan, 1980; Siam et al., 1980; El-Gibaly et al., 1981; El-Refaie et al., 1981) and summarized by Meegan et al. (1981). Four clinical forms of human RVF disease were documented virologically and serologically. All patients experienced an acute febrile disease characterized by sudden onset of fever, headache, severe myalgia, and retroorbital pain. Most patients recovered from this form of illness in 4 to 7 days, but some experienced more severe clinical signs. The majority of the 598 deaths recorded during the outbreak were caused by a hemorrhagic-like disease associated with jaundice, hematemesis, melena, and petechial skin lesions developed 2–4 days after the febrile episode. Alternatively, a meningoencephalitic disease with neurological symptoms, including disorientation, hallucination, and vertigo, developed in some patients 5–15 days after onset of fever. A fourth form observed was an ocular disease that developed in patients 5–15 days after the initial symptoms and was characterized by a well-demarcated, exudate-like lesion in the macular area of the retina resulting in loss of central vision. Although recovery can be complete, frequently some loss of visual acuity has occurred. During a 3-year follow-up, no distinct improvement was seen in severe cases; no iris or pupillary abnormalities, cataracts, or secondary glaucoma were recorded (Siam, 1981).

A mild disease suspected as RVF was reported by El-Gibaly et al. (1981) from two localized outbreaks in Egypt. All the 24 patients observed developed sudden onset of fever from 37.5 to 39°C with flushing of face and congestion of conjunctiva; no complications or death occurred. Diagnosis was based on serological examinations with relative rise in HI and CF titers, as well as one RVFV isolate, which was defined as "a weak variant of RVF."

3. Clinical Pathology

Data that had been obtained in various laboratory animals and experimentally infected domestic animals were reviewed by Easterday (1965). Leukopenia that tended to be more severe in younger animals was seen; the lowest counts were recorded 3–4 days after inoculation, corresponding with peak temperature and viremia, followed by leukocytosis. Icterus index and hematocrit values seemed to change during prolonged infections; liver function disturbance could be demonstrated by various enzymatic tests; clotting time was increased in mice.

Data of the clinical pathology in humans were reported by various investigators. Van Velden et al. (1977) investigated 17 cases. Two encephalitic cases showed leukocytosis of 14,000 to 16,000/μl. Slight thrombocytopenia of 100,000 to 142,000/μl was seen in three patients. Liver function tests on nine patients in the early stage of the illness gave normal values; liver biopsy done at an early stage in two patients did not reveal abnormality. A brain biopsy done in one patient with persistent neurological signs showed perivascular infiltration of lymphocytes. Because patients with hemorrhagic state died soon after admission to hospital, the said data relate to uncomplicated or encephalitic cases. Ten of twelve encephalitic patients recovered.

Boctor (1978) reported data from Egypt that relate mainly to hemorrhagic cases. Most cases showed leukopenia; there were also slight elevation of serum bilirubin levels, decreased prothrombin levels, prolonged coagulation times, and increased urea levels. El-Shinnawi et al. (1978), who also investigated human hemorrhagic cases, reported increased blood levels of bilirubin, urea, aspartate and alaline aminotransferases, and normal levels of total proteins and alkaline phosphatase. El Refaie et al. (1981) reported data from 300 investigated milder cases. Leukopenia was seen in a few cases; bleeding and coagulation times were unchanged.

C. Pathological Changes

1. In Domestic Animals

a. Sheep. The macroscopic lesions and histopathology of RVF in sheep have been described in detail by Daubney et al. (1931), Findlay (1932, 1933), Schulz (1951), Easterday et al. (1962a), and Coetzer (1977), and reviewed by Erasmus and Coetzer (1981). Gross and histological hepatic lesions have been observed in all age groups throughout the years during various outbreaks, and in all susceptible animal species and humans, and are regarded as the most specific lesion of RVF.

i. Gross Lesions of Newborn and Young Lambs. Widespread subcutaneous, visceral, and serosal hemorrhages are evident in newborn and young lambs. Rapid carcass decomposition was reported by Dickson (1951). Slight icterus occurred in about 10% of the lambs (Coetzer, 1977).

The liver is usually moderately enlarged, soft, and friable, the color ranging from yellowish brown to a very dark red. Numerous grayish white necrotic foci, 1–2 mm in diameter, are scattered throughout the hepatic parenchyma. Discoloration might obscure the necrotic foci; they may coalesce into larger foci. Hemorrhages varying in size from petechiae to 2 to 3 cm in diameter are seen, as well as focal congestion that is manifested as large irregular red patches. Fibrinous perihepatitis might be observed. A slight to moderate edema of the gallbladder might be pronounced around the area of attachment to the liver, accompanied by serotic petechiae and ecchymoses. Blood-tinged ascitic fluid was described in some lambs.

There is a slight tumor splenis in some animals; capsular and subcapsular hemorrhages are observed (Schulz, 1951; Coetzer, 1977). Daubney et al. (1931), who did not observe remarkable spleen changes, considered the absence of tumor splenis in RVF for the differential diagnosis of Nairobi sheep disease, heartwater, and bluetongue.

The kidneys were pale but firm with small hemorrhages (Dickson, 1951). Although Coetzer (1977) observed that in most cases kidneys were macroscopically normal, there were also enlarged, congested kidneys noted, with petechiae in the cortex, and also perirenal edema. Infrequently, small hemorrhages occur in the urinary bladder. The adrenals were slightly enlarged in about 20% of the lambs described by Coetzer (1977), and petechiae were present in the cortex.

The alimentary tract showed varying degrees of inflammation, from catarrhal to hemorrhagic–necrotic. Dickson (1951) reported that the entire digestive tract, from abomasum to the colon, was involved. Petechiae and ecchymoses were common on the visceral peritoneum, but most marked in the abomasal mucosa, where the contents was often chocolate-colored with an abnormally large amount of mucus adherent to the folds. In a few cases the Peyer's patches were slightly elevated and enlarged. Daubney *et al.* (1931) described impaction of the colon with "tarry," chocolate-colored feces, in cases of hemorrhagic enteritis. Van der Linde (in Alexander, 1951) observed perforation of abomasum and cecum in lambs.

In the lungs, Coetzer (1977) occasionally found moderate emphysema, congestion, and edema, as well as subpleural petechiae and ecchymoses. Such changes had not been seen in Kenya by Daubney *et al.* (1931), but they described, as a constant finding, small irregular, oval, slightly raised areas on the surface of the lungs. The heart showed subepicardial and subendocardial hemorrhages. A few lambs had a slight hydropericardium. Generalized adenopathy, edema, and congestion of both peripheral and internal lymph nodes was seen, as well as petechiae in the cortex and medulla. Schulz (1951) reported extravasations in the pancreas and thymus.

ii. Gross Lesions in Adult Sheep. The macroscopic changes in adult sheep are slightly different from those described in lambs. Although the liver is the primary organ affected, the lesions differ in severity. According to Daubney *et al.* (1931), Schulz (1951), and J. A. W. Coetzer (unpublished observations, cited by Erasmus and Coetzer, 1981), the liver is usually slightly to moderately enlarged, showing scattered, multifocal pinpoint necrotic foci, and sometimes also disseminated hemorrhages throughout the parenchyma. They describe hemorrhages and edema of the gallbladder wall, frequently associated with blood coagula in the lumen.

Other marked changes in adult sheep were numerous and extensive serosal and visceral hemorrhages, occasionally mild icterus, abomasal edema and hemorrhages, hemorrhagic enteritis, and generalized adenopathy. Schulz (1951) stated that lung changes in adult sheep were more marked than in young lambs and included hyperemia, edema, and emphysema with subpleural and perivascular hemorrhages. Easterday (1961) found diffuse subendocardial hemorrhages in adult sheep but not in young lambs.

iii. Histopathology of Newborn Lambs. The characteristic liver lesions in newborn lambs were described by Daubney et al. (1931) and Schulz (1951). Easterday et al. (1962a) described the gradual development of liver lesions in experimentally infected lambs, related to time of inoculation and to the various amounts of virus inoculated. Coetzer (1977) described in detail histopathological changes of 93 newborn lambs, and summarized the incidence of various hepatic lesions: primary foci of necrosis (100%), pannecrosis (83%), mineralization (62%), intranuclear inclusions (49%), pigmentation of hepatocytes and reticuloendothelial cells (32%), bile stasis (31%), and portal reaction (5%).

The primary lesion of livers of experimentally infected lambs was described by Easterday et al. (1962a) as focal hepatic necrosis; when a larger amount of virus was inoculated, the reaction tended to be general rather than focal. Coetzer (1977) found that well-demarcated foci of severe coagulative necrosis, scattered throughout the liver, were present in 100% of the examined specimens. Combined with pannecrosis, Coetzer regarded them as highly specific changes that hardly can be confused with any other disease of the newborn lamb.

The foci were predominantly centrilobular or midzonal, sometimes involved in the portal areas, causing partial necrosis of the triads; they were infiltrated by histiocytes, lymphocytes, and neutrophils, many with marked pyknosis and karyorrhexis. The whole or part of the cytoplasm of some hepatocytes became more eosinophilic, revealing typical Councilman-like bodies; those bodies were also found free in the sinusoids and were PAS-positive. Daubney and Hudson (1933) described Councilman-like bodies in lambs in Kenya, underlying their resemblance to the structures first described by Councilman in 1880, in hepatocytes of patients who had died of yellow fever. They are acidophilic bodies, probably modified dead hepatocytes.

Extreme pannecrosis was present in 83% of the cases examined by Coetzer (1977), with only the portal triads preserved. In the remaining 17% of the livers, small groups of surviving hepatocytes could be found close to the triads. In 6% of the livers, only the reticulum network remained, as result of disintegration and lysis of all the necrotic hepatocytes in the lobule: the severe destruction of the parenchyma rendered the liver tissue hardly recognizable.

Easterday et al. (1962a) demonstrated that when a larger amount of virus was inoculated, the reaction in lambs tended to be general rather than focal. Experience in Zimbabwe (Lawrence, cited by Swanepoel, 1981) showed that whereas necrosis may be diffuse or focal in fetuses, it tends to be more focal in postnatal animals, but may be extensive and intensely hemorrhagic. Polymorph infiltration was less intense in fetuses than in other animals.

Coetzer (1977) observed mineralization in 62% of the livers examined, involving single or groups of necrotic hepatocytes. In 49% of the cases, intranuclear inclusion bodies were seen in the still recognizable hepatocytes, varying from cigar-shaped through oval to round or ring-shaped. As a rule they were difficult to find, but in 5% of the livers, 80–90% of the nuclei contained inclusions. Those were livers where less advanced necrosis occurred. Swanepoel (1981) reported that in Zimbabwe, eosinophilic intranuclear inclusions are more frequently demonstrated in fetuses and young lambs than in calves or other animals. Coetzer (1977) reported that 32% of the livers showed yellowish brown pigment, positive for iron, in the cytoplasm of the hepatocytes, Kupffer cells, or the reticuloendothelial cells of the portal areas. Bile thrombi were seen in 31% of the cases.

The gallbladder was edematous, in addition to pyknosis and karyorrhexis of the mononuclear cells in the submucosa, and focal hemorrhages in the serosa and submucosa.

The spleen was not found to be significantly affected (Daubney *et al.*, 1931). Schulz (1951) noted necrotic changes in the pulp. Easterday *et al.* (1962a) noted that distinct lymphoid depletion occurred, in 1- to 5-day-old lambs challenged with the van Wyk strain, to a lesser extent in the spleen and lymph nodes than in the lamina propria of the small intestine. Coetzer (1977) reported extensive necrosis of cells of the lymphocytic series, most apparent in the malpighian bodies, in newborn, naturally infected lambs in South Africa. In addition, focal disseminated neutrophilic infiltration ahd hemorrhages were seen in the red and white pulp, as well as capsular hemorrhages.

In the kidneys, Daubney *et al.* (1931) noted mainly tubular degeneration or nephrosis. Schulz (1951) saw also focal congestion and hemorrhages, a marked hemosiderosis in the tubules, and signs of albuminuria. Easterday *et al.* (1962a) found no changes in the kidneys. Coetzer (1977) confirmed the changes described by Schulz, but in addition described perivascular hemorrhages and edema at the corticomedullary junction. In about 10% of the kidneys examined, pyknosis and karyorrhexis of the cellular elements in the glomeruli and a hyalinized appearance of the affected glomeruli were seen. In many cases the glomeruli appeared normal.

Schulz (1951) reported degenerative changes in the adrenal medulla, with cellular hyalin tinted inclusions, as well as cortical and medullary hemorrhages. Varying degrees of necrosis in the adrenal cortex, mainly in the zona fasciculata, and, more frequently, cortical hemorrhages without necrosis, were described by Easterday et al. (1962a). Coetzer (1977) observed focal necrosis and hemorrhages in 30 to 40% of the lambs. Medullar necrosis was confined to individual cells.

In the alimentary tract, Daubney et al. (1931) examined the "tarry" mass filling the lumen and found that it consisted of coagulated blood with embedded epithelial detritus, leukocytes, and bacteria. Schulz (1951) saw varying alimentary changes in animals of various ages, from mucocatarrhal gastroenteritis with localized hyperemia or hemorrhages, to croupous, necrotic enteritis and ulcerations, and not infrequently hemorrhagic gastroenteritis. Coetzer (1977) observed hemorrhages in the submucosa between the gastric pits as well as in the tunica muscularis and serosa of the abomasum, in newborn lambs. In four of eight lambs that were killed for autopsy, necrosis of the tips of the villi in the small intestine was seen. These changes could not be demonstrated in animals presented for autopsy some time after death. The lymphocytes in the Peyer's patches showed varying degrees of pyknosis and karyorrhexis, corresponding in degree of intensity to the changes in other lymphoid tissues in the body.

The lungs, examined by Daubney et al. (1931) in Kenya, showed nothing abnormal, except some distension of the alveolar capillaries with leukocytes, which was macroscopically seen as white raised areas on the surface of the lung. Coetzer (1977) reported a slight congestion, alveolar and interstitial edema with occasional focal hemorrhages, and occasional emphysema. In addition, cell pyknosis and karyorrhexis in the alveolar septae and peribronchial lymphoid tissue were seen.

The peripheral and internal lymph nodes, as seen by Daubney et al. (1931), showed various degrees of hemorrhages and polymorph infiltration, but no distinct necrotic foci. Schulz (1951) saw some necrobiotic foci, focal neutrophilic infiltration, pigmentation, marked karyorrhexis, and catarrh of the sinuses. Easterday et al. (1962a) saw some lymphoid depletion but less than the depletion observed in the lamina propria of the small intestine. Cytolytic foci were seen in the sinuses. Coetzer (1977) saw varying degree of pyknosis and karyorrhexis of the lymphocytes, mainly in the cortex, as well as yellowish-brown pigmentation of the reticuloendothelial medullar cells.

Easterday et al. (1962a) noted that the vertebral, sternal, and costal bone marrow was moderately aplastic.

No changes in the brain were observed by Daubney et al. (1931); this was confirmed by Easterday et al. (1962a). However, Schulz (1951) reported degenerative changes of the neurons in various parts of the brain, especially marked in the hippocampus and the Purkinje cells. Coetzer (1977) reported slight congestion and edema of the brain in some lambs, but no encephalitis was observed, nor were any lesions in the eyes. The neurotropic RVF virus was found to cause inflammatory and degenerative cerebral lesions in lambs (Findlay et al., 1936a), and hydranencephaly or micranencephaly in fetal lambs (Coetzer and Barnard, 1977).

No changes were observed in other organs, specifically regarding the urinary bladder, testis, uterus, thyroid gland, salivary glands, thymus, tongue, skeletal muscles (Coetzer, 1977), and retina (Easterday et al., 1962a).

iv. Histopathology in Adult Sheep. The microscopic lesions in older animals have been reviewed by Erasmus and Coetzer (1981), who state that the main difference is the hepatic picture. The microscopic liver lesions, as seen by all investigators, were less severe in older animals. The necrosis is confined as a rule to focal areas in individual liver lobules, whereas in newborn lambs whole lobules throughout the liver are practically destroyed. Daubney et al. (1931) indicated that hepatic foci persisted sometimes for 8 weeks after reaction but were not found after 10 weeks. Swanepoel (1981) reported the less frequent demonstration of eosinophilic intranuclear inclusions in older animals. Lawrence (cited by Swanepoel, 1981) reported that although necrosis may be diffuse or focal in fetuses, it tends to be more focal in postnatal animals but may be extensive and intensely hemorrhagic; polymorph infiltration is less intense in fetuses than in older animals.

Daubney et al. (1931) reported more definite tubular nephrosis in adult sheep than in hyperacute cases in lambs, where death occurs too rapidly to permit the development of any extensive lesion.

b. Cattle. Daubney et al. (1931) reported that postmortem lesions in cattle resembled those produced in adult sheep. The similarity of bovine and ovine lesions was demonstrated when the first diagnosis of RVF was made in South Africa on the basis of the postmortem examination of a bull. The practitioner (Meare, cited by Gear, 1975), who carried out the autopsy in Bloemfontein in April 1951, in a country where this disease had never been diagnosed before, described his findings: "The intestinal mucosa, especially of the small intestine and caecum, was reddened. The contents were bloody. The wall of the gall bladder was oedematous and bloody. Focal necrosis of the hepatic lobules was evident throughout the liver. Multiple petechial haemorrhages, ecchymoses and extravasations were present under the pericardium, endocardium, pleura and peritoneum [p. 221]." Later on, RVF was diagnosed on the basis of histological examinations, and mice inoculated with liver suspension of the bull died, with typical hepatic nuclear eosinophilic inclusions.

Dickson (1951) and Schulz (1951) were involved in the further diagnosis and evaluation of the outbreak in South Africa; they reported that lesions in cattle and sheep were very similar. However, Schulz reported that some RVF cases in cattle resembled bluetongue, namely, acute catarrhal stomatitis associated with mucosal erosions, necrosis of some parts of the skin (particularly on the udder and scrotum), hemorrhages in the light-colored portions of the skin, laminitis, coronitis, and sometimes a very marked ascites. Such lesions had not been reported from Kenya. He also observed that subepicardial, subendocardial, and myocardial hemorrhages were comparatively more pronounced and extensive in bovines than in ovines.

Easterday et al. (1962b) observed extensive hepatic changes in calves after experimental infection; he stated that the macroscopic and microscopic changes were similar to those seen in lambs. Erasmus and Coetzer (1981) reported that the hepatic lesions in aborted bovine fetuses, in calves, and in adult cattle, although not identical, are very similar to those described for the newborn lamb and for adult sheep. Swanepoel (1981) reported from Zimbabwe that eosinophilic intranuclear inclusions are less frequently demonstrable in calves than in young lambs and fetal lambs.

c. *Goats.* Findlay (1932) described hemorrhages of the submucosa in the cardia and abomasum in one goat, and also one case of enteritis.

Easterday et al. (1962b) reported that gross and histological liver lesions in experimentally infected kids were similar to those described for lambs (Easterday *et al.*, 1962a). The hepatic necrosis tended to remain focal and did not become diffuse as in the livers of most lambs.

d. *Dogs and Cats.* Mitten *et al.* (1970) described in detail the pathological changes in 27 pups and kittens experimentally infected with the van Wyk RVFV strain. The gross and histological hepatic lesions were very similar to those described in other species, although there was relative lack of definite Councilman-like bodies, as well as eosinophilic intranuclear inclusions. Significant histological changes were found in the heart. Acute and chronic myocarditis were seen in the heart; in most animals, small focal areas of a mixed inflammatory cell infiltrate were present between hyalinized muscle fibers. In several hearts, multiple large focal areas of necrosis were seen.

In the brain, focal gliosis and necrosis were found; meningitis was always present in severely affected animals. Those changes were essentially like changes caused by other viral encephalitides. Moderate congestion was evident in the spleens of most animals. In some animals, focal alveolar edema in the lungs, and focal degeneration of renal tubular epithelial cells were visible. No lesions were found in eyes, gastrointestinal tract, adrenals, lymph nodes, bladder, ovaries, uterus, prostate, epididymis, or testis.

2. In Rodents

The hepatic lesions in mice and hamsters appeared to be extensive and diffuse, resembling the changes in newborn lambs (Findlay, 1932, 1933). Hemorrhagic enteritis was also noted in the mice. Mims (1957) described in detail the development of histologic changes in mice liver in relation to viral multiplication; similar changes in mice were shown by McGavran and Easterday (1963). Findlay (1932) found laboratory piebald adult rats to be highly susceptible to the Kenya strain of RVFV, with extensive liver necrosis and also hemorrhagic enteritis and stomach submucosal hemorrhages. Later, Findlay and Howard (1952) demonstrated extensive liver necrosis following inoculation with the same virus strain, only in rats under 15 days of age, not in adult rats. The rats they used in this experiment were Glaxo albino rats. The histological changes in the suckling rats were exactly like those seen in adult mice infected with the hepatotropic RVFV strain.

Peters and Anderson (1981) observed three different reactions in inbred *Rattus norvegicus* strains, which they defined as "susceptible," "resistant," and "encephalitic" rat strains. The susceptible strains developed early focal involvement that later became confluent, histologically manifested as total hepatic necrosis as a fatal lesion. Vasculitis and focal lymphoid necrosis are also evident. Viral antigen was located mainly in the liver, and to a lesser extent in the renal glomeruli and some tubules, foci of adrenal cortical cells, most areas of the spleen except the T-dependent periarteriolar sheaths, some littoral macrophages in lymph nodes, and scattered small vessel walls.

In "encephalitic" strains, dying rats do not have any gross lesions; the only microscopic changes are seen in the brain. The pathological changes in a group of 42 inoculated "encephalitic" rats were described by Bucci et al. (1981). Lesions were present only in the brains of rats that died or were killed between Days 9 and 14 postinoculation. Most rats did not show clinical signs; one that was well when killed on Day 10 postinoculation had microscopic encephalitis. The major changes were patchy neuronal necrosis, focal malacia, and infiltration by neutrophils, lymphoid cells, and plasma cells. There were endothelial hyperplasia and inflammatory cell cuffing of small blood vessels in affected areas. The most prominent lesions were observed about the third and fourth ventricles, primarily in the white tracts and nuclei of the midbrain, brain stem, and cerebellum.

Various species were compared by Peters and Anderson (1981) with regard to their response to RVFV. Syrian hamsters, Sprague-Dawley rats, and ICR Swiss mice developed hepatic necrosis. Cotton rats (*Sigmodon hispidus*), lauchas (*Calomys callosus*), and gerbils (*Meriones unguiculatus*) developed encephalitis without hepatitis after inoculation with RVFV (Peters and Anderson, 1981).

3. In Humans

Gross pathological changes have been reported by Van Velden et al. (1977) in four cases from South Africa, by Yassin (1978) in five cases from Egypt, and by Swanepoel et al. (1979) in one case from Zimbabwe. Histological changes were described in detail by Van Velden et al. (1977) in four cases; El-Shinawi et al. (1978) examined four cases and Swanepoel et al. (1979) two.

Van Velden et al. (1977) described four cases who died during the major epizootic in South Africa in 1975; three had a hemorrhagic state and one had encephalitis. The three first patients had similar pathological findings. Evidence of extensive submucosal petechial and ecchymotic hemorrhages was found throughout the gastrointestinal tract. The ecchymoses were most marked in the stomach, extending through the wall to the subserosa, as well as on the visceral and parietal peritonea, the respiratory tract, and the pericardial and pleural surfaces. Extensive hemorrhages and pronounced icterus were the prominent external finding from a case in Zimbabwe (Swanepoel et al., 1979). The liver was found by Van Velden et al. (1977) to be enlarged in all four cases, wtih mottled yellowish-brown surface and underlying petechiae; the cut surface showed congestion, the lobular pattern slightly obscured by necrotic areas. The extent and location of the necrosis as well as the cytopathic and nuclear changes were in accordance with RVF changes in lambs. Councilman-like cytoplasmic inclusions were observed. There was only a slight inflammatory cell infiltration, mostly of lymphocytes and histocytes. Bile stasis was not noted.

El Shinnawi et al. (1978) noted similar changes; in some specimens he observed massive necrosis with complete absence of liver cells over wide areas. Schistosomal infestation was identified in three of four cases examined.

The spleen, as described by Van Velden et al. (1977), had clearly defined malpighian corpuscles and congested pulp. Few lymphocytes showed nuclear pyknosis, and megakaryocyte-like cells were observed.

Yassin (1978) observed tumor splenis in all cases, and some with scattered petechial subcapsular hemorrhages. El Shinnawi et al. (1978) observed fibrocongestive changes. Swanepoel et al. (1979) saw slight hyaline changes in the splenic arteries, and a small infarct. The kidneys, as described by Van Velden et al. (1977), showed subcapsular hemorrhages and swelling of some glomeruli associated with slight cell infiltration. The proximal tubules were degenerate, and many contained amorphous hyaline eosinophilic material and round hyalinic eosinophilic bodies. The adrenals showed some medullar degeneration. The gastrointestinal tract contained blood, and on microscopical examination showed foci of hemorrhagic mucosal necrosis with extravasation of blood in the muscularis and subserosa. Yassin (1978) reported that in three of five cases the stomach was full of blood; the small intestine was not affected, but the descending colon and sigmoid were full of blood with severe mucosal congestion. No esophageal varices were detected.

Congestion of tracheal and bronchial mucosa was reported by Van Velden et al. (1977), and there were hemorrhages in the lungs. The interalveolar capillaries were dilated; some of the alveoli had small hemorrhages and edema. A few subepicardial hemorrhagic petechiae were noted in the heart. Microscopically, few muscle fibers showed fragmentation, which was regarded as artifactual. Yassin (1978) reported dilated and flabby hearts. In one case, slight pericardial hemorrhagic effusion was seen.

Van Velden et al. (1977) reported that the anatomical pattern of the lymph nodes was preserved. Pyknotic changes and nuclear fragmentation were observed in the cortex. Numerous monocytic cells, some with chromatin margination or nuclear fragmentation, were seen in the medullar sinuses. Blood vessels were dilated and congested with hemorrhagic areas.

The brain, in one case, showed focal areas of necrosis, associated with infiltration of round cells, mostly lymphocytes and macrophages. In two other cases, perivascular cuffing was the only sign of encephalitis. Yassin (1978) reported scattered endodural and subarachnoid petechiae in all the cases. The brain substance was normal in four cases, and in one it was very congested and edematous. No histological changes were observed by El Shinnawi et al. (1978).

D. Differential Diagnosis

A history of a disease among ruminants, characterized by abortions, neonatal death, and necrotic liver lesions, combined with a self-limited acute febrile disease in humans, must be regarded as highly suspicious of RVF.

Daubney et al. (1931) mentioned that four common viral sheep diseases in Kenya could be differentiated from RVF, namely Nairobi sheep disease, bluetongue, heartwater, and sheep pox. They stated that the only disease of cattle with which RVF could be clinically confused was ephemeral fever. However, it should be noted that during the said outbreak in Kenya, bluetongue was suspected when abortions occurred in the ewe flocks, and on two occasions, blood taken from aborting ewes produced bluetongue on inoculation into susceptible sheep at the laboratory.

The diagnosis of RVF was established in 1951 in South Africa only several months after the reporting of the first outbreaks; many of these outbreaks were attributed to enterotoxemia and bluetongue. Alexander (1951) described symptoms observed in cattle in Orange Free State that might readily be confused with bluetongue. These included hyperemia of the buccal mucosa, erosions on tongue, lips, and cheeks, lameness, coronitis, and hyperemia of the skin around the dewclaws; the unpigmented skin, particularly in areas such as the teats, the udder, and the scrotum, was dry, hard, and cracked.

Enterotoxemia and lamb dysentery were suspected in South Africa, because many of the RVF cases studied manifested a marked hemorrhagic gastroenteritis. Histological examinations of the liver, serum neutralization, and mouse inoculation eliminated the possible involvement of those diseases, however.

Weiss (1957) discussed the possible confusion between RVF and Wesselsbron disease (WBD), which had many clinical, pathological, or epidemiological similarities. Definite diagnosis could be made only by laboratory methods, such as isolation and identification of the virus, serology, and histological examination of the liver. Coetzer et al. (1978) studied the gross pathological and histological differences between RVF and WBD in newborn lambs. The hepatic lesions were of much more diffuse nature in WBD and failed to reveal the prominent, well-defined primary foci of coagulative necrosis that characterize RVF; they concluded that these lesions could be easily and definitely distinguished. In addition, icterus seemed to be a fairly consistent gross finding in WBD, and less marked in RVF in newborn lambs. Mortality seemed to be higher in RVF. Wesselsbron disease in animals and humans is regarded as a milder disease than RVF (Coetzer, 1981).

A comparative study of experimental infection of nonpregnant adult sheep with RVFV and Nairobi sheep disease (NSD) virus was reported by Scott (1981), revealing higher pathogenicity of the latter. Because diarrhea, the prominent symptom of NSD, is also a frequent symptom in RVF, epidemiological differentiation might be based also on the wide host range and widespread occurrence of RVF, in addition to the laboratory examinations. Human infection with NSD was recorded (Weiss et al., 1956).

Coetzer and Barnard (1977) discussed the effects of various viruses on brain teratology in ruminants. The RVF vaccine strain caused changes that were related to those caused by Akabane and WBD (vaccine strain and wild-type) viruses, and could be differentiated from changes caused by bluetongue and bovine virus diarrhea–mucosal disease viruses.

Other infectious animal diseases might be taken into consideration when RVF is suspected. They include zoonotic abortifacient diseases such as Q fever, leptospirosis, brucellosis, toxoplasmosis, listeriosis, and salmonellosis, as well as the nonzoonotic abortifacient diseases campilobacteriosis (bovine and ovine), trichomoniasis, chlamydiasis, Akabane disease, and ephemeral fever. The possibility of rinderpest should also be considered in differential diagnosis.

Since the Egyptian epidemic in 1977, which was the first in RVF history to come to official attention because of considerable human illness rather than epizootic domestic animal illness (Darwish and Hoogstraal, 1981), special attention should be paid to the differential diagnosis of RVF in humans. Daubney et al. (1931) noticed that RVF presented certain similarities to yellow fever, dengue fever, and sandfly fever in humans.

Gear (1975, 1977) reviewed the medical aspects of some zoonoses responsible for dengue-like illnesses or hemorrhagic fevers in humans. He listed 13 viral, 3 ricketsial, 2 bacterial, and 2 protozoal infections including, in addition to RVF, the arboviruses chicungunya fever, Sindbis fever, yellow fever, dengue fever, and West Nile fever. He mentioned also rodent-associated infections: Lassa, as well as Korean, Argentinian, and Bolivian hemorrhagic fevers. McIntosh (1975) mentioned additional arboviruses, pathogenic for humans, namely Bunyamwera, Banzi, Spondweni, and Germiston. Gear (1977) described RVF and Marburg disease in an account of outbreaks in South Africa.

The medical and veterinary significance of Crimean-Congo hemorrhagic fever was discussed by Darwish and Hoogstraal (1981); this tickborne arbovirus had been responsible for some serious epidemics in various countries, and is known to cause viremia in domestic animals. They mention six additional arboviruses that are known to cause viremia and antibodies in domestic animals in Egypt and are closely associated with the animals and their characteristic tick parasites.

Shousha (1978), describing human cases of RVF in Egypt, added malaria, influenza, and infectious hepatitis as diseases that should also be considered.

The differential diagnosis of RVF ocular lesions was discussed by Siam (1981). Many similar fundus lesions, retinitis, and chorioiditis, could be readily mistaken for RVF. Fluorecein angiography was found to be superior to ophthalmoscopy, revealing the specific fluorographic RVF pattern.

IV. Epidemiological Features

A. Epizootiology and Epidemiology

Rift Valley fever has been reported from 20 sub-Saharan African countries prior to the outbreak in Egypt (Table IV). Epizootics were mostly associated with excessively heavy seasonal rains, particularly after prolonged periods of drought (Davies, 1981a; McIntosh and Jupp, 1981; Swanepoel, 1981).

Extensive studies of possible maintenance, incidental, amplifying, and link hosts of RVF have been carried out in South Africa, Kenya, and Zimbabwe. McIntosh and Jupp (1981) reported that the epizootic area in South Africa coincides with the main sheep-farming regions; the true enzootic area is situated in the subtropical, coastal lowlands of Natal, where sheep are absent, human infection is minimal, and RVF is of minor economic significance. Evidence of the enzootic situation in this part was obtained by isolation of the virus from vectors and a progressive increase in the number of immune animals over a number of years without any clinical evidence of the disease (Kaschula, 1953; McIntosh, 1972). Maintenance hosts could not be demonstrated in wild mammals, in birds, or in arthropods; RVFV isolation rate from mosquitoes was low, and no transovarial passage could be confirmed in experimental infection trials, carried out in seven mosquito species that had been found to transmit RVFV (McIntosh and Jupp, 1981). There is a reasonably good correlation between the excessive rainy periods, which show in South Africa a regular quasi–20-year oscillatory pattern, and the occurrence of outbreaks in the epizootic area. It was suggested that outbreaks on the plateau originate in summers from the enzootic foci by some unknown means, when climatic conditions favor the breeding of large numbers of mosquitoes (Barnard, 1981; McIntosh and Jupp, 1981). *Culex theileri* was found to be the most effective vector, readily infected even at $10^{4.0}$ MIC $LD_{50}/0.02$ ml, and transmitted the virus to mice, hamsters, and sheep (McIntosh and

TABLE IV

GEOGRAPHIC DISTRIBUTION AND CHRONOLOGY OF RVF IN AFRICA

Country	Year	Reported evidence	Reference
Angola	1960	Antibodies in humans	Kokernot et al. (1965b)
Botswana	1955	Antibodies in humans and animals	Weiss (1957); Food and Agriculture Organization (1957)
	1959	Antibodies in humans	Kokernot et al. (1965a)
Cameroon	1968	Antibodies in animals	Food and Agriculture Organization (1969)
Chad	1968	Antibodies in animals	Food and Agriculture Organization (1969)
Egypt	1977	Extensive epizootic, virus isolations	Imam and Darwish (1977); World Health Organization (1977)
	1978	Extensive epizootic, virus isolations	Johnson et al. (1978); Meegan (1979)
Ethiopia	1962	Suspected, not confirmed	Food and Agriculture Organization (1963)
Gabon	1936	Antibodies in humans	Findlay et al. (1936b)
Kenya	1912	Clinically diagnosed epizootic?	Montgomery (1912)
	1930–1931	Extensive epizootic, virus isolations	Daubney et al. (1931)
	1936–1954	Limited outbreaks	Scott et al. (1956)
	1968	Extensive epizootic	Davies (1975)
	1978	Extensive epizootic	Davies (1981a,b)
Lesotho	1969	Clinically suspected	Food and Agriculture Organization (1970)
Malawi	1969	Clinically recognized	Food and Agriculture Organization (1970)
	1974–1975	Antibodies in animals	Klastrup and Halliwell (1977)
Mali	1936	Antibodies in humans	Findlay et al. (1936b)
Mozambique	1969	Extensive epizootic, virus isolations	Valdaão (1969); McIntosh (1972, 1975)
	1976	Moderate incidence	Food and Agriculture Organization (1977)
Namibia	1955	Extensive epizootic	Weiss (1957)
	1974	Extensive epizootic	Schneider (1977)
Nigeria	1959	Virus isolation, antibodies in animals	Ferguson (1959)
	1967–1970	Virus isolations from mosquitoes and *Culicoides*	Lee (1970, 1979)
	1970–1972	Antibodies in animals	Fagbami et al. (1973)
	1980	Antibodies in humans	Tomori (1980)

(*continued*)

TABLE IV (Continued)

Country	Year	Reported evidence	Reference
Somali	1979	Enzootic situation	Brès (1981)
South Africa	1950–1951	Extensive epizootic, virus isolations	Alexander (1951); Mundel and Gear (1951)
	1953	Limited epizootic	Van der Linde (1953)
	1956	Limited epizootic	Weiss (1957)
	1969	Limited epizootic	McIntosh (1972)
	1974–1976	Extensive epizootic	Barnard and Botha (1977)
Sudan	1936	Antibodies in humans	Findlay et al. (1936b)
	1973	Extensive epizootic, virus isolations	Eisa et al. (1977)
	1976	Limited epizootic	Eisa et al. (1980)
Tanzania[a]	1978–1979	Epizootic; antibodies in animals	Davies and Highton (1980)
Uganda	1936	Antibodies in humans	Findlay et al. (1936b)
	1944–1967	Virus isolations from mosquitoes and humans	Smithburn et al. (1948); Knight et al. (1968)
	1968	Limited epidemic in humans	Henderson et al. (1972)
Zaire	1936	Antibodies in humans	Findlay et al. (1936b)
	1954	Antibodies in humans and in subhuman primates	Pellissier (1954) Pellissier and Rousselot (1954)
Zambia	1973–1974	Extensive epizootic in cattle	Akafekwa (1975)
	1978	Extensive epizootic, antibodies in animals	Food and Agriculture Organization (1979) Davies and Highton (1980)
Zimbabwe	1955	Antibodies in animals	Shone (1958)
	1957–1958	Extensive epizootic; virus isolations	Shone (1958); Swanepoel (1981)
	1969–1970	Extensive epizootic, antibodies in animals	Christie (1969); Swanepoel (1976)
	1978	Extensive epizootic	Swanepoel (1981)

[a]Limited enzootic situation, confined to certain regions, reported annually to FAO–WHO–OIE Animal Health Yearbook since 1955.

Jupp, 1981). Other species were also shown to be potential transmitters (see Table IV).

In Kenya, quite a similar epidemiological situation was observed, with excessive rainy periods predisposing to epizootics (Daubney et al., 1931; Scott et al., 1956). The epizootic area was confirmed to be forest-derived grassland, bush savannah, and acacia grassland (Davies, 1975). The coastal forest was regarded as the true enzootic area, with enzootic foci within the epizootic area. No activity of the virus could be demonstrated within epizootic areas during the interepizootic period, and no maintenance host could be demonstrated. It was suggested that certain bats might be significant as reservoir hosts (Addy and Tukei, 1975, cited by Davies and Onyango, 1978), but no evidence has been available. Seroconversions in cattle, held at forest edge situations are postulated as part of the interepizootic maintenance cycle (Davies, 1975) Isolation of RVFV from trapped mosquitoes and *Culicoides* have been reported (Table V).

The virus is enzootic in Zimbabwe within the epizootic area, where epizootics occur when rain exceeds the norm for the area, following intensification of virus activity in an area where it is already present, rather than lateral spread from cryptic enzootic foci. The outbreaks appear simultaneously in locations hundreds of kilometers apart. Serological examinations of various mammals and humans have yielded little evidence of RVF outside the main watershed plateau, regarded as the enzootic area. Cattle are, so far, the main amplifier host recognized in Zimbabwe during epizootics (Swanepoel, 1981).

In Zimbabwe (Swanepoel, 1976), Kenya (Davies, 1975), and Malawi (Klastrup and Halliwell, 1977), RVFV has been found to be etiologically involved with subclinical abortions and infertility in cattle. In Uganda, and probably in Nigeria, human involvement seems to be unrelated to animal infection (Williams *et al.*, 1960; Tomori, 1980).

The epizootic in Egypt that was diagnosed in October 1977 followed epizootics in Sudan in 1973 and 1976 (Eisa *et al.*, 1977, 1980). The virus entered into an ecosystem totally different from all previously reported outbreaks, being rapidly established in a riverine or delta irrigated area edging the desert, with a major human and animal involvement. Mortality rates were reported to be high among sheep and cattle, intermediate or low among buffalo, camels, goats, donkeys, and rodents (Meegan, 1981). Hemagglutination inhibition antibodies were found in sheep (36%), cattle (30.7%), humans (26.9%), buffalo (21.9%), camels (21.5%), goats (8.7%), donkeys (3.7%), and four rodent species (3.1–14.3%). The morbidity in humans in 1977 was estimated at 20,000–200,000 and higher, with at least 598 fatalities (El-Akkad, 1978; Meegan, 1981). The disease continued throughout 1978, involving at least 400 officially recorded acute cases in humans, but the morbidity data were presumably higher; sporadic cases in humans and at least three virus isolations from animal fetuses were recorded in 1979 and 1980 (Darwish and Hoogstraal, 1981), indicating the disease might have become enzootic. The titers of virus in sera of infected humans ranged from $10^{4.2}$ to $10^{8.6}$ and in sheep from $10^{8.9}$ to $10^{10.0}$

TABLE V
Rift Valley Fever Virus Isolations from Field-Collected Arthropods

Species	Location	Year	Reference
Aedes africanus	Uganda; Lunyo Forest	1956	Weinbren et al. (1956)
A. caballus	South Africa; inland plateau	1953	Gear et al. (1955)
A. cinereus	South Africa; inland plateau	1974–1975	McIntosh et al. (1980a)
A. circumluteolus	South Africa; coastal lowlands	1956	Smithburn and Kokernot (1980)
	Uganda; Lunyo Forest	1955	Weinbren et al. (1956)
A. dentatus	Zimbabwe; highlands	1969	McIntosh (1972)
A. dendrophilus[a]	Uganda; Semliki Forest	1948	Smithburn et al. (1948)
A. juppi	South Africa; inland plateau	1974–1975	McIntosh et al. (1980a)
A. lineatopennis	Zimbabwe; highlands	1969	McIntosh (1972)
	Kenya; bushed grasslands	1978	Davies and Highton (1980)
A. tarsalis	Uganda; Semliki Forest	1948	Smithburn et al. (1948)
Anopheles cinereus	South Africa; inland plateau	1974–1975	McIntosh et al. (1980a)
A. coustani	Zimbabwe; highlands	1969	McIntosh (1972)
	Kenya; bushed grassland	1978	Davies and Highton (1980a)
Coquillettidia fuscopennata[b]	Uganda; Entebbe area	1960	Williams et al. (1960)
Culex antennatus	Nigeria; Ibadan	1967–1970	Lee (1970)
Cx. pipiens	Egypt; Nile Delta	1978	Hoogstraal et al. (1979)
Cx. theileri	South Africa; inland plateau	1953	Gear et al. (1955)
	South Africa; inland plateau	1956	Smithburn and Kokernot (1980)
	South Africa; inland plateau	1970	McIntosh (1972)
	South Africa; inland plateau	1974–1975	McIntosh et al. (1980a)
	Zimbabwe; highlands	1969	McIntosh (1972)
Eretmapodites spp.	Uganda; Semliki Forest	1948	Smithburn et al. (1948)
E. quinquevittatus	South Africa; coastal lowlands	1971	McIntosh (1972)
Mansonia africana	Uganda; Entebbe area	1959	Williams et al. (1960)
	Uganda; Lunyo Forest	1968	Henderson et al. (1972)
Culicoides spp.	Nigeria; Ibadan	1967–1970	Lee (1979)
	Kenya; bushed grassland	1978	Davies and Highton (1980)
Simulium spp.	South Africa; Orange River	1953	Van Velden et al. (1977)

[a] As *Aedes deboeri*.
[b] As *Mansonia fuscopennata*.

(Meegan, 1979). The potential role of rodents as maintenance and amplifying hosts was examined by experimental infection trials; they developed a short viremia of 10^2 to 10^3. The ubiquitous *Culex pipiens*, being the predominant mosquito species in the epizootic area, was shown to be the chief candidate for consideration as the RVF vector in Egypt; Virus isolation rate was rather low, but it transmitted RVFV in experimental trials for periods of up to 36 days postfeeding (Hoogstraal *et al.*, 1979; Meegan, 1981).

The manner in which RVF penetrated into Egypt has been widely discussed and remains speculative. Serological evidence indicates that the virus was not present in Egypt prior to 1977 (Darwish, 1980). Hoogstraal *et al.* (1979) regarded camels as having introduced RVF from Sudan; 30% of Sudanese camels demonstrated HI antibodies immediately after crossing the border into Egypt. Sellers *et al.* (1982) discussed the alternative routes of RVF penetration, underlining the possible spread by hematophagous insects carried from the Sudan on winds in the Intertropical Convergence Zone into the Aswan area, where amplification and further spread could have occurred.

No wild vertebrate hosts have so far been shown to be involved with the Egyptian outbreak, though ongoing observations in rodents (*Rattus alexandrinus*) have shown that phleboviruses, so far undefined, could be isolated with the RVF enzootic area (World Health Organization, 1982a).

Meegan (1981) compiled data reported by various investigators that implicated domestic animals and humans as amplifying hosts or reservoirs; viremias with peak titers of 10^8–10^{10} were reported in humans with duration of 3 to 10 days, and in sheep, cattle, and goats with duration of 2 to 5 days. Rift Valley fever virus could be detected in spleens of experimentally infected sheep for periods of 11 to 21 days postinoculation (Yedloutschnig *et al.*, 1981c).

The possible potential spread of RVF by viremic humans or animals to other continents was demonstrated by reports of serological evidence, acquired in countries outside Africa, indicating infections that have been acquired shortly beforehand in endemic–enzootic areas (Mahdy *et al.*, 1979; Niklasson *et al.*, 1979; Shimshony *et al.*, 1981a). In this respect, Kaschula (1957) could be cited: "If this virus were introduced into the United States in the summer or fall, it would probably spread rapidly. The type of country in South Africa, in which the disease occurs extensively, closely resembles the prairieland of this country [p. 220]."

Major epizootics involving domestic ruminants and humans have been reported up until now in eight southern and eastern African countries (Fig. 1).

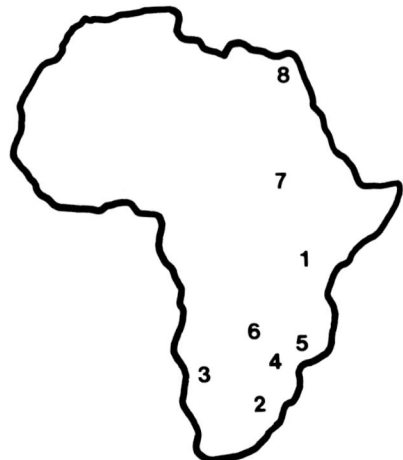

FIG. 1. Map showing major RVF epizootics. 1. Kenya; 2. South Africa; 3. Namibia; 4. Zimbabwe; 5. Mozambique; 6. Zambia; 7. Sudan; 8. Egypt. For details see Table IV.

The epidemiology of RVF in humans seems to be closely linked with the epizootical situation. For many years it was thought that RVF infected only people who came into close contact with contaminated animal tissues. Daubney et al. (1931) believed that about 200 dengue-like, nonfatal cases occurred in people during the 1930 outbreak in Kenya. According to K. H. Schulz (1951, cited by Henning, 1956), ~70% of the 32,000 people exposed to infection during the 1950–1951 epizootic in South Africa became infected to some degree. No fatalities were recorded, but a number of patients developed retinitis and loss of vision (Freed, 1951). During the said outbreak, about 100,000 sheep and cattle died from the disease (Henning, 1956). During the South African epizootic of 1974 and 1975, numerous cases of serious complications in humans were recorded (McIntosh et al., 1980b). Most of them developed retinitis with temporary vision defects, but in a few the defect was permanent. Several patients developed nonfatal meningoencephalitis. Laboratory confirmation of 110 cases was obtained. All 7 of the fatal cases that were recorded were characterized by hemorrhagic state associated with hepatitis. Most of the people involved were farmers, farm laborers, and veterinary surgeons. The overall immunity rate among residents on affected farms was 14.5%.

The 1977 outbreak in Egypt is the largest epidemic in humans with the most extensive clinical complications yet observed. Morbidity estimates range between 20,000 and 200,000 cases, and at least 600 fatalities were recorded (Meegan et al., 1980a). The area involved in the epizootic had an estimated human population of 1 to 3 million (Meegan, 1979). Further estimates of the mortality rate are 0.2% in the military (El-Gibaly, 1978), 3.3% in the general population (El-Akkad, 1978), and 14% in hospitalized patients (Madkour, 1978). Attack rates, rates of each of the three described disease complication syndromes (i.e., encephalitis, liver involvement, and retinitis), and total number of cases remain unknown, though 26.9% of human sera were found positive in the epizootic center (Meegan, 1981). Abdel-Aziz *et al.* (1980) could not find evidence of abortogenic activity of RVFV in humans.

During an epizootic in Zimbabwe in 1978, RVF was suspected to have caused five fatalities. Laboratory confirmation was achieved in three cases (Swanepoel *et al.*, 1979). Many infections occurred in two abattoirs, most of them on the slaughterfloor and particularly in the section where condemned carcasses were handled (Chambers and Swanepoel, 1980).

Cases of RVF in humans that were seemingly unrelated to epizootics have been reported from Uganda (Williams *et al.*, 1960), Tanzania (Deutman and Klomp, 1981), and Nigeria (Tomori, 1981). In other countries, antibodies were found in human populations without recorded clinical symptoms (Findlay *et al.*, 1936b; Pellissier, 1954; Kokernot *et al.*, 1965a). A serological survey in Sudan was carried out after the 1973 and 1976 epizootics. Of 846 sera tested, 3.2% were found to be RVF-positive by the CF test (Saleh *et al.*, 1981).

B. Vectorial Transmission

1. Diptera (Mosquitoes)

Daubney *et al.* (1931) assumed that the disease was transmitted by biting insects. They observed that Rift Valley fever was most prevalent during rainy seasons, especially in low-lying areas, and that it could be controlled by moving flocks to pastures situated at higher altitudes or by confining animals in mosquito-proof stables. The great majority of the mosquitoes that prevailed during the outbreak were found by these workers to be *Culex pipiens* and *Cx. fatigans;* small numbers of three anophelines were also collected. No infection in susceptible lambs was obtained by inoculation of collected culex mosquitoes; they incriminated a species of *Taeniorrhynchus* as a possible vector. First positive proof of arthropod transmission was obtained by Smithburn *et al.* (1948), who isolated the virus from wild-caught mosquitoes in the uninhabited Semliki Forest of western Uganda. The virus was isolated from at least six species of the genus *Eretmopodites* and three species of

Aedes. They found that the *Aedes* species were not actively involved in transmission, because virus was isolated sporadically and in low concentrations. However, the *Eretmopodites* species contained higher level of virus in each of three successive 5-day catches. Subsequently, they transmitted the virus with *E. chrysogaster* from lamb to lamb, lamb to mouse, mouse to lamb, and mouse to mouse (Smithburn *et al.*, 1949a).

Following the observations in Uganda and the epizootic in South Africa in 1950 and 1951, numerous virus isolation attempts from field-collected arthropods have been carried out, resulting in the isolation of the virus from 18 mosquito species belonging to six genera as well as from *Culicoides* and *Simulium* spp. These results are summarized in Table V.

The ability of 17 mosquito species to transmit RVFV to susceptible laboratory or domestic animals after an extrinsic incubation has been studied by various laboratories. In addition to 10 species that had been found to be infected in the field, 7 species have been incorporated in the studies to test their transmission potential, although they had not been found infected in the field or were not included in trappings. The results of those studies are represented in Table VI. It has been found that 14 species can transmit the virus experimentally. McIntosh *et al.* (1980a) could not confirm the previously observed transmission of RVFV by *Aedes caballus*. They explain this by the possible confusion with the newly described *A. juppi* species, because both species coexist over areas where the earlier studies were carried out.

It has been found that *Culex theileri* was the most efficient vector: 92–100% of females were infected by 6.5 to 8.5 log LD_{50} of virus; 11 of 20 mosquitoes transmitted virus from hamsters to 6-day-old mice. Lower infection and transmission rates were recorded with other mosquitoes (McIntosh *et al.*, 1973a,b).

On the basis of field observations and experimental infection and transmission trials, it was concluded (McIntosh and Jupp, 1981) that *Cx. theileri* is the main epizootic vector in southern Africa; *A. juppi*, *A. lineatopennis,* and possibly other mosquito species are vectors in a minor capacity. Apart from having shown the highest natural infection rate and experimental transmission rate, there are other factors implicating *Cx. theileri*. It is by far the most prevalent and widespread mosquito in the epizootic area, adult populations persist from early summer to midwinter, and it is relatively resistant to aridity. It feeds mainly on sheep and cattle but also readily on humans, and commonly enters houses; therefore it can be regarded as an important vector of

TABLE VI

Rift Valley Fever Virus Experimental Transmissions with Arthropods

Species	Natural infection	Experimental transmission	References
Aedes aegypti		+	Mims and Gillet (1956); Weinbren *et al.* (1957); Easterday *et al.* (1962c); McIntosh *et al.* (1980a)
A. caballus	+	+	Gear *et al.* (1955)
		−	McIntosh *et al.* (1980a)
A. circumluteolus	+	−	McIntosh *et al.* (1973a)
A. coustani	+	+	McIntosh *et al.* (1973a)
A. juppi	+	+	McIntosh *et al.* (1980a)
A. lineatopennis	+	+	McIntosh *et al.* (1980a)
A. triseriatus		+	Easterday *et al.* (1962c)
Anopheles coustani	+	−	McIntosh *et al.* (1973a)
Culex neavei		+	McIntosh *et al.* (1973a)
Cx. pipiens	+	+	Meegan *et al.* (1980b)
Cx. quinquefasciens		+	McIntosh *et al.* (1980a)
Cx. rubinotus		−	McIntosh *et al.* (1980a)
Cx. theileri	+	+	McIntosh *et al.* (1973a)
Cx. univittatus		+	McIntosh *et al.* (1980a)
Cx. zombaensis		+	McIntosh *et al.* (1973a)
Eretmapodites chrysogaster		+	Smithburn *et al.* (1949a)
E. quinquevittatus	+	+	McIntosh *et al.* (1973a)

RVF in animals but also suspect as a cause of at least some human infections. McIntosh *et al.* (1980a) have also underlined their statement by successful transmission trials with sheep.

Moderate to high experimental infection (86.7%) and transmission (40%) rates were obtained in Egypt with laboratory-reared *Cx. pipiens*, though only two pools of field-collected female mosquitoes of 1174 were found to be infected. *Cx. pipiens* constituted over 95% of the total number collected. The transmission was carried out after 7 to 12 days of extrinsic incubation (Meegan *et al.*, 1980b). In a former study, transmission was obtained after 12 to 36 days of extrinsic incubation (Hoogstraal *et al.*, 1979).

Cx. pipiens is frequently observed to feed avidly on humans in Egypt; precipitin tests there show that domestic mammals serve as hosts. From these results, it was suggested that *Cx. pipiens* was a vector of RVFV during the 1977–1978 epizootics in Egypt. No evidence was obtained to suggest that mosquitoes are involved in the maintenance of the virus. Infected lots of seven mosquito species, including *Cx. theileri*, have been reared and tested for virus by McIntosh *et al.* (1980a). Virus was not isolated from any life stage, indicating that RVFV does not pass transovarially or transstadially in mosquitoes. Meegan *et al.* (1980b) observed a decreasing ability of mosquitoes to transmit RVFV after several generations in the laboratory.

The molecular basis of oral transmission of bunyaviruses by mosquitoes has been examined by Beaty *et al.* (1981). They found that the M-RNA segment, which codes for the virion glycoproteins, may be a major determinant of oral transmission of bunyaviruses by mosquitoes. Because RVFV belongs to the same family, sharing the same segmented RNA genome, it might also have similar determinants for oral transmission by mosquitoes.

2. *Diptera (*Culicoides*)*

Culicoides (family Ceratopogonidae; biting midges) are vectors of various arboviruses. Various attempts have been carried out to evaluate their role in the transmission of Rift Valley fever. The most extensive studies have been carried in southern Africa. No virus was isolated from a total of 14,158 insects, collected during 1969 and 1970 and during 1974 and 1975 (McIntosh, 1972; McIntosh *et al.*, 1980a). During the 1974–1975 extensive epizootic in South Africa, 16 mixed pools of *Culicoides*, including 12,368 insects, were collected on infected farms and found negative; in contrast, 18 isolations were obtained from 536 pools of various mosquitoes, including 21,722 insects, collected on the same premises. In Zimbabwe, a large number of *Culicoides* from infected farms were found negative (Taylor and Swanepoel, 1980). A limited study in Egypt, including 300 *Culicoides* of various species has yielded no virus (Meegan *et al.*, 1980b).

Two successful attempts to isolate the virus vrom *Culicoides* have been reported. Lee (1979) carried out vectors collection during the period 1967–1970 in Ibadan, Nigeria. A total of 269,580 *Culicoides*, in mixed pools of 100 to 250 gnats, were processed for viral assay. They isolated RVFV from one pool of unfed and one pool of engorged insects. The pools included 14 *Culicoides* spp.; the most abundant were *C. austeni, C. krameri, C. imicola (C. pallidipenis)*, and *C. shulzei*. The isolated virus was later found to be indistinguishable from the Lunyo strain (Uganda) by cross-neutralization test, and antigenically similar, although not identical by complement fixation (Fagbami *et al.*, 1975).

Davies and Highton (1980) isolated RVFV from one mixed pool of

Culicoides of four pools, each containing 250 unengorged gnats, collected in 1979 during an epizootic on an infected farm. They regard *Culicoides* as the most numerous and aggressive insects feeding on cattle in Kenya and consider it possible that contaminated mouthparts may have been the source of the isolated virus.

Jennings *et al.* (1982) demonstrated that *C. varriipennis* females were not susceptible to laboratory oral infection with RVFV.

Although additional work on *Culicoides* is needed to determine their potential as vectors of RVF, the presently collected data, mainly in South Africa, do not indicate that they have a major role in the epidemiology of the disease (Peters and Meegan, 1981; World Health Organization, 1982b).

3. Other Possible Arthropod Vectors

Simuliidae (black flies) were included in studies carried out in southern Africa: in 1969 and 1970, 4 pools of *Simulium* spp. (including 476 insects), and in 1974 and 1975, 16 pools (including 1131 insects) were found negative (McIntosh, 1972; McIntosh *et al.*, 1980a). There is no circumstantial evidence concerning their abundant prevalence during epizootics in infected areas. However, Van Velden *et al.* (1977) reported one isolate from a batch of Simuliidae collected in the vicinity of the Orange River, South Africa, in 1953.

During the 1974–1975 epizootic in South Africa, pools of collected Tabanidae and Muscidae (*Stomoxys*) were collected on infected farms and tested for RVFV with negative results (McIntosh *et al.*, 1980a).

Acarina (ticks) have not been circumstantially found to be involved in the epidemiology of RVF. Daubney and Hudson (1933) reported the infection of *Rhipicephalus appendiculatus*. McIntosh *et al.* (1980a) tested the vector competence of *Ornithodoros savignyi*, in which no virus multiplication was obtained. This tick was studied because of its potential to serve as a viral maintenance host due to its distribution in animal burrows.

During the epizootic in Egypt in 1977 and 1978, Meegan *et al.* (1980b) studied 276 collected ticks of various species with negative results.

There are very few observations concerning the role of biting flies (*Phlebotomus*) during the 50 years following the first isolation of RVFV in 1930. A limited study was carried out in Natal, South Africa during the period 1972–1979; no RVFV was isolated from 391 *Phlebotomus* in 46 pools, as well as from 71,561 mosquitoes in 2414 pools, also collected in the same area, which is regarded as an enzootic area (McIntosh *et al.*, 1980a). *Phlebotomus papatasii* is common in localized areas in Egypt, but no virus isolation trials from this species have been reported during the outbreak in Egypt in 1977 and 1978.

Since the discovery of the close relationship between RVFV and other members of the *Phlebovirus* genus (Shope *et al.*, 1980), the possible role of *Phlebotomus* in the transmission or maintenance of RVF has been the subject of various discussions (Brès, 1981; Peters and Meegan, 1981; Prozeski, 1981). Studies concerning the maintenance of the virus in epizootic areas and during interepizootic periods, the possible role of *Phlebotomus* and other arthropods in transmitting it horizontally or vertically, and the interrelationship with wild vertebrates, will undoubtedly be undertaken in the near future.

Larval *Taenia crassicolis* from infected mice were found to absorb RVFV (Findlay and Howard, 1951).

C. Nonvectorial Transmission

There is good evidence to show that the primary means of virus transmission to humans is close contact with infected animal tissue during slaughter, food preparation, postmortem examinations, or laboratory studies (Daubney *et al.*, 1931; Smithburn *et al.*, 1949b; Gear *et al.*, 1951; Van Velden *et al.*, 1977; Swanepoel *et al.*, 1979). Vector-transmitted RVF has not been clearly demonstrated in humans, although it might well occur (Schrire and Gear, 1956; McIntosh and Jupp, 1981) and was thought to have played a role during the outbreak in Egypt in 1977 and 1978 (Hoogstraal *et al.*, 1979). Spread from patient to patient has never been encountered (Kaschula, 1957; Peters and Meegan, 1981).

In the absence of insect vectors, RVF usually does not spread in animals. Daubney *et al.* (1931), who reported that mosquitoes were suspected to be the vectors, failed to infect lambs by drenching them with infected blood; they also reported that lambs remained healthy although nursed by actively infected ewes. Findlay (1932) could not infect mice and rats by feeding them with infected livers and spleens.

Attempts to demonstrate virus in various excretions, such as urine, feces, and milk from several species, have been unsuccessful (reviewed by Easterday, 1965). However some accumulated data might indicate potential virus shedding. Wedum (cited by Walker *et al.*, 1970a) reported that virus was shed in the saliva of infected puppies but not in the urine. Harrington *et al.* (1980) isolated $10^{5.3}$ PFU/ml virus from the saliva of sheep, collected 5 days after challenge with the ZH-501 RVFV strain, at which time there was a PRN_{80} antibody titer of 1:20 and no detectable viremia. Barnard (1981) reported that milk of artificially infected ewes contained traces of RVFV, and that the said ewes excreted virus in their blood-stained nasal discharge. Excretion of virus in cow's milk had been reported by Alexander (1951).

High levels of RVFV in aborted fetuses and fetal membranes have been reported by Yedloutschnig et al. (1981a); amniotic fluid of infected sheep has been found to contain very high titers of hemaglutinating and complement-fixing RVF antigen (Imam et al., 1981b). Human throat washings contained RVFV (Francis and Magill, 1935).

Experimental contact transmission trials in domestic and laboratory animals have been carried out by various workers, mostly with negative results (reviewed by Easterday, 1965). Easterday et al. (1962b) could infect sheep by swabbing the buccal mucosa with gauze pads soaked in RVFV, but not by lengthy contact between infected sheep and goats and susceptible lambs. Kaschula (1957) stated that "susceptible sheep or mice can be together without danger of transmission from one to the other." Mims (1956c) reported infection in cannibalistic mice, as well as in mice that had a fairly large amount of virus in their drinking water. Weiss (1957) reported that the virus could be readily spread from infected mice to susceptible suckling mice by attendant handling. Easterday et al. (1962c) could not infect lambs when virus was given in capsules.

There are contradictory data from various additional observations. Keefer et al. (1972) reported that puppies and kittens were not infected after ingesting skim milk containing as much as $10^{6.4}$ MIC LD_{50} of the van Wyk RVFV strain. Bucci et al. (1981) could not demonstrate any contact transmission between infected and susceptible rats kept together. The rats were of a strain that is highly susceptible to parenteral infection. Barnard (1981) reported that susceptible lambs of artificially infected ewes were not infected, although the ewes excreted virus in nasal discharge and milk. Henning (1952) reported that calves were not infected by contaminated milk. Kruse and Wedum (1970) reported that cross-infection among caged laboratory monkeys inoculated with the van Wyk strain occurred only if the inoculation was done by the "whole-body exposure" or "head-only exposure," but not after inoculations by the im, ip, iv, or sc routes. Mice inoculated ic or ip did not infect their susceptible cagemates.

In contrast, Walker et al. (1970a,b) reported both horizontal and ascending transmissions in puppies and kittens with the van Wyk strain. Barzilai and Ben-Nathan (1982b) indicated ascending and descending, but no horizontal transmissions in suckling mice inoculated with the neuroadapted Smithburn strain. Yedloutschnig et al. (1981a) reported direct transmission of the ZH-501 strain in sheep kept under crowded conditions in an isolation unit with infected aborting sheep. Harrington et al. (1980) reported contact transmission in a sheep under similar conditions.

Suspected airborne transmission of RVFV was reported by Francis and Magill (1935), who described three cases in humans whom they believed to have been infected in the laboratory via the respiratory tract. Hoogstraal et al. (1979) reported that six people possibly became infected by inhalation of the virus from blood droplets discharged from a dying sheep.

Experimental infection by intranasal inoculation was demonstrated by Findlay (1932) and Easterday (1961) in rhesus and cynomolgus monkeys, and by Francis and Magill (1935) in ferrets. Contrary to the monkeys, which reacted subclinically, the ferrets developed pneumonia, hepatitis, hemorrhagic diarrhea, and death.

Aerosol infection was experimentally induced by various investigators (Table VII); it should be borne in mind that various infection techniques and virus assays were used. Brown et al. (1981) compared the respiratory infectivity in mice of a recently isolated RVFV strain from Egypt with isolates less pathogenic for humans. The virulence and the respiratory infectivity of the Egyptian isolate were no greater than those expressed by the other strains. Initial virus replication occurred in the lungs of the exposed mice, but no evidence of pneumonia could be determined histologically. The ultimate outcome of the infection was a fulminant and fatal hepatic necrosis. The high suscep-

TABLE VII

EXPERIMENTAL AEROSOL INFECTION WITH RVFV

Species	RVFV strain	$\sim ID_{50}$	References
Lamb	van Wyk	1.0–9.0 MIP LD_{50}	Easterday et al. (1962c)
Rhesus monkey	van Wyk	<1.0 MIP LD_{50}	Easterday (1961)
Rhesus monkey	Pantropic	76 MIP LD_{50}	Miller et al. (1963)
Cynomolgus monkey	van Wyk	<1.0 MIP LD_{50}	Easterday (1961)
Hamster	van Wyk	1.0–10.0 MIP LD_{50}	Easterday and Murphy (1963b)
Hamster	Pantropic	0.525 MIP LD_{50}	Miller et al. (1963)
Puppies	van Wyk	25.0 MIC LD_{50}	Keefer et al. (1972)
Kittens	van Wyk	5.0–7.0 MIC LD_{50}	Keefer et al. (1972)
Mice (ICR)	ZH-501	$10^{2.2}$ PFU	Brown et al. (1981)
Mice (ICR)	Entebbe	$10^{1.9}$ PFU	Brown et al. (1981)
Mice (ICR)	SA-51	$10^{2.6}$ PFU	Brown et al. (1981)
Mice (ICR)	SA-75	$10^{1.9}$ PFU	Brown et al. (1981)

tibility of mice to infectious aerosols of the van Wyk strain had been demonstrated also by Easterday and Murphy (1963b).

The role of contact and aerosol transmission in animals in the field is probably negligible, because most evidence supports the concept that epizootic RVF infection of domestic animals is transmitted by mosquitoes (Peters and Meegan, 1981); the nonarboviral route seems to play a role only when the viral load is already high (Prozesky, 1981). Most of the published evidence shows that nonvectorial transmission (contact or respiratory) may be the predominant cause of RVF morbidity in humans. The potential spread by animal products was reviewed by the World Health Organization (1982b), stating that although little or no information is available concerning the possible role of wool, bones, skins, hides, and manure, the use of fresh, unpasteurized milk should be avoided. However, direct contact with meat of freshly slaughtered sick animals might cause infection in humans. A significant example was recorded in two abattoirs in Zimbabwe, where numerous human infections occurred on the slaughterfloor, and particularly in the by-products section where diseased carcasses are processed. Infection rates were significantly lower in people who had only contact with cold or frozen tissue that was 24 hr old or more, or had no contact with meat at all; no outbreaks were observed in urban consumer populations (Chambers and Swanepoel, 1980; Swanepoel, 1981). It was concluded that the virus content of the meat decreases rapidly after slaughter.

D. Virus Maintenance in Mammals

1. Rodents

Daubney and Hudson (1932) discussed the heavy mortality in two murid species, *Arvicanthus abyssinicus nairobiae* and *Rattus rattus kijabius,* on farms affected during the 1930 epizootic in Kenya, but they could not prove that RVF was etiologically involved. Consequently, various observations have been carried out to try to assess the role of rodents in the maintenance and epidemiology of RVFV, including serological examinations, virus isolation attempts, histological examinations, and experimental infection.

Mims (1956e) found neutralization antibody in one serum sample from an *Arvicanthus abyssinicus nubilans* rat of 102 sera of murids collected in an epizootic area in Uganda. Hemagglutination inhibition titers were detected in an unstated number of 1145 examined sera from nonspecific rodents from Kenya, tested in South Africa (Anonymous 1961), and in 31 of 106 pooled sera of murids, shrews, and dormice (Anonymous, 1962). Swanepoel et al. (1978) examined 867 sera of wild-caught rodents in enzootic areas in Zimbabwe; 16 were HI-positive, including the murids *Praomys natalensis* (12 of 736), *Aethomys chrysophilus* (2 of 45), and *Saccostomys campestris* (1 of 15), as well as the shrew *Crocidura hirta* (1 of 7). But on examination for neutralization antibodies, only one *P. natalensis* rat of 1038 examined was found positive; 222 murids, shrews, and dormice of 13 species were found negative.

Hoogstraal et al. (1979) examined HI reactions in four rodent species trapped in Egypt during the Egyptian epizootic in 1977 and 1978. Positive reactions were observed in the Nile grass rat, *Arvicanthus niloticus* (26 of 121), the spiny mouse *Acomys cahirinus* (4 of 49), and the house rat *Rattus rattus* (5 of 161) but not in 21 trapped house mice (*Mus musculus*).

Negative serological findings were recorded in other observations involving a large number of murids, shrews, dormice, and nonspecific rodents (Gear *et al.*, 1951, 1955; Davis, 1957; Anonymous, 1958, 1961; Scott and Heisch, 1959; Henderson *et al.*, 1972) in East Africa and South Africa.

Numerous virus isolation attempts from rodents have been carried out in enzootic and epizootic areas, involving a large number of various African species of murids (rats and mice), shrews, and dormice, with negative results (Gear *et al.*, 1951; Davis, 1957; Anonymous, 1958, 1959, 1961, 1962; Scott and Heisch, 1959; Henderson *et al.*, 1972; Davies, 1975; Swanepoel *et al.*, 1978). Hoogstraal *et al.* (1979) failed to isolate RVFV from 352 trapped rodents during the epizootic in Egypt, but Imam *et al.* (1979) reported the isolation of RVFV from the brain of one of eight *Rattus rattus* from Sharqiya in Egypt.

Experimental infection in various rodent species was carried out and reported. Weinbren and Mason (1957) demonstrated that viremia titers of up to $10^{8.0}$ M LD$_{50}$/0.3 ml occurred in *A. abyssinicus nubilans* rats, infected ic or by peripheral routes. The rats did not readily succumb to infection by any route, and therefore the species was regarded as a potential reservoir host. In South Africa, McIntosh (1961) found that at least two of five species that he infected, namely *Saccostomys campestris* and *Aethomys chrysophilus*, developed viremia of an intensity sufficient to infect mosquitoes, which he found to be $10^{6.5}$–$10^{8.5}$ LD$_{50}$ of the virus (McIntosh *et al.*, 1973a). *Aethomys namaquensis*, a murid that is widely distributed but not abundant in Zimbabwe, was shown in limited observations to be capable of circulating moderate amounts of virus; *Rhabdomys pumilio, S. campestris, A. chrysophilus,* and *Lemniscomys griselda* were found to circulate large amounts of virus (Swanepoel *et al.*, 1978), compared to *Praomys natalensis* and *Tatera leucogastea*, which had lower viremia titers, not sufficient for mosquito infection; *Leggada minutoides* exhibited minimal viremia in a single observation. Keogh and Isaacson (1978) report that *S. campestris* is used in South Africa for RVF research, being the only field rodent to die when tested for susceptibility to RVF.

Hoogstraal *et al.* (1979) infected eight serologically negative rodents, two of each of the four species prevalent in Egypt, with 2000 MIC LD_{50} RVFV. The titer of the resulting viremia in each case was low (10^2–10^3 MIC LD_{50}/ml) and of short duration. Thirty-six virus isolates, belonging to the *Phlebovirus* genus but not yet further differentiated, from 90 rodents were reported from Egypt (World Health Organization, 1982a). The isolates were made during 1981 from rodents, mainly *Rattus alexandrinus*, captured in areas where RVF strains had been isolated from humans some time before. Further differentiation of the isolates might implicate the role of the rats in RVF epidemiology.

Histological examinations were carried out by Gear *et al.* (1955) in livers of 77 murids and shrews from an epizootic area with negative results. Swanepoel *et al.* (1978) concluded that murids fail to encounter infection in nature and are unlikely to play a role in circulation and dissemination. Further knowledge about the genetic susceptibility of various wild rodents, as indicated by Peters and Anderson (1981), and the duration of viremia in various species, should be acquired. Kasahara and Koyama (1973) demonstrated that RVFV could be isolated over a period as long as 62 days from the spleen, thymus, and lymph nodes of immune mice.

2. Wild Ruminants

During the 1951 RVF outbreak in South Africa, mortality and abortion among game was reported from the affected area but not confirmed as being due to RVF (Dickson, in Alexander, 1951). Maurice (1967) demonstrated HI antibodies in the sera of wild ruminants in Chad and Cameroun. Davies (1975) tested 498 sera of 11 wild ruminant species in an enzootic area in Kenya; only 7 were positive with mouse NT and FAT, compared with 514 positive cattle sera of 3669 in the same area. He concluded that wild ruminants played no role in the maintenance of RVFV.

3. Primates

Pellissier and Rousselot (1954) reported the presence of antibody to RVFV in 12 of 122 monkeys kept in captivity in Brazzaville. In contrast, 72 wild monkeys (Smithburn et al., 1948), 333 baboons (Davies et al., 1972), and 1304 green monkeys (Davies and Onyango, 1978) from enzootic areas in East Africa were found negative. Davies (1981a) concluded that primates do not appear to be involved. In addition, 464 primates, belonging to 7 species, have been serologically examined in Kenya. Antibodies were found among vervet monkeys (2 in 136), baboons (3 in 184), and grivet monkeys (1 in 56) (Johnson et al., 1982).

4. Birds

Davies and Addy (1979) tested 171 sera of birds from forest and forest edge situations in Uganda; three ploceus weavers were found to contain low RVF PRN antibody. Alexander (1958) suggested that the Sudan dioch (*Quelea quelea*) produced outbreaks on its migration route, but further details are not available.

5. Other Animals

Gear (1953, cited by Weiss, 1957) reported the isolation of RVFV from a skunk that had died in the field. Weinbren and Hewitt (1958) reported finding RVFV-neutralizing antibody in hippopotamus serum.

Addy and Tukei (1975, cited by Davies and Onyango, 1978) suggested that bats may be significant as reservoir hosts. Bucci et al. (1980) could not demonstrate CF antibodies in 179 bat sera in Egypt. Ten *Rosettus* bats were inoculated with an Egyptian strain that was lethal to control hamsters without clinical response, but all produced CF antibodies within 14 days of inoculation.

V. Prevention and Control Measures

The two classical forms of vaccines, based on inactivated virus or on a live modified strain, were developed quite early in the history of RVF and were shown to prevent RVF. Thus far, both types have been successfully employed in livestock, whereas only inactivated vaccines have been used for human immunization.

The reader is referred to an evaluation concerning the use, production, and standard requirements of veterinary RVF vaccines (World Health Organization, 1983b).

A. Live Vaccines

All live RVF vaccines contain a virus strain that has undergone some modification of its pantropic properties. The main modification is a reduced infectivity by extraneural inoculation. The modified virus, however, retains its potential for causing a fulminant disease if able to reach susceptible locations for growth, such as the brain or embryonal tissues. Because the vaccine strains are by no means completely attenuated, the terms "modified virus" vaccines or "neurotropic" vaccines should be used preferentially.

The immunizing potential of the first neurotropic RVFV strain to be developed (MacKenzie and Findlay, 1936) was readily recognized (MacKenzie and Findlay, 1936; also Findlay and MacKenzie, 1936; Findlay et al., 1936a). The 92nd mouse brain (MB) passage of this strain was put to field use as early as 1937, during the 1936–1937 RVF epizootic in Kenya (Davies, 1981b). During this field trial it was noted by Mulligan (1937) that the vaccine was innocuous for nonpregnant ewes and lambs over 6 months old, but caused abortions in pregnant animals, and encephalitis and death among neonatal lambs.

Much more information has been accumulated concerning vaccination with the Smithburn neurotropic strain of RVFV. Already in the initial study Smithburn (1949) reported that ip inoculation of mice or sheep with the 83rd–85th MB passage of the neurotropic strain protected these animals when challenged with the pantropic strain. He also noted that his vaccine had abortifacient properties, that maternal immunity could be transferred to lambs, and that this passive immunity lasted for about 5 months.

An extensive field trial of the Smithburn strain was carried out in South Africa after the 1951–1952 RVF epizootic there (Barnard and Botha, 1977). The vaccine material was a brain suspension from mice inoculated with the 102nd passage of the Smithburn strain. Again, excessive abortion rate was noticed.

Several attempts, made to further attenuate the virus strain in mouse brains and in embryonated eggs, yielded vaccines with various degrees of immunogenicity and side effects (Kaschula, 1953; Weiss, 1957). The overall superiority of all these derivatives, however, was somewhat questionable, and since 1958 all the live vaccines in South Africa were produced from the original 102nd MB passage of the Smithburn strain (Weiss, 1962; Barnard and Botha, 1977). Until 1971, the vaccine material was a suspension of infected mouse brains. Since 1971, the vaccine has been prepared from virus propagated in BHK cells (ibid). In Kenya, the MB-propagated Smithburn strain (106th MB passage) has been used for the vaccination of sheep and cattle since 1960 (Capstic and Gosden, 1962; Coackley et al., 1967b). Although cattle respond usually with low NI levels (Coackley et al., 1967b;

Howell, cited by Coetzer and Barnard, 1977), vaccinated cattle were shown to resist infection by the pantropic strain under experimental conditions or during RVF outbreaks (Coackley et al., 1967b; Davies, 1981a,b). Barnard (1979) demonstrated that on challenge of Afrikander-type cattle with a pantropic strain, 1 year after vaccination, neither pyrexia nor viremia was induced despite the low NI levels. The postchallenge NI levels were unrelated to the prechallenge levels.

In 1967, Coackley et al. (1967b) investigated the efficacy and safety of the IB 8 neurotropic strain. This strain was derived from a local isolate of a pantropic virus (Coackley, 1965). Because this strain exhibited no substantial superiority over the Smithburn strain, its use has been discontinued. The accumulated experience with the vaccination with neurotropic strains revealed additional effects. Shep acquire lifelong immunity (Barnard, 1981). Goats are good responders and develop NI of higher values than cattle or sheep (Barnard, 1981). One-day-old lambs can be vaccinated if born to nonimmune ewes (Weiss, 1962). Passive immunity is induced in lambs via the colostrum of immunized ewes. Immunization of pregnant ewes may cause passive as well as active immunization of prenatal lambs, or may cause intrauterine infections. In addition to the abortifacient properties of the neurotropic vaccine, it was shown to be also teratogenic and to cause hydrops amnii (Coetzer and Barnard, 1977; Coetzer, 1979).

The neuromodified vaccine has been widely used in various African countries; 18 million doses were used in South Africa during the epizootic of 1975 (Barnard and Botha, 1977); lambs of immune ewes were vaccine, it was shown to be also teratogenic and to cause hydrops amnii (Coetzer and Barnard, 1977).

The neurotropic strain has been incriminated as pathogenic to humans (Smithburn, 1949) and therefore hazardous to unimmunized persons. In Smithburn's report of 1949, it is stated, however (footnote to Table I) that the infective virus was of the 22nd MB passage, and thus by no means completely neurotropic. Weiss (1957) concluded from the reported cases (Smithburn, 1949; Kitchen, 1950) that a low-brain-passage neurotropic virus is infectious to humans and may readily revert to pantropism during such an infection. An unsettled issue, of some concern to epidemiologists, is whether the neurotropic vaccine induces viremia in the recipient animal. Smithburn (1949) and Kitchen (1950) failed to detect viremia in extraneurally inoculated animals. Findlay et al. (1936a) found viremia in ip inoculated sheep. Findlay and Howard (1951) found circulating virus of the 85th MB passage after ip inoculation in mice. Coackley et al. (1967b) reported viremia in two of eight sheep inoculated with the 107th MB passaged Smithburn strain.

B. Inactivated Vaccines for Humans

The first experimental immunization by an inoculation with inactivated preparation of a pantropic RVFV strain was reported by MacKenzie (1935). The virus source was plasma from mice infected with the pantropic strain. Virus inactivation was achieved either by (a) formalin or by (b) methylene blue and light. This work was not followed by a field study.

Randall et al. (1962) and Binn et al. (1963a,b) compared the immunogenicity of formalin-inactivated vaccines of two RVFV strains. The pantropic virus was the Entebbe strain, and the neurotropic strain was Kaschula's high-passage $NRVF_2$ as modified by Weiss with additional 12 MB passages (Weiss, 1957). Various virus-propagating systems were employed, including MB and embryonated eggs. Animal studies and trials in human volunteers indicated that the best immunogen was the pantropic Entebbe strain, propagated in monkey cells. The rhesus-derived cells were later replaced by similar cells from African green monkey, a species with far less prevalence of natural SV_{40} infection (Randall et al., 1963).

During the 1960s, semiindustrial production of the Randall vaccine was attained in the United States. The product, known as NDBR-103, was proven to be safe and immunogenic in humans according to a large-scale clinical trial with over 1000 participants (Eddy et al., 1981). Lyophilized lots of NDBR-103 retained their full potency after over 10 years of storage at $-20°C$. During May through December of 1979, 973 soldiers of the Swedish battalion stationed in the Sinai DMZ were effectively immunized with NDBR-103 produced in 1968 (Niklasson, 1982). The serious side effects (one case each) were herpes zoster activation, cardiac arrhythmia, and a presumptive Guillain-Barré syndrome.

Eddy et al. (1981) reported that attempts were made since 1976 to produce an even safer vaccine for human use. The virus was the same pantropic strain. Also, the procedures for harvest and inactivation remained unchanged. The primary cultures of monkey kidney cells, however, were replaced by the FRhL-2 cell line for virus propagation. This cell line (derived from the lungs of a rhesus embryo) is certified by the FDA for production of human vaccines. Little has been reported about the TSI-GSD-200 vaccine.

C. Inactivated Veterinary Vaccines

The live RVF vaccine was proven teratogenic and abortifacient. Reportedly, its immunogenicity in cattle was poor. It has been regarded as pathogenic to humans by several investigators. All these drawbacks to the live vaccine led Barnard and Botha (1977) to explore other means of immunization. The virus they used was a local pantropic strain, isolated from cattle. The virus was propagated in MB and in BHK cells. According to the propagation system, two types of formalin-inactivated vaccines were produced: graded by the NI elicited in recipient sheep, the BHK vaccine was slightly better than the MB vaccine. Both types induced lower NI than live vaccines derived from BHK or MB. Irrespective of the vaccine status (live or inactivated) and the vaccine source, the recipient adult merino sheep were refractory to experimental challenge. However, both vaccines could not prevent viremia in 30 to 40% of experimentally challenged sheep. The immunogenic efficacy of the inactivated vaccine was proven during an outbreak of RVF. Records were taken from over 400 immunized ewes and over 100 nonimmunized controls, all in advanced stages of pregnancy. Immunized sheep displayed the following reductions: 17-fold in ewe mortality, 10-fold in lamb mortality, and 3-fold in abortions (Barnard and Botha, 1977).

Barnard (1979) studied the effects of varying doses and combinations of live and inactivated vaccines in cattle. Both NI and HI levels were poor after initial vaccination of Afrikander-type young cattle with both vaccine types, but a booster dose of inactivated vaccine evoked pronounced rise in antibody levels in cattle that had been inoculated for the first time 3 months earlier with either of the vaccines. Levels of HI in vaccinated ruminants were studied also in Israel, where more than 2 million doses of the Onderstepoort inactivated vaccine were used during the 1978–1980 period. Klopfer-Orgad *et al.* (1981) reported that high HI levels were demonstrated in sheep and cattle for more than a year after booster vaccination. Results in goats did not differ significantly, but a limited observation in vaccinated camels failed to detect HI titers 6 and 14 months postvaccination. Consequently, it was concluded (Shimshony *et al.*, 1981b) that the first revaccination should be carried out within 3 to 6 months after the initial vaccination, to be followed by annual vaccinations. It was reported that the inactivated vaccine could be inoculated simultaneously with inactivated foot and mouth disease vaccine.

The South African experience with inactivated vaccines coincided with the Egyptian RVF outbreak in 1977 and 1978. Consequently, renewed interest in inactivated RVF vaccine became apparent. Several investigators in the United States tried to immunize sheep and cattle with the inactivated NDBR-103 human RVF vaccine (Harrington *et al.*, 1980; Reynolds *et al.*, 1980; Yedloutschnig *et al.*, 1979).

All claimed some sort of immunity being evoked by as little as one inoculation of NDBR-103. The attained immunity prevented clinical disease and death on challenge with the Egyptian ZH-501 pantropic strain (Yedloutschnig et al., 1979; Harrington et al., 1980). However, a single dose of NDBR-103 did not prevent viremia or abortions after ZH-501 challenge in significant numbers of the immunized animals. Yedloutschnig et al. (1980, 1981d) tried to immunize sheep and cattle with an inactivated vaccine produced from the Entebbe pantropic strain grown in BHK cells. A single dose failed to protect ewes from high-level (10^8 M LD_{50}) viremia or abortions after ZH-501 challenge (Yedloutschnig et al., 1981d). Cattle that received booster doses were better protected from the ZH-501 challenge, as shown by lack of abortions, viremia, and febrile response (Yedloutschnig et al., 1980). Meanwhile, Egyptian investigators began to produce various inactivated vaccines, differing in virus strain and propagation system (Imam and El-Karamany, 1978; Abdel-Ghaffar et al., 1980). The most promising combination found in Egypt was a pantropic RVFV isolate from sheep, propagated in CER cells and inactivated by formalin (El-Karamany et al., 1981).

In contrast to the orthodox inactivated vaccines for human uses, some innovations were introduced to the veterinary vaccine. β-Propiolactone was introduced for virus inactivation (El-Karamany et al., 1981). Adjuvants were studied and incorporated into inactivated vaccine preparations. Barnard and Botha (1977) reported somewhat higher NI with aluminium hydroxide as adjuvant, and also that alum was better in this respect than mineral oil adjuvants. El-Karamany et al. (1981) imparted similar information for his vaccine. Reynolds et al. (1980) announced a new metabolizable lipid adjuvant. This new adjuvant elicited higher NI levels in sheep and monkeys.

Harrington et al. (1980) claimed that better serological responses were attained when a poly(ICLC) adjuvant was used. B. A. Peleg, N. Kuper-Ron, and K. Hornstein (personal communication, 1982) were able to induce HI titers in the 10^4–10^5 levels by an investigational adjuvant, used in experimental vaccination of indigenous sheep in Israel. The same inactivated vaccine without adjuvant induced HI levels of 20 to 640.

D. Unorthodox Vaccines

In the late 1970s at least two new avenues for prospective vaccines were opened. It has been demonstrated that members of the Bunyaviridae may exchange segments of genomic RNA even at an interspecific level (Bishop and Shope, 1979). Eddy et al. (1981) pointed out that such a reassortant may be created, having immunogenicity of RVFV and the innocuousness of another phlebovirus; however, the immunogenicity and the pathogenicity of a bunyavirus may both reside in the same M-RNA segment, so this approach is not straightforward. Another avenue entertained is the use of recombinant DNA technology in order to generate an immunogenic, RVFV-specific, noninfectious protein. This has been achieved for FMD virus (Kleid et al., 1981). Again, as Eddy et al. (1981) pointed out, the immunogenic components of RVFV are probably glycoproteins; no glycoprotein has yet been produced by recombinant DNA technique, and the immunogenicity of nonglycosylated glycoproteins is not known yet. Another approach for attenuation could have been the generation of a stable temperature-sensitive mutant (Prozeski, 1972).

E. Treatment and Laboratory Safety Precautions

Passive antibody treatment was discussed by Henning (1956) and found effective in mice and in 1- to 3-day-old lambs (Bennet et al., 1965). Findlay and Howard (1951) studied the effect of BAL (2,3-dimercaptopropanol) on the course of RVF in mice, with negative results. They also tried oral treatment of infected mice with aureomycin and terramycin, with similar results.

Eddy et al. (1981) reported the screening of various antiviral drugs for their curative value. Three products were compared (ribavirin, poly(ICLC), and immune serum), and all three were highly effective in treatment of mice aged 4–5 weeks that had been infected sc with 10^6 PFU of the ZH-501 RVFV strain; the treatment was successful even if begun 3 days postinfection, in protecting the liver. Late encephalitis occurred in some mice. In the mouse model, there was no clear-cut advantage to any of the therapies, singly or combined. Treatment of ic inoculated mice was unsuccessful.

In rhesus monkeys, as little as 0.025 ml/kg of immune serum prevented detectable viremia. On the basis of both experiments, the writers suggest that immune globulin could be stockpiled and used to provide immediate, temporary protection for exposed laboratory workers or nonimmune populations in epidemic areas. Interferon, poly(ICLC), or ribavirin could also be used, but their potential for preventing encephalitis is questionable.

The various guidelines for handling RVFV have been reviewed by international organizations, and the recommendations have been summarized and published (World Health Organization, 1982b), referring to the measures to be taken in enzootic as well as nonenzootic areas. Special care should be taken to ensure that human cases suspected of being cases of RVF with hemorrhagic complications are handled with extreme caution until their illness has been shown not to be other hemorrhagic diseases, such as Ebola or Marburg fevers. It is recommended that all laboratory personnel be vaccinated and shown to have the antibody. In nonenzootic areas, manipulations should be carried out in a physically protected containment and in biosafety cabinets. The RVF virus should never be imported into any area free of RVF or handled there without the permission and the periodical review of the national authorities.

F. Prevention and Control

The control of RVF during the periodic epizootics in the enzootic–endemic countries in sub-Saharan Africa consisted of vaccinating the principal disease hosts either with live modified or with inactivated vaccines; control of arthropod vector populations has not often been feasible. Protection of exposed humans was carried out by applying safety precautions in laboratory and field, vaccination being an exception.

Following the penetration of RVF into Egypt, neighboring countries and the international public and veterinary health organizations applied special measures and prepared contingency plans to prevent the spread of RVF outside the African continent. This included the resolution of the Office International des Epizootics (OIE) to add RVF to List A of notifiable epizootic diseases, and the establishment of an FAO–WHO working group on RVF. The strategy of international and national activities to prevent spread and to deal with future outbreaks, both within and outside the enzootic area, were summarized and published (World Health Organization, 1982b). The contingency plans for five categories of countries were outlined: enzootic endemic, receptive neighboring, nonreceptive neighboring, receptive nonneighboring, and penetration-prone, nonreceptive countries. The measures outlined were legislative, extension, diagnosis, surveillance, prevention, and applied research, and they included animal movement restrictions, meat inspection, import control, and vaccination.

Vaccination recommendations for countries beyond and in the enzootic sub-Saharan range have been considered and summarized (World Health Organization, 1982c). The recommended vaccination policies of enzootic countries differ from those of nations beyond the enzootic range. In sub-Saharan Africa, annual vaccination was recommended for all exotic cattle, sheep, and goats in known epizootic areas; those were defined according to their ecological characterization. Vaccination in face of an epizootic was recommended for marginal or rarely affected RVF areas. Only use of killed vaccine is recommended in infected areas beyond the enzootic range, and in similar adjacent ecological zones. In emergency situations, mosquito control measures, both environmental and insecticidal, are recommended (World Health Organization, 1982b).

The reader may refer to other publications in respect to RVF prevention and control measures (Van Tongeren, 1979; Mussgay, 1980; Brès, 1981; Peters et al., 1981; Prozesky, 1981; Shimshony et al., 1981a,b; Shope et al., 1982; Swartz and Costin, 1981).

REFERENCES

Abdel-Aziz, A. A., Meegan, J. M., and Laughlin, L. W. (1980). Trans. R. Soc. Trop. Med. Hyg. **74,** 685–686.
Abdel-Ghaffar, S., Ayoub, N. N., Mohsen, A. Y., El-Nimr, M., Nafeh, E. K., and Malik, S. K. (1980). Bull. Off. Int. Epizoot. **92,** 845–849.
Abdel Wahab, K. S. E., Elbaz, L. M., Eltayeb, E. M., Omar, H., Ossman, M. A. M., and Yasin, W. (1978). Trans. R. Soc. Trop. Med. Hyg. **72,** 392–396.
Addy, P. A. K., and Tukei, P. M. (1975). Cited by Davies and Onyango (1978).
Akafekwa, G. I. (1975). Bull. Off. Int. Epizoot. **83,** 843–863.
Alexander, R. A. (1951). J. S. Afr. Vet. Med. Assoc. **22,** 105–109.
Alexander, R. A. (1958). Proc. 4th Annu. Meet. IACED p. 29 (cited by Davies and Addy, 1979).
Andrewes, C. H., and Horstman, D. M. (1949). J. Gen. Microbiol. **3,** 290–297.
Anonymous (1958). "Annual Report of The Arthropod-borne Virus Research Unit." South African Institute for Medical Research, Johannesburg.
Anonymous (1959). "Annual Report of the Arthropod-borne Virus Research Unit." South African Institute for Medical Research, Johannesburg.
Anonymous (1961). "Annual Report of the Arthropod-borne Virus Research Unit." South African Institute for Medical Research, Johannesburg.
Anonymous (1962). "Annual Report of the Arthropod-borne Virus Research Unit." South African Institute for Medical Research, Johannesburg.
Ayoub, N. N. K., and Allam, L. H. (1981). J. Egypt. Public Health Assoc. **56,** 454–462.
Barnard, B. J. H. (1979). J. S. Afr. Vet. Assoc. **50,** 155–157.
Barnard, B. J. H. (1981). Rift Val. Fever, Tech. Ser. **1,** 27–33.
Barnard, B. J. H., and Botha, M. J. (1977). J. S. Afr. Vet. Assoc. **48,** 45–48.
Barzilai, R., and Ben-Nathan, D. (1982a). Isr. J. Med. Sci. **18,** 24–24.
Barzilai, R., and Ben-Nathan, D. (1982b). Refu. Vet. **39,** 57.
Beaty, B. J., Holterman, M., Tabachnik, W., Shope, R. E., Rozohn, E. J., and Bishop, D. H. L. (1981). Science **211,** 1433–1435.
Bennett, D. G., Glock, R. D., and Gerone, P. J. (1965). Am. J. Vet. Res. **26,** 57–62.
Berge, T. O., ed (1975). "International Catalogue of Arboviruses," 2nd ed., Publ. No.

(CDC) 75–8301. Public Health Service, U.S. Department of Health, Education and Welfare, Atlanta, Georgia.
Binn, L. N., Randall, R., Harrison, C. J., Gibbs, C. J., Jr., and Aulisio, C. G. (1963a). *Am. J. Hyg.* **77,** 160–168.
Binn, L. N., Randall, R., Harrison, C. J., Gibbs, C. J., Jr., and Aulisio, C. G. (1963b). *Am. J. Trop. Med. Hyg.* **12,** 236–238.
Bishop, D. H. L. (1979). *Curr. Top. Microbiol. Immunol.* **86,** 1–33.
Bishop, D. H. L., and Shope, R. E. (1979). *Compr. Virol.* **14,** 1–156.
Bishop, D. H. L., Calisher, C. H., Casals, J., Chumakov, M. P., Gaidamovich, S. Ya., Hannoun, C., Lvov, D. K., Marshall, I. D., Oker-Blom, N., Pettersson, R. F., Porterfield, J. S., Russel, P. K., Shope, R. E., and Westaway, E. G. (1980). *Intervirology* **14,** 125–143.
Boctor, W. M. (1978). *J. Egypt. Public Health Assoc.* **53,** 177–180.
Bouloy, M., and Hannoun, C. (1976). *Virology* **69,** 258–264.
Boyle, J. J. (1965). *Am. J. Vet. Res.* **26,** 190–191.
Boyle, J. J. (1967). *Am. J. Vet. Res.* **28,** 1027–1031.
Brès, P. (1981). *Contrib. Epidemiol. Biostat.* **3,** 178–190.
Broom, J. C., and Findlay, G. M. (1932). *Lancet* **222,** 609–611.
Broom, J. C., and Findlay, G. M. (1933). *Br. J. Exp. Pathol.* **14,** 179–181.
Brown, J. L., Dominik, J. W., and Morrissey, R. L. (1981). *Infect. Immun.* **33,** 848–853.
Bucci, T. J., Wood, O. L., Gaines, J. F., and Meegan, J. M. (1980). *Int. Conf. Impact Viral Dis. Devl. Afr. & Middle East Countries, 2nd, 1980* Abstracts, p. 54.
Bucci, T. J., Moussa, I. M., and Wood, O. L. (1981). *Contrib. Epidemiol. Biostat.* **3,** 60–67.
Capstick, P. B., and Gosden, D. (1962). *Nature (London)* **195,** 583–584.
Casals, J. (1963). *Ann. Microbiol. Enzimol.* **11,** 13–34.
Casals, J. (1967). *Methods Virol.* **3,** 113–198.
Casals, J. (1971). *In* "Comparative Virology" (K. Maramorosch and E. Kurstak, eds.), pp. 307–333. Academic Press, New York.
Casals, J. (1978). *J. Egypt. Public Health Assoc.* **53,** 209–215.
Cash, P., Robeson, G., Erlich, B. J., and Bishop. D. H. L. (1981). *Contrib. Epidemiol. Biostat.* **3,** 1–20.
Chambers, P. G., and Swanepoel, R. (1980). *Cent. Afr. J. Med.* **26,** 122–126.
Christie, G. J. (1969). *Rhod. Sci. News* **3,** 238–240 (cited by Swanepoel, 1981).
Clarke, D. H., and Casals, J. (1958). *Am. J. Trop. Med. Hyg.* **7,** 561–573.
Coackley, W. (1963). *J. Pathol. Bacteriol.* **86,** 530–532.
Coackley, W. (1965). *J. Pathol. Bacteriol.* **89,** 123–131.
Coackley, W., Pini, A., and Gosden, D. (1967a). *Res. Vet. Sci.* **8,** 399–405.
Coackley, W., Pini, A., and Gosden, D. (1967b). *Res. Vet. Sci.* **8,** 406–414.
Coetzer, J. A. W. (1977). *Onderstepoort J. Vet. Res.* **44,** 205–212.
Coetzer, J. A. W. (1981). *J. S. Afr. Vet. Assoc.* **52,** 349.
Coetzer, J. A. W., and Barnard, B. J. H. (1977). *Onderstepoort J. Vet. Res.* **44,** 119–126.
Coetzer, J. A. W., Theodoridis, A., and Van Heerden, A. (1978). *Onderstepoort J. Vet. Res.* **45,** 93–106.
Craig, D. E., Thomas, W. J., and DeSanctis, A. N. (1967). *Appl. Microbiol.* **15,** 446–447.
Darwish, M. A. (1980). *Zentralbl. Bakteriol., Parasitenkd., Infektionskr. Hyg., Abt. 1, Suppl.* **9,** 101–110.
Darwish, M. A., and Hoogstraal, H. (1981). *J. Egypt. Public Health Assoc.* **56,** 46–84.
Daubney, R., and Hudson, J. R. (1932). *Lancet* **1,** 611–612.
Daubney, R., and Hudson, J. R. (1933). *East Afr. Med. J.* **10,** 2–19.

Daubney, R., Hudson, J. R., and Garnham, P. C. (1931). *J. Pathol. Bacteriol.* **34**, 545–579.
Davies, F. G. (1975). *J. Hyg.* **75**, 219–229.
Davies, F. G. (1981a). *The Rift Valley Fever, Technical Series* **1**, 49–53.
Davies, F. G. (1981b). *J. Egyp. Public Health Assoc.* **56**, 490–494.
Davies, F. G., and Addy, P. A. K. (1979). *Trans. R. Soc. Trop. Med. Hyg.* **73**, 584–585.
Davies, F. G., and Highton, R. B. (1980). *Trans. R. Soc. Trop. Med. Hyg.* **74**, 815–816.
Davies, F. G., and Karstad, L. (1981). *Trop. Anim. Health Prod.* **13**, 185–188.
Davies, F. G., and Onyango, E. (1978). *Trans. R. Soc. Trop. Med. Hyg.* **72**, 213–214.
Davies, F. G., Clausen, B., and Lund, L. J. (1972). *Trans. R. Soc. Trop. Med. Hyg.* **66**, 363–365.
Davis, D. H. S. (1957). *S. Afr. J. Med. Sci.* **22**, 55–61.
Deutman, A. and Klomp, H. J. (1981). *Am. J. Ophthalmol.* **92**, 38–42.
Dickson, J. L. (1951). In Alexander (1951, pp. 110–111).
Easterday, B. C. (1961). Ph.D. Thesis, University of Wisconsin, Madison (cited by Easterday, 1965).
Easterday, B. C. (1965). *Adv. Vet. Sci.* **10**, 65–127.
Easterday, B. C., and Jaeger, R. F. (1963). *J. Infect. Dis.* **112**, 1–6.
Easterday, B. C., and Murphy, L. C. (1963a). *Cornell Vet.* **53**, 3–11.
Easterday, B. C., and Murphy, L. C. (1963b). *Cornell Vet.* **53**, 423–433.
Easterday, B. C., McGavran, M. H., Rooney, J. R., and Murphy, L. C. (1962a). *Am. J. Vet. Res.* **23**, 470–479.
Easterday, B. C., Murphy, L. C., and Bennett, D. G. (1962b). *Am. J. Vet. Res.* **23**, 1224–1230.
Easterday, B. C., Murphy, L. C., and Bennett, D. G. (1962c). *Am. J. Vet. Res.* **23**, 1231–1240.
Eddy, G. A., Peters, C. J., Meadors, G., and Cole, F. E., Jr. (1981). *Contrib. Epidemiol. Biostat.* **3**, 124–141.
Eisa, M. (1981). *Rift Valley Fever, Technical Series* **1**, 2–13.
Eisa, M., and Obeid, H. M. A. (1977). *Bull. Anim. Health Prod. Afr.* **25**, 349–355.
Eisa, M., Obeid, H. M. A., and El-Saei, A. S. A. (1977). *Bull. Anim. Health Prod. Afr.* **25**, 343–347.
Eisa, M., Kheir el Sid, E. D., Shomein, A. M., and Meegan, J. M. (1980). *Trans. R. Soc. Trop. Med. Hyg.* **74**, 417–419.
El-Akkad, A. M. (1978). *J. Egypt. Public Health Assoc.* **53**, 123–128.
El-Gibaly, M. R. (1978). *J. Egypt. Public Health Assoc.* **53**, 137–146.
El-Gibaly, M. R., Imam, I. Z. E., El-Karamany, H. M., Mansoury, H. M., and Omar, F. (1981). *J. Egypt. Public Health Assoc.* **56**, 415–426.
El-Karamany, R., Imam, I. Z. E., Farid, A. H., and Saber, M. S. (1979). *J. Egypt. Public Health Assoc.* **54**, 105–114.
El-Karamany, R., Imam, I. Z. E., Farid, A. H., Saber, M. S., Moustafa, A. F., Zaki, M., and Bashandy, A. (1981). *J. Egypt. Public Health Assoc.* **56**, 495–525.
Ellis, D. S., Simpson, D. I. H., Stamford, S., and Abdel Wahab, K. S. E. (1979). *J. Gen. Virol.* **42**, 329–337.
El-Mekki, A. A., and van der Groen, G. (1981). *J. Virol. Methods* **3**, 61–69.
El-Refaie, M., El-Sheikh, N., Sami, H., and Fahmi, I. (1981). *Armed Forces Med. J.* **23**, 5–20 (Egypt).
El-Shinnawi, B. M., Sobhy, F., and El-Zawahry, A. (1978). *J. Egypt. Public Health Assoc.* **53**, 187–189.
Endo, M. (1951). *Virus* **1**, 42–50.

Erasmus, B. J., and Coetzer, J. A. W. (1981). *Contrib. Epidemiol. Biostat.* **3**, 77–82.
Fagbami, A. H., Tomori, O., and Kemp, G. E. (1973). *Niger. Vet. J.* **2**, 45–48.
Fagbami, A. H., Tomori, O., Fabiyi, A., and Isoun, T. T. (1975). *Res. Vet. Sci.* **18**, 334–335.
Ferguson, W. (1959). *Bull. Epizoot. Dis. Afr.* **7**, 317–318.
Findlay, G. M. (1932). *Trans. R. Soc. Trop. Med. Hyg.* **25**, 229–265.
Findlay, G. M. (1933). *Br. J. Exp. Pathol.* **14**, 207–219.
Findlay, G. M. (1936). *Br. J. Exp. Pathol.* **17**, 89–104.
Findlay, G. M., and Daubney, R. (1931). *Lancet* **2**, 1350–1351.
Findlay, G. M., and Howard, E. M. (1951). *Arch. Gesamte Virusforsch.* **4**, 411–423.
Findlay, G. M., and Howard, E. M. (1952). *Ann. Trop. Med. Parasitol.* **46**, 33–37.
Findlay, G. M., and MacKenzie, R. D. (1936). *Br. J. Exp. Pathol.* **17**, 431–441.
Findlay, G. M., MacKenzie, R. D., and Stern, R. O. (1936a). *Br. J. Exp. Pathol.* **17**, 431–441.
Findlay, G. M., Stefanopoulo, G. J., and MacCallum, F. O. (1936b). *Bull. Soc. Pathol. Exot.* **29**, 986–996.
Food and Agriculture Organization (1957). "FAO-OIE, Animal Health Yearbook, 1957," pp. 5A-5A (Note C). FAO, Rome.
Food and Agriculture Organization (1963). "FAO-WHO-OIE, Animal Health Yearbook, 1962," pp. 83–83. FAO, Rome.
Food and Agriculture Organization (1969). "FAO-WHO-OIE, Animal Health Yearbook, 1968," pp. 49–49. FAO, Rome.
Food and Agriculture Organization (1970). "FAO-WHO-OIE, Animal Health Yearbook, 1969," pp. 83–83. FAO, Rome.
Food and Agriculture Organization (1977). "FAO-WHO-OIE, Animal Health Yearbook, 1976," pp. 42–42. FAO, Rome.
Food and Agriculture Organization (1979). "FAO-WHO-OIE, Animal Health Yearbook, 1978," pp. 10–10. FAO, Rome.
Francis, T., and Magill, T. P. (1935). *J. Exp. Med.* **62**, 433–448.
Freed, I. (1951). *S. Afr. Med. J.* **25**, 930–932.
Gear, J. H. S. (1975). *J. S. Afr. Vet. Assoc.* **46**, 221–225.
Gear, J. H. S. (1977). *J. S. Afr. Vet. Assoc.* **48**, 5–8.
Gear, J. H. S., de Meillon, B., Measorch, V., Harwin, R., and Davis, D. H. S. (1951). *S. Afr. Med. J.* **25**, 908–912.
Gear, J. H. S., de Meillon, B., Le Roux, A. F., Kofski, R., Rose-Inns, R., Steyn, J. J., Oliff, W. D., and Schulz, K. H. (1955). *S. Afr. Med. J.* **29**, 514–518.
Gentsch, J. R., and Bishop, D. H. L. (1978). *J. Virol.* **28**, 417–419.
Gentsch, J. R., and Bishop, D. H. L. (1979). *J. Virol.* **30**, 767–770.
Gentsch, J. R., Rozhon, E. J., Klimas, R. A., El-Said, L. H., Shope, R. E., and Bishop, D. H. L. (1980). *Virology* **102**, 190–204.
Hahon, N. (1969). *Am. J. Vet. Res.* **30**, 1007–1014.
Hahon, N., and Zimmerman, W. D. (1969). *Appl. Microbiol.* **17**, 775–776.
Haig, D. A., and Kaschula, V. R. (1952). Unpublished data (published by Weiss, 1957).
Harrington, G., Lupton, H. W., Crabbs, C. L., Peters, C. J., Reynolds, A., and Slone, T. W. (1980). *Am. J. Vet. Res.* **41**, 1559–1564.
Henderson, B. E., McCrae, A. W. R., Kirya, B. G., Ssenkubuge, Y., and Sempala, S. D. K. (1972). *Ann. Trop. Med. Parasitol.* **66**, 343–355.
Henning, M. W. (1952). *J. S. Afr. Vet. Med. Assoc.* **23**, 65–78.
Henning, M. W. (1956). "Animal Diseases of South Africa," 3rd ed., pp. 1105–1127. Central News Agency Ltd., Pretoria.

Hess, W. R., May, H. J., and Patty, R. E. (1963). *Am. J. Vet. Res.* **24**, 59–64.
Hoogstraal, H., Meegan, J. M., Khalil, G. M., and Adham, F. K. (1979). *Trans. R. Soc. Trop. Med. Hyg.* **73**, 624–629.
Horning, E. S., and Findlay, G. M. (1934). *J. R. Microsc. Soc.* **54**, 1–9.
Imam, I. Z. E., and Darwish, M. A. (1977). *J. Egypt. Public Health Assoc.* **52**, 417–418.
Imam, I. Z. E., and El-Karamany, R. (1978). *J. Egypt. Public Health Assoc.* **53**, 245–248.
Imam, I. Z. E., El-Karamany, R., and Kasem, S. (1978). *J. Egypt. Public Health Assoc.* **53**, 273–280.
Imam, I. Z. E., El-Karamany, R., and Darwish, M. A. (1979). *Bull. W.H.O.* **57**, 441–413.
Imam, I. Z. E., El-Karamany, R., Zaki, M., and Omar, F. M. (1981a). *J. Egypt. Public Health Assoc.* **56**, 435–443.
Imam, I. Z. E., El-Karamany, R., Omar, F., Bashandy, A., and Zaki, M. (1981b). *J. Egypt. Public Health Assoc.* **56**, 484–489.
Iwasa, S. (1959). *Jpn. J. Exp. Med.* **29**, 323–334.
Jennings, M., Platt, G. S., and Bowen, E. T. W. (1982). *Trans. R. Soc. Trop. Med. Hyg.* **76**, 587–589.
Johnson, B. K., Chanas, A. C., El-Tayeb, E., Abdel-Wahab, K. S. E., Sheheta, F. A., and Mohamed, A. E. D. (1978). *Lancet* **2**, 745–745.
Johnson B. K., Gitau, L. G., Gichogo, A., Tukei, P. M., Else, J. G., Suleman, M. A., Kimani, R., and Sayer, P. D. (1982). *Trans. R. Soc. Trop. Med. Hyg.* **76**, 307–310.
Johnson, R. W., and Orlando, M. D. (1968). *Am. J. Vet. Res.* **29**, 463–471.
Kamel, S. (1981). *The Rift Valley Fever, Technical Series* **1**, 41–48.
Karabatsos, N., ed. (1978). *Am. J. Trop. Med. Hyg.* **27**, 372–440.
Kasahara, S., and Koyama, H. (1973). *Kitasato Arch. Exp. Med.* **46**, 105–112.
Kaschula, V. R. (1953). Ph.D. Thesis, University of Pretoria, South Africa (cited by Weiss, 1957).
Kaschula, V. R. (1957). *J. Am. Vet. Med. Assoc.* **131**, 219–221.
Keefer, G. V., Zebarth, G. L., and Allen, W. P. (1972). *J. Infect. Dis.* **125**, 307–309.
Keog, H. J., and Isaäcson, M. (1978). *J. S. Afr. Vet. Assoc.* **49**, 229–231.
Kitchen, S. F. (1934). *Am. J. Trop. Med.* **14**, 547–564.
Kitchen, S. F. (1950). *Ann. Trop. Med. Parasitol.* **44**, 132–145.
Klastrup, N. O., and Halliwell, R. W. (1977). *Nord. Veteringer Med.* **29**, 325–330.
Kleid, D. G., Yansura, D., Small, B., Dowbenko, D., Moor, D. M., Grubman, M. J., McKercher, P. D., Morgan, D. O., Robertson, B. H., and Bachrach, H. L. (1981). *Science* **214**, 1125–1129.
Klein, F., Walker, J. S., Mahlandt, B. G., Carter, R. C., Orlando, M. D., Weirether, F. J., and Lincoln, R. E. (1969). *Appl. Microbiol.* **17**, 427–434.
Klein, F., Mahlandt, B. G., Eyler, S. L., and Lincoln, R. E. (1970). *Proc. Soc. Exp. Biol. Med.* **134**, 909–914.
Klein, F., Johns, W. I., Jr., Mahlandt, B. G., and Lincoln, R. E. (1971). *Appl. Microbiol.* **21**, 265–271.
Klopfer-Orgad, U., Peleg, B. A., Braverman, Y., Ron, N., and Ianconescu, M. (1981). *Contrib. Epidemiol. Biostat.* **3**, 172–177.
Knight, E. M., Henderson, B. E., Tukei, P. M., Lule, M., and West, R. (1968). *Annu. Rep., East Afr. Virus Res. Inst.* **17**, 14–15.
Kokernot, R. H., Szlamp, E. L., Levitt, J., and McIntosh, B. M. (1965a). *Trans. R. Soc. Trop. Med. Hyg.* **59**, 553–562.
Kokernot, R. H., Casaca, V. M. R., Weinbren, M. P., and McIntosh, B. M. (1965b). *Trans. R. Soc. Trop. Med. Hyg.* **59**, 563–570.
Koyama, H., and Higashihara, M. (1974). *Kitasato Arch. Exp. Med.* **47**, 201–210.

Kruse, R. H., and Wedum, A. G. (1970). *Lab. Anim. Care* **20**, 511–560.
Laughlin, L. W., Meegan, J. M., Starusbaugh, L. J., Morens, D. M., and Watten, R. H. (1979). *Trans. R. Soc. Trop. Med. Hyg.* **73**, 630–633.
Lacatsas, G., and Weiss, K. E. (1968). *Arch. Gesamte Virusforsch.* **25**, 58–64.
Lee, V. H. (1970). *Univ. of Ibadan Arbovirus Res. Proj., 1970 Annu. Rep.* pp. 29–30.
Lee, V. H. (1979). *J. Med. Entomol.* **16**, 76–79.
Levitt, J. (1964). *S. Afr. Med. J.* **40**, 108–108.
Levitt, J., and Polson, A. (1964). *J. Hyg.* **62**, 239–256.
Levitt, J., Naudè, W. du T., and Polson, A. (1963). *Virology* **20**, 530–533.
Lewis, J. C., Botros, B. A. M., and Meegan, J. M. (1978). *J. Egypt. Public Health Assoc.* **53**, 271–272.
Lindsey, H. S., Climas, R. A., and Obijeski, J. F. (1977). *J. Clin. Microbiol.* **6**, 618–626.
Maar, S. A., Swanepoel, R., and Gelfand, M. (1979). *Cent. Afr. J. Med.* **25**, 8–11.
McGavran, M. H., and Easterday, B. C. (1963). *Am. J. Pathol.* **42**, 587–607.
McIntosh, B. M. (1961). *Trans. R. Soc. Trop. Med. Hyg.* **55**, 63–68.
McIntosh, B. M. (1972). *J. S. Afr. Vet. Assoc.* **43**, 391–395.
McIntosh, B. M. (1975). *Entomol. Mem.—S. Afr., Dep. Agric. Tech. Ser.* **43**, 1–19.
McIntosh, B. M., and Jupp, P. G. (1981). *Contrib. Epidemiol. Biostat.* **3**, 92–99.
McIntosh, B. M., Jupp, P. G., Anderson, D., and Dickinson, D. B. (1973a). *J. S. Afr. Vet. Assoc.* **44**, 57–60.
McIntosh, B. M., Dickinson, D. B., and Dos Santos, I. (1973b). *J. S. Afr. Vet. Assoc.* **44**, 167–169.
McIntosh, B. M., Jupp, P. G., Dos Santos, I., and Barnard, B. J. H. (1980a). *S. Afr. Med. J.* **58**, 127–132.
McIntosh, B. M., Russell, D., Dos Santos, I., and Gear, J. H. S. (1980b). *S. Afr. Med. J.* **58**, 803–806.
MacKenzie, R. D. (1933). *J. Pathol. Bacteriol.* **37**, 75–79.
MacKenzie, R. D. (1935). *J. Pathol. Bacteriol.* **40**, 65–73.
MacKenzie, R. D., and Findlay, G. M. (1936). *Lancet* **1**, 140–141.
MacKenzie, R. D., Findlay, G. M., and Stern, R. O. (1936). *Br. J. Exp. Pathol.* **17**, 352–361.
Madkour, S. E. D. (1978). *J. Egypt. Public Health Assoc.* **53**, 163–172.
Mahdy, M. S., Bansen, E., Joshua, J. M., Parker, J. A., and Stuart, P. F. (1979). *Can. Dis. Week. Rep.* **5**, 189–190.
Matumoto, M., Iwasa, S., and Endo, M. (1950). *Jpn. J. Exp. Med.* **20**, 501–508.
Matumoto, M., Saburi, Y., and Nishi, I. (1959). *J. Immunol.* **82**, 219–225.
Maurice, Y. (1967). *Rev. Elev. Med. Vet. Pays Trop.* **20**, 395–405.
Meegan, J. M. (1979). *Trans. R. Soc. Trop. Med. Hyg.* **73**, 618–623.
Meegan, J. M. (1981). *Contrib. Epidemiol. Biostat.* **3**, 100–113.
Meegan, J. M., Hoogstraal, H. and Moussa, A. (1979). *Vet. Rec.* **105**, 124–125.
Meegan, J. M., Hoogstraal, H. and Laughlin, L. W. (1980a). *Zentralbl. Bakteriol., Parasitenkd., Infektionskr. Hyg., Abt. 1, Suppl.* **9**, 179–183.
Meegan, J. M., Khalil, G. M., Hoogstraal, H., and Adham, F. (1980b). *Am. J. Trop. Med. Hyg.* **29**, 1405–1410.
Meegan, J. M., Watten, R. H., and Laughlin, L. W. (1981). *Contrib. Epidemiol. Biostat.* **3**, 114–123.
Meegan, J. M., Digoutte, J. P., Peters, C. J. and Shope, R. E. (1983). *Lancet* **1**, 641–641.
Miller, W. S., Demchak, P., Rosenberger, C. R., Dominik, J. W., and Bradshaw, J. L. (1963). *Am. J. Hyg.* **77**, 114–121.
Mims, C. A. C. (1956a). *Br. J. Exp. Pathol.* **37**, 99–109.

Mims, C. A. C. (1956b). *Br. J. Exp. Pathol.* **37,** 110–119.
Mims, C. A. C. (1956c). *Br. J. Exp. Pathol.* **37,** 120–128.
Mims, C. A. C. (1956d). *Br. J. Exp. Pathol.* **37,** 129–143.
Mims, C. A. C. (1956e). *East Afr. Virus Res. Inst. Annu. Rep.* **6,** 25–25.
Mims, C. A. C. (1957). *Aust. J. Exp. Biol. Med. Sci.* **35,** 595–604.
Mims, C. A., and Gillet, J. D. (1956). *East Afr. Virus Res. Inst. Annu. Rep.* **6,** 20–21.
Mims, C. A., and Mason, P. J. (1956). *Br. J. Exp. Pathol.* **37,** 423–433.
Mitten, J. Q., Remde, N. S., Walker, J. S., Carter, R. C., Stephen, E. L., and Klein, F. (1970). *J. Infect. Dis.* **121,** 25–31.
Montegomery, E. R. (1912). *Vet. Pathol., Annu. Rep.* p. 37 (cited by Henning, 1956).
Moussa, M. I. Wood, D. L., and Abdel Wahab, K. S. E. (1982) *Trans. R. Soc. Trop. Med. Hyg.* **76,** 482–486.
Mulligan, E. J. (1937). Cited by Henning (1956).
Mundel, B., and Gear, J. H. S. (1951). *S. Afr. Med. J.* **25,** 797–800.
Murphy, F. A., Harrison, A. K., and Whitfield, S. B. (1973). *Intervirology* **1,** 297–316.
Mussgay, M. (1980). *Dtsch. Med. Wochenschr.* **105,** 1265–1266.
Naudè, W. du T., Madsen, T., and Polson, A. (1954). *Nature (London)* **173,** 1051–1052.
Niklasson, B. (1982). *Scand. J. Infect. Dis.* **14,** 105–109.
Niklasson, B., Meegan, J. M., and Bengtsson, E. (1979). *Scand. J. Infect. Dis.* **11,** 313–314.
Ohder, H., Lund, L. J., and Whitland, A. P. (1970). *Arch. Gesamte Virusforsch.* **29,** 127–138.
Orlando, M. D., DeLauter, R. D., and Riley, J. M. (1967). *Appl. Microbiol.* **15,** 594–596.
Pellisier, A. (1954). *Bull. Soc. Pathol. Exot.* **47,** 223–227.
Pellisier, A., and Rousselot, R. (1954). *Bull. Soc. Pathol. Exot.* **47,** 228–231.
Peters, C. J., and Anderson, G. W., Jr. (1981). *Contrib. Epidemiol. Biostat.* **3,** 21–41.
Peters, C. J., and Meegan, J. M. (1981). *CRC Handb. Ser. Zoonoses, Sect. B* **1,** 403–420.
Peters, C. J., Bailey, C. L., and Eddy, G. A. (1981). *J. Egypt. Public Health Assoc.* **56,** 384–402.
Pini, A., Lund, L. J., and Davies, F. G. (1970). *Res. Vet. Sci.* **11,** 82–85.
Pini, A., Lund, L. J., and Davies, F. G. (1973). *J. S. Afr. Vet. Assoc.* **44,** 161–165.
Plowright, W., and Ferris, R. D. (1957). *East Afr. Vet. Res. Org., Annu. Rep.* pp. 28–29.
Polson, A. (1953). *Nature (London)* **172,** 1154–1155.
Porterfield, J. S. (1957). *Nature (London)* **180,** 1201–1202.
Provost, A. (1981). *Red. Med. Vet.* **157,** 255–258.
Prozeski, O. W. (1972). *S. Afr. Med. J.* **46,** 820–820.
Prozeski, O. W. (1981). *Contrib. Epidemiol. Biostat.* **3,** 151–158.
Randall, R., Gibbs, C. J., Aulisio, C. G., Binn, L. N., and Harrison, V. R. (1962). *J. Immunol.* **89,** 660–671.
Randall, R., Binn, L. N., and Harrison, V. R. (1963). *Am. J. Trop. Med. Hyg.* **12,** 611–615.
Ranki, M., and Pettersson, R. (1975). *J. Virol.* **16,** 1420–1425.
Reed, L. J., and Muench, H. (1938). *Am. J. Trop. Med. Hyg.* **27,** 493–496.
Reynolds, J. A., Harrington, D. G., Crabbs, C. L., Peters, C. J., and DiLuzio, N. R. (1980). *Infect. Immun.* **28,** 937–943.
Rice, R. M., Erlick, B. J., Rosato, R. R., Eddy, G. A., and Mohanty, S. B. (1980). *Virology* **105,** 256–260.
Rosebrock, J. A., and Peters, C. J. (1982). *In Vitro* **18,** 308–308.
Sabin, A. B., and Blumberg, R. W. (1947). *Proc. Soc. Exp. Biol. Med.* **64,** 385–389.
Saddington, R. S. (1934). *Proc. Soc. Exp. Biol. Med.* **31,** 693–694.
Saleh, A. S., Mohammed, K. A., Hassan, M. M., Bucci, T. J., and Meegan, J. M. (1981). *Trans. R. Soc. Trop. Med. Hyg.* **75,** 129–130.

Schneider, H. (1977). Ph.D. Thesis pp. 170–171. University of Giessen, West Germany.
Schrire, L. (1951). *S. Afr. Med. J.* **25**, 926–930.
Schrire, L. and Gear, J. (1956). *Cent. Afr. J. Med.* **2**, 237–240.
Schulz, K. C. A. (1951). *J. S. Afr. Vet. Med. Assoc.* **22**, 113–120.
Schwentker, F. F., and Rivers, T. M. (1933). *J. Exp. Med.* **59**, 305–313.
Scott, G. R. (1963). *Nature (London)* **200**, 919–920.
Scott, G. R. (1981). *Trans. R. Soc. Trop. Med. Hyg.* **75**, 329–329.
Scott, G. R., and Heisch, R. B. (1959). *East Afr. Med. J.* **36**, 665–667.
Scott, G. R., Weddell, W., and Reid, D. (1956). *Bull. Epizoot. Dis. Afr.* **4**, 17–25.
Scott, G. R., Coackley, W., Roach, R. W., and Cowdy, N. R. (1963). *J. Pathol. Bacteriol.* **86**, 229–231.
Sellers, R. F., Pedgley, D. E., and Tucker, M. R. (1982). *Vet. Rec.* **110**, 73–77.
Shimshony, A., Klopfer-Orgad, U., Bali, S., and Chaimovitz, M. (1981a). *Contrib. Epidemiol. Biostat.* **3**, 159–171.
Shimshony, A., Braverman, Y., Peleg, B. A., and Kuper-Ron, N. (1981b). *The Rift Valley Fever, Technical Series* **1**, 55–62.
Shone, D. K. (1958). *Cent. Afr. J. Med.* **4**, 284–286.
Shope, R. E. (1978). *J. Egypt. Public Health Assoc.* **53**, 235–242.
Shope, R. E., Peters, C. J., and Walker, J. S. (1980). *Lancet* **1**, 886–887.
Shope, R. E., Meegan, J. M., Peters, C. J., Tesh, R. B., and Travassos da Rosa, A. A. (1981). *Contrib. Epidemiol. Biostat.* **3**, 342–352.
Shope, R. E., Peters, C. J., and Davies, F. G. (1982). *Bull. W. H. O.* **60**, 299–304.
Shousha, E. S. A. (1978). *J. Egypt. Public Health Assoc.* **53**, 195–199.
Siam, A. L. (1981). *J. Egypt. Public Health Assoc.* **56**, 403–407.
Siam, A. L., and Meegan, J. M. (1980). *Trans. R. Soc. Trop. Med. Hyg.* **74**, 539–541.
Siam, A. L., Meegan, J. M., and Gharbawi, K. F. (1980). *Br. J. Ophthalmol.* **64**, 366–374.
Smithburn, K. C. (1949). *Br. J. Exp. Pathol.* **30**, 1–16.
Smithburn, K. C., and Kokernot, R. H. (1980). Unpublished data (cited by McIntosh *et al.*, 1980a).
Smithburn, K. C., Haddow, A. J., and Gillett, J. D. (1948). *Br. J. Exp. Pathol.* **29**, 107–121.
Smithburn, K. C., Haddow, A. J., and Lumsden, W. H. R. (1949a). *Br. J. Exp. Pathol.* **30**, 35–47.
Smithburn, K. C., Mahaffy, A. F., Haddow, A. J., Kitchen, S. F., and Smith, J. F. (1949b). *J. Immunol.* **62**, 213–217.
Stordy, R. J. (1913). *Dep. Agric. Br. East Afr. Annu. Rep.* p. 13. (cited by Henning, 1956).
Struthers, J. K., and Swanepoel, R. (1982). *J. Gen. Virol.* **60**, 381–384.
Swanepoel, R. (1976). *J. S. Afr. Vet. Med. Assoc.* **47**, 93–94.
Swanepoel, R. (1981). *Contrib. Epidemiol. Biostat.* **3**, 83–91.
Swanepoel, R., and Blackburn, N. K. (1977). *J. Gen. Virol.* **34**, 557–561.
Swanepoel, R., Blackburn, N. K., Lander, K. P., Vickers, D. B., and Lewis, A. R. (1975). *Rhod. Vet. J.* **6**, 42–55.
Swanepoel, R., Blackburn, N. K., Efstrathiou, S., and Condy, J. B. (1978). *J. Hyg.* **70**, 183–196.
Swanepoel, R., Manning, B., and Watt, J. A. (1979). *Cent. Afr. J. Med.* **25**, 1–8.
Swartz, T. A., and Costin, C. (1981). *Contrib. Epidemiol. Biostat.* **3**, 142–150.
Swartz, T. A., Klinberg, M. A., and Goldblum, N., ed. (1981). "Rift Valley Fever," Contribu. Epidemiol. Biostat. Vol. III. Karger, Basel.
Takemori, N., Nakano, M., Hemmi, M., Ikeda, H., Yanagida, S., and Kitaoka, M. (1954). *Nature (London)* **174**, 688–700.
Takemori, N., Nakano, M., Hemmi, M., and Kitaoka, M. (1955a). *Virology* **1**, 58–82.

Takemori, N., Nakano, M., and Hemmi, M. (1955b). *Virology* **1**, 250–251.
Taylor, P., and Swanepoel, R. (1980). *Zimbabwe Vet. J.* **11**, 44–49.
Tesh, R. B., Peters, C. J., and Meegan, J. M. (1982). *Am. J. Trop. Med. Hyg.* **31**, 149–155.
Theiler, M. (1957). *Proc. Soc. Exp. Biol. Med.* **96**, 380–382.
Thomas, W. J., O'Neil, T. W., Craig, D. E., De Meio, J. L., and DeSanctis, A. N. (1978). *J. Biol. Stand.* **6**, 51–58.
Tomori, O. (1979a). *Res. Vet. Sci.* **26**, 152–159.
Tomori, O. (1979b). *Res. Vet. Sci.* **26**, 160–164.
Tomori, O. (1980). *J. Med. Virol.* **5**, 343–350.
Tomori, O., and Kasali, O. (1979). *Br. J. Exp. Pathol.* **60**, 417–422.
Valadaão, F. G. (1969). *Vet. Mocambicana* **2**, 13–20.
Van der Linde, N. T. (1953). *J. S. Afr. Vet. Med. Assoc.* **24**, 145–150.
Van Tonder (1975). *Vet. Med. Rev.* **75**, 109–138.
Van Tongeren, H. A. E. (1979). *Tijdschr. Diergeneeskd.* **104**, 659–673.
Van Velden, D. J. J., Meyers, J. D., Olivier, J., Gear, J. H. S., and McIntosh, B. (1977). *S. Afr. Med. J.* **51**, 867–871.
Walker, J. S., Carter, R. C., Klein, F., Snowden, S. E., and Lincoln, R. E. (1969). *App. Microbiol.* **17**, 658–664.
Walker, J. S., Remmele, N. S., Carter, R. C., Mitten, J. Q., Schuh, L. G., Stephen, E. L., and Klein, F. (1970a). *J. Infect. Dis.* **121**, 9–18.
Walker, J. S., Stephen, E. L., Carter, R. C., Mitten, J. Q., Schuh, L. G., and Klein, F. (1970b). *J. Infect. Dis.* **121**, 19–24.
Weinbren, M. P., and Hewitt, L. E. (1958). *East Afr. Virus Res. Inst., Annu. Rep.* **9**, 13.
Weinbren, M. P., and Mason, P. J. (1957). *S. Afr. Med. J.* **31**, 424–430.
Weinbren, M. P., Williams, M. C., and Haddow, A. J. (1956). *East Afr. Virus Res. Inst., Annu. Rep.* **6**, 21–22.
Weinbren, M. P., Williams, M. C., and Haddow, A. J. (1957). *S. Afr. Med. J.* **31**, 951–957.
Weiss, K. E. (1956). Unpublished data (cited by Weiss, 1957).
Weiss, K. E. (1957). *Bull. Epizoot. Dis. Afr.* **5**, 431–458.
Weiss, K. E. (1962). *Onderstepoort J. Vet. Res.* **29**, 3–9.
Weiss, K. E., Haig, D. A., and Alexander, R. A. (1956). *Onderstepoort J. Vet. Res.* **27**, 183–195.
Williams, M. C., Woodall, J. P., Corbet, P. S., and Haddow, A. J. (1960). *East Afr. Virus Res. Inst., Annu. Rep.* **10**, 23–28.
World Health Organization (1977). *Week. Epidemiol. Rec.* **50**, 401–401.
World Health Organization (1982a). *Week. Epidemiol. Rec.* **27**, 207–207.
World Health Organization (1982b). *W.H.O. Offset Publ.* **63**.
World Health Organization (1983). *Bull. W.H.O.* (in press).
Yassin, W. (1978). *J. Egypt. Public Health Assoc.* **53**, 191–194.
Yedloutschnig, R. J., Dardiri, A. H., Walker, J. S., Peters, C. J., and Eddy, G. A. (1979). *Proc. 83rd Annu. Meet. U.S. Anim. Health Assoc.* pp. 253–260.
Yedloutschnig, R. J., Dardiri, A. H., Walker, J. S., Peters, C. J., and Eddy. G. A. *Proc. Int. Congr. Dis. Cattle, 11th, 1980* pp. 530–539.
Yedloutschnig, R. J., Dardiri, A. H., and Walker, J. S. (1981a). *Contrib. Epidemiol. Biostat.* **3**, 53–59.
Yedloutschnig, R. J., Dardiri, A. H., and Walker, J. S. (1981b). *Contrib. Epidemiol. Biostat.* **3**, 68–71.
Yedloutschnig, R. J., Dardiri, A. H., and Walker, J. S. (1981c). *Contrib. Epidemiol. Biostat.* **3**, pp. 72–76.
Yedloutschnig, R. J., Dardiri, A. H., Mebus, C. A., and Walker, J. S. (1981d). *Vet. Rec.* **109**, 383–384.

Note Added in Proof

Recently, Meegan *et al.* (1983) demonstrated using monoclonal antibodies that Zinga virus was virtually identical to RVFV in its antigenic structure; through preliminary mouse and hamster inoculation studies, they indicated that it is a classic pantropic, virulent strain of RVFV. These findings extend the range of known RVFV circulation into West and Central Africa and add the mosquitoes *Aedes dalzieli* and *A. palpalis* group to the list of mosquitoes implicated as possible vectors of RVFV in Africa.

Heartwater (*Cowdria ruminantium* Infection): Current Status

GERRIT UILENBERG

Institute for Tropical Veterinary Medicine and Protozoology, Faculty of Veterinary Medicine, State University of Utrecht, Utrecht, The Netherlands

I.	Introduction	428
	A. General	428
	B. Unpublished Data	429
II.	The Causal agent	430
	A. In the Mammalian Host	430
	B. In the Tick Vector	435
	C. Classification	436
	D. *In Vitro* Culture	438
III.	Transmission	440
	A. Natural Transmission	440
	B. Artificial Transmission	442
IV.	Distribution	444
V.	Susceptibility	445
	A. Domestic Animals	445
	B. Wild Animals	446
	C. Laboratory Animals	447
VI.	Epidemiology	452
VII.	The Disease	457
	A. Symptoms and Course	457
	B. Postmortem Findings	459
	C. Pathogenesis	460
VIII.	Diagnosis	460
IX.	Immunity	464
X.	Therapy	467
XI.	Prevention	469
	A. Tick Control	469
	B. Immunization	469
XII.	Heartwater in the Western Hemisphere	473
	References	475

I. Introduction

A. General

Heartwater, or cowdriosis, is an African infectious disease of ruminants, transmitted by ticks of the genus *Amblyomma,* caused by the rickettsia *Cowdria ruminantium.* It is still relatively neglected even in many African countries where it occurs, for reasons that will be discussed further on.

For the early history, the reader is referred to Alexander (1931) and Henning (1956). The disease has been known in South Africa since 1838, but it was not until almost a century later that heartwater was recognized as the first rickettsial disease of animals (Cowdry, 1925a).

It is probably true that heartwater is usually a latent infection in indigenous breeds of cattle in endemic areas, subjected to natural selection over centuries and benefiting to some extent from endemic stability as well. It emerges as a significant disease problem when animals are introduced from areas free from the disease. For susceptible populations of cattle it is second in importance only to East Coast fever (*Theileria parva* infection) and tsetse-transmitted trypanosomiasis, as far as vector-borne infections are concerned, but it has a wider distribution than either of these. Neitz (1968) in South Africa wrote "From observations made over a number of years in an anaplasmosis, babesiosis and heartwater enzootic area, it was determined that mortality due to the latter was three times as great as that from the former two diseases [p. 332]." These words, correct as far as exotic and crossbred cattle are concerned, put the disease into proper perspective for those who are familiar with tick-borne diseases. The virulence for exotic goats and sheep is even greater, and before systematic acaricidal dipping was introduced, exotic small ruminant farming was practically impossible in certain parts of South Africa (Spreull, 1922). The disease is generally not a problem in indigenous breeds of sheep and goats in endemic countries, but there may be some exceptions.

Because exotic breeds of ruminants were first brought into contact with cowdriosis in South Africa, it is in that country that most research has been carried out. After initial progress, especially since the causal agent was discovered in 1925, further advances in the control of the disease proved to be elusive because of the failure to cultivate *C. ruminantium in vitro,* to adapt it permanently to laboratory animals, and to develop a serological test. Research on heartwater has been largely neglected for a long period, even in South Africa. However, since several developing endemic countries have started to import susceptible breeds of ruminants, thus creating an overt disease problem, and also because scientific progress made attempts at new approaches possible, interest in the disease has seen a renewal. The demonstration of its occurrence in the western hemisphere (Perreau et al., 1980) has solicited interest outside Africa as well.

It is not the intention of this review to cover every aspect of cowdriosis in detail, but to highlight recent developments and pinpoint important gaps in our knowledge. Well-known aspects such as clinical symptoms and postmortem lesions will only be noted superficially. The reader also is referred to reviews by Spreull (1922), Alexander (1931), Curasson (1943), Haig (1955), Magimel (1955), Henning (1956), Neitz (1968), Rajaonarison (1970), Andreasen, (1974a), Ilemobade (1976), Uilenberg (1977, 1981), and Scott (1978).

B. Unpublished Data

This article is essentially a review of selected aspects of heartwater, but it has been augmented with unpublished results of research in our institute at Utrecht. General methods used are those reported previously (Jongejan et al., 1980; van Winkelhoff and Uilenberg, 1981; Uilenberg, 1982; Uilenberg et al., 1982). All ruminants used, mainly goats belonging to different breeds, were born and bred in the Netherlands.

Five strains of *C. ruminantium* have been used in these experiments: (a) a Nigerian strain isolated in 1974 as strain D 225 (Ilemobade, 1976; Ilemobade and Leeflang, 1977), (b) the South African Ball 3 strain, used for many years for immunization purposes and known already to Haig (1952), (c) the South African Zeerust strain isolated in 1979 (Jongejan et al., 1980), (d) a Sudanese strain isolated in 1981 from a clinical case of heartwater in a sheep at Umm Banein, Blue Nile Province (F. Jongejan, personal communication, 1981), and (e) a strain from the West African island of São Tomé, isolated in 1981 (Uilenberg et al., 1982).

Amblyomma ticks used in some of the experiments were reared on the ears of rabbits (larvae, nymphs) or the ears and sometimes the tail of ruminants (adults). For transmission experiments all tick stages were fed on the ears and sometimes the tail of ruminants. Engorged ticks were held at 27°C and a relative humidity of 90%, but were transferred to 20°C and the same relative humidity after having moulted or hatched.

II. The Causal Agent

A. IN THE MAMMALIAN HOST

Heartwater has long been believed to be due to an ultravisible virus, at one time thought to be identical with the virus of African horse sickness. At Sir Arnold Theiler's suggestion that the disease might be caused by a rickettsia, a visiting American scientist in South Africa showed in a series of studies that this is indeed the case (Cowdry, 1925a,b, 1926a,b,c). Practically all his findings are still valid.

In the mammalian host, *Cowdria ruminantium* is found in the cytoplasm of vascular endothelial cells, in which it occurs in groups, also called colonies or clusters. Although Cowdry (1925a, 1926a,c), working with histological sections, noticed differences in particle size, Jackson (1931) first reported on the extensive variation in size and shape as seen in smears. The size of the individual particles varies from 0.2 to >2.5 μm; small, medium-sized, and large organisms are usually distinguished, with intermediate forms between these. The rickettsias in one group are fairly uniform in size, except for those containing very large forms, where a great variation in size may be seen. Groups containing large forms are usually smaller and more densely packed than those made up of small coccoid elements, which may form very large masses (Figs. 1, 2, and 3). In stained smears viewed with the light microscope, the small coccoid forms appear to be uniform, whereas the larger ones are pleomorphic and include rings, horseshoe shapes, and possibly even bacillary forms. Detailed morphological studies with the light microscope are also reported by Cilli and Corazzi (1954), Pienaar (1970), and Ilemobade (1976).

Electron microscopic studies show that even the small forms are pleomorphic. The groups of rickettsias are always situated inside a membrane-lined vacuole in the cytoplasm of an endothelial cell. Pienaar (1970), as well as Stewart and Howell (1981), report that each rickettsia is surrounded by two unit membranes separated by a narrow electron-pale space; electron-dense and electron-pale areas are distinguished within the organism. Pienaar (1970) suggests that the ground substance contains closely packed ribosomes. Multiplication appears to occur mainly by binary fission, although there are indications of multiple budding and endosporulation (Pienaar, 1970).

Apart from vascular endothelial cells, the heartwater organism occurs in the circulating blood of affected animals, which is regularly infective if inoculated intravenously into susceptible ruminants. Conflicting results have been obtained in attempts to localize the organism

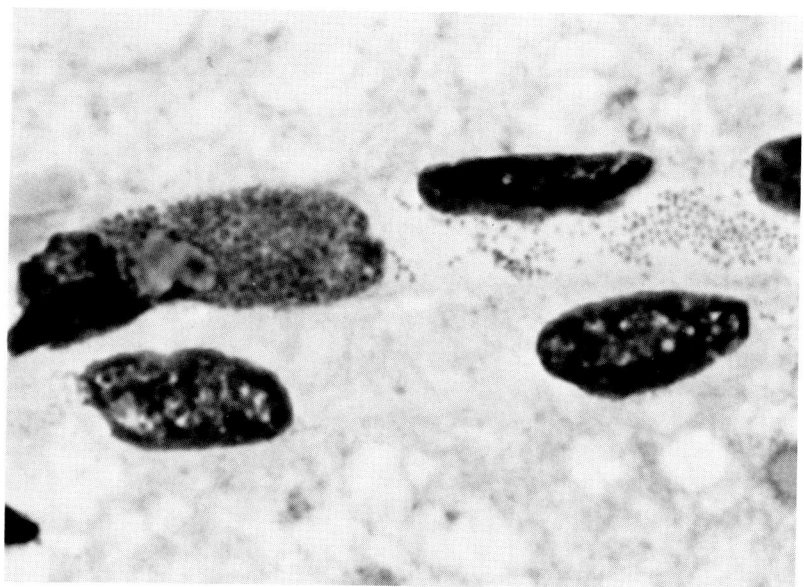

Fig. 1. *C. ruminantium* in brain capillary. Loosely packed and scattered small forms and more dense group of intermediate-sized organisms. ×2000 (original).

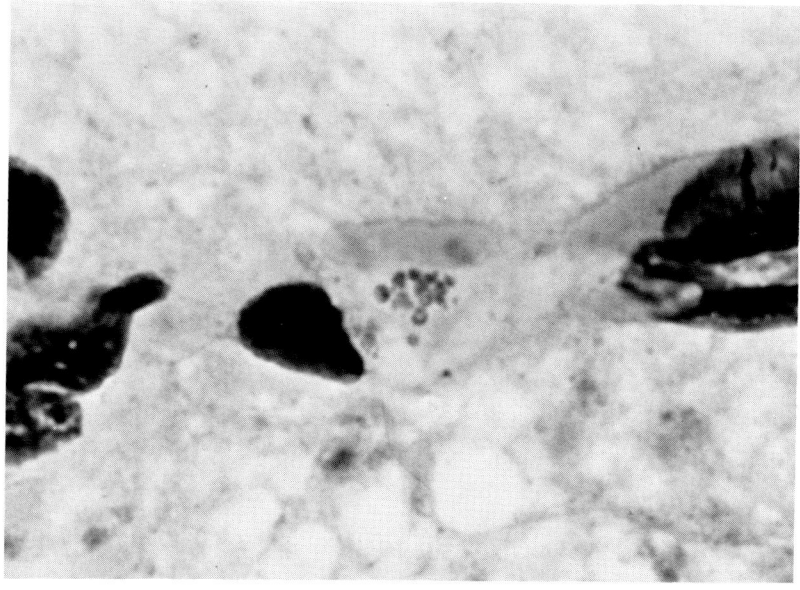

Fig. 2. *C. ruminantium* in brain capillary. Small group of large forms. Note ring-shaped organism. ×2000 (original).

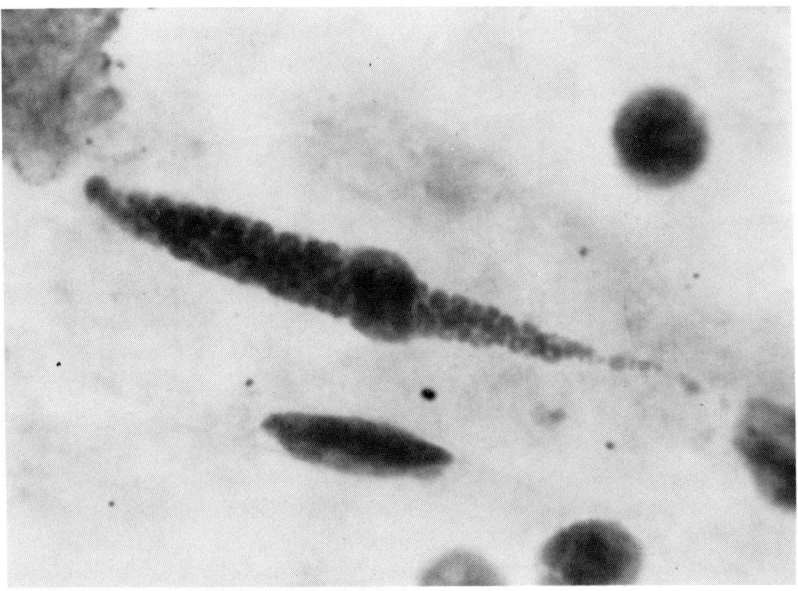

FIG. 3. *C. ruminantium* in brain capillary. Large, predominantly ring-shaped, densely packed organisms on both sides of the endothelial nucleus, which appears to be compressed. ×2000 (original).

in the blood. Infectivity has been associated with the white cell fraction (K. E. Weiss, in du Plessis, 1970a; Ilemobade, 1976; Ilemobade and Blotkamp, 1978a), with the red cell fraction (Fawi *et al.*, 1977), with both these fractions (Alexander, 1931), and also free in the plasma (Ramisse, 1971; Ilemobade, 1976; Ilemobade and Blotkamp, 1978a), but not in the serum (Ramisse, 1971). In our institute, leukocyte fractions from three goats, obtained by separation on Ficoll-Isopaque, proved infective in two cases. The red cell portion, tested with one animal, gave a negative result; this was the same donor as the one with the negative white cell fraction. In one case, plasma containing many thrombocytes was infective; in another case the thrombocyte fraction obtained after centrifugation of the plasma on a Percoll gradient was not (A. J. van Winkelhoff, A. A. M. Spanjer, and N. M. Perié, unpublished data, 1979–1980). Although differences in the methods of separation employed by different authors might account for some of the divergent results, due to greater or lesser contamination of one blood fraction by the other, the diametrically opposed results of Fawi *et al.* (1977) to those of Ilemobade (1976) and Ilemobade and Blotkamp (1978a) are difficult to reconcile. Fawi *et al.* injected each group of 5 goats with whole blood, red cells, white cells, platelets, plasma, or serum; all 10 goats that received whole blood or the erythrocyte fraction contracted fatal heartwater; none of the others reacted, and all proved susceptible on subsequent challenge. Ilemobade (1976), in contrast, found that whole blood and the white cell fraction from four donors was infective in every case; plasma transmitted heartwater in three of four cases, but the red cell fraction gave a negative result in all four attempts.

On the basis of light microscopic observations of the rickettsia in endothelial cells and the knowledge that the circulating blood is infective, Cowdry (1925a, 1926a,c) and Jackson and Neitz (1932) believed that individual rickettsias in the blood enter endothelial cells, where they grow from a single granule to a large group. This causes the cell to rupture and disseminate the organisms once again into the blood, thus repeating the cycle. Cowdry reported having seen rickettsias being discharged from ruptured host cells into the lumen of the vessel, and Jackson and Neitz (1932) claimed to have detected rare organisms free in the blood. Although this last observation has not been repeated, and single rickettsias would be almost impossible to identify with any certainty with the light microscope, Stewart and Howell (1981) did see clusters projecting into the lumen of capillaries, as if about to be discharged. Using the electron microscope, these authors, as well as Pienaar (1970), frequently found rickettsias in the lumen of vessels. Jackson and Neitz postulated that single rickettsias in the blood would enter endothelial cells at random, particularly where the rate of flow is slow, such as the capillaries and the jugular vein of grazing animals. They found no tendency for cells lying in contiguity with infected ones to be involved, contrary to Cilli and Corazzi (1954), who stated that parasite masses may spread beyond the limit of an infected cell and believed that spread by contiguity is likely.

Apart from vascular endothelial cells and circulating blood, some authors have reported the occurrence of *C. ruminantium* in various cell types such as macrophages, monocytes, histiocytes, Kupffer's cells, reticulum cells of lymph nodes, fibroblasts and connective tissue cells of various organs, and in one case the epithelial cells of bronchi (da Graça, 1964, 1966; du Plessis, 1970a, 1975; Ilemobade, 1976; Ilemobade and Blotkamp, 1978a). None of these reports is entirely convincing. The majority are based on observations with the light microscope. Ilemobade (1976) and Ilemobade and Blotkamp (1978a) base their report on the occurrence in lung macrophages on circumstantial evidence. Cells obtained by washing the lungs of animals dead from cowdriosis transmitted the disease; however, apart from macrophages (containing unidentified particles in the cytoplasma), there were also erythrocytes and epithelial cells.

The findings of du Plessis (1970a, 1975) are preliminary and await confirmation. Mesenteric lymph nodes of intravenously infected sheep were swollen during the incubation period; poorly outlined structures in the cytoplasm of reticulum cells and macrophages, not found in control sheep, were suspected of being initial developmental stages of the organism. Extracellular bodies containing granules were considered to be free rickettsial colonies in the medullary sinuses. Suspensions of lymph nodes made during the incubation period were infective, and also the blood. Using electron microscopy, du Plessis (1975) found solid, dense bodies without a limiting membrane in intimate contact with the cytoplasm of reticuloendothelial cells of mesenteric lymph nodes of sheep and cattle infected with the Ball 3 strain, and in peritoneal macrophages of mice infected with a mouse-infective strain. Du Plessis hypothesized that the initial development takes place mainly in reticuloendothelial cells, beginning with the formation of dense bodies. These grow and undergo cleavage, resulting in irregular fragments with poorly defined edges, around which double unit membranes develop, giving rise to mature organisms lying free in the cytoplasm. He supposed that membrane-bound colonies in endothelial cells only develop in a second phase, during the febrile period. These surprising findings and conclusions warrant further study.

Pienaar (1970), using electron microscopy, found only two cells appearing to be monocytes to be infected; all others were endothelial cells. Stewart and Howell (1981) were unable to find *C. ruminantium* in lung macrophages or buffy coat material; they showed that certain intracytoplasmic granules resembling *C. ruminantium* were lysosomes. The uniformly negative results of attempts to grow the organism in cells of the leukocyte blood fraction (see Section II, D) would tend to confirm that they are not normally infected.

The only certainty is apparently that *C. ruminantium* lives and multiplies in vascular endothelial cells of ruminants, and occurs in the circulating blood. The findings of du Plessis need to be investigated; confirmation or negation would have important implications for an understanding of the developmental cycle and classification of the causal agent, as well as of the pathogenesis of the disease. It would be logical to carry out similar studies in ruminants infected by ticks, so that the hypothetical initial development can be daily monitored by taking biopsies from superficial lymph nodes, starting with the one draining the site of tick attachment.

B. In the Tick Vector

Cowdry (1925b, 1926b) studied the development in the tick *Amblyomma hebraeum*. His findings still stand today. *C. ruminantium* were found only in epithelial cells of the intestine and also in the lumen of the gut, where they occurred in characteristic densely packed groups. Cowdry was unable to find the organism in the salivary gland and suggested that transmission might occur by regurgitation from the alimentary canal during feeding. Theiler and du Toit (1926, 1928) found that emulsified flat nymphs infected in the larval stage and injected by the intravenous (iv) route, were rarely infective, whereas emulsified engorged infected nymphs virtually always caused the disease. J. D. Bezuidenhout (personal communication, 1979) found that the infectivity of flat infected nymphs is low, and increases during feeding to reach after 3 days a high level that persists during further feeding, through to full engorgement. Large quantities of saliva, pooled from pilocarpine-stimulated engorged females infected in the larval and nymphal stages, were only rarely infective and then only slightly so. Suspensions of the intestine of infected engorged nymphs are highly infective. Because pilocarpine also stimulates the gut of ticks to some extent, there is a possibility that in the few cases where the saliva was infective, contamination by gut contents occurred. Bezuidenhout (1981) summarized this unpublished work by saying that the infectivity of saliva from infected females of *A. hebraeum* was very low compared to ground-up tick suspensions made from the same group of ticks. He also found that the infectivity of fully engorged infected nymphs is so high that a quantity of material corresponding to only 0.0015 homogenized nymph would transmit the disease.

In our institute, salivary glands of adult *Amblyomma variegatum*, unfed or fed for 2 or 3 days, of batches of ticks that had been shown to be infective, did not cause heartwater in goats when inoculated intravenously (A. J. van Winkelhoff, unpublished, 1979). Theiler and du Toit (1926, 1928) found that flat infected adults, incubated at 37°C for $4\frac{1}{2}$ days, were not infective when homogenized and injected intravenously. In our institute, four groups of nymphs of *A. variegatum* from one batch infected in the larval stage were compared. Group 1, fed on a goat, transmitted heartwater; groups 2, 3, and 4 were homogenized and injected intravenously into goats after being fed for 3 days on a rabbit (group 2), incubated unfed at 37°C for 3 days (group 3), or maintained continuously unfed at 20°C (group 4); only the homogenate of ticks fed for 3 days on the rabbit was infective (A. J. van Winkelhoff, unpublished, 1979). However, in a later experiment we did succeed in one trial in transmitting heartwater with homogenized unfed *A. hebraeum* females, incubated at 37°C for 4 days (R. H. Dwinger, unpublished, 1981). Attempts to infect engorged nymphs of *A. variegatum* and *A. hebraeum* by parenteral injection of infective blood or brain into the intestine did not succeed (A. J. van Winkelhoff and T. A. Niewold, unpublished, 1979, 1981); this method has been used successfully to infect engorged nymphs of *A. variegatum* with *Theileria mutans* (Schreuder and Uilenberg, 1976) and *T. velifera* (Van Vorstenbosch *et al.,* 1978).

All known vectors of cowdriosis are three-host *Amblyomma* species in which the infection is transstadial, from larva to nymph, from nymph to adult, or from larva through nymph to adult, but not transovarial (see Section III).

Analyzing what is known about the development and localization of *C. ruminantium* in the tick, it appears likely that, after having been ingested in blood, the rickettsia invades the epithelial cells of the tick, where it multiplies, especially after the tick has moulted and starts to feed again. The infection spills over into the lumen of the gut, from where it is regurgitated into the mammalian host. The higher temperature during the stay of the tick on the host does not appear to be a major factor in stimulating the tremendous increase in infectivity during feeding, as is known to be the case in some other tick-borne infections (reviewed by Kocan *et al.,* 1982), but there have not been enough experiments to warrant definite conclusions. During the ecdysis of nymphs that have transmitted the infection, it appears that most of the rickettsias are lost with the old intestinal cells, but a low infectivity persists in the new epithelium.

C. CLASSIFICATION

In the eighth edition of Bergey's Manual (Philip, 1974), *Cowdria ruminantium* (Cowdry, 1925) is the sole representative of the genus *Cowdria* Moshkovski, 1947 (synonyms *Ehrlichia (Cowdria)* Moshkovski, 1945; *Nicollea* Macchiavello, 1947; and *Kurlovia* Zhdanov, 1953). Cowdry (1925a) originally named the organism *Rickettsia ruminantium.* It is placed in order Rickettsiales, family Rickettsiaceae, and tribe Ehrlichieae. It seems logical to suggest a taxonomic position near to that of *Ehrlichia (sensu lato,* including *Cytoecetes,* considered by some authors as a separate genus). Both are tick-borne rickettsias; both occur in colonies situated in vacuoles in the host cell, where they multiply by binary fission, whereas members of the genus *Rickettsia* grow free in the cytoplasm and sometimes the nucleus of the host cell (with the exception of *R. sennetsu,* which grows in vacuoles; Anderson *et al.,* 1965) and should certainly be removed from this genus, as it has moreover been shown to be closely related to *Ehrlichia canis* (Ristic *et al.,* 1981; Hoilien *et al.,* 1982). In at least two species of *Ehrlichia,* pleomorphism similar to that of *Cowdria* has been observed (Tuomi and von Bonsdorff, 1966; Gribble, 1969), and the aspect in electron micrographs is strikingly similar. This is apparent when the pictures of Pienaar (1970) are compared to those of Tuomi and von Bonsdorff (1966) and Hildebrandt *et al.* (1973). However, this does not necessarily mean that the inclusion of tribe Ehrlichieae in family Rickettsiaceae is correct. The organisms now placed by Storz and Page (1971) as a single genus in a separate order, the Chlamydiales, share with *Cowdria* and *Ehrlichia* a position in membrane-lined vacuoles in the host cell cytoplasm and also are pleomorphic, although forms comparable to the "elementary bodies" of *Chlamydia* apparently have no counterpart in the other genera. Rake *et al.* (1945) suggested that the heartwater agent should be classified between typical representatives of *Rickettsia* and the psittacosis– lymphogranuloma–trachoma group, now called *Chlamydia.* Tuomi (1966) and Tuomi and von Bonsdorff (1966) share this opinion. Mohan (1968) goes so far as to synonymize *Cowdria* with *Chlamydia.* It is not necessary to go to this extreme to realize that the taxonomy of the Rickettsiales is far from settled. According to Coles (1953, p. 458),

> I have failed to discern any possible dividing line between the Rickettsiaceae and the Chlamydozoaceae. It is easy to put a single colony of organisms, stained with Giemsa, under the microscope, and defy anybody to identify them as *Coxiella burnetii, Cowdria ruminantium, R. canis, R. bovis,* or one of the accepted causal agents of salmon 'poisoning,' ovine enzootic abortion, psittacosis, trachoma, and conjunctivitis of cattle.

In spite of the extensive use of the electron microscope since that time, nothing much seems to have changed. Using the electron microscope, one would be hard pressed to tell the difference between vacuole-contained colonies of *C. ruminantium, E. canis, E. (Cytoecetes) phagocytophila, Rickettsia (= Ehrlichia) sennetsu,* or even *Anaplasma* spp. and *Coxiella burnetii.* If it were to be shown conclusively that the spherical bodies of homogeneously high electron density, without a limiting membrane, in intimate contact with the host cytoplasm of cells of lymph nodes of ruminants and peritoneal macrophages of mice are really part of the developmental cycle of *C. ruminantium,* as suspected by du Plessis (1975), the classification of the organism might have to be drastically revised. Confirmation of these observations is needed, as du Plessis admitted. Apart from this, if one admits that *Cowdria* and *Ehrlichia* appear to be related, and to share also characters of *Chlamydia* as well as of *Rickettsia,* the logical decision is to abolish the order of the Chlamydiales and reintegrate *Chlamydia* into the Rickettsiales.

D. *In Vitro* Culture

So far, all attempts at culturing *C. ruminantium in vitro* have failed, although South African scientists have tried to propagate the organism in all kinds of mammalian cells (J. D. Bezuidenhout, personal communication, 1979).

Haig (1955) reported that the organism remained alive in the developing chicken embryo for 9 days, but attempts at serial passage failed. Haig has been unable to repeat this.

Ramisse and Uilenberg (1971) and Ramisse (1971, 1972), besides inoculating chicken embryos with negative results, tried to culture the rickettsia in white blood cells of reacting animals. Ramisse (1971, 1972) attempted its culture also in fetal ovine cells from various organs (spleen, amnion, choroid plexus, stomach, testis, and skin), as well as peritoneal macrophages and spleen cells of adult sheep, to which virulent blood was added. None of these cultures was infective to susceptible sheep. Attempts have been made in our laboratory to cultivate the heartwater organism in buffy coat cells according to a technique developed for the diagnosis of African swine fever (Hess and DeTray, 1960).* Three different strains of *C. ruminantium* were used. Buffy coat cultures from four different goats reacting to cowdriosis were tested after 4 to 7 days for infectivity by intravenous inoculation into susceptible goats. Three of these cultures were tested once; goat inoculation with the other was done 5, 6, and 7 days after initiation. None of the inoculated goats reacted, and all proved subsequently susceptible to challenge. No structures resembling *C. ruminantium* were found in Giemsa- or Castaneda-stained smears prepared from the buffy coat cultures of these four goats, as well as of two others that were not tested for infectivity. In another case, monocyte culture of a reacting goat was initiated according to the method of Nyindo *et al.* (1971) for *E. canis.* The culture was injected into a susceptible goat after 5 days, with a negative result. The use of dextran sulfate was not found to be of

---

*The technique was suggested by Dr. A. H. Dardiri, Plum Island Animal Disease Center, USDA/ARS, Greenport, New York.

advantage for the separation of goat monocytes (F. F. J. Franssen, R. H. Dwinger, and N. M. Perié, unpublished data, 1982).

Andreasen (1974a,b) established primary cultures of tick cells initiated from moulting nymphs of two species of African *Amblyomma* ticks. As many as three subpassages could be made from the primary monolayer. After virulent blood was added, subcultures were infective 9 days later but not after 4 days. He also observed granules similar to *C. ruminantium* in some of the cells 4 days, and in most cells 9 days, after the blood was added. Culturing was at 26°C. These results have not been confirmed.

Jongejan *et al.* (1980) were able to maintain the infectivity of primary kidney cell cultures from reacting goats for as long as 13 days. Further studies in our laboratory have examined different variables in the system, such as the source of the serum used to supplement the medium (fetal or newborn calf, or adult goat), adding or omitting penicillin and streptomycin, rolling or stationary culture flasks, increasing the calcium concentration, varying the quantity of culture inoculated into goats to test infectivity and different strains of *C. ruminantium*. Indications were as follows:

1. Dissociation of the kidney cells before initiating the cultures and removing the cells attached to the flasks appeared to give better results when done by trypsin than by mechanical means.
2. Large quantities of culture (totaling 900 cm^2 of flask surface) were more reliably infective after a week than small quantities (150 cm^2).
3. No culture remained infective for longer than 14 days.
4. Cultures without penicillin and streptomycin were not more reliably infective than those containing the antibiotics.

Haig (1955) believed that the *in vitro* contact with penicillin was harmful to *Cowdria*. *Cowdria ruminantium* was not seen in Giemsa-stained preparations made from these cultures; of two cultures showing suspected granules in cells, only one proved to be infective (A. Starink, F. Jongejan, T. A. Niewold, and F. F. J. Franssen, unpublished data, 1980–1981). Attempts at culturing the organism in primary-cell cultures from brain cortex of reacting goats also gave negative results; the resulting monolayers of fibroblast-like cells were not infective (F. Jongejan and A. J. van Winkelhoff, unpublished, 1980).

Bell (1980) developed a method for cultivating *Theileria parva* in backless tick explants. Attempts have been made in our laboratory to cultivate *C. ruminantium* in this way (T. A. Niewold, unpublished data, 1981). The dorsal tegument of infected flat adult *A. hebraeum* was removed after the ticks had been surface-sterilized. The backless ticks were maintained in Leibowitz L-15 medium with caprine or newborn calf serum and tryptose phosphate broth at 37 and/or 28°C. Groups of particles resembling *C. ruminantium* were found in the cytoplasm of intestinal cells after 1 to 2 days. They were not seen in nonincubated infected control ticks and in incubated noninfected control ticks. Intestinal material of backless infected ticks, harvested after 4 days incubation, proved infective to a goat. Multiplying cells from infected backless ticks detached and could be maintained *in vitro* for several months, but they were not infective to goats.

So far *C. ruminantium* has not been cultured *in vitro* and has only survived for 2 weeks. The negative results of buffy coat cultures might indicate that circulating macrophages and monocytes are not used by the organism as host cells or at least not as favorite host cells. The preliminary attempts at culturing *C. ruminantium* in backless ticks should be followed up and might possibly lead to a way of obtaining small quantities of antigen for a serological test.

III. Transmission

A. Natural Transmission

It became apparent early that heartwater was an infectious but not a contagious disease. The role of the tick *Amblyomma hebraeum*, suspected before, was proven by Lounsbury (1900). Since then, the disease has been transmitted experimentally by 11 species of *Amblyomma* (9 African and 2 American), all three-host ticks (Table I). Transmission is transstadial. Attempts of transovarial transmission have invariably failed, apart from one report on one single occasion (Bezuidenhout, in Uilenberg, 1981). Ticks infected as larvae transmit the disease as nymphs, and for some vectors it has been shown that the infection may be carried from the larval stage through the nymphal stage (even when the nymph feeds on a nonsusceptible animal) through to the adult (Table I). Ticks infected as nymphs transmit in the adult stage. Male ticks, although capable of transmitting heartwater (Alexander, 1931), appear to be poor vectors (Ilemobade, 1976; Ilemobade and Leeflang, 1977).

Some other African *Amblyomma* species are likely candidates for a vector role, such as *A. splendidum,* and *A. eburneum*. Experiments with *A. marmoreum,* a parasite of reptiles in southern Africa of which immatures are sometimes found on domestic animals, have given negative results (du Toit, in Alexander, 1931; Alexander, 1931, Nor-

TABLE I

PROVEN EXPERIMENTAL VECTORS OF HEARTWATER

Amblyomma spp.	Proven way of transmission[a]	First reference
African		
A. hebraeum	I, II, III	Lounsbury (1900)
A. variegatum	I, II, III	Daubney (1930)
A. pomposum	I, II	Neitz (1947)
A. gemma	?	Lewis (1949)[b]
A. lepidum	I, II	Karrar (1966)
A. tholloni	I, II, III	Mackenzie and Norval (1980)
A. sparsum	I[c]	Norval and Mackenzie (1981)
A. astrion	I[d]	Uilenberg and Niewold (1981)
A. cohaerens	I, II, III[e]	G. Uilenberg, unpublished, 1982
American		
A. maculatum	I, II, III	Uilenberg (1982)
A. cajennense	I[c]	G. Uilenberg (unpublished, 1982)

[a]I, From larval to nymphal stage; II, from nymphal to adult stage; III, from larval through nymphal to adult stage.

[b]The quotation "Lewis (1945)" by Neitz (1947, 1956) does not appear to be supported by any literature record.

[c]Transmission experiments from nymph to adult and from larva through nymph to adult failed (A. sparsum, A. cajennense).

[d]One unpublished transmission experiment with A. astrion from larva through nymph to adult failed. Adults collected on cattle have been shown to be infected (Uilenberg et al., 1982).

[e]A. cohaerens appears to be an efficient vector; all three transmission attempts were successful.

val, 1975). One experiment with a similar, more widely distributed species, *A. nuttalli,* was also unsuccessful (Alexander, 1931). The potential role of Asian *Amblyomma* species is unknown. Transmission by American species should be further investigated. *A. maculatum* has been shown to be an efficient vector; *A. cajennense* would appear to be a poor one. After initial negative results obtained with the latter species (Uilenberg, 1982), transmission was finally obtained in only one experiment, using nymphs infected in the preceding larval stage (Table I); the infection was not carried through to the adult stage, and transmission from the nymphal stage to the adult did not succeed (although the nymphs had fed on the same donor at the same time as the larvae giving rise to the single positive outcome).

Not all proven African vectors are of equal significance. *A. variegatum* is the most important one, being perfectly adapted to domestic livestock, being a very efficient vector, and having the widest distribution, including most of tropical sub-Saharan Africa, Madagascar, La Réunion, Mauritius and other islands near Africa, southern parts of the Arabian peninsula, and several islands in the Caribbean region. *A. hebraeum,* another good vector and also adapted to livestock, is limited to southeastern Africa. Of the other species common on domestic ruminants, *A. lepidum* and *A. gemma* inhabit dry areas of eastern and northeastern sub-Saharan Africa, and *A. pomposum* occurs in Angola and other parts of southern-central Africa. *A. cohaerens* normally infests savannah buffalo of central and eastern Africa but has also become common on cattle in parts of Ethiopia (Pegram *et al.,* 1981). *A. tholloni,* widely distributed in tropical Africa, is in the adult stage a rather strictly specific parasite of the African elephant; it would not appear to be important for domestic stock, which is seldom maintained in significant numbers in areas inhabited by elephants (Mackenzie and Norval, 1980). *A. sparsum* of eastern Africa is seldom found on domestic animals, but could have a role in maintaining a reservoir in wild animals, as could *A. tholloni* and *A. astrion.* The latter, normally rather strictly limited to the wild buffalo in the Central African Republic, Zaire, and Angola, is only known to have adapted to livestock on the islands of São Tomé and Príncipe, where it transmits heartwater. A most useful survey of the distribution of African ticks, visualized in maps, has been prepared by Morel (1969).

There is no evidence of adaptation of local heartwater strains to local *Amblyomma* vectors. *C. ruminantium* from São Tomé was as easily transmitted by South African *A. hebraeum* as were South African *Cowdria* strains, and Nigerian and South African strains were easily transmitted by *A. astrion* from São Tomé. Several more examples could be given. *C. ruminantium* does not lose its capability of being biologically transmitted by ticks even after very numerous serial mechanical passages in mammals; some organisms with a more complicated developmental cycle in the vector and a less simple structure, such as trypanosomes and babesias, are well known to lose the power of developing in the vector under these circumstances.

B. Artificial Transmission

Heartwater can be transmitted by parenteral injection of infected blood or homogenized tissues from various organs. Even milk from reacting animals can be infective (Spreull, 1922).

Alexander (1931) summarized South African experiments. Although the intravenous inoculation of as little as 0.1 ml of virulent blood may produce fatal heartwater, comparatively large quantities of blood must be used for reliable results. Alexander's arbitrary standard of 5 ml for small ruminants and 10 ml for cattle is generally still followed. Ramisse (1971) could transmit the infection with 0.5 ml of blood, but not with 0.1 ml, injected intravenously (iv) into sheep. Later he succeeded with 0.02 ml (Ramisse, 1973).

Aside from the quantity of blood, the route of inoculation is very important. Blood injected subcutaneously will not infect more than 25% of susceptible animals (Alexander, 1931; Uilenberg, 1971a; Ilemobade, 1976; Ilemobade and Blotkamp, 1978a). According to Alexander, iv injection of 5 to 10 ml infective blood causes heartwater in over 98% of sheep and goats, but only 9 of 12 susceptible cattle. Weiss et al. (1952) also believed that cattle do not react as reliably to iv injection as do sheep. In contrast, Haig (1955) stated that about 5% of cattle would not react but were susceptible on subsequent inoculation. Uilenberg (1971a) found that 38 of 38 cattle reacted to iv infection, 52 of 53 sheep, and 7 of 7 goats. Van der Merwe (1979) had only 7 nonreactors among 2743 cattle given two doses of virulent blood with an interval of a week. Du Plessis and Bezuidenhout (1979) stated that it is "common experience" that only 60–70% of susceptible cattle show a reaction, but practically 100% of sheep. They found a highly significant inverse relationship between the severity of the reaction and the serum levels of natural conglutinins in the cattle. J. L. du Plessis (personal communication, 1979) believed that many zebu cattle cannot be infected. The results of du Plessis and Bezuidenhout (1979) are difficult to interpret. Although they stated that no final conclusions could be drawn from the conglutinin determinations because of the way the sera were stored, the absence of reaction in some of their cattle may have been due to subclinical infections or to previously acquired immunity as the experiments were carried out in an endemic area and a few infected ticks were present in spite of regular dipping. The severity of the reaction in cattle is variable, from subclinical to peracutely fatal. Absence of apparent reaction may be due to the reaction being subclinical in the individual susceptible animal, to previously acquired immunity, or to failure of the animal to become infected. The latter category will usually react to a subsequent injection. In my experience this category is very small, as is also apparent from the challenge results by du Plessis and Bezuidenhout (1979). Although the conglutinin level might possibly influence the severity of the reaction in cattle, so far there appears to be very little hard evidence for the occurrence of any cattle refractory to infection without previous exposure to heartwater.

Organ emulsions also will only reliably establish infection if they are injected iv. The only exception known is brain cortex homogenate of infected animals, which is infective by the subcutaneous route in most cases (Ilemobade, 1976; Ilemobade and Blotkamp, 1978a). Its infectivity was first shown in Kenya (Anonymous, 1952). In our laboratory such brain material proved infective to the majority of subcutaneously injected goats, but somewhat less reliable than iv injection of blood or tick material (A. J. van Winkelhoff, A. Starink, and G. Uilenberg, unpublished data, 1979–1981).

Because ticks transmit heartwater by the inoculation of minute quantities of material into the skin, Uilenberg (1977) suggested that the possibility of using tick-derived stabilates for infection by the subcutaneous route should be investigated. However, in spite of the high infectivity of filtrate of homogenized engorged infected ticks when administered iv, subcutaneous inoculation of this material was not successful, except when uninfected sheep brain filtrate was added (Bezuidenhout, 1981). Intradermal injection of tick filtrate also failed to transmit the disease (J. D. Bezuidenhout, personal communication, 1979). Experiments with two batches of similar tick homogenate were carried out in our institute (A. J. van Winkelhoff, unpublished, 1979). Identical quantities of each batch were inoculated into three goats, in one iv, in the others subcutaneously; one of the latter two received the tick material alone, the other the tick material mixed with uninfected brain homogenate. In the first experiment only the goat inoculated iv was infected; in the second all three goats contracted heartwater.

Alexander (1931) reported that blood inoculated intradermally did not cause heartwater, and the intraperitoneal route was rarely positive. Later Balozet (1936) appears to have transmitted fatal cowdriosis in a sheep by the intraperitoneal inoculation of infected brain material, and possibly in another by the intracerebral route; his further experiments in laboratory animals using the intracerebral and intraperitoneal routes cannot be taken into account, as he was almost certainly not transmitting heartwater by then (see Section V,C).

The importance of the route of inoculation has also been shown in mice, in which certain strains have been serially passaged (see Section V,C).

IV. Distribution

The disease is known to occur throughout most of Africa south of the Sahara, from the Cape Province in South Africa to as far north as Kassala in the Sudan, from Senegal in the West to Somalia in the East.

Neitz (1968) estimated the endemic area at about 5 million square miles (13 million km^2). Its distribution includes the island of Madagascar, and it has recently been diagnosed on other islands near Africa, La Réunion and Mauritius to the East (Perreau et al., 1980) and São Tomé in the Atlantic Ocean (Uilenberg et al., 1982). Perreau et al. (1980) also confirmed its existence on the island of Guadeloupe in the Caribbean area, where it had been suspected for some time, associated with *A. variegatum,* introduced in the nineteenth century (see Section XII). Its distribution is likely to cover approximately that of the African *Amblyomma* vectors, and may well include the southern parts of the Arabian peninsula, where *A. variegatum* is known to be established (Hoogstraal and Kaiser, 1959; Hoogstraal, 1980).

Reports of its possible occurrence elsewhere are unconfirmed. Heartwater has been suspected to occur in Iran on the strength of the resistance to the disease in South Africa of a breed of sheep erroneously called Persian, but which is in fact a black-headed African breed apparently originating from heartwater-endemic areas in East Africa (Uilenberg, 1981). Lestoquard (1932) diagnosed heartwater in sheep in Turkey on the basis of suspect symptoms and lesions, and the belief that heartwater occurred in Iran. Aleraj et al. (1956), Cvjetanovic (1956), and Cvjetanovic and Berberovic (1958) reported a disease in sheep, goats, and cattle in Yugoslavia, which they suspected to be heartwater because rickettsia-like bodies (transmissible to the chicken embryo and to laboratory rodents) were seen in endothelial cells. Thuraisingham (1963, quoted by Mohan, 1968) found rickettsias in endothelial cells of domestic buffalo in Malaysia affected with a disease of unknown etiology. These and similar observations must be substantiated by further evidence before they can be taken as indications for the occurrence of heartwater, which does appear to be a truly African disease, so far associated with African *Amblyomma* spp. only. This does not exclude the possibility that *C. ruminantium* might become established elsewhere, transmitted by suitable non-African *Amblyomma* ticks, in the Americas (Uilenberg, 1982) or in southern Asia.

V. Susceptibility

A. Domestic Animals

All Bovidae can probably be infected. Apart from sheep, goats, and cattle, the classical victims, Asian domestic buffalo may also contract fatal heartwater (Mammerickx, 1961, quoted by Mohan, 1968; Bück, 1965, quoted by Cockrill, 1974). David Livingstone's account (quoted by Cockrill, 1974) of the sudden deaths of working buffalo is more indicative of heartwater than of tsetse-transmitted disease, to which it was attributed by Livingstone.

There are no real indications for the receptivity of other domestic animals. The evidence for the susceptibility of the camel (Karrar, 1960) is insufficient. Once the early confusion concerning the different identities of the agents of heartwater and African horse sickness had been defined, it was shown that the horse was not receptive (Alexander, 1931). Details of the experiments by D. T. Mitchell (unpublished, quoted by Alexander, 1931) do not offer support for the claim that *C. ruminantium* was passaged eight times in dogs, and Alexander could not duplicate these results; he concluded that the heartwater agent is not infective for dogs. Curasson and Delpy (1928) could not induce clinical disease in pigs.

B. Wild Animals

Several species of wild Bovidae living in the endemic areas can be infected. Naturally contracted fatal heartwater has been found in springbok (*Antidorcas marsupialis*) and eland (*Taurotragus oryx*) (Neitz, 1944; Young and Basson, 1973). Artificially infected young springbok developed temperature reactions but recovered with tetracycline treatment (Young, 1970); however, young elands from heartwater-free regions did not show any reactions to artificial infection and survived in a heavily infected area (Grosskopf, 1958). Blesbok (*Damaliscus dorcas albifrons*) and black wildebeest (*Connochaetes gnou*) could be experimentally infected (Neitz, 1933, 1935, 1937). The infections were subclinical in the wildebeest, and their blood was infective. Blood of the blesbok also became infective; some died, but only in one animal could an association between heartwater and death be established by finding rickettsias in intima smears. Heartwater has been implicated, without proof, in mortality in bushbuck in South Africa (J. Webb, 1877, quoted by Henning, 1956). Curasson and Delpy (1928) were unable to cause disease in bushbuck (*Tragelaphus scriptus*) and in duiker (*Cephalophus* sp.), but there is no evidence to show whether subclinical infection was perhaps established, or whether the animals had been exposed to natural infection previously and perhaps were immune. Gradwell *et al.* (1976) inoculated the Ball 3 strain into captive impalas (*Aepyceros melampus*), blue wildebeest (*Connochaetes taurinus*), a kudu (*Tragelaphus strepsiceros*), a buffalo (*Syncerus caffer*), a giraffe (*Giraffa camelopardalis*), and a sheep living with these animals. The sheep contracted heartwater; none of the other animals reacted.

Wild Bovidae and also Cervidae exotic to sub-Saharan Africa have been known to contract fatal heartwater: Indian nylghaie (*Boselaphus tragocamelus*), Barbary sheep (*Ammotragus lervia*), Himalayan tahr (*Hemitragus jemlahicus*), and fallow deer (*Dama dama*) in South Africa (Young and Basson, 1973), and Java deer (*Cervus timorensis*) in Mauritius (Poudelet et al., 1982). An artificially infected Indian blackbuck (*Antilope cervicapra*) died of heartwater, as did a fallow deer and a moufflon (*Ovis musimon*) (Hofmeyr, 1956). Young (in Gradwell et al., 1976) reported typical symptoms of heartwater in moufflon, Barbary sheep, and fallow deer.

Warthog (*Phacochoerus aethiopicus*) did not develop clinical disease after artificial infection (Curasson and Delpy, 1928; Gradwell et al., 1976).

C. Laboratory Animals

Many attempts at establishing *C. ruminantium* infection in various laboratory animals have been carried out. Numerous early attempts are summarized by Alexander (1931) and Mason and Alexander (1938, 1940). Some experiments are reported by Ramisse and Uilenberg (1971). These negative results concern guinea pigs, rabbits, rats, and mice, subjected to various immunosuppressive treatments and infected by various routes using various tissues and blood from infected ruminants.

The results of other experiments were not substantiated by microscopical examination and/or subinoculation of susceptible ruminants. Balozet (1936) reported successful infection in guinea pigs, rats, and rabbits, whereas mice were refractory; however, he did not carry out microscopic examination, either in the laboratory animals or in subinoculated sheep. These sheep showed a temperature reaction after inoculation with material from the laboratory animals, but remained fully susceptible to real heartwater. Balozet quoted a personal communication from P. J. du Toit, who had similar findings in guinea pigs and sheep. Mason and Alexander (1938) found an intercurrent infection in laboratory animals, not heartwater but apparently related to rat typhus. This "X-disease" is also similar to that which Balozet reported as heartwater in laboratory animals. Pellissier et al. (1950) studied a disease in crossbred cattle at Brazzaville, associated with rickettsialike inclusions in endothelial cells of large vessels. They could infect guinea pigs, rabbits, a vervet monkey, and sheep, whereas rats and mice appeared to be refractory. Fatal disease could be induced in a calf after three passages in guinea pigs; direct transmission between cattle was not attempted. The authors did not think they were dealing with heartwater because of the atypical chronic disease picture and also the bacilliform shape of the rickettsias, quite unlike *C. ruminantium*. Hughes (1953) reported an acute disease typical of heartwater in goats imported from the United Kingdom into Ghana, but he apparently isolated another rickettsial infection in subinoculated guinea pigs that may have been murine typhus.

Mason and Alexander (1938, 1940) claimed to have observed the survival of *C. ruminantium* in the brain of a guinea pig and a rat, but gave no details. The first success in infecting laboratory animals with *C. ruminantium* was reported by Mason and Alexander (1940), who were able to make five serial passages in ferrets. The infection was lost after the fifth passage. Haig (1955) and Henning (1956), quoted a personal communication from Adelaar, who found that the virulence for ferrets increased with continued passage, and that no attenuation for sheep occurred.

Hudson and Henderson (1941) first observed the possible survival of the heartwater agent during 2 weeks in vitamin-deficient rats and in wild rodents (*Rhabdomys pumilio*). Haig (1952) demonstrated the infectivity of spleen emulsion of white mice, injected up to 90 days previously with infected brain, spleen, or blood from sheep and cattle, using four different strains, including the Mara and Ball 3 strains. He did not succeed in carrying the infection through two successive mouse passages, but could accomplish nine alternating passages between sheep and mice. Similar observations were made by Ramisse and Uilenberg (1971), who made a few alternating passages with a Malagasy strain between sheep and mice, but did not succeed in passing the infection through two consecutive mouse passages. Abdel Rahim and Shommein (1978a) could maintain, like Haig, (Sudanese) *C. ruminantium* for 3 months in laboratory mice; the incubation period in the subinoculated goats was longer than usual. K. E. Weiss (personal communication to du Plessis and Kumm, 1971) supposedly obtained three successive passages of the Ball 3 strain in mice. No microorganisms were found in the mice, and no mortality or signs of disease resulted; the infectivity of mouse material could only be demonstrated by subinoculation into ruminants. Ramisse (1970, 1972, 1973), using the same strain as Ramisse and Uilenberg (1971) (the K2 strain, Uilenberg, 1971a) was able to make up to 100 successive passages in cortisone-treated mice, but only after he adopted the iv route of injection, using blood, instead of intraperitoneal inoculation of spleen material. There was no clear evidence for the necessity of cortisone treatment. One of the uses that Ramisse made of successful mouse passage was to eliminate intercurrent *Eperythrozoon ovis*.

Totally different results were obtained in South Africa, where first du Plessis and Kumm (1971) and later Mackenzie and van Rooyen (1981) isolated strains of *C. ruminantium* from small ruminants that were not only mouse-infective and could be passaged serially in mice, but were highly pathogenic for them. These strains are quite different from each other, however.

The strain isolated from a goat by du Plessis and Kumm (1971) was easily established and passed serially in mice using spleen and liver material inoculated intraperitoneally. The mice died in 10 to 14 days, showing splenomegaly and hydrothorax, with rickettsial groups detectable in Kupffer's cells, in reticulum spleen cells, and in alveolar capillary endothelial cells of the lungs. They also are found in peritoneal macrophages (du Plessis, 1975) and a few in the brain (J. L. du Plessis, personal communication, 1979). The infection is latent in rats (J. L. du Plessis, personal communication, 1979). After 120 serial passages in mice, no loss of pathogenicity for mice occurred (du Plessis, in Mackenzie and van Rooyen, 1981). Mouse material was infective to sheep, causing high mortality with lesions similar to those of heartwater, although less pronounced, and scanty, small, and often poorly defined rickettsial colonies in brain smears of the sheep. Sheep that recovered from the mouse strain were partially immune to infection with the Ball 3 strain, but sheep that recovered from the Ball 3 strain showed no immunity to challenge with the mouse strain. The mouse strain causes atypical mild reactions in cattle, and cattle recovered from infection are not protected against the Ball 3 strain (J. L. du Plessis, personal communication, 1979). These various differences with "normal" strains have even caused doubts as to whether the mouse strain could be considered as *C. ruminantium* (Ramisse and Uilenberg, 1971; Andreasen, 1974a; Uilenberg, 1977, 1981).

The Kwanyanga strain isolated from sheep by Mackenzie and van Rooyen (1981) was also infective to mice, in which case it could be passaged serially and caused a mortality of 99% after 6 to 22 days (average 10). There are important differences with the du Plessis strain, however. High mortality (99%) was only caused if the mice were inoculated iv, using homogenate of infected mouse liver or blood; intraperitoneal injection with these inocula only killed a few mice, although it was not stated whether the survivors had actually been subclinically infected. A second difference is that no rickettsias could be found microscopically in smears made from moribund mice. Third, the cross-immunity between the Kwanyanga and the Ball 3 strains, although not solid, was far better than between the du Plessis and the Ball 3 strains. All five sheep that recovered from the Ball 3 strain showed only moderate febrile reactions on challenge with Kwanyanga mouse material. One of five sheep that recovered from infection with Kwanyanga mouse material succumbed to challenge with the Ball 3 strain; the others showed slight to moderate thermal response. All five sheep that recovered from a substrain of the Kwanyanga strain passaged in sheep, survived on challenge with the Ball 3 strain, showing moderate to pronounced febrile reactions. Furthermore, in cross-immunity tests in mice between the Kwanyanga and the du Plessis strains, the only evidence of slight reciprocal protection was an increase in the mean survival time on heterologous challenge.

The cross-immunity experiments need to be supplemented with further experimental data before definite conclusions on these immunological comparisons can be made, because no homologous challenge was given to prove the existence of solid homologous immunity prior to the heterologous challenge. The mice and sheep recovered from the initial infection by Gloxazone treatment, and, as far as mice are concerned, latent infection can reportedly be eliminated by treatment with Gloxazone whereas the immunity in mice is associated with persistence of the rickettsias in the tissues of the animals, according to du Plessis (1981b) (see Section X). Another difference is the response of infected mice to Gloxazone treatment: 100% of mice infected with the du Plessis strain were cured by a single dose of 20 mg/kg given iv, as contrasted to 50% of mice infected with the Kwanyanga strain (Mackenzie and van Rooyen, 1981). The Kwanyanga strain was also highly pathogenic for sheep, even after 16 serial mouse passages. Cattle could be infected: one of two calves infected with the sheep-passage substrain died of heartwater; four of four calves inoculated with mouse-passage material showed moderate temperature reactions, and all survived. Another interesting point is that the Kwanyanga substrain passaged in sheep was not infective to mice after 15 or 19 sheep passages. Later P. K. I. Mackenzie (personal communication, 1981) established a second strain in mice from another part of South Africa. This strain, named Nonile, was also highly pathogenic to mice and sheep; 100% of mice injected iv died, against only 30% of intraperitoneally infected mice.

Andreasen (1974a) compared the behavior of the Malagasy K2 strain passaged serially in mice by Ramisse (see earlier) in homozygotic congenitally athymic (*nude*) mice, heterozygotic *nude* mice, and homozygotic normal mice, injecting blood by the iv route that had been successfully used by Ramisse. After eight attempted serial passages, blood from normal mice was not infective to sheep, but blood from homozygotic and heterozygotic *nude* mice transmitted heartwater. Andreasen observed mortality, which he attributed to heartwater, only in the homozygotic *nude* mice, and reported the occurrence of purple granules, thought to be *C. ruminantium,* in endothelial cells, especially of the spleen, fewer in the liver, and a few in the brain. No such granules were found in the other groups of mice. In a second series of serial passages in homozygotic *nude* mice, the infection was carried through six passages.

Results of work in our institute (A. J. van Winkelhoff, A. Starink, T. A. Niewold, F. F. J. Franssen, D. Zivkovic, A. A. M. Spanjer, and G. Uilenberg, unpublished work, 1979–1982) may be summarized as follows: the Nigerian D 225 strain could not be passaged in either homozygotic nude mice or normal Swiss mice, using infected sheep or goat brain intramuscularly, or infected ruminant blood intravenously, the attempts at serial mouse passage being done iv with blood. Blood from the mice was inoculated iv and in one case also brain was inoculated subcutaneously into susceptible goats after various intervals (9–43 days); heartwater was not transmitted. Single passages in normal Swiss mice could be achieved with the South African Zeerust strain. Two serial passages could be made with this strain in corticosteroid-treated Swiss mice and nude mice; three serial passages could not be attained. No disease or mortality attributable to the infection was noted in mice, and no rickettsias were found on microscopic examination. The small number of experiments does not allow the conclusion that immunosuppressive treatment or the use of nude mice enhances the chance of success. Goat blood infected with the Umm Banein strain or the São Tomé strain did not cause symptoms or mortality in Swiss mice injected intravenously; the infectivity to ruminants of material from these mice was not verified.

It is becoming apparent that there may be a spectrum of strains as to infectivity for mice: (*a*) strains such as the Nigerian D 225 that are entirely noninfective and nonpathogenic, (*b*) strains such as the Ball 3 and the Zeerust that are nonpathogenic but may be passaged once or exceptionally two or three times in succession, (*c*) strains such as the Malagasy K2 that are nonpathogenic but can be serially passaged indefinitely if the iv route is used, (*d*) the Kwanyanga strain, which is highly infective and pathogenic when inoculated iv but not intraperitoneally, and which, like the preceding types, is not seen microscopically in mouse cells, and (*e*) the strain of du Plessis and Kumm, which is highly infective and pathogenic even when inoculated intraperitoneally and is microscopically demonstrable in mouse cells. The situation may not be static: the Kwanyanga strain lost its infectivity for mice after 15 serial passages in sheep, but this observation also could be explained by assuming that the original isolate comprised two strains, one "normal," one mouse-infective, of which the latter was lost during the passages in sheep. The opinion of du Plessis that his mouse-infective organism is *C. ruminantium* appears to be vindicated by new evidence: serum of sheep recovered from infection with the Ball 3 strain gave similar titers to mouse-derived antigen of the du Plessis strain in an indirect fluorescent antibody test, as did sera of sheep recovered from the mouse strain (du Plessis, 1981a). Moreover, J. L. du Plessis (personal communication, 1979) has found that the mouse strain is transmissible by *A. hebraeum*.

A problem is that heartwater strains from geographically widely separated areas have been shown to be entirely cross-protective (van Winkelhoff and Uilenberg, 1981; see also Section VI), but there is only limited unilateral cross-immunity between the du Plessis strain and the Ball 3 strain, better but still incomplete cross-immunity between the Kwanyanga and the Ball 3 strains, and hardly any between the Kwanyanga and the du Plessis strains. Some of these results need confirmation where homologous challenge is given before the heterologous one (see earlier). An explanation might be that antigenic changes occur during passages in mice. Du Plessis and Kumm (1971) suggested this possibility in quoting a personal communication of K. E. Weiss, who found that sheep recovering from the Ball 3 strain that had exceptionally been passaged serially three times in mice were only partially immune to the original strain. Cross-immunity tests between the Ball 3 strain and the du Plessis mouse-infective strain, after numerous passages of the latter in sheep, might indicate whether there may be any truth in this suggestion. If antigenic changes do occur in mice, then mouse-infective strains offer little promise for immunization purposes, even if they were to become attenuated for ruminants. The main importance of mouse-infective strains may lie in their possible use as a source of antigen for serological tests, as a laboratory model for chemotherapeutic screening, and for the study of the immunology of heartwater and possibly of its pathogenesis—although this may be quite different in mice and in ruminants.

VI. Epidemiology

The epidemiology of heartwater is determined by several factors such as the infection rate of the vector population, the age resistance in young ruminants, the genetically determined susceptibility of the ruminant population, possible immunological strain differences, the presence or absence of wild reservoirs for the heartwater organisms or the vector, seasonal climatic changes influencing tick activity, and the intensity of tick control.

The infection rate of the *Amblyomma* population appears to be generally low, as evidenced by the long period during which susceptible ruminants may escape infection in endemic regions, several months (Curasson and Delpy, 1928; Alexander, 1931; Bonsma, 1944) or years (Neitz and Alexander, 1945; Uilenberg, 1971a). The infection rate in a batch of larvae or nymphs fed together on an infective ruminant is probably high, but the three-host *Amblyomma* vectors are indiscriminate feeders, especially in the immature stages, so that many ticks never acquire the infection, having fed in the preceding stages on some nonsusceptible animal. The absence of transovarial transmission helps to limit the infection rate. Another factor is that blood of infected ruminants is only infective for a limited period during the clinical reaction and for an average of only 2–3 weeks after that; reinfections may cause the blood to become temporarily infective again, even in solidly immune animals (see Section IX).

Young calves and lambs possess a reverse age resistance, quite independent of the immune status of the dam (Neitz and Alexander, 1941; Alexander *et al.*, 1946; Uilenberg, 1971a). This resistance is short-lived, according to Neitz and Alexander (1941), lasting up to 4 weeks in calves and at least 7 days in lambs. Later Alexander *et al.* (1946) indicated an age resistance of about 3 weeks in both calves and lambs. The resistance is not absolute, because calves infected at less than 3 weeks of age and, lambs at 10 days are known to have died (Neitz and Alexander, 1941; Uilenberg, 1971a). The latter inoculated merino lambs, all born to susceptible dams not exposed to infection. The youngest seven (ages 3–9 days) survived; two aged 10 and 16 days succumbed. Little is known about an age resistance in goat kids. Thomas and Mansvelt (1957) concluded that kids appear to have some natural resistance that is probably not as high as that of calves.

It might be imagined that when ticks are not intensively controlled, a stable endemic situation might result, as is known to be possible in similar circumstances in bovine babesiosis and anaplasmosis. However, the combination of a low infection rate in the tick population and the very short duration of the age resistance does not allow all or even a majority of the young animals to become infected before the resistance wanes. In an endemic area in Tanzania without tick control, susceptible calves contracted fatal heartwater up to the end of an exposure period of 60 days (Uilenberg *et al.*, 1977). Fatal heartwater may occur in animals that have lived for years in an endemic area. A stable endemic situation without apparent disease problems can probably not be attained in populations that are genetically susceptible to the disease. The large numbers of *Amblyomma* ticks required for a stable situation would be unacceptable because they would cause or predispose to other harmful effects, such as a deterioration of the general condition, bacterial infections such as abscesses, dermatophilosis and bovine farcy, and parasitic infestations such as screwworm.

Great differences in susceptibility occur between different populations of cattle, sheep, and goats. These differences do not appear to be linked to any particular breed or species and probably depend mainly or exclusively on inherited resistance acquired by local livestock through long, natural selection. It is a resistance against severe reaction to infection, so that heartwater commonly is not an apparent disease until exotic stock is introduced. Bonsma (1944) showed differences in mortality due to heartwater between local Afrikanders and European breeds of beef cattle, although these findings were at first not accepted by Neitz and Alexander (1945) and Alexander *et al.* (1946). The great differences in susceptibility between local and exotic breeds of cattle have been confirmed on many occasions, but even though most local cattle in endemic areas are zebu (*Bos indicus*) or sanga (African breeds resulting from crossing humped and humpless cattle), inherited resistance has nothing to do with zebu influence. Exotic zebu cattle such as Brahman or Sahiwal are as highly susceptible as European cattle; however, local African humpless breeds in the endemic areas, such as the N'dama and Dahomey, are highly resistant. In all comparisons, innate resistance should be distinguished from acquired immunity, and different groups of cattle can only be compared when they have had the same previous history.

Matters may be somewhat less simple where small ruminants are concerned. Although the uniformly high susceptibility of exotic breeds of sheep and goats is undisputed, there is no general agreement on the innate resistance of local breeds in endemic country. Theiler (1905) stated that in the lower parts of the Transvaal only local goats and sheep were found in any number, and exotic animals could not be kept. Curasson and Delpy (1928) found, in what was then called French West Africa, that the peracute form of the disease was seen only after the introduction of merino sheep and Angora goats. Alexander (1931) noticed that local sheep in South Africa had a natural resistance in contrast to imported breeds, of which "Persian" sheep were the sole exception, erroneously as has been discovered (see Section IV). Hornby (1935), in Tanzania, saw that heartwater completely eliminated within a year a flock of merino sheep introduced into an area where its existence had not been suspected in the native sheep. Neitz (1939a) and Henning (1956) also found that indigenous sheep and goats suffered little mortality compared to exotic breeds, although Alexander et al. (1946) surprisingly denied breed differences in susceptibility. In Madagascar, 9 of 17 merinos, aged 6 months and over, died following artificial infection, as compared to none of 9 sheep of the local breed of comparable age that had almost certainly not been exposed to the disease before (Uilenberg, 1971a).

In contrast, Curasson and Delpy (1928) reported high mortality in local breeds, although the course of the disease was slower than in imported ones. Cilli and Corazzi (1954) found that heartwater caused high mortality in sheep in Erithrea, as did Evans (1963) in northern Somalia, and Karrar (1960, 1968) in the Sudan, where goats were also badly affected. Aklaku (1980) reported in Ghana considerable mortality by peracute heartwater in local West African dwarf goats and sheep, particularly in young animals of 4 to 6 months of age. Ilemobade (1977) found in endemic areas of northern Nigeria that only 4 of 28 local cattle, aged 2–4 years, were susceptible; only 3 of 6 sheep aged 15–30 months were susceptible, but as many as 39 of 43 goats. Rousselot (in Girard and Rousselot, 1947), Rousselot (1953), Karrar et al. (1963), Karrar (1968), and Ilemobade (1977) attributed the difference in susceptibility of local cattle and small ruminants to the fact that cattle are the favorite hosts of adult *Amblyomma* ticks, resulting in early immunity in cattle, but persisting susceptibility of many small ruminants. The method of animal husbandry may also be important in explaining these differences; in northern Nigeria a substantial proportion of the goats are maintained in villages and are thus less exposed to ticks, besides not being preferential hosts of adult *Amblyomma* (Ilemobade, 1977). Although these explanations are somewhat plausible, many questions remain. For instance, Karrar (1968) found that numerous local sheep and goats in the Sudan died, but the study by Karrar et al. (1963) would seem to indicate that sheep are very good hosts of adult *A. lepidum*. In the Sudan, the disease was well known to the stock owners (Karrar, 1960), whereas it appeared to be new in northern Somalia (Evans, 1963). Edelsten (1975) attributed the heavy losses by widespread tick-associated disease in local small ruminants in northern Somalia for over 90% to Nairobi sheep disease, but heartwater was difficult to separate from the various diseases encountered in the field and appeared to be sporadic.

If marked immunological strain differences occur, they could greatly influence the epidemiology because individual animals would have to overcome more than one disease attack in order to acquire a solid immunity. At first it was believed that complete immunity to all strains could only be gradually acquired through repeated reinfections with different strains (Spreull, 1922; Alexander, 1931). Some of the early findings may have been due to intercurrent infections such as *Eperythrozoon ovis* in sheep, an unidentified infection called "virus A," bluetongue, *Ehrlichia* (Neitz, 1939a), and *Borrelia theileri* and *Anaplasma ovis* (Uilenberg, 1971a). In cattle various blood parasites may simulate heartwater. Moreover, Alexander's opinion (1931) is not supported by the details of the experiments he reports, carried out by du Toit. Alexander's experiments appear to indicate a surprisingly low immunity to homologous challenge rather than to prove immunological strain differences (see Section IX). Neitz (1939a) found no immunological differences among 10 strains isolated in the Transvaal. All recovered sheep were solidly immune to challenge, whether heterologous or homologous, for at least 6 months after recovery, and only 10 of 121 responded by a febrile reaction to homologous or heterologous challenge 7–34 months after recovery. Complete cross-protectivity between different strains in sheep was confirmed by Neitz *et al.* (1947). Karrar (1960) noted no significant differences in cross-immunity tests with two Sudanese strains, only mild thermal response in two animals. Van Winkelhoff and Uilenberg (1981) found that strains from South Africa and Nigeria were completely cross-protective.

In experiments in our institute, the South African Ball 3 and Zeerust strains are being compared in cross-immunity tests in goats to strains from the Sudan and São Tomé (D. Zivkovic, R. H. Dwinger, A. A. H. M. ter Huurne, N. M. Perié, and G. Uilenberg, unpublished, 1981–1982). The reaction to first infection is controlled by oxytetracycline; a homologous challenge is first given after 1 to 2 months, followed by heterologous challenge after another interval of 1 to 2 months. Homologous reinfection prior to heterologous challenge has proved essential, because mild febrile reactions to homologous challenge sometimes occur and might be erroneously attributed to strain differences if homologous challenge was omitted. So far seven goats have had the full series of homologous and heterologous infections; all were solidly immune to heterologous challenge. They include goats immune to the São Tomé strain challenged with South African strains or the Sudanese one, goats immune to a South African strain challenged with the Sudanese one, and goats immune to the Sudanese strain challenged with a South African or the São Tomé strain. So far, there are no indications of immunological differences between randomly obtained strains originating from geographically widely separated countries; all strains isolated in the field, tested in the way indicated, apparently belong to one antigenic type. Only the mouse-infective strains isolated in South Africa (du Plessis and Kumm, 1971; Mackenzie and van Rooyen, 1981) have given very different results, the du Plessis strain appearing to be the least related to a "normal" strain such as the Ball 3. These differences may possibly be due to antigenic changes during passage in mice; cross-immunity tests with the Kwanyanga strain should be repeated using homologous challenge prior to heterologous infection (see Section V,C).

Heartwater does not require a wildlife reservoir to maintain itself in domestic ruminants (Neitz, 1967), as has been shown in Madagascar, on Guadeloupe, and on São Tomé where susceptible wild hosts are absent or rare. It is only when the eradication of the vector and the disease is attempted that wild ruminants may constitute a real problem. In Zimbabwe, *A. hebraeum* and heartwater were virtually eradicated except for the areas where wild ungulates occurred in appreciable numbers (Norval and Lawrence, 1979). Ilemobade (1976), Ilemobade and Leeflang (1977), and Mackenzie and van Rooyen (1981) speculated that rodents might serve as a reservoir for heartwater. This would seem unlikely, because it has only exceptionally been possible to infect rodents and also because larvae of *Amblyomma,* the usual stage found on rodents, are not infective in the absence of transovarial transmission. Small mammals and birds may be responsible for bringing infected nymphs into well-fenced ranches, and the rapid spread of the tick and the disease in Zimbabwe following the breakdown of dipping appeared to be due to the lack of specificity of the immature ticks, feeding on hosts that were not restricted by fences (Norval, 1978, 1979). The tick vector itself also constitutes a reservoir, the infection surviving in adult ticks for over 15 months (Ilemobade, 1976). One tick generation, infected in the larval stage, is able to maintain the infection for over 3 years (Neitz, 1968).

Seasonal climatic changes affect the vector population. Although cases of heartwater do occur throughout the year, more are seen in the season when the adult ticks are more active, the rainy summer and autumn in regions with a pronounced dry season (Neitz, 1968; Perreau, 1973; Ilemobade, 1976; Norval, 1979).

VII. The Disease

A. Symptoms and Course

For detailed descriptions of the clinical disease, the reader is referred to reviews by Alexander (1931), Curasson (1943), Rousselot (1953), Henning (1956), Neitz (1968), Ilemobade (1976), and Uilenberg (1981).

The incubation period after natural transmission by ticks varies from 1 to 5 weeks, with an average of about 2. After artificial infection by iv inoculation of virulent material, small ruminants show a febrile reaction between 5 and 35 days with a mean of 9 to 10 days; it is slightly longer in cattle, about 12 days. There appears to be an inverse relation with the size of the dose when minimal quantities are used. The average incubation period may vary to some extent according to the strain.

Typical acute cowdriosis starts with a sudden rise in temperature, which usually rises above 41°C within 1 or 2 days. It may remain high, dropping to subnormal shortly before death. Loss of appetite and cessation of rumination gradually set in. Cyanosis of the mucous membranes and dyspnea may be noted. In the majority of cases nervous symptoms commence within a few days, ranging from rapid blinking of the eyes, rapid protruding of the tongue, twitching of individual muscles, and hypersensitivity to the touch, to a staggering, often high-stepping gait, circling, abnormal postures, and aggressive behavior in cattle. Once nervous symptoms appear, the disease normally progresses rapidly and recovery is rare. Fits and convulsions occur, during which the animal in lateral recumbency makes pedaling movements and exhibits nystagmus, opisthotonus, chewing movements, and often frothing at the mouth. Temporary recovery may occur, followed by renewed fits. Death usually occurs during these attacks, or the animal may linger for a few days in a state of virtual nonreactivity, as if irreversible cerebral damage had occurred (Clark, 1962). Marked nervous symptoms may be absent in some cases of acute heartwater in cattle; a profuse and often hemorrhagic diarrhea is frequent and may sometimes be the only major sign. A moist cough is frequently noticed, associated with bronchial rales.

Peracute cases are rather common in exotic breeds of cattle and goats, less so in sheep. The animal collapses and dies in convulsions without premonitory symptoms, although pyrexia is usually present. At the other extreme, mild and even subclinical forms are common in very young animals, animals of genetically resistant populations, and partially immune individuals. The only symptoms may be fever and an increase in the respiration rate.

The mortality rate is high in susceptible populations. Losses of 90% are common in infected Angora goats; as many as 60% of susceptible cattle may die; the mortality of merino sheep is intermediate. Neitz (1964) reports a mortality in calves in endemic areas of as much as 40% during the first 8 months of life, but such figures depend on the morbidity rate, which is greatly affected by tick control, immunization, and treatment. Stampa (1969) observed that 280 of 900 sheep died within 3 months of being introduced onto an infected farm, in spite of weekly dipping. Losses in local breeds in the endemic areas usually are low, below 5 or 10%, but in small ruminants the picture may be different (see Section VI). The virulence of the strain greatly influences the mortality rate in the laboratory (Neitz et al., 1947), varying in merino sheep from a low of 5 to a high of 95% (Neitz, 1964, 1968). In the field, strains of both low and high virulence might occur in one site.

Hematological findings in heartwater have been fairly divergent and, in general, do not appear to be spectacular, apart possibly from a significant drop in eosinophilic granulocytes (see Section VIII). Anemia is common. The reader is referred for details to Graf (1933), Clark (1962), Owen et al. (1973), Synge (1976, quoted by Synge and Scott, 1978), Abdel Rahim and Shommein (1978b), and Ilemobade and Blotkamp (1978b).

B. Postmortem Findings

Descriptions of macroscopic lesions are given by Steck (1928), Alexander (1931), Curasson (1943), Henning (1956), Pienaar et al. (1966), Uilenberg (1971b, 1981), Ilemobade (1976), and Shommein and Abdel Rahim (1977a).

In typical cases, accumulations of liquid are present in the pericardial sac and also in the thoracic and peritoneal cavities. Other frequent lesions include edema of the lungs, froth in the respiratory passages, edema of the mediastinal and sometimes the perirenal tissues, congestion of the liver with distension of the gallbladder, petechiae and large hemorrhages in various mucosae and serous membranes, hyperemia of the abomasal mucosa, enteritis (sometimes hemorrhagic, especially in cattle), swelling of the spleen and lymph nodes, and degeneration of the kidneys and the heart muscle. The brain does not usually show any striking macroscopic lesions apart from congestion of the meningeal blood vessels and occasionally edema of the meninges. These different lesions never occur together. Hydropericardium is more common in sheep than in cattle and goats. The longer the disease persists, the more frequently the exudates and several of the other lesions are found. In peracute cases, a marked edema of the lungs is frequently the only striking lesion. The pathological picture is believed to vary with the strain of *Cowdria* responsible for death.

Histopathological lesions have been described by Steck (1928), Daubney (1930), Pienaar et al. (1966), Isoun et al. (1974), Ilemobade (1976), and Shommein and Abdel Rahim (1977a). Pienaar et al. and

Isoun et al. concentrate on the lesions in the brain. Many of the cases examined included accumulation of white cells in small blood vessels and perivascular and interstitial cellular infiltration. In the brain, common lesions also included focal necrosis of blood vessels, hemorrhages, glial changes, edema, swollen axis cylinders, microcavitation, focal necrosis of the granular layer of the cerebellum, and subarachnoidal cellular exudation. "Brain swelling" appeared an appropriate description in some cases (Pienaar et al., 1966), whereas Isoun et al. (1974) used the term acute hemorrhagic meningoencephalitis.

C. Pathogenesis

The pathogenesis of heartwater is poorly understood. The extent of the lesions show no correlation with the numbers of rickettsias, and cellular infiltration is not a local reaction to the presence of the organisms. Cowdry (1926c) noted that the infected endothelial cell showed no lesions, except that the nucleus might be flattened or pushed to one side by the pressure of the growing cluster of rickettsias. It is difficult to reconcile the various findings of Clark (1962), Pienaar et al. (1966), Owen et al. (1973), Abdel Rahim and Shommein (1978b), and Ilemobade and Blotkamp (1978b). Owen et al. (1973) suggested that the pathogenesis of heartwater may be different in animals with different postmortem findings. Pronounced hydropericardium could contribute to cardiac insufficiency, and edema of the lungs is sometimes so pronounced, especially in peracute cases in bovines, that death is explained by simple asphyxiation. A sudden terminal drop in blood pressure and plasma volume has been associated with the accumulation of the characteristic exudates, and explained by an increase in the permeability of the capillaries (Clark, 1962; Owen et al., 1973). Increased capillary permeability has been ascribed to a toxin (Neitz, 1968), but such a toxin has never been demonstrated. Toxins have also been invoked, without evidence, to explain the nervous symptoms in heartwater, the lesions in the brain being generally considered insufficiently constant and serious as explanation. Nevertheless, the conclusion drawn by Pienaar et al. (1966), Isoun et al. (1974), and Ilemobade (1976) may make it necessary to reconsider this opinion.

VIII. Diagnosis

In the live animal, diagnosis is never a certainty. There is no way of demonstrating the organism during life (other than subinoculation of blood into susceptible ruminants, or microscopic examination of brain material obtained by biopsy according to the method of Synge, 1978). Blood smears are of no value; the claim of Jackson and Neitz (1932) that they were able to distinguish single large rickettsias in blood smears has not been confirmed, and such findings would not have any practical significance in diagnosis because of their great rarity. The finding that eosinophilic granulocytes in the circulating blood decrease considerably during the disease (Clark, 1962; Owen et al., 1973; Ilemobade, 1976) may be of help. Clark (1962) also reported that the color of the blood plasma becomes progressively darker during cowdriosis, often reaching a deep orange. The nature of this pigment is unknown, but the phenomenon is not due to bilirubinemia; it probably also accounts for the frequently yellow color of the transudates seen at autopsy. Gruss (1981a,b) found that in all cases of heartwater in Angora goats an orange-yellow pigment appeared in the plasma with the commencement of the febrile phase. The pigment also was found in the plasma of sheep (Gruss, 1981b). Gruss believes this color to be of diagnostic value. In our laboratory, after it was noticed on one occasion that the plasma of a goat reacting to experimental heartwater was exceptionally dark yellow in color, the plasma of four more infected goats was examined during the clinical disease, and in three of the animals at frequent intervals from 3 days after infection until death or recovery. The "Clark–Gruss phenomenon" did not occur in a single animal (G. Uilenberg, unpublished data, 1982). The animals were Dutch goats of different breeds but did not include any Angoras. An investigation of this point should compare different breeds of cattle, sheep, and goats. The serological tests reported by Ilemobade and Blotkamp (1976) and du Plessis (1981a), even if their value were to be confirmed, are of no help during clinical disease.

Diagnosis is based on clinical symptoms, aided by herd or flock history, including the presence of known *Amblyomma* vectors. The disease may sometimes be diagnosed as a near certainty when typical nervous symptoms are present, but the clinical signs are variable and very often not typical. Because the course of the disease is rapid, treatment must be given quickly and on clinical suspicion only. The differential diagnosis includes rabies, cerebral babesiosis in cattle, cerebral theileriosis in cattle, tetanus, strychnine poisoning, poisoning by certain plants (cf. Mettam, 1928), and hypomagnesemic tetany in the event that nervous disorders are present. Peracute cases may simulate anthrax, especially when there is a combination of high fever, blood-tainted feces, and sudden death. Hemorrhagic diarrhea, not uncommon in cowdriosis in cattle, is also indicative of coccidiosis, arsenical poisoning, and poisoning by certain plants. When pulmonary signs dominate, the disease may resemble peracute hemorrhagic septicemia (pasteurellosis).

Heartwater can usually be diagnosed after death by microscopic demonstration of the rickettsia in suitable postmortem samples. If a laboratory examination is impossible, the postmortem lesions, combined with observations made before death, may be of help in arriving at a tentative diagnosis. However, often typical lesions such as a hydropericardium are absent, and commonly there are no striking macroscopical lesions.

Following the discovery of the causal rickettsia by Cowdry, microscopic diagnosis was at first based on examination of histological sections of organs, especially the cortex of the brain and kidney, according to most authors the richest in infected endothelial cells. Jackson (1931) showed that groups of *C. ruminantium* can also be found in smears made from scrapings of the intima of large blood vessels. Purchase (1945) examined smears from the brain cortex. The search in histological sections can be lengthy and uncertain, because the rickettsial groups may be confused with host cell nuclei (Jackson, 1931; Burdin, 1962), and, in addition, the chances of finding a group in a section are far less than in brain smears where capillaries can be scrutinized lengthwise; this also makes brain smears superior to intima smears (Purchase, 1945; Rousselot, 1953; Uilenberg, 1971a; Ilemobade, 1976).

Smears made from the brain cortex are the method of choice, and Purchase (1945) found smears from the cerebrum best. Some workers believe the smears should be made from hippocampus material, but in our experience the site is immaterial as long as cortex (gray matter) is used. The difficulty in obtaining brain specimens and the fiction, started by Cowdry (1925a, 1926a), that the rickettsias can only be stained for a very short period after death, is one of the main causes that the disease goes in many cases unrecognized. Uilenberg (1971a) showed that the organisms could be demonstrated in the brain until putrefaction is far advanced, a matter of 3 weeks in the refrigerator or over 2 days at room temperature; fixed or unfixed brain smears left at room temperature could be satisfactorily stained for at least a month. Schreuder (1980) demonstrated that cerebellar cortex can be obtained with a sharp spoon introduced through the foramen magnum following removal of the head. Cerebellum is as suitable as cerebral cortex. Smears made from the medulla oblongata were less satisfactory; Purchase found spinal cord preparations very suitable. It has been confirmed in our laboratory that cerebellar cortex provides satisfactory smears for the diagnosis of heartwater. A small fragment of gray matter (no larger than a matchhead) is crushed between two slides that are drawn over each other lengthwise so that two smears are obtained (Uilenberg, 1972). There are variants of the method. Purchase (1945) advocated the use of a spreader slide, lifted at a slight angle. Haig (1955) and Leeflang (1972) preferred wavy smears, with alternating thick and thin areas. After fixation and staining, areas containing networks of capillaries are located and these are searched with the oil-immersion objective.

Romanovsky-type stains, particularly Giemsa stain, are used for staining *C. ruminantium* after fixation in methanol or absolute ethanol (Cowdry, 1925b, 1926b). In brain smears, the groups of *Cowdria* are reddish purple (small forms) to blue (large forms) and can be distinguished from the endothelial nuclei by their morphology (Figs. 1–3). Prolonged (15 min) washing of the stained smears in tap water may improve the result of staining (unpublished, 1982). In Giemsa-stained histological sections, the color of *Cowdria* is dependent on the fixative that is used (Alexander, 1931). Castaneda's method is also suitable (Donatien and Lestoquard, 1938) and has been used on brain smears by Karrar (1960). In our laboratory, Castaneda's procedure has been found to produce faintly stained brain smears, with a good differentiation between the blue rickettsias and the red nuclei and protoplasm of the host cells. Purchase (1945) found Macchiavello's method unsatisfactory for staining rickettsias. Preliminary results in our laboratory indicate that basic fuchsin is retained to some extent by *Cowdria*. Giménez' modification was not useful. Burdin (1962) found methyl green–pyronin Y staining suitable, according to the method of Kurnick (1955), both for methanol-fixed brain smears and for paraffin sections fixed with Carnoy's fluid; *C. ruminantium* stained red and the cell nuclei took the methyl green.

Diagnosis of heartwater is different in countries where it has not been found previously. The disease was recently discovered on Guadeloupe (Perreau *et al.*, 1980). In this situation it is necessary to determine the presence or absence of the disease. Although brain smears from suspected cases should be examined, and blood from suspected animals may be subinoculated into susceptible ruminants, faster results may be expected by exposing and monitoring susceptible sentinel animals, by subinoculating pooled blood taken at random, and by collecting engorged *Amblyomma* larvae and nymphs from ruminants and feeding the next stage following moulting on susceptible animals.

A reliable serological test would be a great value in a survey. So far, the lack of suitable antigen has hampered the development of serological tests for heartwater. Du Plessis (1970b) reported negative results of an indirect fluorescent antibody test (IFAT), using infected brain smears as antigen. Ilemobade (1976) was not successful using the IFAT and brain material. Ilemobade and Blotkamp (1976) reported on a capillary flocculation test, using antigen prepared from infected brain. The test was positive during 1 to 4 weeks, beginning 1–2 weeks after recovery, so that it would not be useful either as an aid to clinical diagnosis or in field surveys. Its usefulness would be limited to laboratory studies. It has not been possible to reproduce these results in South Africa (J. D. Bezuidenhout, personal communication, 1979). Du Plessis (1981a) has developed an IFAT test using peritoneal cells of mice infected with the mouse-infective strain isolated by du Plessis and Kumm (1971). Antibodies appeared 2 weeks after infection of sheep with either the mouse strain or the Ball 3 strain, corresponding with the height of the febrile reactions. High levels were attained shortly after recovery, followed by a decline starting 6 weeks postinoculation. Heterologous challenge caused a distinct rise in titer after 3 weeks, followed by a decline 10 weeks after challenge, but significant titers were still present 18 months after challenge. Cattle infected with the Ball 3 strain showed somewhat lower titers to the mouse antigen, detectable for at least 10 weeks postinoculation. This IFAT is not ready to be released for general use (J. L. du Plessis, correspondence, 1982). Antigen obtained from liver and spleen of mice infected with the mouse strain has been used in a complement fixation test; a low titer was found in serum of sheep recovered from infection with the Ball 3 strain, whereas there was no cross-reaction with sera containing antibodies to various other rickettsias and *Chlamydia* (J. L. du Plessis, personal communication, 1979).

IX. Immunity

All strains of *C. ruminantium* examined so far appear to be completely cross-protective, apart from two South African mouse-infective strains where the differences might perhaps be due to rodent passage and in one case to the method of cross-immunity testing (see Section VI).

There are widely differing opinions on the duration of the immunity after recovery from heartwater, and the results of experiments are difficult to reconcile.

Alexander (1931) reported that of 34 recovered sheep, 2 died, 5 had a severe reaction, and only 2 had no febrile response to homologous challenge (apparently given between 14 days and 11 months after recovery). Unrecognized intercurrent infections may have influenced these and other early experimental results (Neitz, 1939a; see also Section VI). In the experiments of Neitz (1939a), all recovered sheep were solidly immune if tested within 6 months of recovery, and only 10 of 121 responded by a febrile reaction, without any further clinical symptoms, to homologous or heterologous challenge 7–34 months after recovery. Neitz et al. (1947) found that immunity was solid if the sheep were challenged within 2 months of recovery, and that afterwards a gradual, progressive decrease in immunity followed that remained sufficient to protect against a fatal outcome of challenge for at least 4 years. In fact, only 1 of 148 sheep succumbed to challenge, 25 responded only by a febrile reaction, and all others were solidly immune to challenge after varying intervals following recovery. In contrast, du Plessis (1981b) reported that four of nine immunized sheep reacted with a febrile response to homologous challenge after 6 months, whereas three of eight sheep did so after being similarly challenged after 9 months.

The duration of immunity in goats is not well documented. Ilemobade (1976) found that 10 goats given homologous challenge 2–8 weeks after oxytetracycline-induced or spontaneous recovery were immune, although a few febrile reactions occurred (the exact number is impossible to deduce from the publication, but was at most three), lasting 1–2 days. Six animals that were challenged a second time had no febrile reactions. In the cross-immunity experiments in our institute (see Section VI), 12 goats were given a homologous challenge 1–2 months after the initial infection. Nine of the animals did not react, one had a slight pyrexia that lasted for 4 days, with a maximum of 40°C on Day 16. Hyperthermia in the other two goats was probably not due to heartwater: one had a pyrexia lasting 5 days, with a peak of 40.8°C as late as Day 23 after challenge; the other goat started a moderate pyrexia, which responded to ampicillin treatment, as early as 3 days after challenge.

Immunity in cattle is considered by some authors to be short-lived unless it is reinforced by repeated reinfection. The data of Neitz and Alexander (1945) indicated the occurrence of fatal heartwater in up to 12% of cattle in the $3\frac{1}{2}$ years following immunization. Haig (1955) stated that immunity in cattle may wane considerably earlier than in sheep, many instances being reported where there was little or no immunity after 4 months. Henning and Haig (in Henning, 1956), in contrast, found that the protection in cattle was generally sufficient to prevent severe clinical symptoms or death when challenged from 12 to 18 months after immunization. Chabeuf (1976) reported that 5 of 15

Friesian cattle, immunized by the infection and treatment method, died of naturally contracted cowdriosis within 2 years after being exposed to natural infection in Madagascar. Arnold and Asselbergs (1981) reported that the protection afforded to adult exotic bulls by immunization against field exposure appeared to be good. Of some 400 bulls, mainly Brahmans, the death of only 2 could be ascribed to cowdriosis; one of these died nearly 2 months after immunization, the other 2 years later.

The nature of the immunity is unknown. Serum or large quantities of γ-globulins from immune or hyperimmunized animals, whether given simultaneously with the infection, during the incubation period, or during the clinical reaction, do not influence the outcome of infection (Alexander, 1931; du Plessis, 1970b). A mixture of infective blood and γ-globulins lost its infectivity within 2 hr at room temperature, whether γ-globulins from a susceptible or an immune sheep were used (du Plessis, 1970b). This single experiment has not been confirmed. Ramisse (1971) could not neutralize the infectivity of blood by hyperimmune serum. Du Plessis (1981a) found no relationship between the antibody titers found in the indirect fluorescent antibody test and the resistance to heterologous challenge. Alexander (1931) suggested that the immunity was probably cellular and not humoral.

It is still not known whether the immunity is linked to the persistence of *Cowdria* in the host, or whether sterile immunity occurs. Infection cannot usually be demonstrated to persist for more than 2–3 weeks by subinoculating blood into susceptible ruminants. Alexander (1931) reported an average of 17 days after the return of the temperature to normal; sometimes the blood was not infective as soon as 8 days after the height of the fever reaction; sometimes the infection could be transmitted up to 35 days after recovery. All attempts to demonstrate the presence of *C. ruminantium* in the blood for longer than 2 months after recovery have failed, and Neitz (1939a) also could not transmit heartwater with organ emulsions and endothelial scrapings of sheep recovered for more than 60 days. Donatien and Lestoquard (1937) were unable to transmit the disease with very large quantities of blood from a sheep recovered for 105 days, but claimed that homogenized blood vessels of the sheep caused fatal heartwater after a long incubation period (23 days); the diagnosis of heartwater was apparently carried out on clinical reaction and gross post mortem lesions only.

Ilemobade (1978) found that blood could be infective up to 50 days following recovery or challenge. *C. ruminantium* has also persisted in the brain of goats dying of heartwater up to 9 weeks after oxytetracycline treatment, but the blood was not infective (Ilemobade,

1976). Reinfections may cause the blood to become temporarily infective in partially immune animals (Neitz, 1939a) and solidly immune ones (Neitz et al., 1947). There are no convincing indications of a permanent carrier state in ruminants. Du Plessis (1981b) stated that his mouse-infective strain was found (in unpublished experiments) to persist in mouse tissues over almost the entire 18 months during which the mice were immune and suggests that the immunity in mice is associated with latent infection. His attempts to demonstrate the same mechanism in sheep with the Ball 3 strain were inconclusive. Support of the possibility that a carrier state follows recovery comes from field observations. Animals occasionally come down with fatal heartwater when they are submitted to stress such as vaccinations, dipping, or transportation. This might indicate a relapse of latent infection, but equally possibly could be the stress factor aggravating a mild or subclinical primary infection or a reinfection. Neitz (1968) wrote that recovered animals might relapse during the period the carrier state could be demonstrated (up to 2 months) if stressed by tick toxicosis. Splenectomy has no influence on the course of the disease and causes no relapse, even when there are rickettsias in the blood (Neitz, 1939a).

X. Therapy

An effective drug was not available prior to 1939. Curasson and Delpy (1928) thought that neoarsphenamine might somewhat prolong the course of heartwater, but Neitz (1940a) reported that arsenical compounds appeared to aggravate the disease. Ramisse (1970) did not note any influence of the drug on the course of the disease.

The sulfonamides were the first drugs shown to have a curative effect. Neitz (1939b, 1940b) found that uleron [4-(4'-aminobenzolsulfonamide)benzolsulfonedimethylamide] was active if administered early in the disease. Other sulfonamides such as sulfapyridine and sulfadimidine were also used later.

These drugs have been almost completely abandoned since the activity of tetracyclines was discovered, first chlortetracycline (Simpson and Wiley, 1951; Weiss et al., 1952), followed by oxytetracycline (Haig et al., 1954) and rolitetracycline (Poole, 1961b). Immelman and Dreyer (1982) recently found that doxycycline was effective.

Penicillin and streptomycin do not influence the infectivity of tick-derived heartwater vaccine (Bezuidenhout, 1981), nor do colistin and vancomycin (J. D. Bezuidenhout, personal communication, 1979). Haig (1955) also states that neither penicillin nor chloramphenicol have any effect. Experiments using spiramycin were not promising (Uilenberg, 1971b). Continuous administration of high doses of ampicillin during the incubation period and throughout the course of the disease did not prevent death (D. Zivkovic and G. Uilenberg, unpublished experiment, 1982).

A dithiosemicarbazone, α-ethoxyethylglyoxal dithiosemicarbazone, Gloxazone (Synge and Scott, 1976, Shommein and Abdel Rahim, 1977b; Synge, 1976, quoted by Scott, 1978), known to be active in other rickettsial diseases such as anaplasmosis (Brown *et al.*, 1968), is as effective as the tetracyclines. Mackenzie and van Rooyen (1981) reported differences in response to Gloxazone between two mouse-infective strains. Du Plessis (1981b) stated that Gloxazone may eliminate latent persistent infection by a mouse-infective strain in mice. There have been toxicity problems and the drug is apparently not being marketed.

Imidocarb has been found inactive against heartwater, including du Plessis' mouse-infective strain (N. McHardy, personal communication, 1979). Results of its use against another rickettsial disease, canine ehrlichiosis, are conflicting (Price and Dolan, 1980; van Heerden and van Heerden, 1981). Its activity against anaplasmosis is well documented.

The best available drugs are the tetracycline antibiotics. They are successfully used in the infection and treatment method of immunization when administered in the earliest stage of the disease, as soon as the febrile reaction begins. A single treatment is not reliable, and a second injection is often needed to bring about a return of the temperature to normal and prevent death. Temperature relapses may occur after initial improvement, and require further treatment. Animals can be saved if treated twice, either on consecutive days or with an interval of 1 day, starting on the first or second day of the febrile reaction, using one of the tetracyclines at a dosage rate of 5 to 10 mg/kg, or less with doxycycline (Immelman and Dreyer, 1982). No proper comparisons have been made between various formulations and routes of administration or between different tetracyclines. Poole (1961a,b) did use various tetracyclines and various formulations and routes of injections without conclusive results. The use of a long-acting formulation of oxytetracycline (Terramycin L. A.), administered intramuscularly at 20 mg/kg, does not always offer advantages over a normal formulation, given by the same route at 10 mg/kg, because two or more treatments may also be necessary with Terramycin L. A. (numerous unpublished observations in our laboratory, 1980–1982). Differences in the blood level of antibiotics administered in muscles of the thigh or rump as opposed to the neck should be taken into account (Groothuis *et al.*,

1980; Rutgers *et al.*, 1980). Karrar and El Hag Ali (1965) reported good results with oral oxytetracycline treatment for several days if started early in the course of the disease.

The situation is different if disease symptoms other than fever have developed, especially marked nervous symptoms or a hemorrhagic diarrhea. In those cases tetracycline treatment is usually of no avail. Cassard (1957) could not save any of 12 Friesian cattle suffering from naturally contracted heartwater, using chlortetracycline intravenously at 5 to 20 mg/kg.

Treatment with tetracyclines does not interfere with the establishment of immunity (Simpson and Wiley, 1951).

In addition to specific antibiotic treatment, supportive symptomatic therapy may help. All excitation of the animal should be avoided so as not to precipitate a fit of convulsions, and tranquilizers and muscle-relaxing drugs may be useful.

XI. Prevention

A. Tick Control

In areas where there are no alternate hosts for the tick, virtual elimination of *Amblyomma hebraeum* can be achieved locally (Norval and Lawrence, 1979). The prospects for the eradication in Africa of ticks in general, and of *Amblyomma* spp. in particular, are dim (Uilenberg, 1980). Emerging acaricide resistance in African species of the genus also poses an increasing problem.

When tick control is the only measure taken against heartwater, it should be as intensive as possible where susceptible breeds are concerned, with the disadvantage that precious endemic stability as regards babesiosis and anaplasmosis may be lost. This disadvantage may have to be accepted, even if the prevention of heartwater is supplemented by immunization, because *Amblyomma* ticks are also very harmful by their more direct effects (see Section VI).

Research in the creation of *Amblyomma*-resistant breeds, in analogy with *Boophilus*-resistant Australian cattle (Utech *et al.*, 1978), is unlikely to lead to great success (Uilenberg, 1980).

B. Immunization

When the causal agent was unknown, attempts at immunization (summarized by Alexander, 1931) met with little success.

Neitz and Alexander (1941, 1945) introduced a method based on inoculating young calves iv with virulent blood, making use of their innate age resistance. With the discovery of a specific chemotherapeutic treatment, immunization was extended to older cattle as well as sheep and goats, but this entailed close monitoring of animals in order to allow initiation of treatment at the first rise of temperature.

The infection and treatment method is expensive, laborious, time-consuming, and to some extent risky because of peracute reactions, especially in cattle and goats, and failures of treatment. It also requires spacious deep-freezing facilities, good transportation, expertise, and good laboratory facilities. Roughly 100,000 doses are issued annually in the Republic of South Africa (J. D. Bezuidenhout, personal communication, 1979), and it is not applied on a significant scale elsewhere.

Strains vary greatly in virulence, and because the degree of immunity does not depend on the severity of the reaction, a mild strain should be selected, although there is no guarantee that virulence will not change. However, it is important to use a strain that causes well-defined febrile reactions. This last criterion appears to have been satisfied in South Africa, where the highly virulent Ball 3 strain is used.

Blood is normally used as the infective material. Merino sheep are the usual donors, because they tend to have marked but predictable reactions. Skilled supervision and good isolation facilities should guarantee that the blood is free from other transmissible diseases or disease agents, such as bluetongue, Nairobi sheep disease, *Anaplasma,* or *Babesia.* The blood is withdrawn at the height of the temperature rise, using an anticoagulant. Fresh blood kept on ice must be used within 24 hr or preferably less. At room temperature the infectivity is often lost within 12 hr according to Alexander (1931). If a delay is expected, it should be sent deep-frozen (in dry ice or liquid nitrogen) or the live donor taken to the site of immunization.

Blood must be injected iv to be infective, which is a great disadvantage in the field. Another disadvantage is that large quantities are used (5–10 ml/dose), requiring bulky deep-freezing equipment for any large-scale stocking. The intravenous injection of blood sometimes induces shock, although this is rarely fatal. In Nigeria small quantities of homogenized infective brain are injected subcutaneously (A. A. Ilemobade, personal communication, 1979). This is obviously a great improvement over iv administration of blood, but it is still not certain whether the reliability of transmission is good (see Section III,B). In South Africa the use of filtrate of homogenized engorged infected nymphs is currently advocated (Bezuidenhout, 1981). The material is so highly infective that 1 ml can be diluted to give 20 doses, solving the storage problem of deep-frozen material. The cost of the tick-derived vaccine is also said to be much less than blood. This material is injected intravenously. Bezuidenhout advises that the injection take place over a period of 3 min, as is also usual with the blood vaccine, in order to avoid possible shock. Shock is not likely to occur with the highly diluted material. The reaction is similar whether blood, brain, or tick-derived vaccine is used.

In calves and lambs less than 3 weeks old, the reaction is often not monitored, but some mortality can be expected. The resistance of goat kids may not be adequate for this method (Thomas and Mansvelt, 1957). It is safer, especially in the case of highly susceptible purebred exotic stock, to use the infection and treatment method, and this is necessary in older animals. The immunization of pregnant animals is dangerous. The safest method is daily monitoring of the temperature and applying treatment as soon as the febrile reaction commences (see Section X). Taking daily temperatures limits the number of animals that can be handled at one time, and in the case of sheep it is probably safe to initiate tetracycline treatment systematically on Days 10 and 12 after infection (Poole, 1962a). Certain strains may vary in their average incubation period (Neitz *et al.*, 1947), so different strains may require different intervals between infection and treatment. Poole (1962b) also immunized young goats by giving systematic treatment (Days 11 and 13), but as peracute cases are more common in goats than sheep, the method is likely to be risky. Peracute cases are also relatively common in cattle, and the incubation period is rather variable. A single systematic oxytetracycline treatment given on Day 14 appeared to prolong the incubation period (Uilenberg, 1971b), but it is likely that two systematic treatments would give better results. For these reasons, it is safest to monitor the temperature once or twice per day, and treat as soon as it rises. Even then, some mortality is to be expected. Fick and Schuss (1952) and Barnard (1953) lost more than 5%, Sutton (1960) more than 4%. The results of van der Merwe (1979) were better, possibly because she treated at least twice on 2 consecutive days; she lost less than 1%. The use of sulfadimidine gave good results in severe reactions that persisted in spite of repeated oxytetracycline treatments. Close clinical supervision helped to detect beginning reactions, including petechiae of mucous membranes, hypersensitivity, and edema of the lungs, in about 3% of the animals before the febrile reactions commenced. Arnold and Asselbergs (1981) immunized cattle imported into Mozambique. The ear vein of Brahman cattle was used for inoculation of 5 ml of blood. Reacting animals were either treated for 3 consecutive days or given systematic oxytetracycline treatment. Losses due to vaccination were rare. Additional articles on heartwater immunization include those by Thomas (1957), Maré (1972), and Erasmus (1976).

The protection against field exposure is not well documented and has been discussed (see Section IX). Several authors believe that immunity wanes rather quickly, especially in cattle, if not maintained by reinfections. If, however, annual revaccination is considered on farms with light tick challenge, the possibility of shock by a second injection of foreign blood (or tick material) is a possibility.

Spickett et al. (1981) irradiated infected ticks and found that more organisms were killed by higher levels of irradiation, but attenuation did not occur.

C. ruminantium has been cryopreserved for many years at the temperature of dry ice, but few details have been published (Weiss et al., 1952; Thomas and Mansvelt, 1957). Ramisse and Uilenberg (1970) maintained the infectivity of snap-frozen blood at $-75°C$ or in liquid nitrogen, using sodium citrate, versene, or heparin as an anticoagulant, and dimethylsulfoxide (DMSO) at a final concentration of 10% as a cryoprotectant. The infectivity of snap-frozen blood was lost with or without 20% DMSO. Although Ilemobade et al. (1975) were successful in cryopreserving rapidly frozen infected blood with or without DMSO at 10%, Abdel Rahim and Shommein (1978a) could not maintain the infectivity of blood frozen without a cryoprotectant. Bezuidenhout (1981) could not detect a difference in infectivity between a freshly prepared filtrate, obtained from homogenized engorged nymphs of A. hebraeum, and snap-frozen filtrate with 10% DMSO; the infectivity of the latter was significantly decreased after being frozen and thawed four times. The infectivity of tick filtrate frozen without DMSO is far lower than when DMSO has been added (J. D. Bezuidenhout, personal communication, 1979). Brain homogenate also retains it virulence at low temperatures (Ilemobade and Blotkamp, 1978a) if preserved with DMSO (Uilenberg, 1981). Comparisons between brain material with and without cryoprotectant have not been reported. Ramisse and Uilenberg (1970) believed that glycerol as a cryoprotectant might be too toxic for the rickettsia as a result of the findings of Foggie et al. (1966) with *Ehrlichia phagocytophila,* the agent of tick-borne fever of ruminants in Europe. Mackenzie and van Rooyen (1981) found a marked loss of infectivity in cryopreserved blood with glycerol at 10% as a cryoprotectant, but not in supernatant of homogenized (mouse) liver frozen with glycerol. The toxicity of glycerol to C. ruminantium was known to Alexander (1931), who quoted experiments by P. J. du Toit and H. Graf.

Because C. ruminantium has not been grown in culture and, until recently, no strains infective for laboratory animals were available, no large-scale infectivity titrations to determine the most suitable methods of cryopreservation have been reported. Nevertheless, from the various publications it appears that (*a*) glycerol is unsuitable as a cryoprotectant, (*b*) the use of DMSO (at no more than 10%) should be strongly advised, and (*c*) rapid freezing gives good results, although no proper comparative studies between rapid and slow freezing have been reported.

An alternative approach to the prevention of heartwater, so far academic, is using animals with an innate resistance to the disease. In this way, the disease could become the latent problem that it was before the introduction of exotic stock. It is not suggested that exotic animals in Africa should be phased out and replaced by less productive local stock, but rather that an effort be made to combine disease resistance and productivity by judicious crossing. But the day is probably far off when cattle, sheep, and goats that combine good productivity with tick and disease resistance will roam the heartwater-endemic regions of Africa without immunization and tick control. Game farming or game ranching, making use of resistant wild animals, may in certain circumstances be considered.

XII. Heartwater in the Western Hemisphere

African zebu cattle were imported from Senegal into the Caribbean region in 1830 (Curasson, 1943), and West African N'dama cattle were shipped from Senegal to the Virgin Islands in 1860 or 1880, to contribute to the creation of the Senepol breed of cattle (Rouse, 1973; Hupp, 1978). It is likely that *A. variegatum* was introduced into the area on one or possibly both of these occasions. On Guadeloupe the tick is called *la tique sénégalaise* ("the Senegalese tick") (Neumann, 1899; Bück, 1966). In addition to Guadeloupe, *A. variegatum* is known to have invaded Antigua, Martinique, St. Kitts, Nevis, St. Croix, Puerto Rico, Vieques, St. Lucia, and St. Martin (Hoogstraal, 1956; Morel, 1966; Hourrigan *et al.,* 1969; Butler, 1975; Anonymous, 1976; Maldonado Capriles and Medina Gaud, 1977; Uilenberg, 1982). It recently has been found on Anguilla (G. D. Thye, personal communication, 1982). The reports of the tick in Guatemala, French Guyana, Surinam, and Venezuela (Neumann, 1899; Maldonado Capriles and Medina Gaud, 1977) are unconfirmed. Becklund (1968) reported, among exotic ticks found on animals imported into the United States, the presence of known vectors of heartwater, such as *A. gemma* on giraffe, zebra, and rhinoceros, *A. hebraeum* on rhinoceros, *A. pomposum* on topi (*Dama-*

liscus korrigum), *A. tholloni* on elephant, and *A. variegatum* on rhinoceros. Only males of these five species were collected so that there was no danger of their permanent establishment, apart from the unsuitable climatic conditions in most of the sites where they were found.

Nouval (1932) reported a decimating disease of cattle on Guadeloupe, which he called *folie du boeuf* ("cattle madness"), associated with fury and sudden death, or fever, trembling, and sometimes hemorrhagic diarrhea, followed by death in 1 or 2 days. Mauzé and Montigny (1954) and Floch *et al.* (1972) also observed a fatal disease in cattle on Guadeloupe, associated with *A. variegatum* and nervous disorders. Retrospectively, this disease was undoubtedly heartwater, as suspected by Bück (1966) and Morel (1967). The existence of heartwater on Guadeloupe was confirmed by Perreau *et al.* (1980).

The question was asked by the U.S. delegation to a meeting on tick-borne diseases (Anonymous, 1956) whether American *Amblyomma* spp. were potential vectors of heartwater. Because Perreau *et al.* (1980) did confirm its presence, a study of the potential vector role of American *Amblyomma* ticks has been started. It has been shown that *A. maculatum* is an efficient vector (Uilenberg, 1982); *A. cajennense* appears to be a poor one (see Section III,A), and experimental transmission using *A. americanum* has so far been unsuccessful.

Research on heartwater in the Caribbean area is about to commence. The first necessity is to determine the distribution of *A. variegatum* and that of *C. ruminantium,* and also that of potential American *Amblyomma* vectors. As long as the problem remains confined to some of the islands, a concerted effort may lead to success. If the mainland were to be invaded in a suitable climatic zone, the problem would become uncontrollable and could lead to a catastrophe for the cattle industry in large parts of tropical and even subtropical America.

Acknowledgments

Sincere thanks are extended to Ms. M. A. Pesman for typing the manuscript and maintaining her cheerfulness throughout. I am also grateful to the various persons acknowledged in the text as contributors to the unpublished experiments, and who also maintained their good humor during the often frustrating exercise of studying heartwater.

Addendum

After the manuscript of this article was completed and submitted, a copy was obtained of a D. V. Sc. thesis by J. L. du Plessis: "Mice infected with a *Cowdria ruminantium*–like agent as a model in the study of heartwater," University of Pretoria, 1981 (157 pages). The reader is referred to this thesis for further details on the mouse-infective organism discovered by du Plessis and Kumm (1971).

REFERENCES

Abdel Rahim, A. I., and Shommein, A. M. (1978a). *Bull. Anim. Health Prod. Afr.* **26**, 148–149.
Abdel Rahim, A. I., and Shommein, A. M. (1978b). *Bull. Anim. Health Prod. Afr.* **26**, 232–235.
Aklaku, I. K. (1980). *Bull. Off. Int. Epizoot.* **92**, 1227–1231.
Aleraj, Z., Audi, S., and Topolnik, E. (1956). *Vet. Arh.* **26**, 111–119; summary in *Vet. Bull. (London)* **28**, 185–186 (1958).
Alexander, R. A. (1931). *Rep. Dir. Vet. Serv. Anim. Ind., Onderstepoort* **17**, 89–150.
Alexander, R. Neitz, W. O., and Adelaar, T. F. (1946). *Farm. S. Afr.* **21**, 548–552.
Anderson, D. R., Hopps, H. E., Barile, M. F., and Bernheim, B. C. (1965). *J. Bacteriol.* **90**, 1387–1404.
Andreasen, M. P. (1974a). Ph.D. Thesis, Royal Veterinary and Agricultural University, Copenhagen.
Andreasen, M. P. (1974b). *Acta Pathol. Microbiol. Scand., Sect. B* **82B**, 455–456.
Anonymous (1952). "Annual Report for 1950. Veterinary Department, Kenya," pp. 16–18. Gov. Printer, Nairobi.
Anonymous (1956). *Rep. Jt. FAO/OIE Meet. Control Tick-borne Dis. Livestock* Meet. Rep. No. 1956/18.
Anonymous (1976). *U.S., Dep. Agric., Agric. Handb.* **485.**
Arnold, R. M., and Asselbergs, M. (1981). *World Anim. Rev.*, (40), 23–29.
Balozet, L. (1936). *Arch. Inst. Pasteur Tunis* **25**, 251–271.
Barnard, W. G. (1953). *Bull. Epizoot. Dis. Afr.* **1**, 300–313.
Becklund, W. W. (1968). *J. Parasitol.* **54**, 622–628.
Bell, L. J. (1980). *Acta Trop.* **37**, 319–325.
Bezuidenhout, J. D. (1981). *In* "Tick Biology and Control" (G. B. Whitehead and J. D. Gibson, eds.), pp. 41–45. Tick Research Unit, Rhodes University, Grahamstown.
Bonsma, J. C. (1944). *Farm. S. Afr.* **19**, 71–96.
Brown, C. G. D., Wilde, J. K. H., and Berger, J. (1968). *Br. Vet. J.* **124**, 325–334.
Bück, G. (1966). Note d'information sur des actions d'élevage aux Antilles, "No. 1/Doc. Institut d'Elevage et de Médecine Vétérinaire des Pays Tropicaux, Maisons-Alfort.
Burdin, M. L. (1962). *Vet. Rec.* **74**, 1371–1372.
Butler, M. C. (1975). *State Vet. J.* **30**, 279–283.
Cassard, H. (1957). *Rev. Elev. Med. Vet. Pays Trop.* **10**, 371–372.
Chabeuf, N. (1976). *Rev. Elev. Med. Vet. Pays Trop.* **29**, 259–266.
Cilli, V., and Corazzi, G. (1954). *Riv. Parassitol.* **15**, 337–352.
Clark, R. (1962). *Onderstepoort J. Vet. Res.* **29**, 25–33.
Cockrill, W. R. (1974). *In* "The Husbandry and Health of the Domestic Buffalo" (W. R. Cockrill, ed.), pp. 662–675. FAO, Rome.
Coles, J. D. W. A. (1953). *Ann. N. Y. Acad. Sci.* **56**, 457–483.
Cowdry, E. V. (1925a). *J. Exp. Med.* **42**, 231–252.
Cowdry, E. V. (1925b). *J. Exp. Med.* **42**, 253–274.
Cowdry, E. V. (1926a). *Rep. Dir. Vet. Educ. Res., Onderstepoort* **11/12**, 161–177.

Cowdry, E. V. (1926b). *Rep. Dir. Vet. Educ. Res., Onderstepoort* **11/12,** 181–196.
Cowdry, E. V. (1926c). *J. Exp. Med.* **44,** 803–814.
Curasson, G. (1943). *In* "Traité de Protozoologie Vétérinaire et Comparée" (G. Curasson, ed.), Vol. III, pp. 359–378. Vigot Frères, Paris.
Curasson, G., and Delpy, L. (1928). *Bull. Acad. Vet. Fr.* **81,** 231–244.
Cvjetanovic, V. (1956). *Vet. Arh.* **26,** 135–141; summary in *Vet. Bull. (London),* **27,** 125–126 (1957).
Cvjetanovic, V., and Berberovic, M. (1958). *Veterinaria (Sarajevo)* **7,** 215–220; summary in *Vet. Bull. (London),* **29,** 191 (1959).
da Graça, H. M. (1964). *Bull. Off. Int. Epizoot.* **62,** 963–969.
da Graça, H. M. (1966). *Bull. Off. Int. Epiz.* **66,** 751–756.
Daubney, R. (1930). *Parasitology* **22,** 260–267.
Donatien, A., and Lestoquard, F. (1937). *Arch. Inst. Pasteur Algérie* **15,** 147–187.
Donatien, A., and Lestoquard, F. (1938). *Acta Conv. Tert. Trop. Malar. Morbis* Part 1, pp. 557–564.
du Plessis, J. L. (1970a). *Onderstepoort J. Vet. Res.* **37,** 89–96.
du Plessis, J. L. (1970b). *Onderstepoort J. Vet. Res.* **37,** 147–150.
du Plessis, J. L. (1975). *Onderstepoort J. Vet. Res.* **42,** 1–14.
du Plessis, J. L. (1981a). *In* "Tick Biology and Control" (G. B. Whitehead and J. D. Gibson, eds.), pp. 47–52. Tick Research Unit, Rhodes University, Grahamstown.
du Plessis, J. L. (1981b). *Onderstepoort J. Vet. Res.* **48,** 175–176.
du Plessis, J. L., and Bezuidenhout, J. D. (1979). *J. S. Afr. Vet. Assoc.* **50,** 334–338.
du Plessis, J. L., and Kumm, N. A. L. (1971). *J. S. Afr. Vet. Med. Assoc.* **42,** 217–221.
Edelsten, R. M. (1975). *Trop. Anim. Health Prod.* **7,** 29–34.
Erasmus, J. A. (1976). *J. S. Afr. Vet. Assoc.* **47,** 143.
Evans, S. A. (1963). *Bull. Epizoot. Dis. Afr.* **11,** 232–234.
Fawi, M. T., Karrar, G., Obeid, H. M., and Campbell, R. S. F. (1977). *Bull. Anim. Health Prod. Afr.* **25,** 45–47.
Fick, J. F., and Schuss, J. (1952). *J. S. Afr. Vet. Med. Assoc.* **23**(1), 9–14.
Floch, H., Capponi, M., and Giroud, P. (1972). *Bull. Soc. Pathol. Exot.* **65,** 194–198.
Foggie, A., Lumsden, W. H. R., and McNeillage, G. J. C. (1966). *J. Comp. Pathol.* **76,** 413–416.
Girard, H., and Rousselot, R. (1947). *Encycl. Vet. Period.* **4,** 403–418.
Gradwell, D. V., van Niekerk, C. A. W. J., and Joubert, D. C. (1976). *J. S. Afr. Vet. Assoc.* **47,** 209–210.
Graf, H. (1933). *Onderstepoort J. Vet. Sci.* **1,** 285–334.
Gribble, D. H. (1969). *J. Am. Vet. Med. Assoc.* **155,** 462–469.
Groothuis, D. G., Werdler, M. E. B., van Miert, A. S. J. P. A. M., and van Duin, C. T. M. (1980). *Res. Vet. Sci.* **29,** 116–117.
Grosskopf, J. F. W. (1958). *J. S. Afr. Vet. Med. Assoc.* **29,** 329–330.
Gruss, B. (1981a). *In* "Tick Biology and Control" (G. B. Whitehead and J. D. Gibson, eds.), pp. 135–136. Tick Research Unit, Rhodes University, Grahamstown.
Gruss, B. (1981b). *J. S. Afr. Vet. Assoc.* **52,** 338.
Haig, D. A. (1952). *J. S. Afr. Vet. Med. Assoc.* **23**(3), 167–170.
Haig, D. A. (1955). *Adv. Vet. Sci.* **2,** 307–325.
Haig, D. A., Alexander, R. A., and Weiss, K. E. (1954). *J. S. Afr. Vet. Med. Assoc.* **25**(4), 45–48.
Henning, M. W. (1956). *In* "Animal Diseases in South Africa" (M. W. Henning, ed.), 3rd ed., pp. 1155–1178. Central News Agency, South Africa.
Hess, W. R., and DeTray, D. E. (1960). *Bull. Epizoot. Dis. Afr.* **8,** 317–320.

Hildebrandt, P. K., Conroy, J. D., McKee, A. E., Nyindo, M. B. A., and Huxsoll, D. L. (1973). *Infect. Immun.* **7**, 265–271.
Hofmeyr, C. F. B. (1956). *J. S. Afr. Vet. Med. Assoc.* **27**(4), 263–282.
Hoilien, C. A., Ristic, M., Huxsoll, D. L., and Rapmund, G. (1982). *Infect. Immun.* **35**, 314–319.
Hoogstraal, H. (1956). *In* "African Ixodoidea. Vol. 1. Ticks of the Sudan" (H. Hoogstraal, ed.), pp. 263–266. Department of the Navy, Bureau of Medicine and Surgery, U.S. Gov. Printing Office, Washington, D.C.
Hoogstraal, H. (1980). *J. Oman Stud., Spec. Rep.* No. 2, pp. 265–272.
Hoogstraal, H., and Kaiser, M. N. (1959). *Fieldiana, Zool.* **39**, 297–322.
Hornby, H. E. (1935). *Annu. Rep. Dep. Vet. Sci. Anim. Husb., Tanganyika, 1934* pp. 14–15.
Hourrigan, J. L., Strickland, R. K., Kelsey, O. L., Knisely, B. E., Crago, C. D., Whittaker, S., and Gilhooly, D. J. (1969). *J. Am. Vet. Med. Assoc.* **154**, 540–545.
Hudson, J. R., and Henderson, R. M. (1941). *J. S. Afr. Vet. Med. Assoc.* **12**(2), 39–49.
Hughes, M. H. (1953). *Ann. Trop. Med. Parasitol.* **47**, 299–303.
Hupp, H. D. (1978) "History and Development of Senepol Cattle," Rep. No. 11. Agricultural Experiment Station, St. Croix.
Ilemobade, A. A. (1976). Ph.D. Thesis, Ahmadu Bello University, Zaria.
Ilemobade, A. A. (1977). *Trop. Anim. Health Prod.* **9**, 177–180.
Ilemobade, A. A. (1978). *Trop. Anim. Health Prod.* **10**, 170.
Ilemobade, A. A., and Blotkamp, J. (1976). *Res. Vet. Sci.* **21**, 370–372.
Ilemobade, A. A., and Blotkamp, C. (1978a). *Trop. Anim. Health Prod.* **10**, 39–44.
Ilemobade, A. A., and Blotkamp, C. (1978b). *Tropenmed. Parasitol.* **29**, 71–76.
Ilemobade, A. A., and Leeflang, P. (1977). *Rev. Elev. Med. Vet. Pays Trop.* **30**, 149–155.
Ilemobade, A. A., Blotkamp, J., and Synge, B. A. (1975). *Res. Vet. Sci.* **19**, 337–338.
Immelman, A., and Dreyer, G. (1982). *J. S. Afr. Vet. Assoc.* **53**, 23–24.
Isoun, T. T., Akpokodje, J. U., Ikede, B. O., and Fayemi, O. (1974). *Bull. Anim. Health Prod. Afr.* **22**, 331–334.
Jackson, C. (1931). *Rep. Dir. Vet. Serv. Anim. Ind., Onderstepoort* **17**, 161–173.
Jackson, C., and Neitz, W. (1932). *Rep. Dir. Vet. Serv. Anim. Ind., Onderstepoort* **18**, 49–70.
Jongejan, F., van Winkelhoff, A. J., and Uilenberg, G. (1980). *Res. Vet. Sci.* **29**, 392–393.
Karrar, G. (1960). *Br. Vet. J.* **116**, 105–114.
Karrar, G. (1966). *Sudan J. Vet. Sci. Anim. Husb.* **6**, 83–85.
Karrar, G. (1968). *Sudan J. Vet. Sci. Anim. Husb.* **9**, 328–343.
Karrar, G., and El Hag Ali, B. (1965). *Br. Vet. J.* **121**, 28–33.
Karrar, G., Kaiser, M. N., and Hoogstraal, H. (1963). *Bull. Entomol. Res.* **54**, 509–522.
Kocan, K. M., Barron, S. J., Holbert, D., Ewing, S. A., and Hair, J. A. (1982). *Am. J. Vet. Res.* **43**, 32–35.
Kurnick, N. B. (1955). *Stain Technol.* **30**, 213–230.
Leeflang, P. (1972). *Aust. Vet. J.* **48**, 72.
Lestoquard, F. (1932). *Arch. Inst. Pasteur Alger.* **10**, 265–293.
Lewis, E. A. (1949). "Annual Report for 1947. Department of Veterinary Services, Kenya," p. 51. Gov. Printer, Nairobi.
Lounsbury, C. P. (1900). *Agric. J. Cape Good Hope* **16**, 682–687.
Mackenzie, P. K. I., and Norval, R. A. I. (1980). *Vet. Parasitol.* **7**, 265–268.
Mackenzie, P. K. I., and van Rooyen, R. E. (1981). *In* "Tick Biology and Control" (G. B. Whitehead and J. D. Gibson, eds.), pp. 33–39. Tick Research Unit, Rhodes University, Grahamstown.

Magimel, J. (1955). Thèse Doct. Vét., Alfort.
Maldonado Capriles, J., and Medina Gaud, S. (1977). *J. Agric. Univ. P.R.* **61**, 402–404.
Maré, C. J. (1972). *Trop. Anim. Health Prod.* **4**, 69–73.
Mason, J. H., and Alexander, R. A. (1938). *Acta Conv. Tert. Trop. Malar. Morbis* Part 1, pp. 526–550.
Mason, J. H., and Alexander, R. A. (1940). *J. S. Afr. Vet. Med. Assoc.* **11**(3), 98–107.
Mauzé, J., and Montigny, C. (1954). *Bull. Soc. Pathol. Exot.* **47**, 504–505.
Mettam, R. W. M. (1928). *Kenya East Afr. Med. J.* **5**(3), 68–76; summary in *Trop. Vet. Bull.* **17**, 37–38. (1929).
Mohan, R. N. (1968). *Vet. Bull. (London)* **38**, 567–576.
Morel, P. C. (1966). *Rev. Elev. Med. Vet. Pays Trop.* **19**, 307–321.
Morel, P. C. (1967). *Rev. Elev. Med. Vet. Pays Trop.* **20**, 291–299.
Morel, P. C. (1969). D. Sci. Thesis, Université de Paris.
Neitz, W. O. (1933). *J. S. Afr. Vet. Med. Assoc.* **4**(1), 24–26.
Neitz, W. O. (1935). *Onderstepoort J. Vet. Sci.* **5**, 35–40.
Neitz, W. O. (1937). *Onderstepoort J. Vet. Sci.* **9**, 37–46.
Neitz, W. O. (1939a). *Onderstepoort J. Vet. Sci.* **13**, 245–283.
Neitz, W. O. (1939b). *Berl. Muench. Tieraerztl. Wochenschr.* **9**, 134–136.
Neitz, W. O. (1940a). *J. S. Afr. Vet. Med. Assoc.* **11**(1), 11–14.
Neitz, W. O. (1940b). *J. S. Afr. Vet. Med. Assoc.* **11**(1), 15.
Neitz, W. O. (1944). *Onderstepoort J. Vet. Sci.* **20**, 25–27.
Neitz, W. O. (1947). *S. Afr. Sci.* **1**, 83.
Neitz, W. O. (1956). *Onderstepoort J. Vet. Res.* **27**, 115–163.
Neitz, W. O. (1964). *Bull. Off. Int. Epizoot.* **62**, 607–625.
Neitz, W. O. (1967). *J. S. Afr. Vet. Med. Assoc.* **38**, 129–141.
Neitz, W. O. (1968). *Bull. Off. Int. Epizoot.* **70**, 329–336.
Neitz, W. O., and Alexander, R. A. (1941). *J. S. Afr. Vet. Med. Assoc.* **12**(4), 103–111.
Neitz, W. O., and Alexander, R. A. (1945). *Onderstepoort J. Vet. Res.* **20**, 137–158.
Neitz, W. O., Alexander, R. A., and Adelaar, T. F. (1947). *Onderstepoort J. Vet. Sci.* **21**, 243–252.
Neumann, G. (1899). *Mem. Soc. Zool. Fr.* **12**, 107–294.
Norval, R. A. I. (1975). *J. Parasitol.* **61**, 737–742.
Norval, R. A. I. (1978). *Rhod. Vet. J.* **9**, 9–16.
Norval, R. A. I. (1979). *J. S. Afr. Vet. Assoc.* **50**, 289–292.
Norval, R. A. I., and Lawrence, J. A. (1979). *Zimbabwe Rhod. Agric. J.* **76**, 161–166.
Norval, R. A. I., and Mackenzie, P. K. I. (1981). *Vet. Parasitol.* **8**, 189–191.
Nouval, (1932). *Recl. Med. Vet. Exot.* **5**, 112–115.
Nyindo, M. B. A., Ristic, M., Huxsoll, D. L., and Smith, A. R. (1971). *Am. J. Vet. Res.* **32**, 1651–1658.
Owen, N. C., Littlejohn, A., Kruger, J. M., and Erasmus, B. J. (1973). *J. S. Afr. Vet. Assoc.* **44**, 397–403.
Pegram, R. G., Hoogstraal, H., and Wassef, H. Y. (1981). *Bull. Entomol. Res.* **71**, 339–359.
Pellissier, A., Troquereau, P., and Trinquier, E. (1950). *Bull. Soc. Pathol. Exot.* **43**, 168–176.
Perreau, P. (1973). *In* "Maladies tropicales du bétail" (P. Perreau, ed.), pp. 161–170. Presses Univ. de France, Paris.
Perreau, P., Morel, P. C., Barré, N., and Durand, P. (1980). *Rev. Elev. Med. Vet. Pays Trop.* **33**, 21–22.
Philip, C. B. (1974). *In* "Bergey's Manual of Determinative Bacteriology" (R. E.

Buchanan and N. E. Gibbons, eds.), 8th ed., 893–897. Williams & Wilkins, Baltimore, Maryland.
Pienaar, J. G. (1970). *Onderstepoort J. Vet. Res.* **37**, 67–78.
Pienaar, J. G., Basson, P. A., and van der Merwe, J. L. de B. (1966). *Onderstepoort J. Vet. Res.* **33**, 115–138.
Poole, J. D. H. (1961a). *J. S. Afr. Vet. Med. Assoc.* **32**, 361–365.
Poole, J. D. H. (1961b). *J. S. Afr. Vet. Med. Assoc.* **32**, 523–527.
Poole, J. D. H. (1962a). *J. S. Afr. Vet. Med. Assoc.* **33**, 35–41.
Poole, J. D. H. (1962b). *J. S. Afr. Vet. Med. Assoc.* **33**, 357–362.
Poudelet, M., Poudelet, E., and Barré, N. (1982). *Rev. Elev. Med. Vet. Pays Trop.* **35**, 23–26.
Price, J. E., and Dolan, T. T. (1980). *Vet. Rec.* **107**, 275–277.
Purchase, H. S. (1945). *Vet. Rec.* **57**, 413–414.
Rajaonarison, J. J. (1970). Thèse Doct. Vèt., Toulouse.
Rake, G., Alexander, R., and Hamre, D. M. (1945). *Science* **102**, 424–425.
Ramisse, J. (1970). *Rapp. Annu. Lab. Cent. Elev., Tananarive* pp. 14–19.
Ramisse, J. (1971). *Rapp. Annu. Lab. Cent. Elev., Tananarive* pp. 12–26.
Ramisse, J. (1972). *Rapp. Annu. Lab. Cent. Elev., Tananarive* pp. 17–24.
Ramisse, J. (1973). *In* "Rapport Annuel de l'Institut d'Elevage et de Médecine Vétérinaire des Pays Tropicaux, Maisons-Alfort," pp. 39–40.
Ramisse, J., and Uilenberg, G. (1970). *Rev. Elev. Med. Vet. Pays Trop.* **23**, 313–316.
Ramisse, J., and Uilenberg, G. (1971). *Rev. Elev. Med. Vet. Pays Trop.* **24**, 519–522.
Ristic, M., Huxsoll, D. L., Tachibana, N., and Rapmund, G. (1981). *Am. J. Trop. Med. Hyg.* **30**, 1324–1328.
Rouse, J. E. (1973). *In* "World Cattle III. Cattle of North America" (J. E. Rouse, ed.), pp. 466–470, 481. Univ. of Oklahoma Press, Norman.
Rousselot, R. (1953). *In* "Notes de parasitologie tropicale. Tome I. Parasites du sang des animaux" (R. Rousselot, ed.), pp. 75–87, 149. Vigot Frères, Paris.
Rutgers, L. J. E., van Miert, A. S. J. P. A. M., Nouws, J. F. M., and van Ginneken, C. A. M. (1980). *J. Vet. Pharmacol. Ther.* **3**, 125–132.
Schreuder, B. E. C. (1980). *Trop. Anim. Health Prod.* **12**, 25–29.
Schreuder, B. E. C., and Uilenberg, G. (1976). *Tropenmed. Parasitol.* **27**, 422–426.
Scott, G. R. (1978). *In* "Tick-borne Diseases and their Vectors" (J. K. H. Wilde, ed.), pp. 451–473. University Press, Edinburgh.
Shommein, A. H., and Abdel Rahim, A. I. (1977a). *Sudan J. Vet. Sci. Anim. Husb.* **18**, 60–64.
Shommein, A. M., and Abdel Rahim, A. I. (1977b). *Sudan J. Vet. Sci. Anim. Husb.* **18**, 65–69.
Simpson, R. M., and Wiley, A. J. (1951). *Annu. Rep. Vet. Dep. Kenya, 1949* pp. 23–27.
Spickett, A. M., Bezuidenhout, J. D., and Jacobsz, C. J. (1981). *Onderstepoort J. Vet. Res.* **48**, 13–14.
Spreull, J. (1922). *J. Dep. Landbou (Suidafrika)* **4**, 249–258; English version reported to exist: *J. Dep. Agric. (S. Afr.)* **4**, 236–245 (1922).
Stampa, S. (1969). *In* "The Biology and Control of Ticks in Southern Africa," pp. 133–150. Institute of Social and Economic Research, Rhodes University, Grahamstown.
Steck, W. (1928). *Rep. Dir. Vet. Educ. Res., Onderstepoort* **13/14**, 283–305.
Stewart, C. G., and Howell, P. G. (1981). *In* "Tick Biology and Control" (G. B. Whitehead and J. D. Gibson, eds.), pp. 29–32. Tick Research Unit, Rhodes University, Grahamstown.

Storz, J., and Page, L. A. (1971). *Int. J. Syst. Bacteriol.* **21**, 332–334.
Sutton, G. D. (1960). *J. S. Afr. Vet. Med. Assoc.* **31**, 285–288.
Synge, B. A. (1978). *Trop. Anim. Health Prod.* **10**, 45–48.
Synge, B. A., and Scott, G. R. (1976). *Annu. Rep. Cent. Trop. Vet. Med.* p. 20.
Synge, B. A., and Scott, G. R. (1978). *In* "Tick-borne Diseases and their Vectors" (J. K. H. Wilde, ed.), pp. 519–522. University Press, Edinburgh.
Theiler, A. (1905). *Annu. Rep. Dir. Agric., Transvaal, 1903–1904* pp. 190–202.
Theiler, A., and du Toit, P. J. (1926). *Bull. Soc. Pathol. Exot.* **19**, 725–737.
Theiler, A., and du Toit, P. J. (1928). *Rep. Dir. Vet. Educ. Res., Onderstepoort* **13/14**, 17–44.
Thomas, A. D. (1957). *Farm. S. Afr.* **33**(5), 19, 25.
Thomas, A. D., and Mansvelt, P. R. (1957). *J. S. Afr. Vet. Med. Assoc.* **28**, 163–168.
Tuomi, J. (1966). *Suom. Elainlaakaril.* **72**, 415–422.
Tuomi, J., and von Bonsdorff, C.-H. (1966). *J. Bacteriol.* **92**, 1478–1492.
Uilenberg, G. (1971a). *Rev. Elev. Med. Vet. Pays Trop.* **24**, 239–249.
Uilenberg, G. (1971b). *Rev. Elev. Med. Vet. Pays Trop.* **24**, 355–364.
Uilenberg, G. (1972). *Aust. Vet. J.* **48**, 534.
Uilenberg, G. (1977). "Second FAO Expert Consultation on Research on Tick-borne Diseases and their Vectors," AGA:TD/77/3. FAO, Rome.
Uilenberg, G. (1980). In "Ticks and Tick-borne Diseases" (L. A. Y. Johnston and M. G. Cooper, eds.), pp. 1–3. Australian Veterinary Association, Sydney.
Uilenberg, G. (1981). *In* "Diseases of Cattle in the Tropics" (M. Ristic and I. McIntyre, eds.), pp. 345–360. Martinus Nijhoff Publishers, The Hague.
Uilenberg, G. (1982). *Am. J. Vet. Res.* **43**, 1279–1282.
Uilenberg, G., and Niewold, T. A. (1981). *Rev. Elev. Med. Vet. Pays Trop.* **34**, 267–270.
Uilenberg, G., Silayo, R. S., Mpangala, C., Tondeur, W., Tatchell, R. J., and Sanga, H. J. N. (1977). *Tropenmed. Parasitol.* **28**, 499–506.
Uilenberg, G., Corten, J. J. F. M., and Dwinger, R. H. (1982). *Vet. Q.* **4**, 106–107.
Utech, K. B. W., Wharton, R. H., and Kerr, J. D. (1978). *Aust. J. Agric. Res.* **29**, 885–895.
van der Merwe, L. (1979). *J. S. Afr. Vet. Assoc.* **50**, 323–325.
van Heerden, J., and van Heerden, A. (1981). *J. S. Afr. Vet. Assoc.* **52**, 173–175.
van Vorstenbosch, C. J. A. H. V., Uilenberg, G., and van Dijk, J. E. (1978). *Res. Vet. Sci.* **24**, 214–221.
van Winkelhoff, A. J., and Uilenberg, G. (1981). *Trop. Anim. Health Prod.* **13**, 160–164.
Weiss, K. E., Haig, D. A., and Alexander, R. A. (1952). *Onderstepoort J. Vet. Res.* **25**(4), 41–50.
Young, E. (1970). *Zool. Afr.* **5**, 167–177.
Young, E., and Basson, P. A. (1973). *J. S. Afr. Vet. Assoc.* **44**, 185–186.

Diagnosis and Control of Bovine Paratuberculosis (Johne's Disease)

HANS P. RIEMANN AND BABIKER ABBAS

Department of Epidemiology and Preventive Medicine, University of California, Davis, California

I. Introduction 481
II. The Host–Parasite Relationship in Johne's Disease 483
    A. The Agent 483
    B. Mode of Infection and Pathogenesis 483
III. The Diagnosis of Johne's Disease 485
    A. Cultivation of the Agent 485
    B. Methods of Microscopy 486
    C. Immunological and Serological Tests 486
    D. Trends in the Diagnosis 488
    E. Problems in the Diagnosis of Subclinical Johne's Disease 491
IV. Efforts toward Control of Johne's Disease 495
    A. The Removal of Infected and Suspect Animals 495
    B. Vaccination 497
    C. General Recommendations 500
V. Summary 501
    References 502

I. Introduction

The failure to formulate an effective control program for bovine paratuberculosis, or Johne's disease, despite efforts starting as early as the first decades of this century, has served to maintain an interest in research on this disease. The major problem encountered to date has been the low accuracy of laboratory diagnostic procedures to identify infected animals.

Johne's disease is predominantly a subclinical infection (Reinders, 1963). Unknown factors cause approximately 5% of the infected animals to exhibit clinical Johne's disease signs, whereas the majority of infected animals show no signs (Jensen, 1948).

Despite its low incidence, Johne's disease is known to cause significant economic losses in dairy cattle (Buergelt and Duncan, 1980), sheep (Stamp and Watt, 1954), and goats (Baas, 1976). In cattle, the disease has been associated with infertility, long intercalving intervals, and extensive culling (Buergelt and Duncan, 1980). Johne's disease also has been reported to cause significant losses in revenue as a result of lower milk production and shorter life expectancy of affected cattle (Sorensen and Flint, 1967; Anonymous, 1971; Merkal et al., 1975). A study conducted by the Food and Agricultural Organization (FAO) of the United Nations (Worthington, 1963) concluded that Johne's disease was one of the most serious diseases affecting the cattle industry. A survey in England and Wales based on culture of mesenteric lymph nodes from cattle indicated that 11% of all cattle were infected (Withers, 1959). Other surveys revealed that 20–30% of cattle sent to knackeries or casualty slaughter were infected (Peck, 1957). In Canada, Julian (1975) stated that the disease was a cause of serious economic losses in individual herds despite its low clinical incidence. Johne's disease is also widespread in the United States (Kopecky, 1973), and it would probably be found wherever good efforts were undertaken toward its diagnosis (Larsen, 1972). Studies in Wisconsin (Kopecky, 1977) and California (Riemann et al., 1979) showed that the majority of selected herds studied had occurrences of Johne's disease. There are no reliable prevalence estimates of clinical or subclinical Johne's disease in the United States.

Denmark had an experimental control program with indemnity paid to farmers from 1974 to 1975. During this period paratuberculosis was detected in 5% of herds at risk, but the real prevalence was undoubtedly higher because many subclinical cases probably were not reported. The real prevalence is assumed to be about 20%. The detected infected herds had an average prevalence of clinical cases of 8% (J. C. Flensburg, personal communication, 1979).

Bovine Johne's disease has been the subject of extensive studies, and reviews of the disease have also been published (Julian, 1975; Katic, 1969, 1977; DeLisle, 1978). The main emhasis in this article will be on the diagnosis of Johne's disease and the efforts undertaken toward control and eradication.

II. The Host—Parasite Relationship in Johne's Disease

A. THE AGENT

Mycobacterium paratuberculosis, the causative agent of Johne's disease, is a short, slender rod, 1–2-μm-long and 0.5-μm-wide, generally straight, nonmotile, gram-positive and, strongly acid-fast (Merchant and Berner, 1971).

After its initial isolation from diseased cattle (Johne and Frothingham, 1895), *M. paratuberculosis* was subsequently isolated from a variety of domestic and wild animals. Natural infection was reported in mule deer (Katic, 1961), bighorn sheep, and Rocky Mountain goats (Williams *et al.,* 1979), white-tailed deer (Libke and Walton, 1975), roe deer (Hellermark, 1966), European red deer (Vance, 1961), moose (Soltys *et al.,* 1967), axis deer and fallow deer (Riemann *et al.,* 1979), and elk (Jessup *et al.,* 1981). Although Johne's disease is of chief importance in ruminants, investigators have reported the presence of the infection in monogastric animals. The disease was reported in a captive pygmy ass (Van Ulsen, 1970) and was suspected in pigs (Ringdal, 1963). Experimental infection resulted in clinical signs in chickens (Larsen and Moon, 1972), and both lesions and clinical disease in horses (Larsen *et al.,* 1974). No reliable laboratory model was found, although a variety of laboratory animals can readily be infected (Harding, 1959). The main problem with laboratory animal models for Johne's disease is probably that the incubation period required to obtain expression of clinical signs is too long to allow practical use of small laboratory animals (Lominiski *et al.,* 1956). However, because pathological lesions develop quite readily in experimental animals (e.g., mice and hamsters), these animals could probably be used in drug or vaccine trials, or in evaluating the pathogenicity of strains of *M. paratuberculosis* (Larsen and Miller, 1978; Abbas, 1983).

B. MODE OF INFECTION AND PATHOGENESIS

Under natural conditions, infection is acquired predominantly by ingestion of the organism in contaminated feed or water. Pasture contamination leads to the persistence of the organism in the environment of animals, because *M. paratuberculosis* can survive about 270 days in pond water (Larsen *et al.,* 1956), at least 246 days in bovine feces (Lovell *et al.,* 1944), and as long as 252 days in cattle slurry (Jorgensen, 1977).

The high prevalence of infection in young animals in one study (Riemann et al., 1979) suggested vertical spread of infection. It is known that congenital infection is possible (Kopecky et al., 1967). Uterine and fetal infections have been reported from cattle not showing clinical signs of Johne's disease (Pearson and McClelland, 1955; Doyle, 1958), and in one instance, placentitis and abortion followed clinical disease in a cow (Omar et al., 1967).

The intestinal tract is the main site of primary infection and bacterial proliferation (Gilmour, 1965a). In calves (Gilmour, 1965b) as well as in adults given the organism for the first time (Payne and Rankin, 1961), lesions appeared within 1 to 2 months in the intestinal mucosa and lymph nodes, and large numbers of organisms were then shed for varying lengths of time. After the development of lesions (Nisbet et al., 1962; Jubb and Kennedy, 1970; Buergelt et al., 1978a), the organism may be transported from the intestinal mucosa and adjacent lymph nodes to almost every organ (Hole, 1958; Kluge et al., 1968). M. paratuberculosis has been shown to resist degradation by macrophages (Bendixen et al., 1981), and the latter are most likely the vehicles by which the organisms migrate to secondary target organs.

In Johne's disease, not only the extensive tissue destruction, but also immediate hypersensitivity mediated by histamine, have been suggested as causative of initial diarrhea. Merkal et al. (1970), who first suggested this association, were able to reduce the severity of clinical signs in experimentally infected cattle through the administration of large amounts of antihistamines. The findings of Buergelt et al. (1978a) seem to further implicate hypersensitivity-mediated mechanisms in the pathogenesis of Johne's disease. From their detailed cytologic work on naturally infected cattle, they noted that mast cells, in the form of "globule leukocytes," were closely associated with intestinal lesions in clinical cases of disease. Globule leukocytes are mast cells loaded with vesicles of pharmacologically active amines. This, however, is circumstantial evidence, and further work is needed to substantiate the hypothesis of immune mechanisms in the pathogenesis of Johne's disease. The disease has been widely accepted as a malabsorption syndrome, resulting in protein loss and subsequent starvation (Patterson et al., 1967, 1968; Patterson, 1968). Hole and McClay (1959) expressed the view that familial susceptibility is a significant factor in the development of clinical signs, but other investigators have indicated that age at the time of first infection may be the most important factor (Hagen, 1938; Taylor, 1953; Doyle, 1956a). Rankin (1962a,b) found no difference in the development of clinical signs of Johne's disease in calves exposed to infection at 6 months of age or cows naturally exposed at 4 years of age. In infected herds, it has been estimated that carrier animals were up to 20 times as common as clinical cases (Withers, 1959). The carrier state in Johne's disease will be discussed further in the section dealing with diagnosis. Shorthorn and Jersey breeds of cattle were reported to have a higher incidence of infection with *M. paratuberculosis* (Doyle, 1956a; Sorensen and Flint, 1967; Jorgensen, 1972), but age of animals might have been a confounding factor in comparing incidence among breeds in these studies.

III. The Diagnosis of Johne's Disease

A. Cultivation of the Agent

In the first successful effort to isolate *M. paratuberculosis,* Twort and Ingram (1913) used the following method: cultures of *Mycobacterium phlei* (intended to supply growth-potentiating factor) were killed by moise heat and the growth was scraped off and dried. The bacilli were then ground in a mortar and added in 0.5 to 1.0% concentration to Dorset's egg medium containing 4% glycerine. On this medium, primary cultures of *M. paratuberculosis* consisted of tiny dull-white colonies, rarely visible to the naked eye before 4 weeks had elapsed. Twort and Ingram stated that the growth factor was not specifically present in acid-fast bacilli but could be obtained by alcohol extraction from a variety of sources, including various vegetable substances such as currant grapes, figs, oats, linseed, and the fungus *Cantherellus aurantiacus*. Minett (1942) was able to isolate *M. paratuberculosis* from fecal and tissue samples of clinical cases of Johne's disease after using 20% antiformin as an agent to eliminate contaminants. Among several media tested for ability to support growth, he suggested a medium composed of whole egg, 1% *M. phlei* extract, and 4% glycerol added. Taylor (1950) reported that the best results were obtained with a medium containing over 50% egg yolk with *M. phlei* extract. The growth-potentiating factor was a matter of some debate until Francis *et al.* (1956) isolated in pure form from *M. phlei* a compound with iron-sequestering capacity and named it mycobactin. Part of the mycobactin dependence of newly isolated strains of *M. paratuberculosis* on such complex media as egg yolk or serum agar was attributed to the inability of the organisms to extract sufficient ferric iron from such media (Nemeto, 1969). The need for mycobactin could be eliminated if 0.1% ferric ammonium citrate was added to the medium; growth was equal to that on mycobactin-supplemented media (Morrison, 1965; Merkal and Curran, 1974).

Considerable improvement of the culture procedure as well as of the bacteriological diagnosis of Johne's disease has been introduced by Merkal and co-workers (Larsen and Merkal, 1961; Merkal and Larsen, 1962; Merkal et al., 1964; Merkal and Richard, 1972). Their method is as outlined here: suspected tissues are digested with 0.5% trypsin for 20 to 30 min; the digest is decontaminated with benzalkonium chloride and allowed to settle for 18 to 24 hr. Then 0.1 ml of sediment is inoculated on four slants of modified Herrold's egg yolk medium, three of the slants containing 0.2% mycobactin and one without mycobactin. The cultures are incubated for 12 to 14 weeks and inspected every 2 weeks. Fecal samples are treated similarly except for digestion. The fecal sample (1 gm) is shaken in 40 ml of water, and 5 ml of the supernatant are treated with a disinfectant to kill contaminants. This method of culture has become the method of choice for most laboratories and is fairly standardized (U.S. Department of Agriculture, 1974). In primary isolation the organism may take 9–12 weeks to develop visible colonies. However, in practice, cultures are not discarded until after 14 weeks of incubation. Growth occurs at 20 to 43°C, with the optimum growth rate at 39°C.

Biochemical tests useful in other mycobacteria have not been useful in the identification of *M. paratuberculosis* (Merkal and Thurston, 1966; Gunnarson and Fodstad, 1979a). The identification of this organism relies on slow growth (9–14 weeks) and mycobactin dependence on initial isolation.

B. Methods of Microscopy

Microscopic methods of diagnosis include the histologic examination of biopsy material obtained from the mesenteric lymph nodes (most commonly iliac lymph nodes) and the staining of rectal scrapings with the Ziehl–Neelsen acid-fast procedure (Merkal et al., 1968b). Rectal scrapings may not correctly identify a diseased animal except in severe long-standing infections, and instead a liver biopsy has been recommended (Buergelt et al., 1978a).

C. Immunological and Serological Tests

Allergic tests for bovine paratuberculosis have been used extensively, they were discarded because of unsatisfactory performance. There were consistently large numbers of false-positive and false-negative reactors (Green, 1941; Hole, 1953; Larsen et al., 1963a; Merkal et al., 1968a), and despite efforts to improve the purity of the allergens (Annau, 1959; Ross et al., 1967), the improvements, particularly in specificity, were small. The skin test utilizes Johnin (Johnson and Cox, 1942) purified protein derivatives (PPD) prepared from *M. paratuberculosis* or from *M. avium*, 0.2 ml of which is injected intradermally (Hagen and Zeissig, 1929; Minett, 1935). In a sensitized animal a localized cellular response occurs (delayed hypersensitivity), with swelling of the skin at the injection site (Knost and Watson, 1943). The test is usually read after 48 hr. This test is less satisfactory than what would be imagined from its current widespread use. Systemic tests using intravenous Johnin have been widely used and are still used to a limited extent. There are two forms of intravenous Johnin testing: the temperature response and the white blood cell response. In the former, an elevation of body temperature of 1.5°F 6 hr after injection of 2 to 4 ml of Johnin is considered significant, whereas in the latter a positive result is indicated when the ratio of neutrophils to lymphocytes 6 hr after injection is more than twice the ratio of neutrophils to lymphocytes before injection (Larsen and Kopecky, 1965; Kopecky *et al.*, 1971). Both tests are of most value in the differentiation of clinical Johne's disease from other causes of chronic diarrhea (Larsen, 1972). The greatest problem with the allergic test is the lack of persistence of the reaction; reactors often become anergic (Green, 1941; Larsen and Johnson, 1949; Larsen *et al.*, 1963a). In an overall comparison with cultural and histological methods of diagnosis the intradermic Johnin test was shown to have a specifity of 35 to 40% and a sensitivity of 50 to 55% (Colburn and Cutright, 1977).

The complement fixation test (CFT) for Johne's disease has been consistently found to be unreliable in detecting subclinical cases of the disease (Jensen, 1956; Larsen *et al.*, 1963b; Thoen, 1979). Also, its agreement with culture or microscopic diagnosis of the disease was not great (Merkal *et al.*, 1968b; Merkal, 1970). It has been used in Europe as the official screening test, but subsequent evidence showed that it is not suitable for that purpose (Rankin, 1961; Goudswaard *et al.*, 1976). The test is positive in advanced cases of the infection, but this seropositive state is transient and the level of antibody usually diminishes after the development of clinical disease (Merkal *et al.*, 1968b). It has been suggested that antibodies may combine with antigen in the intestine. Sigurdsson (1956) suggested that the problem with the complement fixation test was related to the impurity of antigen preparations employed at that time. However, subsequent efforts utilizing more highly purified preparations met with similar results (Rice *et al.*, 1959, 1960; Yugi *et al.*, 1966a,b). In some subsequent applications of the complement fixation test, specificity has ranged between 50 and 55%, with sensitivity ranging between 60 and 63% (Colburn and Cutright,

1977). The hemagglutination test was adapted for Johne's disease by Larsen et al. (1953) and was evaluated with sera from naturally infected cattle. It was found to be inferior to the complement fixation and allergic tests, despite its enhanced sensitivity (Larsen et al., 1965; Merkal, 1973; Goudswaard et al., 1976).

The gel diffusion precipitin test was first used by Parlett and Youmans (1958) to detect antibodies against mycobacterial antigens. Long and Topp (1964) performed the test with serums from tuberculous cattle, but they failed to obtain positive test results from tuberculin-reactor cattle that at necropsy had tuberculous lesions. The applicability of this test for Johne's disease was demonstrated with sera of sheep that were inoculated with whole cells, cell walls, or protoplasm of *M. paratuberculosis* in incomplete Freund's adjuvant. The test was of excellent quality in classifying exposed and unexposed sheep, and with sera of high titer, 5–10 precipitin bands were formed (Merkal et al., 1968a). The test also was found to be satisfactory for the detection of Johne's disease in naturally infected goats (Sherman and Gezon, 1980). Application of the precipitin test to the diagnosis of Johne's disease in cattle was not satisfactory, however. Goudswaard et al. (1976) found it relatively insensitive for the detection of subclinical and clinical cases of the disease as compared to complement fixation, hemagglutination, or fluorescent antibody tests.

D. Trends in the Diagnosis

Beginning with the 1970s, the literature reflects efforts to adapt old tests or to develop new ones, and to evaluate them for the diagnosis of Johne's disease. This period featured reevaluation of the fluorescent antibody technique, the leukocyte migration and lymphocyte immunostimulation tests, and also the adaptation of enzyme-linked immunosorbent assay (ELISA) and radioimmunoassay.

The fluorescent antibody test was adapted for mycobacterial diagnosis by Bennedsen (1969). The test was subsequently adopted for Johne's disease and evaluated by Gilmour and other investigators (Gilmour 1968, 1971; Gilmour and Gardiner, 1969; Gilmour and Angus, 1976a,b). Of particular interest is the finding that, using homologous sera produced in rabbits, the test could distinguish between *M. avium* and *M. paratuberculosis* (Gilmour, 1971). Otherwise, the test still suffered from a lack of sensitivity and specificity (Gilmour, 1968). In one field trial, however (Gilmour and Angus, 1976a), the test was positive for only 4 cattle of 100 that did not have bacteriological or pathological evidence of infection, as compared to 20 animals positive by the complement fixation test. In 26 infected animals from another herd, the fluorescent antibody test was positive in 16, whereas the complement fixation test was positive in 12. In another 92 cattle with no evidence of *M. paratuberculosis* infection, the fluorescent antibody test was positive in 7 and complement fixation in 22. In a comparison of five serological tests, the fluorescent antibody and complement fixation tests were both equally sensitive in detecting subclinically infected cattle, whereas other tests were found to be insensitive. It was concluded that the complement fixation and fluorescent antibody tests should be used together for the best results in screening cattle for Johne's disease (Goudswaard et al., 1976). Hence, there is at least some evidence in favor of further evaluating one surveillance test for Johne's disease.

In vitro assays of cellular immunity have included the migration inhibition test and the lymphocyte transformation test. Migration inhibition tests measure the production of lymphokine (migration inhibition factor, MIF) by its effect on a target cell population (other lymphocytes or macrophages). The reaction of sensitized lymphocytes from an infected animal with the antigen releases into the medium the MIF that inhibits the migration of macrophages (David et al., 1964; Clausen, 1971). The lymphocyte transformation test measures the blastogenic response of lymphocytes to specific antigen stimulation (Dutton, 1967). The reaction can be detected with a microscope, but more quantitative results can be obtained by measuring the amount of a DNA precursor taken up by these cells for DNA replication (Ferket et al., 1971).

The migration inhibition test was first evaluated for Johne's disease by Bendixen (1977). It was found to perform very well on some of the clinical cases but was not satisfactory for the detection of subclinical infections. Such animals showed weak responses to antigenic stimulation of their lymphocytes. The author explained this reaction of preclinically infected cows as a result of immunological tolerance. However, false-positive reactions were explained on the basis of an earlier experience with *M. paratuberculosis* followed by a termination of the infection by the lymphoreticular system, resulting in primed immunocompetent cells that reacted to the test. It was concluded that any diagnostic test using antigenic stimulation *in vivo* or *in vitro* will often be positive without the presence of bacteria.

Buergelt et al. (1977) applied the lymphocyte stimulation test to a group of experimentally infected cattle and were able to follow the extent of infection with a sensitivity of 90% and a specificity of 84%. However, in a subsequent report from a study of a naturally infected herd, also using the lymphocyte stimulation test, the same authors (Buergelt et al., 1978b) were not able to confirm the previous findings despite the enhanced sensitivity of the test in comparison to other test procedures. In three test series from the same herd, the test was positive in 68, 40, and 45% of the animals, and fecal culture was positive in 6, 2.4, and 2.6% of the animals, respectively. Because the only way of evaluating a test for Johne's disease is by comparison to fecal culture, the lymphocyte transformation test was not recommended as a means of surveillance for Johne's disease. Alhaji et al. (1974) reported that they were able to differentiate by the lymphocyte stimulation test between a cow infected with *M. bovis* and another infected with *M. paratuberculosis,* but their data are too limited to permit an inference with respect to recommending this test for diagnostic purposes. Colburn and Cutright (1977) applied the lymphocyte stimulation test to 57 cattle among which there were 9 diseased animals; the test identified only 3 cattle as such and reacted in a false-positive manner in 11 cattle (25% false positive).

Enzyme-linked immunosorbent assay (ELISA) has been developed largely by Engvall and Perlmann (1971). The test detects specific antigen–antibody binding via an enzyme-labeled antispecies antibody, the reaction being optically detected by the effect of the label enzyme on its substrate. A review of the utility of the test indicates that it has been both sensitive and specific for a variety of diseases (Schuurs and Van Weemen, 1977). Nassau et al. (1976) found the test to be potentially useful in the diagnosis of tuberculosis in human patients. Jorgensen and Jensen (1978) used ELISA for the detection of antibodies to *M. paratuberculosis* in cattle. They reported that one test could detect all of the bacteriologically positive animals, with titers as high as two to four times those detected by complement fixation. For bacteriologically negative cows, ELISA was also negative. This report indicates that ELISA is both sensitive and specific for Johne's disease. The results of this work are, however, based on experimentally infected animals, and an evaluation of the test under field conditions is necessary before definitive statements can be made concerning its reliability in diagnosing subclinical infections in cattle. Ocadiz (1981) recently evaluated ELISA in a herd of goats in California and found a great disparity between ELISA and complement fixation, with an enhanced sensitivity on the part of ELISA. The author concluded that ELISA may be a useful test provided that purer antigens of *M. paratuberculosis* are employed. The lack of agreement between ELISA and complement fixation also has been encountered in an effort to evaluate ELISA for the surveillance of Johne's disease in cattle (Abbas, 1981). It is clear from the foregoing that more work on ELISA in Johne's disease is needed.

Radioimmunoassay (RIA) relies on competition for antibody between a radioactive indicator ligand and its unlabeled counterpart in the test sample: the higher the level of unlabeled antigen in the test sample, the less labeled antigen is bound (Farr, 1960). The concentration of the antigen in the test sample is determined by comparison with a calibration curve prepared with purified ligand at known concentrations. The solid-phase version of this test is an economical, rapid, and sensitive procedure. In one popular version, antibodies to the ligand are easily adsorbed to the walls of plastic tubes. When the labeled ligand is introduced it binds to the antibody; and in the presence of unlabeled ligand, less of the former is specifically bound and the excess is decanted (Rose and Friedman, 1976). This latter procedure was adopted by Warsaae (1978), who evaluated the diagnostic features of RIA employing ^{125}I-labeled purified protein derivative from *M. paratuberculosis*. The test was shown to be promising as judged by a high sensitivity (97%) and a specificity of 74%, together with ease of performance and rapidity. In this test there is a need for special equipment. Also, the test needs evaluation under field conditions, because Warsaae (1978) used complement fixation test results as the state of nature.

O. Aalund (unpublished data, 1982) analyzed extensive data from 12 infected and 20 noninfected herds that were monitored by fecal culture, lymphocyte transformation, complement fixation, RIA, and ELISA, and concluded that immunological results could only "render vague circumstantial evidence for the infectious status of an animal in regard to *M. paratuberculosis* infection." Statistical analysis indicated that ELISA and lymphocyte transformation may have a potential value when conducted simultaneously on Johne's disease-affected cattle.

E. Problems in the Diagnosis of Subclinical Johne's Disease

From the foregoing it is evident that the diagnosis of subclinical infections with *M. paratuberculosis* is problematic. An analysis of the situation is thus necessary in order to understand the origin of the problem.

From the outset, the status of a clinically affected animal need not be of great concern. First, there may be little difficulty in diagnosing a case of clinical Johne's disease in the usual situation (Smythe, 1935). Differential diagnosis and unresponsiveness of the condition to symptomatic antidiarrheal treatment are readily resorted to, with rather definite conclusions. Also, there is usually little or no difficulty in this situation in deciding what should be done with the particular animal; a clinically sick animal is usually a poor performer and can be economically disposed of.

In control or eradication programs, the intention is to destroy the infective reservoir of the etiological agent, and in Johne's disease this usually resides in the subclinical carriers, animals that show no obvious signs of being infected (Gilmour, 1965a; Blood and Henderson, 1968). The predominance of subclinical cases of Johne's disease in an infected herd maintains the organism indefinitely (Melechov, 1967), and the persistence of *M. paratuberculosis* in the soil for as long as a year further increases its spreading potential (Larsen, 1970). In considering the performance of a diagnostic test, there are several outcomes. The tests may be negative although the animal is actually infected. This is reflected in the number of false-negative reactions and limits the sensitivity of the test, a feature encountered in most tests when used in the field on naturally infected animals. Alternatively, the tests may be positive, although the animal is not infected. This is reflected in the number of samples reacting in a false-positive manner. This has also been encountered as a feature of various tests evaluated for Johne's disease.

A diagnostic test could fail to disclose the status of a subclinical *M. paratuberculosis* infection for several reasons. Absence of antibodies (or other material) sought by the test procedure in the specimen is one cause of false-negative reactions. Thus fecal samples may not contain culturable bacilli because of their irregular shedding by an infected animal (Minett, 1942; Payne and Rankin, 1961; Merkal, 1970). This will result in a misclassification of the natural state of the animal. Likewise, infected animals may not have an immune reaction detectable by the conventional antibody or cellular immunity assays (Merkal, 1973; Goudswaard *et al.*, 1976; O. Aalund, unpublished data, 1982). Because of these observations accumulated over the years, several scholars speculated that Johne's disease is in essence a truly "spectral" disease. Although this notion was implicit in the observations of many former workers, Larsen (1973) gave the first classification of animals on a herd basis to encompass this suggested spectrum. According to that classification, animals in an infected herd could belong in one of four categories: (1) clinically ill, (2) asymptomatic shedders, which include (3) carrier animals, and (4) uninfected. Duncan *et al.* (1978) suggested a classification evolving more from the immunologic experience of the animal. According to this "immune spectrum" of Johne's disease, no serologic or cellular immunity test will identify all animals in the disease spectrum.

1. There are infected resistant animals that control their infections but are unable to rid themselves completely of *M. paratuberculosis*. Such animals do not react in antibody assays, and as they have too small a bacterial load, they shed too few organisms to be detected by routine fecal cultures. Because the circulating lymphocytes of these animals are sensitized to *M. paratuberculosis* antigens, their response to the lymphocyte transformation test will be positive.

2. If the host fails to control the infection, there will be an increase in the bacterial load, antibodies will appear in the serum, and an increasing number of bacilli will be shed in the feces. These animals, the "intermediate" infected, have no or minimal signs of Johne's disease, although they continue to shed moderate to large numbers of organisms.

3. The advanced diseased animals show some variation in antibody level that will be demonstrated by an immunodiffusion test, complement fixation test, and Johnin test.

However, a certain proportion of these animals will not have circulating antibodies and will fail to react positively in a number of tests. Intradermal skin testing of "advanced diseased" animals has indicated that some of them will be anergic. Similarly, some of these animals will not respond on the lymphocyte transformation test, suggesting an impaired cell-mediated immune response.

Bendixen (1978) suggested that three distinct immunological episodes occur in Johne's disease: immunity, tolerance, and hypersensitivity. Immune animals are resistant to the disease, which is attributed to an optimally functioning immune system at the time of exposure. Such animals will probably react positively to *in vivo* and *in vitro* tests for cell-mediated immunity. Whether permanent exposure to the bacteria is necessary to maintain this state is not discussed by Bendixen. Tolerance is postulated to describe animals that are apparently healthy but are harboring and shedding bacteria. Animals in this category will react negatively in cell-mediated immunity tests and may or may not give positive antibody responses. The hypersensitivity state is the condition that signals the onset of clinical disease. This is viewed as a result of a breakdown of tolerance. These animals will react positively in tests for cell-mediated immunity unless under the influence of inhibitory factors, excessive loads of antigen, or *in extremis*. As tolerance begins to wane, antibody synthesis starts, so that most animals are positive in antibody assays.

Other phenomena, apart from the postulated spectral nature of this disease, may come into play to confuse the outcome of a diagnostic test. Davies et al. (1974) found a humoral suppressor of lymphocyte transformation in sera from cows suffering from clinical Johne's disease. The presence of this factor is in agreement with the inability of the animal to mount a delayed hypersensitivity reaction to various antigens to which it had been sensitized. The function of such inhibitory factors was interpreted as a feedback control on cell-mediated immunity, to prevent excessive destruction during chronic intracellular infection.

An immune assay could fail to classify an uninfected animal correctly, because the antigenic material employed in the test is not sufficiently pure to avoid cross-reaction with antibodies directed toward similar but not identical antigens. Even with what may be considered unrelated antigens, low-affinity interactions may occur and become stabilized by nonspecific forces (Chaparas, 1981).

Mycobacteria have four classes or groups of antigens (Grange, 1979);

Group (i)   antigens are common to all mycobacteria, and some are shared with related bacterial genera (nocardia, corynebacteria).
Group (ii) antigens occur in fast growers and also in nocardia.
Group (iii) antigens are restricted to the slow-growing group.
Group (iv) antigens are peculiar to each individual species.

Cross-reactions are thus a possibly significant factor contributing to a low specificity of immune assay procedures. The need for highly purified antigens in the diagnosis of mycobacterial diseases has been stressed several times (Lind, 1965; Closs et al., 1975; Janicki et al., 1976; Chaparas, 1979). Encouraging results have been obtained with M. tuberculosis (Daniel and Anderson, 1977, 1978) and M. bovis (Nagal et al., 1981). When partially purified antigens were used in affinity chromatography against monospecific antisera, antigens of remarkable specificity were isolated.

Few attempts have been made to isolate specific antigens from M. paratuberculosis using chemical extraction agents such as phenol, alcohol, and urea combined with gel filtration methods. The fractions obtained in this way have, however, proved to be deficient with regard to either sensitivity or specificity (Annau, 1959; Rice et al., 1959, 1960; Yugi et al., 1966a,b; Ross et al., 1967).

A considerable amount of effort in this area has been directed toward the perfection of the complement fixation test, but the results have indicated little improvement in the specificity or sensitivity of the test for detection of Johne's disease.

Gunnarson and Fodstad (1979b) found that *M. paratuberculosis* was characterized by 44 different antigens, only 2 and possibly 3 of which were species specific. A considerable amount of cross-reaction was noted with *M. avium* and BCG. Cross-reactions between *M. paratuberculosis* and other organisms were not studied.

The mycolic acids of mycobacteria are closely related to those of nocardia and corynebacteria (Larsen and Johnson, 1947; Minden *et al.*, 1972). This, together with the antigenic relatedness among mycobacteria (Stanford, 1972; Daniel, 1976), makes it necessary to take into consideration the role of cross-reaction in the diagnosis of Johne's disease. Because mycobacteria are widely prevalent in the environment (Fodstad, 1977; Grange, 1979), sensitization could readily occur; thus the use of antigens with high specificity becomes paramount.

IV. Efforts toward Control of Johne's Disease

Despite the relatively long history of Johne's disease, control and preventive measures are still predominantly at the experimental level. Although a few efforts seem to be fairly well evaluated with regard to their outcome, some still await field testing. Several other control strategies are offered on what seems to be pure speculation. The lack of uniformity is noticeable among these, as well as in the whole area of the control of Johne's disease. This admittedly is due to the lack of a standardized, universally acceptable surveillance procedure. Only control programs that have been fairly well evaluated will be presented in this section. Also, because documentation for the various experiences is not always sufficiently detailed, emphasis will be placed on certain control programs that may be considered as typical of a group of similar endeavors. Some of the recommendations for the control of Johne's disease that have been made will also be reviewed.

The various programs examined in this review can be considered under two broad categories: (*a*) removal of suspect and shedder animals (including clinical cases) and (*b*) vaccination. Both programs feature sanitation and management as significant supportive procedures.

A. The Removal of Infected and Suspect Animals

This approach was adopted in several European localities, but the experience in northern Ireland seems to be the best documented (Pearson, 1964; Pearson and Ogg, 1967) and is presented here as an example of methods of control applicable in situations where the disease is not widespread. The Irish program consisted of two voluntary control programs to encourage farmers to identify and slaughter clinical cases and carriers (Pearson and Ogg, 1967). The program was designed to compensate farmers for slaughter of clinically ill cattle. The responsibility for slaughter, disinfection of premises, and so forth, rested with the Ministry of Agriculture (northern Ireland). Suspect nonclinical carriers could not be purchased, and a further Johne's Disease Experimental Program (JDE) was introduced later to detect such animals. Johnin and avian tuberculin skin tests were applied at the time of an initial CFT. Animals with a positive Johnin reaction and/or those suspected of *M. paratuberculosis* contact were then subjected to a second CFT 14–17 days later. A rise in titer was regarded as indicative of an existing *M. paratuberculosis* infection. It was acknowledged that the tests used were not specific and that, consequently, the percentage error may have been high (Pearson, 1964).

Initially, the tests were applied at 6-month intervals for as long as reactors remained, but when these ceased to occur or when postmortem confirmation of *M. paratuberculosis* ceased to be obtained in the herd, the time interval was extended to 12 months. The program also included a propaganda campaign utilizing films, leaflets, broadcasts, and lectures. Other general measures used in control of Johne's disease have included advice on rearing of calves, early segregation and slaughter of reactors, pasture management, and segregation of cattle that were possibly infected. The animal owner did not have to accept the test valuations and was free to retain any suspect animal or dispose of it with all concomitant risks to himself or another person. Pearson and Ogg (1967) remarked that the voluntary nature of these programs has been of considerable value in soliciting the farmers' cooperation. They noted that clinical cases were nearly always slaughtered, as the animals were usually unsalable, and the risk of losing a reputation from the sale of suspected cases has been taken on only rare occasions.

The success of these programs can be judged from the following results. Of the 47 herds whose management adopted the tactics just described, 41 herds were negative on several consecutive tests and no further evidence of the disease could be found in these herds. Because in most instances reactors were rather expediently culled, their absence from these herds should not be surprising. Whether this also indicated disease absence could not be confirmed.

Larsen and Merkal (1968) employed CFT and Johnin tests as survey procedures, followed by the removal of reactors. Although the removal of animals was the owners' option, the authors reported that the disease was in fact not being eradicated from the herds by this means. The tests were characterized by low specificity, and this probably jeopardized the attempt to eradicate the disease.

B. Vaccination

Investigation of vaccination as a means of control of Johne's disease in cattle has been limited. Most of the data presented here come from French and British workers who have evaluated vaccination trials in their respective countries. A few studies were conducted in the United States, and these will also be reviewed.

Valle and Rinjard (1926) made the first effort toward vaccination against Johne's disease in France. The vaccine was composed of nonvirulent strains of living *M. paratuberculosis* grown on the surface of synthetic liquid media. The organisms were suspended in equal parts of olive oil and liquid paraffin to a concentration of 5 mg/1.5 ml; 10 mg of pumice powder were added as an irritant. The principle involved is comparable to Koch's phenomenon of premunition: by vaccinating and creating a state of sensitivity the animal is protected against reinfection as long as sensitivity persists. The vaccine gives rise to a nodule that persists in the vaccination site. Resistance to infection is believed to last only as long as the nodule is present and contains the bacilli.

Valle *et al.* (1941) reported that the safety of the vaccine has been proven by inoculation of 35,000 cattle in 896 herds. No case of the disease occurred among 6850 vaccinated cattle examined for 7 years. Similar results were obtained among 9678 cattle in 260 other herds. Vaccination was claimed to have eliminated clinical infection in 8 of 10 herds. Rinjard (1934) reported that he had never seen an animal with vaccine organisms present in the nodule exhibit clinical symptoms. Doyle (1956b) confirmed the latter view but noted that vaccination does not give complete protection, and perhaps should not be expected to serve as a sole means of control of Johne's disease. Goret (1956) stated that the vaccine is considered by veterinary surgeons and stockowners in France to be the best means of protection against the disease. How the vaccine was judged seems rather obscure. Vallee and Rinjard (1943) considered that immunity tests usually cannot be undertaken under laboratory conditions, because it is not always possible to reproduce the disease in experimental animals. The disease can usually be reproduced in young animals by the administration of heavy infecting doses since these frequently overcome the acquired resistance. They advised that the tests should be made on infected herds in the field and considered the most reliable test would be on two neighboring herds with an approximately similar degree of natural infection: vaccinate one herd and keep the other as a control. The basis of this proposal was that the vaccine confers a strong but gradually fading protection that lasts on the average about 18 months. As protection fades in the vaccinates, natural infection develops in the controls. At 18 to 20 months of age, the vaccinal protection will become weak or may even have been eliminated, while some controls will have become infectious and may transmit the disease to the vaccinates. Sigurdsson (1952), although realizing that artificial infection may not constitute a reliable test for vaccine efficiency, also noted that the prophylactic value of the vaccine cannot be assessed by the method presented by Vallee and Rinjard. Therefore, the issue of vaccine evaluation in bovine Johne's disease remains to be resolved. Postmortem examination was found to be very helpful in evaluating a vaccination scheme in goats (Fodstad, 1980).

Other problems with vaccination include (a) the chances of conversion to tuberculin reactivity and (b) duration of immunity and revaccination.

In regard to the first problem, vaccination with avirulent organisms was found to cause conversion to tuberculin in 90% of the animals (Sigurdsson and Tryggvadottir, 1949; Larsen et al., 1969). However, Doyle (1960) reported that when comparative tests were employed, there was no particular difficulty in interpreting the tuberculosis tests in vaccinated herds. Vaccinated animals reacted to both mammalian and avian tuberculins, but the avian reaction was usually stronger and persisted longer than the mammalian; occasionally the reactions were equal, and on rare occasions the mammalian was slightly stronger.

Regarding the second point, revaccination has been extensively practiced in France (Rinjard, 1934). The original procedure was to vaccinate all animals, irrespective of age, in an infected herd. This usually included some preclinically infected animals that subsequently developed signs. To guard against this, revaccination was recommended. Rinjard (1934) claimed that to ensure permanent protection, revaccination was necessary on regression of the nodule. However, the duration of the nodule was found to vary extensively among the vaccinated individuals, ranging from 15 to 30 months. Revaccination was practiced for some time in England until a modified program of vaccinating calves only within 30 days of birth was adopted (Spears, 1959). Doyle (1964) found that a single dose of vaccine proved sufficient to protect cattle against clinical disease. In one heavily infected herd, only one vaccinated animal became infected over a period of 7 to 12 years.

Noting that field studies of vaccination were suffering from obvious limitations (e.g., the lack of adequate controls, loss of animals to the study, and lack of reliability of responses to questionnaires), Stuart (1965) conducted a controlled study with a living avirulent bacterial vaccine. Bacterial shedding was encountered in both the vaccinates and nonvaccinated controls, but the number of shedders was significantly reduced in the vaccinates. No absolute protection was conferred, although clinical disease was substantially reduced. On revaccination, some of the nonclinical vaccinated shedders became overt cases of Johne's disease. Because this condition was not considered to have originated from increased exposure, Stuart (1965) concluded that revaccination not be recommended. In another controlled study, Larsen *et al.* (1974) vaccinated eight calves at 5 days of age using the live vaccine developed in England; eight other calves were kept as controls. The animals were challenged with virulent *M. paratuberculosis* 26 days after vaccination. The resistance conferred by vaccination was monitored by periodic fecal cultures, by Johnin testing, and eventually by histopathological studies, 5 months after challenge. The authors reported that no differences could be disclosed between the vaccinated and the control animals. In addition, the vaccine produced greater sensitivity to tuberculin than exposure alone, but the authors found that when comparative tests were used it was possible to detect infections with *M. bovis.* Larsen *et al.* (1978) conducted a study on the efficiency of two killed vaccines against Johne's disease in naturally infected herds of cattle. Calves from nine herds of cattle were divided into three groups of approximately equal numbers: one group was vaccinated with whole cells autoclaved at 121°C for 5 min; one group was vaccinated with cells ruptured in a Ribi press; and one group was used as control. All calves were exposed to infection by natural contact with infected adults in the herd. The three groups were monitored by periodic fecal cultures, and intradermal tests were conducted to determine the effect of vaccination on tuberculin hypersensitivity. During the study of 6 years, 146 animals were slaughtered and inspected. Twenty-two controls developed signs of Johne's disease, and nine others were found to be infected with *M. paratuberculosis*. Nine calves given fractionated-cell vaccine developed clinical signs, and five others were found infected at postmortem examination. Two calves given whole-cell vaccine developed clinical signs, and two others were found to harbor organisms on postmortem examination. Hypersensitivity resulting from vaccination did not confuse the comparative tuberculin test results. The authors concluded, on the basis of these findings, that control by vaccination alone cannot be recommended and that all procedures presently recommended for controlling the disease (i.e., removal of clinical and suspect animals, hygiene and sanitation, and management improvements) should be used together with calfhood vaccination.

C. General Recommendations

The programs to be reviewed here are all of an experimental nature. They have been offered in view of the contradictory or unsatisfactory performance of some of the strategies just described. These programs encompass a wide range of maneuvers with the purpose of achieving disease-free herd attestation status, a situation that is seen as the ultimate goal of a Johne's disease control program. There have been three such programs in this category.

In order to help prospective cattle buyers identify herds free of paratuberculosis, Merkal (1973) recommended that the United States Animal Health Association establish an Individual Qualified Herd Plan. To qualify under this plan, the following conditions must be met:

1. There must not have been a clinical case of Johne's disease in the herd within the past 3 years.
2. On two tests, 6 months apart, all cattle 6 months old or older must be negative on intradermal test.
3. At the same time the intradermal tests are conducted, fecal samples must be collected and cultured from each animal over 2 years old.
4. If intradermal tests yield positive results in one or more animals, regardless of the fecal culture results, at least two additional negative fecal samplings are required. Rectal cultures are to be obtained at 6-month intervals, to include all animals 2 years old or older in the herd.

Herds that meet these requirements would be designated "Paratuberculosis Qualified" for 1 year after the report of the last fecal culture. For such a herd to remain qualified, negative fecal cultures would be required of all animals 2 years old and older at 12-month intervals.

A second proposal was made by Julian (1975), who considered Merkal's qualified herd program too elaborate for application. This program, intended mainly for application in Canada, is similar to the programs carried out in Ireland. Julian suggests making Johne's disease subject to notification, so that infected herds are identified and would be quarantined. While under quarantine, cattle could be moved only to slaughter. The identification of positive herds should be made after suspect herds are tested with CFT and intradermal Johnin. Herds would be classified as positive only after histological or bacteriological confirmation of Johne's disease was established. In positive herds, vaccination would be permitted because all animals will go to slaughter. Alternatively, the author suggests that owners should have the choice of doing nothing. Where the owner chooses to vaccinate, this would be continued until the herd was culturally negative. The herd would not be certified free until the last vaccinated animals went to slaughter and were negative on CFT and Johnin test.

The third program originated as a response to the unreliability of diagnostic tests or vaccination in Johne's disease control. It was developed after 7 years of study in dairy herds in Wisconsin and came to be known as the Wisconsin guidelines. These guidelines, put forth by Moyle (1975), consist of a 17-point operational chart with the main emphasis on methods of sanitation and prevention of spread of infection. Young animals should be raised separately. Drainage should be adequate. Fecal contamination of water and feed should be avoided. Unthrifty cattle should be removed from the herd until diagnosis is obtained. Feces from all adult cattle should be cultured twice annually. All culture-positive animals and their offspring should be immediately removed from the herd. Areas of possible contamination should be disinfected with a USDA-approved disinfectant. Replacements from outside the herd should be from paratuberculosis-free herds. Sale of known infected stock for dairy or breeding purposes could subject the owner to civil liability.

Moyle assessed this program in four dairy herds of small sizes. After 2 to 3 years of rigid adherence with the guidelines just described, no cattle with clinical signs of paratuberculosis have been observed over a 5-year period. The author noted that the efficacy of the recommendations will be influenced by several factors:

1. The extent of infection in the population and the length of time the herd has been infected will be influential.
2. Herd size: the disease may be eliminated from small herds faster than from larger ones.
3. The type of husbandry employed: herds kept on well-drained pasture will become free from the disease faster than those kept under crowded housing or feedlot conditions.

V. Summary

The literature on Johne's disease is quite extensive. The disease has been diagnosed throughout the world in a wide range of domestic and wild animals, but mainly ruminants. It is of economic importance only in cattle, sheep, and goats. A diagnostic test that is both sensitive and specific has not yet been found. This failure may be due either to the spectral nature of the immune response in an affected animal or to the impurities of the antigen preparations utilized in the various tests.

Control and eradication of the disease is still in the research stage. Vaccination has been adopted mainly in Europe, with apparently satisfactory results. Vaccine evaluation has not always been correctly carried out. Several other control strategies have been attempted or suggested. None has been finally evaluated, and the disease is still a challenging problem.

References

Abbas, B. (1981). Master of Preventive Veterinary Medicine (MPVM) Paper, University of California, Davis.
Abbas, B. (1983). Ph.D. Thesis, University of California, Davis.
Alhaji, I., Johnson, D. W. Muscaplat, C. C., and Thoen, C. O. (1974). *Am. J. Vet. Res.* **35,** 725–727.
Annau, E. (1959). *Nature (London)* **184,** 1612–1613.
Anonymous (1971). *Hoard's Dairyman* **116,** 896–897.
Appleby, E. C., and Head, K. D. (1954). *J. Comp. Pathol.* **4,** 52–53.
Baas, E. J. (1976). *Proc. Sympo. Sheep Goat Pract. American Association of Sheep and Goat Practitioners, 1976* pp. 26–40.
Bendixen, P. H. (1977). *Am. J. Vet. Res.* **38,** 2027–2028.
Bendixen, P. H. (1978). *Nord. Veterinaer med.* **30,** 163–168.
Bendixen, P. H., Block, B., and Jorgensen, B. (1981). *Am. J. Vet. Res.* **42,** 109–113.
Bennedsen, J. (1969). *Acta Pathol. Microbiol. Scand.* **76,** 245–258.
Blood, D. C., and Henderson, J. A. (1968). "Veterinary Medicine," 3rd ed., Baillière, London.
Buergelt, C. D., and Duncan, J. R. (1980). *J. Am. Vet. Med. Assoc.* **173,** 478–480.
Buergelt, C. D., Hall, C. E., Merkal, R. S., Whitlock, R. H., and Duncan, J. R. (1977). *Am. J. Vet. Res.* **38,** 1709–1715.
Buergelt, C. D., Hall, C. E., McEntee, K., and Duncan, J. R. (1978a). *Vet. Pathol.* **15,** 196–207.
Buergelt, C. D., DeLisle, G., and Hall, C. E. (1978b). *Am. J. Vet. Res.* **39,** 591–595.
Chaparas, S. D. (1979). *Bull. Int. Union Against Tubercul.* **54,** 156–162.
Chaparas, S. D. (1981). *Rev. Infect. Dis.* **3,** 934–943.
Clausen, I. E. (1971). *Acta Allergol.* **26,** 56–59.
Closs, O., Harboe, M., and Wassum, A. M. (1975). *Scand. J. Immunol., Suppl.* **2,** 173–185.
Colburn, E., and Cutright, B. H. (1977). Master of Preventive Veterinary Medicine (MPVM) Paper, University of California, Davis.
Daniel, T. M. (1976). *Am. Rev. Respir. Dis.* **113,** 717–719.
Daniel, T. M., and Anderson, P. A. (1977). *J. Lab. Clin. Med.* **90,** 354–360.
Daniel, T. M., and Anderson, P. A. (1978). *Am. Rev. Respir. Dis.* **117,** 533–539.
David, J. R., Lawrence, H. S., and Thomas, L. (1964). *J. Immunol.* **93,** 264–279.
Davies, D. H., Corbeil, L., Ward, D., and Duncan, J. R. (1974). *Proc. Soc. Exp. Biol. Med.* **145,** 1372–1377.

DeLisle, G. (1978). Ph.D. Thesis, Cornell University, Ithaca, New York.
Doyle, T. M. (1956a). *Vet. Rec.* **68**, 869–886.
Doyle, T. M. (1956b). *In* "Control of Johne's Disease in Cattle, Sheep and Goats," pp. 163, European Productivity Agency (eds. Rowan, B. L., Latteur, J. P., and Durand, V. C.) O.E.E.C., Paris.
Doyle, T. M. (1958). *Vet. Rec.* **70**, 328.
Doyle, T. M. (1960). *Br. Vet. J.* **116**, 294–301.
Doyle, T. M. (1964). *Vet. Rec.* **76**, 73–77.
Duncan, J. R., Hall, C. E., and DeLisle, G. (1978). *Cornell Vet.* **68**, 179–188.
Duntton, R. W. (1967). *Adv. Immunol.* **6**, 253–280.
Engvall, E., and Perlmann, P. (1971). *J. Immunol.* **109**, 129–135.
Farr, R. S. (1960). *J. Infect. Dis.* **107**, 115–123.
Ferket, H., Ledercq, J., and Guebelle, F. (1971). *Acta Allergol.* **26**, 191–196.
Fodstad, F. H. (1977). *Acta Vet. Scand.* **18**, 374–383.
Fodstad, F. H. (1980). "Paratuberculosis (Johne's Disease) and Related Mycobacterial Diseases in Norway." National Veterinary Institute, Oslo, Norway.
Francis, J., Macturk, H. M., Madinavieta, J., and Snow, G. A. (1956). *Biochem. J.* **55**, 586–607.
Gilmour, N. J. L. (1965a). *Vet. Rec.* **77**, 1322–1330.
Gilmour, N. J. L. (1965b). *J. Comp. Pathol.* **75**, 281–286.
Gilmour, N. J. L. (1968). *Proc. 72nd Annu. Meet. U.S. Livestock Sanit. Assoc.* pp. 173–181.
Gilmour, N. J. L. (1971). *Res. Vet. Sci.* **12**, 295–297.
Gilmour, N. J. L., and Angus, K. W. (1976a). *Res. Vet. Sci.* **20**, 6–9.
Gilmour, N. J. L., and Angus, K. W. (1976b). *Res. Vet. Sci.* **20**, 10–21.
Gilmour, N. J. L., and Gardiner, A. C. (1969). *J. Comp. Pathol.* **79**, 71–77.
Goret, P. (1956). *In* "Control of Johne's Disease in Cattle, Sheep and Goats," pp. 159–160. European Productivity Agency (eds. Rowan, B. L., Latteur, J. P., and Durand, V. C.). O.E.E.C., Paris.
Goudswaard, J., Gilmour, N. J. L., Dijkstra, R. G., and Van Beck, J. (1976). *Vet. Rec.* **98**, 461–462.
Grange, J. M. (1979). "Mycobacterial Diseases," p. 111. Arnold, London.
Green, H. H. (1941). *J. Hyg.* **41**, 297–319.
Gunnarson, E., and Fodstad, F. (1979a). *Acta Vet. Scand.* **20**, 122–134.
Gunnarson, E., and Fodstad, F. (1979b). *Acta Vet. Scand.* **20**, 200–215.
Hagen, W. A. (1938). *Cornell Vet.* **28**, 34–40.
Hagen, W. A., and Zeissig, A. (1929). *J. Am. Vet. Med. Assoc.* **27**, 985–994.
Harding, H. P. (1959). *J. Pathol. Bacteriol.* **78**, 157–168.
Hellermark, K. (1966). *Acta Vet. Scand.* **7**, 330–336.
Hole, N. H. (1953). *Proc. Int. Vet. Congr. 15th, 1953* pp. 173–177.
Hole, N. H. (1958). *Adv. Vet. Sci.* **4**, 432.
Hole, N. H., and McClay, M. H. (1959). *Vet. Rec.* **71**, 1145–1149.
Janicki, B. W., Wright, G. L., Good, R. C., and Chaparas, S. D. (1976). *Infect. Immun.* **13**, 425–437.
Jensen, J. (1948). *J. Am. Vet. Med. Assoc.* **112**, 52–54.
Jensen, M. H. (1956). *Nord. Veterinaer med.* **8**, 357–367.
Jessup, D., Abbas, B., Behymer, D., and Cogan, P. (1981). *J. Am. Vet. Med Assoc.* **179**, 1252–1254.
Johne, H. A., and Frothingham, L. (1895). *Dtsch. Z. Tiermed.* **21**, 438–454.
Johnson, H. W., and Cox, B. F. (1942). *Am. J. Vet. Res.* **3**, 131–136.

Jorgensen, J. B. (1972). *Nord. Veterinaer med.* **24**, 297–308.
Jorgensen, J. B. (1977). *Nord. Veterinaer med.* **29**, 267–270.
Jorgensen, J. B., and Jensen, P. T. (1978). *Acta Vet. Scand.* **19**, 310–312.
Jubb, K. V. F., and Kennedy, P. C. (1970). "Pathology of Domestic Animals," Vol. 2, pp. 696–698. Academic Press, New York.
Julian, R. J. (1975). *Can. Vet. J.* **16**, 33–43.
Katic, I. (1961). *Nord. Veterinaer med.* **13**, 205–214.
Katic, I. (1969). "Bibliography of Literature on Johne's Disease (Paratuberculosis) 1895–1964." Royal Vet. and Agric. University, Copenhagen, 162 pp..
Katic, I. (1977). Copenhagen. Royal Vet. and Agric. University Year Book. pp. 110–154.
Kluge, J. P., Merkal, R. S., Monlux, W. S., Larsen, A. B., Kopecky, K. E., Ramsey, F. K., and Lehman, R. P. (1968). *Am. J. Vet. Res.* **29**, 953–962.
Knost, H., and Watson, E. A. (1953). *Am. J. Vet. Res.* **4**, 36–44.
Kopecky, K. E. (1973). *J. Am. Vet. Med. Assoc.* **162**, 787–788.
Kopecky, K. E. (1977). *J. Am. Vet. Med. Assoc.* **170**, 320–324.
Kopecky, K. E., Larsen, A. B., and Merkal, R. S. (1967). *Am. J. Vet. Res.* **28**, 1043–1045.
Kopecky, K. E., Booth, M. S., Merkal, R. S., and Larsen, A. B. (1971). *Am. J. Vet. Res.* **32**, 1343–1349.
Larsen, A. B. (1970). *In* "Bovine Medicine and Surgery" (W. J. Gibbons, E. J. Catcott, and J. F. Smithcors eds.), pp. 135–140. Am. Vet. Publ., Wheaton, Illinois.
Larsen, A. B. (1972). *J. Am. Vet. Med. Assoc.* **161**, 1539–1541.
Larsen, A. B. (1973). *J. Am. Vet. Med. Assoc.* **163**, 902–904.
Larsen, A. B., and Johnson, H. W. (1947). *Am. J. Vet. Res.* **8**, 184–185.
Larsen, A. B., and Johnson, H. W. (1949). *Am. J. Vet. Res.* **10**, 344–346.
Larsen, A. B., and Kopecky, K. E. (1965). *Am. J. Vet. Res.* **26**, 673–675.
Larsen, A. B., and Merkal, R. S. (1961). *Am. J. Vet. Res.* **22**, 1974–1976.
Larsen, A. B., and Merkal, R. S. (1968). *J. Am. Vet. Med. Assoc.* **152**, 1771–1773.
Larsen, A. B., and Miller, J. M. (1978). *Am. J. Vet. Res.* **39**, 1866–1867.
Larsen, A. B., Porter, D. A., and Vardaman, T. H. (1953). *Am. J. Vet. Res.* **14**, 562–565.
Larsen, A. B., Merkal, R. S., and Vardaman, T. H. (1956). *Am. J. Vet. Res.* **17**, 549–551.
Larsen, A. B., Vardaman, T. H., and Merkal, R. S. (1963a). *Am. J. Vet. Res.* **24**, 91–93.
Larsen, A. B., Vardaman, T. H., and Merkal, R. S. (1963b). *Am. J. Vet. Res.* **24**, 949–950.
Larsen, A. B., Vardaman, T. H., and Kopecky, R. E. (1965). *Am. J. Vet. Res.* **26**, 254–257.
Larsen, A. B., Merkal, R. S., and Kopecky, R. E. (1969). *Am. J. Vet. Res.* **30**, 2167–2172.
Larsen, A. B., Moon, H. W., and Merkal, R. S. (1972). *Am. J. Vet. Res.* **33**, 2185–2189.
Larsen, A. B., Merkal, R. S., and Moon, H. W. (1974). *Am. J. Vet. Res.* **35**, 367–369.
Larsen, A. B., Moyle, A. I., and Himes, E. M. (1978). *Am. J. Vet. Res.* **39**, 65–69.
Libke, K. G., and Walton, A. M. (1975). *J. Wildl. Dis.* **11**, 552–553.
Lind, A. (1965). *Am. Rev. Respir. Dis.* **92**, Suppl., 54–62.
Lominiski, I., Cameron, J., and Roberts, G. B. S. (1956). *J. Pathol. Bacteriol.* **71**, 211–231.
Long, K. R., and Topp, F. H. (1964). *Am. Rev. Respir. Dis.* **89**, 49–54.
Lovell, R., Levi, M., and Francis, J. (1944). *J. Comp. Pathol.* **54**, 120–128.
Melechov, P. P. (1967). *Veterinarija Moskova,* **43**, 40–44.
Merchant, I. A., and Berner, R. D. (1971). "Infectious Diseases of Domestic Animals," 3rd ed., Chapter 60. Iowa State Univ. Press, Ames.
Merkal, R. S. (1970). *Proc. 74th Annu. Meet. U.S. Anim. Health Assoc.,* pp. 620–622.
Merkal, R. S. (1973). *J. Am. Vet. Med. Assoc.* **163**, 1100–1102.
Merkal, R. S., and Curran, B. J. (1974). *Appl. Microbiol.* **28**, 276–279.
Merkal, R. S., and Larsen, A. B. (1962). *Am. J. Vet. Res.* **23**, 1307–1309.

Merkal, R. S., and Richard, W. D. (1972). *Appl. Microbiol.* **24**, 205–207.
Merkal, R. S., and Thurston, J. R. (1966). *Am. J. Vet. Res.* **27**, 519–521.
Merkal, R. S., Kopecky, K. E., Larsen, A. B., and Thurston, J. R. (1964). *Am. J. Vet. Res.* **25**, 1290–1293.
Merkal, R. S., Larsen, A. B., Kopecky, K. E., and Ness, R. D. (1968a). *Am. J. Vet. Res.* **29**, 963–969.
Merkal, R. S., Larsen, A. B., Kopecky, K. E., and Ness, R. D. (1968b). *Am. J. Vet. Res.* **29**, 1533–1538.
Merkal, R. S., Larsen, A. R., Kopecky, K. E., and Ness, R. D. (1970). *Am. J. Vet. Res.* **31**, 475–485.
Merkal, R. S., Larsen, A. B., and Booth, G. D. (1975). *Am. J. Vet. Res.* **36**, 837–839.
Minden, P., McClatchy, J. K., Cooper, R., Bardana, E. J., and Farr, R. S. (1972). *Science* **176**, 57–58.
Minett, F. C. (1935). *J. Comp. Pathol. Ther.* **48**, 123–132.
Minett, F. C. (1942). *J. Pathol. Bacteriol.* **54**, 209–219.
Morrison, N. E. (1965). *J. Bacteriol.* **89**, 762–767.
Moyle, A. I. (1975). *J. Am. Vet. Med. Assoc.* **166**, 689–690.
Nagal, S., Matsumoto, J., and Nagasuga, T. (1981). *Infect. Immun.* **31**, 1152–1160.
Nassau, E., Parsons, E. R., and Johnson, G. D. (1976). *Tubercle* **57**, 67–70.
Nemeto, H. (1969). *Natl. Inst. Anim. Health Q.* **9**, 53–54.
Nisbet, D. F., Gilmour, N. J. L., and Brotherston, J. G. (1962). *J. Comp. Pathol.* **72**, 80–91.
Ocadiz, J. G. (1981). Master of Preventive Veterinary Medicine (MPVM) Paper, University of California, Davis.
Omar, A. R., Lim, S. Y., and Retnasabapathy, A. (1967). *Kajian Vet. (Singapore)* **1**, 39–43.
Parlett, R. C., and Youmans, G. R. (1958). *Am. Rev. Tuberc.* **77**, 450–471.
Patterson, D. S. P. (1968). *Vet. Rec.* **83**, 55–57.
Patterson, D. S. P., Allen, W. M., and Lloyed, M. K. (1967). *Vet. Rec.* **81**, 717–718.
Patterson, D. S. P., Allen, W. M., Berret, S., and Sweasey, D. (1968). *J. Med. Microbiol.* **1**, 127–135.
Payne, M. J., and Rankin, J. D. (1961). *Res. Vet. Sci.* **2**, 175–179.
Pearson, J. K. L. (1964). *Br. Vet. J.* **120**, 2–7.
Pearson, J. K. L., and McClelland, T. G. (1955). *Vet. Rec.* **67**, 615–616.
Pearson, J. K. L., and Ogg, J. S. (1967). *Br. Vet. J.* **123**, 31–36.
Peck, E. F. (1957). *Vet. Rec.* **69**, 936–946.
Rankin, J. D. (1961). *Res. Vet. Sci.* **2**, 89–92.
Rankin, J. D. (1962a). *J. Comp. Pathol.* **71**, 10–15.
Rankin, J. D. (1962b). *J. Comp. Pathol.* **72**, 113–117.
Reinders, J. S. (1963). *Vet. Bull. (London)* **33**, 423 (abstr.).
Rice, C. E., Annau, E., and Knost, H. (1959). *Can. J. Comp. Med.* **23**, 369–374.
Rice, C. E., Annau, E., and Knost, H. (1960). *Can. J. Comp. Med.* **24**, 96–105.
Riemann, H., Zaman, M. R., Ruppanner, R., Aalund, O., Jorgensen, B. J., Warsaae, H., and Behymer, D. (1979). *J. Am. Vet. Med. Assoc.* **174**, 841–843.
Ringdal G. (1963). *Nord. Veterinaer med.* **15**, 217–218.
Rinjard, P. (1934). *Bull. Off. Int. Epizoot.* **51**, 1–15.
Rose, N. R., and Friedman, H., eds. (1976). "Manual of Clinical Immunology," pp. 169–259. Am. Soc. Microbiol., Washington, D.C.
Ross, G. W., Singleton, L., and Chanter, K. V. (1967). *J. Comp. Pathol.* **77**, 255–262.
Schuurs, A. H. W. M., and Van Weemen, B. K. (1977). *Clin. Chim. Acta* **81**, 1–40.

Sherman, D., and Gezon, H. M. (1980). *J. Am. Vet. Med. Assoc.* **177,** 1208–1211.
Sigurdsson, B. (1952). *J. Immunol.* **68,** 559–565.
Sigurdsson, B. (1956). *Bacteriol. Rev.* **20,** 1–13.
Sigurdsson, B., and Tryggvadottir, A. G. (1949). *J. Bacteriol.* **58,** 271–278.
Smythe, R. H. (1935). *Vet. Rec.* **15,** 85–86.
Soltys, M. A., Andress, C. E., and Fletch, A. L. (1967). *Bull. Wildl. Dis. Assoc.* **3,** 183–184.
Sorensen, D. R., and Flint, G. J. (1967). *Minn. Vet.* **7,** 5–9.
Spears, H. N. (1959). *Vet. Rec.* **71,** 1154–1156.
Stamp, J. T., and Watt, J. A. (1954). *J. Comp. Pathol.* **64,** 26–40.
Stanford, J. L. (1973). *Ann. Soc. Belge Med. Trop.* **53,** 321–330.
Stuart, P. (1965). *Br. Vet. J.* **121,** 289–318.
Taylor, A. W. (1950). *J. Pathol. Bacteriol.* **62,** 647–650.
Taylor, A. W. (1953). *J. Comp. Pathol.* **63,** 355–367.
Thoen, C. O. (1979). *J. Am. Vet. Med. Assoc.* **174,** 838–840.
Twort, E. W., and Ingram, G. L. Y. (1913). "A Monograph on Johne's Disease," p. 44. Bailliére, Tindall, and Cox. London.
U.S. Department of Agriculture (1974). "Laboratory Methods in Veterinary Microbiology for the Isolation and Identification of Mycobacteria," pp. 34–57. Vet. Serv. Lab., APHIS, USDA, Ames, Iowa.
Valle, H., and Rinjard, P. (1926). *Rev. Gen. Med. Vet.* **35,** 1–11.
Valle, H., and Rinjard, P. (1943). *Rev. Gen. Med. Vet.* **43,** 777–779.
Valle, H., Rinjard, P., and Valle, M. (1941). *Bull. Acad. Med. (Paris)* **125,** 195–198.
Vance, M. N. (1961). *Can. Vet. J.* **2,** 305–307.
Van Ulsen, F. W. (1970). *Tijdschr. Diergeneskd.* **95,** 446–448.
Warsaae, H. (1978). *Acta Vet. Scand.* **19,** 153–155.
Williams, E. S., Sparker, T. R., and Schoonveld, G. S. (1979). *J. Wildl. Dis.* **15,** 221–227.
Withers, R. W. (1959). *Vet. Rec.* **71,** 1150–1153.
Worthington, R. (1963). *FAO Agric. Stud.* **61,** 157–186.
Yugi, H., Hatakeyama, H., and Nemeto, H. (1966a). *Natl. Inst. Anim. Health Q.* **6,** 152–165.
Yugi, H., Hatakeyama, H., and Nemeto, H. (1966b). *Natl. Inst. Anim. Health Q.* **6,** 166–177.

Index

A

Acaricide resistance in ticks, 273–324
  chlorinated acaricides, 280, 282–283
  inorganic acaricides, 277, 280, 282, 288
  major acaricide groups and structures, 276
  management of, 290–293
  mechanisms of, 288–290
  methods for determination of, 284–288
  in multihost ticks, 282–284
  new acaricides, 281, 283
  organophosphorus and carbamate acaricides, 280–281, 283, 288–290
  in single-host ticks, 277–281
Acriflavine, use in fish-parasite control, 307
Akabane virus, role in bovine congenital defects, 205–209
Albinism, as congenital defect in cattle, 244
Anencephaly, as bovine congenital defect, 229
Antibiotics, use in fish-disease control, 312–313
Antierythrocyte agglutinins, immune-mediated, classification of, 168
Antimicrobials, use in fish-disease therapy, 311–314
Arnold–Chiari malformation, in cattle, 232
Arthrogryposis, congenital, in cattle, 225–227
Arthropods, as possible Rift Valley fever vectors, 401–402
Ataxia, cerebellar and progressive, as bovine congenital defect, 235
Avian lymphoid leukosis
  epidemiology of, 340–341
  pathogenesis of, 334–335
Avian lymphoproliferative diseases, 325–346
  avian lymphoid leukosis, 334–335, 340–341
  avian retroviruses, 327–329
  classification of, 327
  clinical and pathological features of, 330–336
  epidemiology, virology, and oncogenesis of, 336–346
  lymphoproliferative disease of turkeys, 330–332, 338–340
  Marek's disease, 335–336, 341–342
  reticuloendotheliosis, 332–334, 338–340

B

B-lymphocyte antigens of dogs, 26–27
Bacterins, use in fish-disease control, 315–318
Birds, Rift Valley fever, virus maintenance in, 408
Blood
  bovine congenital defects of, 250
  immune-mediated diseases of, 163–196
Blood vessels, bovine congenital defects of, 249–250
Bluetongue virus, role in bovine congenital defects, 211–212
Bovine congenital defects, 197–271
  causes of, 203–215
  of body cavity, 251
  of cardiovascular system, 249–250
  of central nervous system, 228–242
  defect description, 217–258
  definitions of, 199
  of digestive system, 250–251
  environmental factors in, 203–212
  of eye, 242–243
  frequency of, 201–203
  genetic factors in, 212–215
  of hair, 247–249
  of joints, 224–225
  Kansas genetic disease program and, 215–217
  of liver, 251

metabolic diseases as, 240–242
of metabolism, 255–256
of muscular system, 225–228
nature and effect of, 199–201
rectal palpation role in, 204–205
of reproductive system, 251–255
of respiratory system, 250
of skeleton, 218–224
of skin, 243–247
toxic plant role, 203–204
viral infection role in, 205–212
Bovine paratuberculosis, *see* Johne's disease
Bovine virus diarrhea virus, role in bovine congenital defects, 209–211
Brain stem, bovine congenital defects of, 232–236
Buffalo, Rift Valley fever in, 373

C

Calcium hydroxide, use in fish-parasite control, 307
Camels, Rift Valley fever in, 373–374
Cardiovascular system, bovine congenital defects of, 249–250
Cats
  histocompatibility systems of, 63
  Rift Valley fever in, 375
Cattle
  BoLA system of
    disease associations, 53–54
    HLA cross-reactivity, 54
  class I antigens of, 45–50
    characterization, 48–50
  class II antigens, 50–52
    B-lymphocyte typing, 51–52
    mixed lymphocyte reactivity, 50–51
  congenital defects in, 192–271
  embryo collection in, 140–144
  embryo storage in, 144–147
  embryo transfer in, 138–147
  erythrocyte antigen expression on lymphocytes, 43–45
  histocompatibility systems of, 43–54
  Rift Valley fever in, 370–372
  superovulation in, 138–140
Cell culture techniques for MHS polymorphisms, 17–18

Cerebellum, bovine congenital defects of, 232–236
Cerebral defects, congenital in cattle, 229–232
Cervidae
  sickled red cells in, 77–98
  common names, 79
Channel catfish virus disease, description and control of, 319
Chrondrodysplasia, congenital, in cattle, 222–223
Class I antigens, function of, 9–10
Class II antigens, function of, 10
Cleft palate
  corticosteroid-induced, 111–123
    embryological characteristics, 117–123
    exposure factors, 111–114
    molecular mechanisms, 114–117
Copper sulfate, use in fish parasite control, 307–308
Corpus callosum, agenesis, as bovine congenital defect, 229
Corticosteroid teratogenicity, 99–128
  abnormalities produced by, 109
  cleft palate produced by, 111–123
  in guinea pigs, 109
  in hamsters, 106–107
  interspecies comparison, 100–111
  in mice, 100–103
  in nonhuman primates, 105–106
  in rabbits, 107–109
  in rats, 103–105
Crooked calf disease, as congenital defect, 224
Culicoides, as Rift Valley fever vectors, 400–401
Curliness of hair, as bovine congenital defect, 247

D

Dandy-Walker syndrome in cattle, 232
Deer, sickling in, 80–81
Di-*n*-butyl tin oxide, use in fish parasite control, 308
Digestive system, bovine congenital defects of, 250–251
DLA antigens of dogs, 18–21

INDEX

Dogs
  cell-mediated lympholysis assays on, 30
  DLA antigens of, 18–21
    canine diseases and, 30–31
    functional studies, 27–30
    genes linked to, 31
    genetic definition, 20–21
    immunogenetics of, 31–32
  MHS of, 18–32
  MLR antigens of, 21–26
  Rift Valley fever in, 374–375
Drugs, effect on immune-mediated blood diseases, 188–189

E

Ectopia cordis, as bovine congenital defect, 249
Edema, neuraxial and brain as bovine congenital defects, 235–236
Embryo transfer in domestic animals, 129–162
  in cattle, 138–147
  current technology, 138–154
  donor-female fertility and, 132–134
  embryo importation and exportation, 135–136
  future developments in, 154–156
  historical aspects, 130–132
  in horses, 147–150
  large animals, 132–138
  in pigs, 152–153
  in production of offspring from infertile females, 134–135
  in sheep, 150–151
  twin induction in, 136–137
  undesirable recessives detection, 137–138
Enteric redmouth disease, therapy of, 317
Epilepsy, hereditary, in cattle, 240
Epitheliogenesis imperfecta, as congenital bovine defect, 245–246
Equine lymphocyte antigen
  immunodeficiency, disease and, 60–61
  serology, 54–56
Eye, bovine congenital defects of, 242–243

F

Fish diseases, 297–324
  control and therapy of, 297–324
    antimicrobials used in, 311–314
    by avoidance, 300–301
    bacterins used in, 315–318
    principles of, 300–303
    by stress control, 303
    therapeutic agents used in, 307–311
  diagnosis of, 299–300
  vaccines used against, 314–315
  veterinarian's role in, 298–299
  virus vaccine potential for control of, 318–321
Fluorescent antibody technique for Rift Valley fever virus assay, 360–361
Formalin, use in fish-parasite control, 308–309
Fragility of skin, as congenital bovine defect, 244–245
Freemartinism in cattle, genetic aspects of, 253
Furunculosis in fish, therapy of, 316–317

G

Gangliosidosis, congenital, in cattle, 240–241
Gel diffusion precipitation, of Rift Valley fever virus, 361–362
Gestation, prolonged, in cattle, 255
Glyconeogenesis, congenital, in cattle, 241
Goats
  embryo collection, storage, and transfer in, 152
  histocompatibility systems of, 62–63
  Rift Valley fever in, 372–373
  superovulation in, 151–152
Goiter, congenital, in cattle, 255–256
Goldfish, ulcer disease of, therapy, 317
Guinea pigs, corticosteroid teratogenicity in, 109

H

Hair, bovine congenital defects of, 247

Hamsters, corticosteroid teratogenecity in, 106-107
Heartwater, 427–480
　causal agent of, 430–440
　　classification, 436–438
　　in vitro culture, 438–440
　diagnosis of, 460–464
　distribution of, 444–445
　epidemiology of, 452–457
　historical aspects, 428–429
　immunity to, 464–467
　immunization for, 469–473
　pathogenesis of, 460
　postmortem findings on, 459–460
　prevention of, 469–473
　susceptibility to, 445–452
　symptoms and course of, 457–459
　therapy of, 467–469
　tick control for, 469
　transmission of, 440–444
　in Western Hemisphere, 473–474
Hermaphroditism in cattle, genetic aspects of, 252–253
HLA antigens, disease associations of, 11
Hormones, effect on immune-mediated blood diseases, 187–188
Horses
　embryo collection in, 148–149
　embryo storage in, 149–150
　embryo transfer in, 147–150
　equine lymphocyte antigen of, 54–56
　immunodeficiency disease and, 60–61
　histocompatibility systems of, 54–61
　pregnancy and, 58–60
　Rift Valley fever in, 374
　superovulation in, 148
Humans
　Rift Valley fever in, 347–378
　　pathological changes caused by, 386–387
Hydranencephy, as bovine congenital defect, 229
Hydrocephalus, as bovine congenital defect, 229–232
Hypertrichosis, as bovine congenital defect, 247
Hypotrichosis, as bovine congenital defect, 247–249

I

Ichthyosis, as congenital bovine defect, 246–247
Immune-mediated diseases of blood, 163–196
　breed predisposition, 181
　clinical signs, 165–166
　clinicopathological tests in, 167–173
　diagnosis of, 166–173
　drug effects on, 188–189
　family and breed histories, 173–178
　findings in, 173–178
　genetic influences, 181–182
　history in, 166–167
　hormonal influences on, 187–188
　increased frequency of, 180
　management and treatment of, 190–194
　　platelet disorders, 193–194
　　red cell disorders, 191–192
　platelet tests in, 169–172
　predisposing factors in, 178–190
　prevention of, 194–195
　red-cell tests in, 167–169
　sex predisposition, 181
　SLE tests, 172
　stress effects on, 189–190
　viral infections and, 182–184
Immune response
　genes, disease associations and, 10–13
　non-MHS-linked genes for, 14–15
Infectious hematopoietic necrosis virus description and control of, 320–321
Infectious pancreatic necrosis virus description and control of, 319–320
Interdigital overgrowth, as bovine congenital defect, 249

J

Jersey cattle, rectovaginal constriction in, 254
Johne's disease, 481–506
　agent of, 483
　control efforts, 495–501
　　recommendations, 500–502
　diagnosis of, 485–495
　　problems in, 491–495

host-parasite relationship in, 483–485
mode of infection and pathogenesis, 483–485
vaccination for, 497–500
Joint defects, congenital, in cattle, 224–225

K

Kansas genetic disease program, bovine congenital defects studies by, 215–217
Keratogenesis, imperfect, as congenital bovine defect, 246

L

Liver, bovine congenital defects of, 251
Lymphatics, bovine congenital defects of, 250

M

Major histocompatibility system (MHS)
of cats, 63
of dogs, 18–32
genes for, 2–3
genetic structure of, 4–5
of horses, 54–61
immunological function, 9–14
summary, 13–14
molecular structure and tissue distribution, 6–8
nonimmunological functions of, 15
of pigs, 32–42
polymorphisms, detection, 15–18
population structure, 8–9
of sheep and goats, 61–63
structure and function of, 4–18
Malachite green mixtures, use in fish-parasite control, 309
Mannosidosis, congenital, in cattle, 241–242
Marek's disease
epidemiology of, 341–342
pathogenesis of, 335–336
Masoten, use in fish-parasite control, 309–310

Matchstick sickle cells in deer, 85
Meningoencephalocoele, as bovine congenital defect, 232
Metabolic defects, as bovine congenital defects, 255
Metabolic diseases, congenital, in cattle, 240–242
Methylene blue, use in fish-parasite control, 310
Metronidazole, use in fish-parasite control, 310
Mice, corticosteroid teratogenicity in, 100–103
Microcephaly, as bovine congenital defect, 232
Midges, as Rift Valley fever vectors, 400–401
Mixed lymphocyte reactivity (MLR) antigens of dogs, 21–26
Mosquitoes, as Rift Valley fever vectors, 397–400
Mullerian ducts, bovine congenital defects of, 253–254
Muscular hypertrophy, congenital, in cattle, 227–228
Muscular system, congenital defects of, in cattle, 225–228

N

Neonatal spasticity, as bovine congenital defect, 240
Neuronal lipodystrophy, congenital, in cattle, 242

O

Osteopetrosis, congenital, in cattle, 223–224
Ovary, bovine congenital defects of, 253

P

Pasterns, congenital flexure of, in cattle, 225
Penis and prepuce, bovine congenital defects of, 251

Pigs
  antigens shared by erythrocytes and lymphocytes, 40–41
  embryo collection and transfer in, 152–153
  histocompatibility studies on, 37–39
  MHS of, 32–42
  miniature pigs, 35–36
  MLR assays on, 34–35
  SLA antigens of, 32–35
    biochemical characterization, 36–37
    genes linked to, 42
    production traits associated with, 42
    tissue distribution, 39–40
  Rift Valley fever in, 374
  superovulation in, 152
Porphyria, congenital, in cattle, 255
Potassium-permanganate use, in fish-parasite control, 311
Primates, Rift Valley fever virus maintenance in, 407–408
Protoporphyria, as congenital bovine defect, 247

Q

Quaternary ammonium compounds, use in fish-disease control, 313–314

R

Rabbits, corticosteroid teratogenicity in, 107–109
Rats, corticosteroid teratogenicity in, 103–105
Rectal palpation, role in bovine congenital defects, 204–205
Rectovaginal constriction in Jersey cattle, genetic aspects of, 254
Reproductive system, bovine congenital defects of, 251–255
Respiratory system, bovine congenital defects of, 250
Reticulo endotheliosis
  epidemiology of, 338–340
  lymphoproliferative disease comparison to, 342–343
  pathogenesis of, 332–334, 338–340

Rift Valley fever, 347–424
  in animals, 367–375
  clinical disease symptoms, 367–378
  clinical pathology of, 377–378
  differential diagnosis of, 387–390
  epidemiological features of, 390–408
  etiological agent of, 349–366
  host range and susceptibility to, 366–367
  in humans, 375–378, 386–387
  nonvectorial transmission of, 402–405
  pathological changes caused by, 378–387
  prevention and control measures for, 408–416
  vectorial transmission of, 397–402
  vaccines for, 408–414
  virus
    biosynthesis and morphogenesis, 352–354
    classification, 349–350
    immunological identification, 357
    isolation and assay, 354–357
    maintenance in animals, 405–408
    strains, 362–365
    virion of, 350–352
Rodents
  Rift Valley fever in
    pathological changes caused by, 385–386
    virus maintenance in, 405

S

Salt, use in fish-parasite control, 311
Scottish terrier family, immune-mediated blood diseases in, 176–178
Serological assays, of MHS polymorphisms, 16–17
Sheep
  embryo collection, storage, and transfer in, 150–151
  histocompatibility systems of, 61–62
  Rift Valley fever in, 367–370
  pathological changes caused by, 378–384
Sickled red cells
  in the Cervidae, 77–98
    hemoglobin structure and genetics, 90–94

molecular mechanisms, 83–90
production and behavior, 80–81
Skeletal defects, congenital, in cattle, 218–222
Skin, bovine congenital defects of, 243–247
SLE, tests for, 172
Spastic lethal, as bovine congenital defect, 239–240
Spastic paresis, as bovine congenital defect, 237–239
Spastic syndrome, as bovine congenital defect, 239
Spinal cord, bovine congenital defects of, 236–237
Stress
  effects on immune-mediated blood diseases, 189–190
  role in fish diseases, 303
Superovulation
  in cattle, 138–140
  in goats, 151–152
  in horses, 148
  in sheep, 150

T

Teratogens, corticosteroids as, 99–128
Testicles, bovine congenital defects of, 252
Ticks
  acaricide resistance in, *see* Acaricide resistance in ticks.
  importance to livestock industry, 274–275
  pesticide resistance in, 275
Toxic plants, role in bovine congenital defects, 203–204
Turkeys
  lymphoproliferative disease of
    epidemiology, 336–338
    pathogenesis, 330–332
    RE relationship to, 342–343
Twinning, defective, as bovine congenital defect, 256
Twins, induction of, in cattle, 136–137

U

Ulcer disease of goldfish, therapy of, 317

V

Vaccinations, immune-mediated blood diseases and, 184–187
Vaccines, use in fish-disease control, 314–315
Ventricular septal defects, congenital, in cattle, 249
Vibriosis, therapy of, 317–318
Viral hemorrhagic septicemia, description and control of, 321
Viral infections, immune-mediated blood diseases and, 182–184
Virus infection, role in bovine congenital defects, 205–212
Viruses, avian lymphoproliferative diseases and, 325–346
Vizsla family, immune-mediated blood diseases in, 174–176

W

Weaver condition, as bovine congenital defect, 240
Wesselbron disease virus, role in bovine congenital defects, 212
Wolffian duct, bovine congenital defects of, 252

Contents of Recent Volumes

Volume 15

Bluetongue Disease
John G. Bowne

Environmental Influences on Behavior of Domesticated and Laboratory Animals
M. W. Fox

The Effect of the Use of Antibacterial Drugs on the Emergence of Drug-Resistant Bacteria in Animals
H. Williams Smith

The Impact of Antibiotic Drugs and Their Residues
William G. Huber

Parturient Hypocalcemia in Dairy Cows
D. S. Kronfeld

Respiratory Viruses of Cattle
J. I. H. Phillip and J. H. Darbyshire

Allergic Responses Involving the Skin of Domestic Animals
G. S. Walton

Progess in Laboratory Animal Medicine
Alvin F. Moreland

Sheep Pulmonary Adenomatosis (Jaagsiekte)
J. G. Wandera

Veterinary Medical Research, Education and Service in the Republic of South Africa
B. C. Jansen

AUTHOR INDEX–SUBJECT INDEX

Volume 16

Recent Advances in Veterinary and Comparative Ophthalmology
Kirk N. Gelatt

Reticulosis of the Central Nervous System (CNS) in Dogs
R. Fankhauser, R. Fatzer, H. Luginbühl, and J. T. McGrath

The Management of Clinical and Laboratory Data in Veterinary Medicine
William A. Priester

Congenital Defects of Cattle: Nature, Cause, and Effect
H. W. Leipold, S. M. Dennis, and K. Huston

Animal Models of Atherosclerosis
Thomas B. Clarkson

The Ultrastructural Basis of Cell Injury in Viral Infections
A. M. Watrach

Avian Influenza Viruses: In Avian Species and the Natural History of Influenza
Bernard C. Easterday and Bela Tumova

Recent Advances in the Knowledge of Marek's Disease
H. Graham Purchase

Pathogenesis of Ruminant Lactic Acidosis
Robert H. Dunlop

Motility of the Bovine and Porcine Uterus and Fallopian Tube
K. Zerobin and H. Spörri

The Transfer of Antibodies by Neonates and Adults
M. W. Simpson-Morgan and T. C. Smeaton

AUTHOR INDEX–SUBJECT INDEX

Volume 17

Enzootic Pneumonia of Pigs (EPP)
Peter Whittlestone

Epizootiology of Porcine Transmissible Gastroenteritis (TGE)
D. H. Ferris

Moderated Immunologic Responsiveness in Parasitic Infections
Robert J. Hudson

African Trypanosomiases
T. M. Leach

Feline Viral Infections
James H. Gillespie and Frederic W. Scott

Feline Viral Rhinotracheitis (FVR)
Robert A. Crandell
The Lymphoid Apparatus of the Sheep: Its Growth, Development, and Significance in Immunologic Reactions
G. J. Cole and Bede Morris
The Influence of Nutrition on Response to Infectious Disease
Paul M. Newberne
Recent Advances in Scientific Knowledge and Development Pertaining to Diseases of Fishes
S. F. Snieszko
Hog Cholera (European Swine Fever)
H. W. Dunne
Nonhuman Primates in Viral Oncology
Ronald D. Hunt and T. C. Jones
Epidemiology and Control of Gastrointestinal Nematodoses of Ruminants
Hugh McL. Gordon
AUTHOR INDEX–SUBJECT INDEX

Volume 18
Primate Malarias
William E. Collins
The Ecology of Tularemia
Cluff E. Hopla
Veterinary Nuclear Medicine
F. A. Kallfelz, C. L. Comar, and R. A. Wentworth
Venezuelan Equine Encephalitis
Karl M. Johnson and David H. Martin
Comparative Erythrocyte Metabolism
J. Jerry Kaneko
Slow Virus Diseases of the Central Nervous System
R. F. Marsh
Pathogenesis of Enteric Diseases Caused by *Escherichia coli*
Harley W. Moon
The Reemergence of Newcastle Disease
Robert P. Hanson
Advances in Research on Brucellosis, 1957–1972
Margaret E. Meyer
Some Diseases of Zoo Animals
Lynn A. Griner

Bovine Parvovirus 1, Bovine Syncytial Virus, and Bovine Respiratory Syncytial Virus and Their Infections
George T. Woods
SUBJECT INDEX

Volume 19
Mannosidosis of Angus Cattle: A Prototype Control Program for Some Genetic Diseases
R. D. Jolly
Neonatal Isoerythrolysis in Domestic Animals: A Comparative Review
Clyde Stormont
Significant Recent Advances in Biological Control of Vector Insects
Jaroslav Weiser
Landscape Epidemiology (Epizootiology)
I. G. Galuzo
Some Diseases of Free-Living Wildlife
A. McDiarmid
Vitamin E and Seleniuim Deficiencies (VESD) of Domestic Animals
Nils Lannek and Paul Lindberg
Cat Leukemia and Its Viruses
W. F. H. Jarrett
Equine Infectious Anemia
Susumu Ishii and Ruizo Ishitani
Murine Cytomegalovirus (MCMV)
Gilles Lussier
Functional and Fine Structural Relationships of Parathyroid Glands
Charles C. Capen
The Endocrinologic Changes of Gestation and Parturition in the Sheep
R. I. Cox
SUBJECT INDEX

Volume 20
Congenital Defects of the Cardiovascular System of Dogs: Studies in Comparative Cardiology
D. F. Patterson
Comparative Aspects of Canine Hereditary Eye Disease
K. C. Barnett

Developmental Disorders of the Nervous System in Animals
  J. T. Done
Mechanisms of Psychosomatic Disease in Animals
  James P. Henry
Mycotoxic Nephropathy
  Palle Krogh
Periodontal Disease in Dogs and Man
  Lennart Krook
Histologic Classification and Further Characterization of Tumors in Domestic Animals
  W. Misdorp
Therapy of Neoplasia in Domestic Animals
  L. N. Owen
Chronic Bronchitis in the Dog
  H. M. Pirie and E. B. Wheeldon
Immunity to Mycoplasmas Causing Respiratory Diseases in Man and Animals
  Peter Whittlestone
SUBJECT INDEX

Volume 21
Indirect Measurement of Blood Pressure in Animals
  Allen W. Hahn and Harold E. Garner
Myocardial Contractility
  Robert L. Hamlin
Cardiovascular Diseases of the Domestic Cat
  Neil K. Harpster
Chronic Valvular Disease (Endocardiosis) in Dogs
  James W. Buchanan
Heartworm Heart Disease
  David H. Knight
Pulmonary Hypertension in Cattle
  Gerald E. Bisgard
Cardiovascular Effects of Exercise and Training in Horses
  W. v. Engelhardt
The Glomerulus in Health and Disease: A Comparative Review of Domestic Animals and Man
  Carl A. Osborne, Robert F. Hammer, Jerry B. Stevens, Jack S. Resnick, and Alfred F. Michael

Ultrastructure of Muscular Arteries of Animals
  Charles F. Simpson
Oxygen, the Arterial Wall, and Atherosclerosis
  E. R. Jurrus and H. S. Weiss
Atherosclerosis in Nonhuman Primates
  Robert W. Wissler and Dragoslava Vesselinovitch
Comparative Atherosclerosis
  H. Luginbühl, G. L. Rossi, H. L. Ratcliffe, and R. Müller
SUBJECT INDEX

Volume 22
Environmental Impact on Laboratory Animals
  W. Morgan Newton
Congenital Defects due to Hyperthermia
  M. J. Edwards
Perinatal Mortality: Some Problems of Adaptation at Birth
  G. C. B. Randall
Bovine Respiratory Viruses
  Sashi B. Mohanty
Bluetongue and Epizootic Hemorrhagic Disease Viruses: Their Relationship to Wildlife Species
  Gerald L. Hoff and Daniel O. Trainer
Swine Dysentery: A Perspective
  Richard C. Meyer
Sarcocystis and *Sarcocystosis* in Domestic Animals and Man
  Miles B. Markus
Experimental Transplantation and Histocompatibility Systems in the Canine Species
  Felix T. Rapaport and Radoslav J. Bachvaroff
Autoimmune Disease in the Dog
  R. E. W. Halliwell
Farm Animal Disease Data Banks
  Sherwin A. Hall
Taste Perception and Discrimination by the Dog
  R. L. Kitchell
SUBJECT INDEX

Volume 23

Structural and Functional Characteristics of Immunoglobulins of the Common Domestic Species
P. Porter

Primary and Secondary Immune Deficiencies of Domestic Animals
Lance E. Perryman

Mechanisms of Immunity in Bacterial Infections
A. J. Winter

The Immune System and Helminth Infection in Domestic Species
E. J. L. Soulsby

Mechanisms of Viral Immunopathology
Barry T. Rouse and Lorne A. Babiuk

Immunology of a Persistent Retrovirus Infection—Equine Infectious Anemia
Travis C. McGuire and Timothy B. Crawford

Immunology and Pathogenesis of African Animal Trypanosomiasis
J. B. Henson and Jan C. Noel

Tumor Immunology in Domestic Animals
M. Essex and C. K. Grant

Applications of Transplantation Immunology in the Dog
H. M. Vriesendorp

Effects of Environmental Contaminants on the Immune System
Loren D. Koller

SUBJECT INDEX

Volume 24

Bovine Lymphosarcoma
Jorge F. Ferrer

The Epidemiology of Bovine Brucellosis
Paul Nicoletti

Drug Resistance in Coccidia
John F. Ryley

The Economic Impact of Coccidiosis in Domestic Animals
Paul R. Fitzgerald

Biocontrol in Veterinary Entomology
Marshall Laird

Stress and Its Measurement in Domestic Animals: A Review of Behavioral and Physiological Studies under Field and Laboratory Situations
D. B. Stephens

Current Concepts in Reproduction of the Dog and Cat
Victor M. Shille and George H. Stabenfeldt

Banding Techniques in Chromosome Analysis of Domestic Animals
Ingemar Gustavsson

Whole Body Autoradiography in Metabolic Studies of Drugs and Toxicants
A. G. Rico, P. Bénard, J. P. Braun, and V. Burgat-Sacaze

INDEX

Volume 25

New Enteric Viruses in the Dog
L. E. Carmichael and L. N. Binn

African Swine Fever: A Reassessment
William R. Hess

Persistent Virus Infections of Food Animals: Their Relevance to the International Movement of Livestock and Germ Plasm
Edward P. J. Gibbs

Control of Tsetse Flies, *Glossina* spp.
David A. Dame and Anthony M. Jordan

Bovine Mycoplasmal Mastitis
Donald E. Jasper

Contagious Equine Metritis
David G. Powell

Mycotoxins and Animal Health
Allan C. Pier

Screening for Genetic Diseases: Principles and Practice
R. D. Jolly, W. J. Dodds, G. R. Ruth, and D. B. Trauner

Skeletal Deformities in Poultry
Craig Riddell

Epidemiology of the Feline Urological Syndrome
Preben Willeberg

Motor Functions of the Intestine
Yves Ruckebusch

INDEX

Volume 26
Some Functional Consequences of Species Differences in Lung Anatomy
  N. E. Robinson
The Effects of Age on Lung Function and Structure of Adult Animals
  J. L. Mauderly and F. F. Hahn
Metabolic Functions of the Pulmonary Vascular Endothelium
  James W. Ryan and Una S. Ryan
The Mediation of Pulmonary Inflammatory Injury
  David O. Slauson
Viral–Bacterial Interactions in Pulmonary Infection
  George J. Jakab
Interstitial Pulmonary Disease
  D. L. Dungworth
Chemical-Induced Lung Injury in Domestic Animals
  R. G. Breeze and J. R. Carlson
Allergic Respiratory Disease
  B. N. Wilkie
Slow Virus Infections of Ovine Lung
  K. Perk
Respiratory Mycoplasmosis
  R. N. Gourlay and C. J. Howard
SUBJECT INDEX